PERIPHERAL RECEPTOR TARGETS FOR ANALGESIA

PERIPHERAL RECEPTOR TARGETS FOR ANALGESIA

NOVEL APPROACHES TO PAIN MANAGEMENT

Edited by

Brian E. Cairns, RPh, ACPR, PhD
Faculty of Pharmaceutical Sciences
The University of British Columbia

WILEY

A JOHN WILEY & SONS, INC., PUBLICATION

Published by John Wiley & Sons, Inc., Hoboken, New Jersey.
Published simultaneously in Canada.

Library of Congress Cataloging-in-Publication Data:

Peripheral receptor targets for analgesia : novel approaches to pain treatment / edited by Brian E. Cairns.
p. ; cm.
Includes index.
ISBN 978-0-470-25131-7 (cloth)
1. Nociceptors. 2. Nerves, Peripheral. 3. Analgesia. 4. Analgesics. 5. Pain. I. Cairns, Brian E.
[DNLM: 1. Pain–drug therapy. 2. Analgesics–therapeutic use. 3. Drug Delivery Systems. 4. Pain–physiopathology. 5. Receptors, Drug–physiology. WL 704 P4456 2009]
QP451.4.P47 2009
616′.0472–dc22

2009009731

10 9 8 7 6 5 4 3 2 1

CONTENTS

FOREWORD

Knowledge of pain mechanisms has advanced significantly since Wall and Melzack launched the gate control theory in the late 1960s. Since then, an exponential increase in the number of scientific papers on this topic has been seen. This has lead to a significant increase in our understanding of the fundamental aspects of the pain system and its pharmacology, but unfortunately, this has so far not been reflected in the number of new pharmacological compounds available for the treatment of pain. Aspirin, morphine, and lidocaine are still among the most widely used analgesic drugs. However, in more recent years, other centrally acting drugs (e.g., anticonvulsants, antidepressants), not developed or intended for the management of pain, have found their place in modern polypharmacological treatment regimes. Besides lidocaine, antitumor necrosis factor alpha (TNF-α) and, to some degree, nonsteroidal anti-inflammatory drug (NSAID), compounds targeting peripheral sites for pain relief, have been largely neglected. The present book is therefore an important contribution in the process of conceptualizing peripheral sites as possible targets for the development of new pain management treatments. This approach could also potentially reduce the well-known significant adverse effects associated with centrally acting analgesic drugs, such as drowsiness, somnolence, and mental clouding as well as gastrointestinal ulceration that is a problem with chronic use of NSAIDs. Such unintended side effects can significantly impact the quality of life of chronic pain patients.

Despite these apparent advantages of local analgesics for the treatment of pain, many results from this approach, for example, topical application of analgesic drugs, are disappointing. One reason for failures of this approach is a lack of appreciation of the peripheral pain transduction mechanisms and the diversity of receptors that may be involved in these mechanisms. This book, by reviewing the role of peripheral receptor mechanisms in the transduction of pain, should provide a framework for the development of rationally designed treatments with locally applied analgesics and promote further basic and clinical studies on potentially interesting peripheral receptor targets.

LARS ARENDT-NIELSEN, DR MED, PHD

Center for Sensory-Motor Interaction
Department of Health Science and Technology
Aalborg University, Aalborg, Denmark

PREFACE

The main purpose of *Peripheral Receptor Targets for Analgesia: Novel Approaches to Pain Management* is to bring together in one text much of the diverse body of work on peripheral receptor mechanisms of pain. I hoped, by doing this, to allow the reader to compare work done on various receptor targets to determine which targets might be the most useful to pursue in their own research. Thus, the topics I have chosen for the book should be of interest to health sciences researchers and clinicians (physicians, dentists, pharmacists, nurse practitioners, physiotherapists, and others) as well as researchers in the pharmaceutical industry. Nevertheless, I believe that this book will also be attractive to senior undergraduate and graduate students in the health sciences whose research interests include pain. The book is organized into introductory chapters to provide the reader with a general sense of the importance of peripheral mechanism of pain, followed by select topical chapters focusing on specific receptor targets. The book finishes with chapters that discuss avenues for selective delivery of analgesic agents. I intend that this book will not only provide interesting reading but also serve as useful reference for those interested in the field of pain research.

Brian E. Cairns

Faculty of Pharmaceutical Sciences
The University of British Columbia

CONTRIBUTORS

Per Alstergren, Department of Dental Medicine, Karolinska Institutet, Huddinge, Sweden

Ranjinidevi Ambalavanar, Department of Neural and Pain Sciences and Program in Neuroscience, University of Maryland, Baltimore, MD, USA

Lars Arendt-Nielsen, Center for Sensory-Motor Interaction, Department of Health Science and Technology, Aalborg University, Aalborg, Denmark

Christopher J. Benson, Department of Internal Medicine, University of Iowa, Iowa City, IO, USA

Brian E. Cairns, Faculty of Pharmaceutical Sciences, The University of British Columbia, Vancouver, BC, Canada

Theodore R. Cummins, Department of Pharmacology and Toxicology, Stark Neurosciences Research Institute, Indiana University School of Medicine, Indianapolis, IN, USA

Dean Dessem, Department of Neural and Pain Sciences and Program in Neuroscience, University of Maryland, Baltimore, MD, USA

Malin Ernberg, Division of Clinical Oral Physiology, Department of Dental Medicine, Karolinska Institutet

David J. Fink, Department of Neurology, University of Michigan School of Medicine and VA Ann Arbor Healthcare System, Ann Arbor, MI, USA

Luana Fischer, Laboratory of Pain Physiology, Division of Biological Sciences, Department of Physiology, Federal University of Parana

Parisa Gazerani, Faculty of Pharmaceutical Sciences, The University of British Columbia, Vancouver, BC, Canada, and Center for Sensory-Motor Interaction, Aalborg University, Aalborg, Denmark

Urs O. Häfeli, Faculty of Pharmaceutical Sciences, The University of British Columbia, Vancouver, BC, Canada

Akhlaq Waheed Hakim, Faculty of Pharmaceutical Sciences, The University of British Columbia, Vancouver, BC, Canada

Kazutaka Ikeda, Division of Psychobiology, Tokyo Institute of Psychiatry, Tokyo, Japan

Amit Kale, Faculty of Pharmaceutical Sciences, The University of British Columbia

Toru Kobayashi, Division of Psychobiology, Tokyo Institute of Psychiatry, Tokyo, Japan, and Department of Molecular Neuropathology, Brain Research Institute, Niigata University, Niigata, Japan

Ujendra Kumar, Faculty of Pharmaceutical Sciences, University of British Columbia, Vancouver, Canada

Marina Mata, Department of Neurology, University of Michigan School of Medicine, and VA Ann Arbor Healthcare System, Ann Arbor, MI, USA

Jason J. McDougall, Department of Physiology and Biophysics, University of Calgary, Calgary, AL, Canada

Joseph G. McGivern, Amgen Inc., Thousand Oaks, CA, USA

Daisuke Nishizawa, Division of Psychobiology, Tokyo Institute of Psychiatry, Tokyo, Japan

Carlos Amilcar Parada, Department of Physiology and Biophysics, Institute of Biological Sciences, University of Campinas, Campinas, SP, Brazil

Antti Pertovaara, Biomedicum Helsinki, Institute of Biomedicine/Physiology, University of Helsinki, Helsinki, Finland

Pradit Prateepavanich, Department of Rehabilitation Medicine, Siriraj Hospital, Mahidol University, Bangkok, Thailand

Jana Sawynok, Department of Pharmacology, Dalhousie University, Halifax, NS, Canada

Kathleen A. Sluka, Graduate Program in Physical Therapy and Rehabilitation Science, Pain Research Program, Neuroscience Graduate Program University of Iowa, Iowa City, IO, USA

Barry J. Sessle, Faculty of Dentistry, University of Toronto, Toronto, ON, Canada

Peter Svensson, Department of Clinical Oral Physiology, School of Dentistry, University of Aarhus; Department of Oral and Maxillofacial Surgery, Aarhus University Hospital, Aarhus, Denmark; and Orofacial Pain Laboratory, Center for Sensory-Motor Interaction, Aalborg University, Aalborg, Denmark

Arpad Szallasi, Monmouth Medical Center, Long Branch, NJ, and Drexel University College of Medicine, Philadelpia, PA, USA

Claudia Herrera Tambeli, Department of Physiology, Piracicaba Dental School, University of Campinas, Piracicaba, SP, Brazil

Marcello Trevisani, PharmEste, Ferrara, Italy

Roxanne Y. Walder, Graduate Program in Physical Therapy and Rehabilitation Science, Pain Research Program, Neuroscience Graduate Program, University of Iowa, Iowa City, IO, USA

PART I

PERIPHERAL MECHANISM IN CLINICAL PAIN CONDITIONS

CHAPTER 1

Role of Peripheral Mechanisms in Craniofacial Pain Conditions

BARRY J. SESSLE

Faculty of Dentistry, University of Toronto

Content

1.1 INTRODUCTION

The craniofacial region is the site of some of the most common acute and chronic pain conditions [1,2]. There are various types of headaches that are common and specific to this region, and toothaches are one of the most

Peripheral Receptor Targets for Analgesia: Novel Approaches to Pain Management, Edited by Brian E. Cairns

common reasons for people to seek dental treatment. Moreover, a significant proportion (~10%) of the population may suffer from craniofacial musculoskeletal pain (e.g., so-called temporomandibular disorders or TMD), and many of the chronic types of craniofacial pain are more commonly reported by women.

Acute pain is a transient signal that something is wrong and has a significant value to the person as an alert signal of tissue damage or potential damage. In contrast, chronic pain, which is usually considered as pain persisting for 3–6 months or more, may not have this protective and learning value, and the pain may become a disease or disorder in itself. Associated emotional or health-related stresses may also affect the patient by reducing his or her quality of life and can lead to undesirable changes such as loss of appetite and libido, and sleep disturbances, as well as reduced social interactions with the patient's family and friends. In addition to its emotional and social consequences to the patient and others, chronic pain will become an increasing socioeconomic burden as population demographics in most countries change, with more people being middle-aged or elderly, the age span when many chronic pain conditions are prevalent.

These considerations especially apply in the case of pain in the face and mouth because of the special psychological and emotional meaning and importance that this region has in eating, drinking, speech, sexual behavior, and expression of emotions and because the craniofacial tissues are densely innervated by free endings of nociceptive afferents and have an extensive somatosensory representation in the central nervous system (CNS). These various factors also may explain why many people find it unpleasant and painful to go for a routine dental examination.

There is considerable evidence that peripheral mechanisms play a significant role in the etiology or pathogenesis of many of the craniofacial pain conditions, and in recent years, insights have been gained into the neural and nonneural processes involved. This chapter will review these processes and indicate their documented or potential role in these conditions.

1.2 FEATURES OF PERIPHERAL TISSUES IN THE CRANIOFACIAL REGION

The craniofacial region is unique in the multiplicity of sensory functions manifested in this part of the body, for example, pain, temperature, touch, taste, smell, proprioception/kinesthesia, and detection and discrimination of the hardness, texture, and viscosity of substances or objects placed in the mouth. It is also characterized by a wide variety of tissues that include facial skin, cornea, oral mucosa, teeth and periodontal tissues, periosteum, bone, cartilage, muscles, joints (temporomandibular joint [TMJ]), ligaments, and fascia. These tissues have a rich blood supply and most have a dense innervation that subserves the various sensory functions of the craniofacial region.

The craniofacial tissues on the left or right side are innervated almost exclusively by branches of the ipsilateral trigeminal (V) sensory nerve, although some small parts of the craniofacial region are supplied by other cranial nerves or cervical nerves. The ophthalmic branch or first division of the V nerve supplies principally the supraorbital tissues (e.g., forehead skin) and cornea; its maxillary branch or second division mainly innervates the infraorbital skin, upper lip, maxillary mucosa, and teeth; and the mandibular branch or third division supplies mainly the skin of the low jaw, lower lip, mandibular mucosa, and teeth. Many V primary afferent fibers terminate in these tissues as sense organs (receptors) that are quite complex in their structure and that respond to tactile stimulation (e.g., low-threshold mechanoreceptors) or to other forms of mechanical stimuli such as stretch or tension (e.g., proprioceptors). These receptors are mainly associated with large (Aβ)- or medium (Aδ)-sized afferents that convey the tactile or proprioceptive information into the CNS. Other primary afferents may terminate as free nerve endings, many of which respond to noxious stimuli and which are termed *nociceptors*. These nociceptive afferents are either small-diameter, myelinated (Aδ) primary afferent fibers or even smaller (and even slower conducting) unmyelinated (C) afferent fibers, although there is evidence that in some conditions, Aβ-afferents may take on a nociceptive function. It is important to note that not all of the Aδ- and C-fiber afferents conduct nociceptive information: some are associated with receptors that respond to non-noxious cooling, warming, or even tactile stimuli. In addition, there are other types of receptors (e.g., gustatory, olfactory) that are supplied by afferents in other cranial nerves.

1.3 PERIPHERAL NOCICEPTIVE MECHANISMS IN THE CRANIOFACIAL REGION

1.3.1 General Features of Nociceptors and Chemical Mediators

The craniofacial nociceptive Aδ- and C-fiber afferents mentioned above convey sensory information as nerve impulses (so-called action potentials) from the nociceptors into the CNS and thereby provide the brain with sensory-discriminative information about the spatial and temporal qualities of the noxious stimulus. The peripheral basis for coding the intensity and duration of the noxious stimulus is closely related to the frequency of the nerve impulses and the duration of the nerve impulse discharge of the nociceptive afferent fibers. The peripheral feature of particular importance for localization of the stimulus is the receptive field of the fiber, that is, the area of skin, mucosa, or deep tissue from which the afferent fiber and its associated receptors can be excited by a threshold stimulus. The receptive field of most nociceptive afferent fibers is usually less than 1 mm^2, and the threshold for their activation from the receptive field is very high and in the noxious range. Noxious stimuli, particularly in superficial tissues, usually also activate other receptors such as mechanoreceptors that code for touch, and these help determine the location and quality of the sensation perceived. In tissues that appear to have no such low-threshold mechanoreceptors, such as tooth pulp and muscles, noxious stimuli may give rise to a different quality of pain sensation.

The activation of the nociceptive afferent stems from the tissue damage produced by the noxious stimulus causing the release from the tissues of chemical mediators (e.g., prostaglandins, bradykinins) that activate the free nerve endings of the afferent. This can result in the production of action potentials in the Aδ- and/or C-fiber afferents, which are conveyed into the CNS and may elicit the perception of transient or acute pain. It has become evident in recent years that the processes by which the nociceptive endings are activated are extremely complex and varied between endings and that a multitude of factors and mechanisms can influence their excitability. Subsequent chapters in this book deal at length with these, so only a brief overview is provided here, followed by an outline of findings specifically in craniofacial tissues.

Broadly speaking, the activation of nociceptive afferent endings involves subcellular compartmentalization and signaling pathways, extracellular matrix, cytoskeleton, and intracellular organelles as well as extracellular processes (see References 3–7). Briefly, the subcellular elements and signaling pathways involve numerous intracellular second messenger pathways, networks, and cascades that involve cyclic adenosine monophosphate (cAMP), protein kinases A and C (PKC), mitogen-activated protein (MAP) kinases, and nitric oxide just to name a few. These processes are also very much involved in the sensitization (see below) as well as activation of the afferent endings and manifest considerable plasticity. In addition, components of the cytoskeleton and extracellular matrix as well as organelles within the endings (e.g., intracellular and extracellular scaffolding proteins, and mitochondria) are involved in modulating the excitability of the nociceptive afferent endings; sex hormones may also have a role through local regulatory functions and gene transcription.

A number of extracellular factors and chemical mediators can also influence the excitability of the nociceptive afferent endings. These are outlined in Figure 1.1 and include damage to peripheral tissues, which often results in inflammation, and may also involve products released from the cells of the immune system or from the blood vessels. Substances synthesized in and released from the afferent fibers themselves may influence the excitability of the nociceptive afferents, for example, neurotrophins such as nerve growth factor, and neuropeptides such as substance P and calcitonin gene-related peptide (CGRP) may cause platelets, macrophages, mast cells, and other cells of the immune system to release inflammatory mediators such as histamine, serotonin (5-HT), bradykinin, and cytokines. Under certain conditions, the excitability of the nociceptors may also be modulated by substances, such as norepinephrine, that are released from sympathetic efferents innervating the tissues. In some situations, damage to the afferents themselves may occur and may lead to abnormal nerve changes that are associated with ectopic or aber-

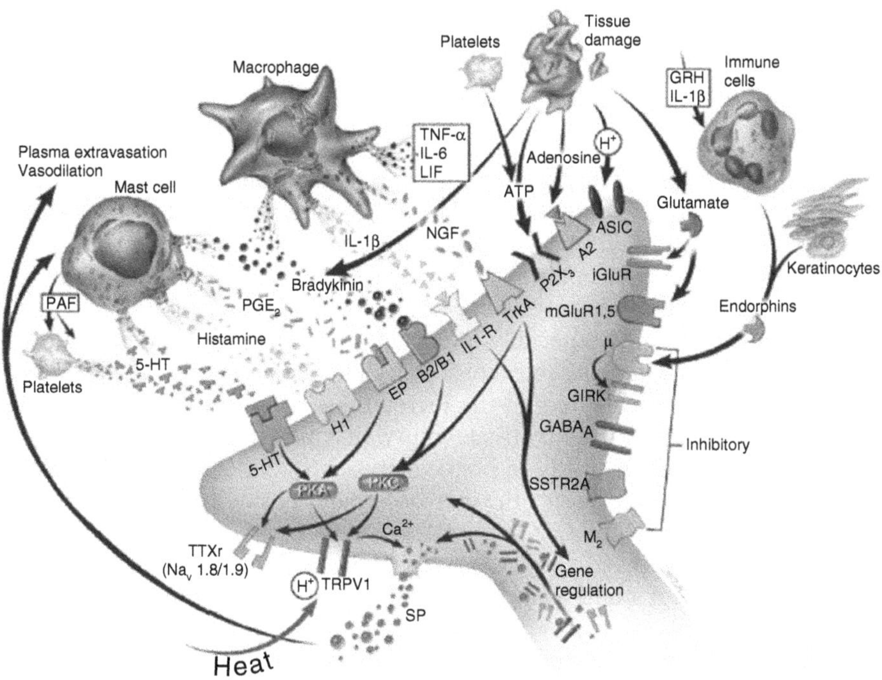

FIGURE 1.1. Peripheral mediators involved in peripheral sensitization following inflammation. Inflammation results in numerous chemicals being released from mast cells, macrophages, immune cells, and injured cells that may alter the sensitivity of peripheral nerve terminals; several of these mediators are shown here. ASIC, acid-sensing ion channel; CRH, corticotropin-releasing hormone; GIRK, G-protein-coupled inward rectifying potassium channel; 5-HT, serotonin; iGluR, ionotropic glutamate receptor; IL-1β, interleukin-1-beta; IL-6, interleukin-6; LIF, leukemia inhibitory factor; μ, mu opioid receptor; M_2, muscarinic receptor; mGluR, metabotropic glutamate receptor; NGF, nerve growth factor; PAF, platelet-activating factor; PGE_2, prostaglandin E_2; PKA, protein kinase A; PKC, protein kinase C; SSTR2A, somatostatin receptor 2A; TNF-α, tumor necrosis factor alpha; TrkA, tyrosine kinase receptor A; TRPV1, transient receptor potential vanilloid 1; TTXr, tetrodotoxin-resistant sodium channel (from Meyer, R.A., Ringkamp, M., Campbell, J.N., Raja, S.N. (2006). Peripheral mechanisms of cutaneous nociception. In: McMahon, S.B., Koltzenburg, M. (eds.). *Wall and Melzack's Textbook of Pain*, 5th ed. Amsterdam: Elsevier, pp. 3–34. [5]). See color insert.

rant neural discharges that are important in neuropathic pain conditions (see below).

Many of these factors increase the excitability of the nociceptors at the site of injury; this is termed *nociceptor or peripheral sensitization*. Sensitized nociceptors exhibit spontaneous activity, lowered activation thresholds, and increased responsiveness to subsequent noxious stimuli that appear to contribute, respectively, to the spontaneous pain, allodynia, and hyperalgesia that are characteristics of many chronic or persistent pain conditions. The inflammatory mediators as well as some of the substances released from the afferent fibers may also cause edema (swelling), redness, and local temperature increases, which, along with pain, are the cardinal signs of inflammation; this process has been termed neurogenic inflammation.

The chemicals may also diffuse through the peripheral tissues and act on the endings of adjacent nociceptive afferents, and so, more nociceptive afferents send their signals into the CNS, thus contributing to the spread and increased size of the painful area. The increased afferent barrage into the CNS from this increased nociceptor activity may also lead to functional changes in central nociceptive processing that contribute to persistent pain. One such series of changes that is especially important in mechanisms underlying pain is *central sensitization*. This central process is involved in the so-called secondary hyperalgesia, which refers to the increased sensitivity to noxious stimuli well beyond the site of original tissue injury. In contrast, peripheral processes involving peripheral sensitization of nociceptive afferent endings at the injury site seem mainly to account for the increased pain sensitivity at the injury site itself (primary hyperalgesia).

These peripheral sensitizing events reflect, in a sense, a form of functional plasticity, and recent studies suggest an added element of complexity in these peripheral plasticity processes. The nociceptive afferent endings may manifest a "primed state" where basal nociceptive thresholds are normal but instead of being sensitized for physical (e.g., mechanical) stimuli, the ending is sensitized against sensitizing agents such that far lower concentrations of inflammatory mediators for instance are sufficient to elicit, in this primed state, much augmented excitability of the ending. This primed state is PKC-dependent and can last for weeks and so could represent an important factor in pain chronicity (see Reference 7).

Also noteworthy is that the nociceptive afferent fibers can undergo phenotypic switches under certain conditions (see References 3, 6, 8, and 9). For example, they can change in response to peripheral inflammation, with alterations in the expression of certain nociceptor receptors or ion channels (e.g., voltage-gated sodium channels). Transcription of neuropeptides, brain-derived neurotrophic factor (BDNF), and ion channels, and translation of transient receptor potential (TRP) channels may occur and enhance peripheral (and central) sensitization. Transcriptional changes may also occur after nerve injury and be involved along with sympathetic efferent sprouting in the development of abnormal, ectopic discharge patterns in the afferents that are often a feature of neuropathic pain. These changes may be manifested in the afferent ganglion cell body as well as in the afferent fiber itself and contribute to the spontaneous nature, allodynia, and hyperalgesia of neuropathic pain.

Compared with studies of spinal nerve fibers, investigations of V afferent endings and ganglion cells have been much fewer but have revealed several analogous changes following V nerve injury or craniofacial inflammation, but some notable differences include the apparent lack of sympathetic efferent sprouting in the V ganglion after nerve injury, time course differences in the abnormal afferent discharge patterns, and differences in the up- or down-regulation of neuropeptide and ion channel expression in the ganglion cells or their peripheral afferent endings (see References 10 and 11).

Additional receptor mechanisms that are involved in pain have been discovered in peripheral nerve endings themselves. They include receptor subtypes for 5-HT, adenosine triphosphate (ATP), bradykinin, nerve growth factor, and opioidergic peptides as well as several TRP receptors such as the transient receptor potential vanilloid 1 (TRPV1) receptor that responds to protons (H^+), heat, and chemicals like capsaicin, the ingredient in hot peppers that produces pain. It should also be noted that chemical mediators long thought to be involved in nociceptive transmission or modulation within the CNS (e.g., the excitatory amino acid glutamate and opioid-related substances such as enkephalins) can also act peripherally on the nociceptive afferent endings. For example, glutamate is synthesized by primary afferent cell bodies. It can excite nociceptive afferents supplying craniofacial musculoskeletal tissues, initiate central sensitization and sustained sensorimotor behavior in animals, and produce a transient pain in humans by activating glutamate receptors (N-methyl-D-aspartate [NMDA] and non-NMDA receptors) located on the afferent endings. These effects in animals and humans are significantly greater in females. In contrast, the well-known centrally acting narcotic analgesic drug morphine also has actions in peripheral tissues as it can depress the activity of nociceptive afferents by interacting with opioid receptors on their afferent endings. In addition, the powerful central inhibitory neurotransmitter gamma-amino butyric acid (GABA) can also act peripherally and depress nociceptive afferent excitability. Several of these chemical mediators may influence afferent excitability indirectly by acting on other cells in these tissues (e.g., mast cells, macrophages, platelets, ketatinoytes, endothelial cells), which themselves have several of the same receptors and ion channels existing in the afferent endings and release many of the mediators mentioned above.

The multiplicity of peripheral chemical mediators, receptors, and ion channels, and intracellular channels involved in peripheral nociceptive activation, sensitization, and related events (e.g., inflammation) are all potential targets for the development of new and more effective therapeutic approaches. Knowledge of the chemical mechanisms involved in the activation or sensitization of the nociceptive afferents has led to the development of therapeutic agents targeting specific peripheral mechanisms. For example, common nonsteroidal anti-inflammatory drugs (NSAIDs) including salicylates such as aspirin, as well as many newly developed analgesics such as cyclooxygenase (COX)-2 inhibitors, have their principal analgesic and anti-inflammatory actions in peripheral tissues (e.g., on prostaglandin E_2 [PGE_2] synthesis). They can reduce inflammation associated with tissue injury, modulate nociceptive afferent excitability, and alter the hyperalgesia associated with short-term craniofacial pain conditions. A cautionary note, however, is warranted to offset any sense of optimism that a peripherally based pharmacological cure for pain is "around the corner." The multiplicity of processes, many of which act in parallel, also means that interception of any one or a few is unlikely to have a major therapeutic impact. The development of effective agents that act further downstream on the consequences of the increased afferent excitability induced by noxious stimulation would seem a more useful and fruitful avenue (see Reference 7).

1.4 PERIPHERAL PROCESSES IN SPECIFIC TISSUES

1.4.1 Facial Skin

The craniofacial region has a dense innervation, especially in the intraoral and perioral region. Three major classes of nociceptive afferent fibers supplying facial skin have been described [12,13]: (i) Aδ mechanothermal nociceptive afferents that respond to intense thermal and mechanical stimuli; (ii) high-threshold mechanoreceptive afferents that respond best to intense mechanical stimuli (most of these conduct in the Aδ range, although some may have conduction velocities in the Aβ- and C-fiber ranges); and (iii) C-polymodal nociceptive afferent fibers that are excited by strong mechanical and thermal, as well as chemical stimuli that include agonists for ATP, 5-HT, bradykinin, and TRP channels. Some chemical stimuli may also act on the Aδ nociceptive afferent endings.

1.4.2 TMJ and Masticatory Muscles

The endings of many of the small-diameter afferents innervating the TMJ and masticatory muscles may respond to a wide range of peripheral stimuli that cause pain in humans. These include heavy pressure, algesic chemicals, and inflammatory agents [12,14] and likely also ischemia especially in the case of muscle nociceptive afferent fibers if it is prolonged and associated with muscle contractions. Several recent studies utilizing immunohistochemical, electrophysiological, and behavioral approaches have provided evidence for peripherally acting agonists for glutamate, TRPV1, GABA, and opioid receptors, just to name a few, as having modulatory effects on these deep craniofacial afferents [14–18]. There is also evidence from animal and human studies that sex differences may exist in some of these effects and have clinical implications (see below).

1.4.3 Cranial Vessels and Meninges

Cranial vessels and the meninges are supplied by small-diameter V afferent fibers that can be activated by noxious stimuli [19,20]. Their activation may also be associated with the subsequent development of vasodilatation related to neurogenic inflammation. The activation and modulation of these afferents by peripheral neurochemical processes (e.g., 5-HT) are thought to be important factors in the initiation and control of certain headaches such as migraine (see below).

1.4.4 Periodontium and Oral Mucosa

As well as a dense innervation supplying low-threshold mechanoreceptors, the periodontal ligament and oral mucosa have free nerve endings, which are associated with Aδ- and C-fiber nociceptive afferents. Although the subject of limited investigation, they have been found to respond to mechanical, thermal, and/or chemical stimuli [12,13] and, in general, appear to have properties similar to nociceptors in other tissues. Interestingly, some periodontal nociceptive afferents branch to innervate the pulp of an adjacent tooth, and the responsiveness of some mucosal nociceptive afferents may be influenced by biomechanical factors in the tissues.

1.4.5 Cornea

Nerve fibers supplying the cornea penetrate into the corneal epithelium and terminate as free nerve endings, which are thus very exposed to changes in the external environment. The most prominent sensations evoked by stimuli of different types applied to the corneal surface are of pain and irritation, although a cooling sensation may also be perceived. These observations are consistent with corneal afferent recordings in experimental animals, which have shown that the cornea contains mechano-nociceptors and polymodal nociceptors as well as low-threshold cold receptors [21].

1.4.6 Tooth Pulp

The tooth pulp is a highly vascular and richly innervated tissue that is exquisitely sensitive to stimulation (for review, see References 22–24). The pulp (the "nerve of the tooth") is encompassed in dentine, which, in the coronal part of the tooth, is itself covered by enamel. Both the pulp and the dentine are innervated, and intradental afferents can respond to a variety of stimuli that predominantly, if not exclusively, produce pain. As well as small-diameter (Aδ- and C-fiber) afferents supplying the tooth, sympathetic afferents and Aβ-fibers also contribute to the innervation. The role of the Aβ-fibers is unclear, but their presence has been used as an argument that pain may not be the only sensation evoked from the pulp. While it appears that a hydrodynamic mechanism is largely responsible for activation of many intradental afferents, thermal and chemical stimuli may directly activate some afferents. The afferents may also manifest peripheral sensitization, and many of the peripheral chemical processes, receptors, and ion channels underlying their activation and sensitization appear to be similar to those identified in other tissues (see 1.3.1 above), including intraneural neuropeptides (e.g., substance P, CGRP, TRP and ATP receptors, and a number of chemical mediators [e.g. histamine, 5-HT, opioids, cytokines, and kinases]); several of these also contribute to pulp inflammatory, repair, and regenerative processes. A special feature of the pulp that should be noted is that while its nociceptive mechanisms are in a dynamic plastic state like that in other tissues (see above), it has a very low compliance because of its encasement in hard tissues. This has been thought to be a factor contributing to the exquisite sensitivity of the tooth in some inflammatory states.

1.5 CRANIOFACIAL PAIN CONDITIONS AND ROLE OF PERIPHERAL MECHANISMS

This section briefly describes some of the most common or intriguing pain conditions in craniofacial tissues and outlines the contribution that peripheral mechanisms may make to each. It is important to note that these pain conditions may in addition or instead involve central neural processes (e.g., central sensitization) that may also contribute (see References 9, 11, 25, and 26). These pain conditions are listed according to the proposed mechanism-based classification of pain (Table 1.1).

1.5.1 Injury and Inflammatory-Related Pain

Trauma and inflammation are not only natural consequences of some dental procedures (e.g., tooth extraction, oral surgery) but can also be associated with

TABLE 1.1. Suggested Classification of Pain according to Underlying Mechanisms.

Transient Pain	Tissue Injury Pain (Inflammatory Pain)	Nervous System Injury Pain (Neuropathic Pain)
Nociceptor specialization*	Primary afferent • Sensitization	Primary afferent • Acquisition of spontaneous and stimulus-evoked activity by nociceptor axons and cell bodies at loci other than peripheral terminals
	• Recruitment of silent nociceptors • Alteration in phenotype • Hyperinnervation	• Phenotype changes
	CNS mediated • Central sensitization recruitment, summation, and amplification	CNS mediated • Central sensitization • Deafferentation of second-order neurons • Disinhibition • Structural reorganization

Note that similar mechanisms may operate in both tissue and nervous system injury pain (from Svensson, P., Sessle, B.J. (2004). Orofacial pain. In: Miles, T.S., Nauntofte, B., Svensson, P. (eds.). *Clinical Oral Physiology*. Copenhagen: Quintessence, pp. 93–139 [43]).

*Specialization refers to specific membrane and neurochemical properties of nociceptors and associated afferent nerve fibers that allows them to be differentially activated by different types of brief noxious stimuli (e.g., mechanical, heat, or chemical).

specific pain conditions, which will be noted below. In addition, trauma normally involves injury of more than one type of tissue, and the clinical manifestation will depend on which tissues are involved, for example, deep pain usually has features quite distinct from those of pain occurring in superficial tissues (e.g., skin, mucosa) in terms of its localizability (diffuse vs. localized) and quality (aching, cramping vs. sharp, burning). Similarly for inflammation, which is a natural consequence of tissue injury, the clinical manifestations may differ depending on the physical properties and functions of the involved tissue; for example, inflammation in the tooth pulp (pulpitis) is associated with clinical characteristics that are different from those associated with gingival inflammation (gingivitis), probably in part due to the relative rigidity of dentine and enamel (also see above).

This leads us to consider one of the most common types of craniofacial pain. The teeth are a common source of pain [27]. *Toothaches* (odontalgias) are usually associated with reversible or irreversible pulpitis. Toothaches can have a "sharp" or a "dull" quality and sometimes a "throbbing" component, and the pain may also be exacerbated by hot and cold stimuli. The pain intensity can be very severe, particularly in the acute stages, with bouts of pain lasting minutes to hours. While the tissue damage is highly localized, the pain may spread and be referred to the ipsilateral face and jaw. *Periapical periodontitis* is also common and is often the consequence of irreversible pulpitis. In the acute stage, periapical periodontitis manifests severe pain that is difficult to localize, and often mechanical and thermal hyperalgesia. Mechanical hyperalgesia but more moderate pain is characteristic of the chronic stage. Other more special types of toothaches are cracked or partially fractured teeth, barodontalgia, and referred pain from remote and other craniofacial sites.

Inflammation can also occur in other craniofacial tissues and cause pain. For example, *gingivitis* and *periodontitis* involve, respectively, inflammation of the gingiva (gums) and periodontal tissues (around the root of the tooth). They are also very common inflammatory conditions, but surprisingly, they usually do not produce symptoms of pain. Why is unclear, but it could be related to the release of peripheral modulators that dampen the excitability of the gingival or periodontal nociceptive afferent endings; this requires further study through the development of specific models. *Maxillary sinusitis* involves inflammation of the lining of the maxillary sinus that often occurs in relation to nasal colds and is associated with cheek pain and tenderness of zygomatic arch tissues and teeth. Inflammatory conditions in the TMJ (*synovitis and capsulitis*) or jaw muscles (*myositis*) can occur after injury, systemic infections or localized inflammatory reactions (e.g., osteoarthritis), or systemic inflammatory states (rheumatoid arthritis) [28].

These many and varied painful conditions associated with local tissue injury and inflammation likely involve some common mechanisms underlying the pain. Studies in animal models of pulpitis, sinusitis, myositis, and arthritis for example, have provided evidence indicating that nociceptive afferents supplying these affected tissues are activated and sensitized in these models by chemical mediators and processes that are generally similar to those noted earlier [14,17,22,24,29]. Mechanisms within the CNS (e.g., central sensitization) have also been shown to be involved [11,25].

1.5.2 Neuropathic Pain

There are several craniofacial pain conditions that are neuropathic in origin [9,30,31]. *Postherpetic neuralgia* is a relatively common complication of acute herpes zoster infection and can affect the V nerve (usually its ophthalmic branch). Damage to or loss of the large peripheral afferent fibers with loss of myelination is a feature of postherpetic neuralgia and is generally thought to lead to changes in central nociceptive transmission and modulation, although peripheral processes may also contribute (e.g., inflammation of the involved cutaneous sites; see Reference 30). *Trigeminal neuralgia* is much less common, fortunately, because it is an excruciatingly painful neuropathic condition. Trigeminal neuralgia has a paroxysmal character, with sudden, unilateral, brief, stabbing, recurrent pain especially in the distribution of the maxillary or mandibular branches of the V nerve. The electric shocklike jolts of pain are usually triggered by light mechanical contact of a specific location in the perioral or intraoral region. Between the pain attacks, the patient is largely asymptomatic, with no clear changes in somatosensory sensitivity. The etiology and pathogenesis of trigeminal neuralgia are still unclear, although it can be secondary to multiple sclerosis, benign or malignant brain tumors, or facial trauma. There is some evidence that it might arise from a mechanical distortion of trigeminal afferents, which induces ectopic discharges of the afferents, but central mechanisms are undoubtedly involved in its pathogenesis [30–32].

Extraction of a tooth and endodontic treatment by their very nature involve deafferentation as well as peripheral nerve injury. Although these procedures are very common in dental practice, it is interesting that only a very low proportion of patients complain about persistent neuropathic pain. It has been suggested that this low incidence of neuropathic pain is because the high vascularization of the orofacial tissues facilitates regeneration and because the injured nerves are usually quite small in number compared with those in the limbs where neuropathic pain following trauma is more common. Pain can also appear when a peripheral branch of the V nerve is injured, for example, during maxillofacial surgery or placement of dental implants, but hypoesthesia and numbness are more common [31,33]. *Atypical odontalgia* and *atypical facial pain* may also represent neuropathic pain conditions due to peripheral events associated with deafferentation (e.g., tooth extraction, endodontic therapy) as well as long-term neuroplastic changes especially in the CNS (e.g., central sensitization). Atypical odontalgia can be difficult to distinguish from conventional odontalgias as pain may be localized to the site or to the tooth where the tooth or tooth pulp used to be before it was removed. As a consequence, the patient may receive excessive and unnecessary dental treatment (e.g., root canal treatments and/or tooth extractions) without any reduction in his or her pain. In the case of so-called atypical facial pain, the pain is more diffuse and often throbbing in character. As the etiology and pathogenesis of both pain conditions are so poorly understood, and because both are difficult to treat successfully, the dentist should not carry out any further dental interventions, unless there are clear signs of tissue pathology, but instead refer the patient to a pain specialist.

Another craniofacial pain that has features suggestive of a neuropathic pain condition is the *burning mouth syndrome* (BMS; also termed stomatodynia). This is a relatively common condition especially in middle-aged and elderly women, particularly after menopause. BMS is characterized by a constant burning pain on the tongue, lips, and/or hard palate, with no clear clinical signs of inflammation or systemic disorders. Like atypical odontalgia and atypical facial pain, its etiology is unclear, although peripheral mechanisms might be involved as loss of some somatosensory and gustatory sensibility has been documented in BMS patients, and there are recent reports of changes in peripheral afferent endings, lending credence to its possible neuropathic origin (see References 34 and 35). Also, like atypical odontalgia and atypical facial pain, BMS is very difficult to manage.

1.5.3 Musculoskeletal and Neurovascular Pain

Although some of the preceding pain conditions may involve musculoskeletal or neurovascular tissues and associated peripheral mechanisms (e.g., myositis, pulpitis), there are two groups of chronic conditions affecting these tissues that are highlighted here: TMD and headaches.

1.5.3.1 TMD. TMD is a collective term for a number of painful conditions in musculoskeletal tissues (e.g., jaw muscles, tendons, TMJ), which may be accompanied by limitations of jaw movements and clicking or grating noises in the TMJ [28,36]. There are three major categories of TMD, namely, myofascial pain affecting predominantly the jaw musculature; disk displacements with or without reduction; and TMJ arthralgia, osteoarthritis, and osteoarthrosis. Some TMD patients may manifest two or all three components. The myofascial and arthralgic forms are usually associated with mechanical hyperalgesia and allodynia, often with referral of pain to other craniofacial tissues on the ipsilateral side. Although the etiology of TMD is unknown, female gender, depression, and the presence of multiple other pain conditions are significant risk factors.

Generally, TMD are viewed as multifactorial problems involving anatomical, neuromuscular and neurobiological, and psychosocial factors, which can act as predisposing, precipitating, or aggravating influences in an individual patient. Concepts of the etiology of TMD have, in the past, focused on the anatomical factors as most important; thus, peripheral processes associated with structural changes in the TMJ or in the dental occlusion were emphasized and provided the basis for therapeutic approaches aimed at correcting "the bite." Such concepts have since been largely discredited and do not seem to apply to most TMD patients, and nowadays, more emphasis is given to neurobiological and psychosocial factors, with therapy tailored to these concepts. The allodynia, hyperalgesia, and pain spread and referral that are characteristic of TMD suggest a role for both peripheral and central sensitization in TMD-associated pain. In the case of peripheral mechanisms, although overt structural changes in the TMJ or dental occlusion do not seem to apply in most cases (see above), injury, inflammation, or even degeneration of the TMJ or muscle is still often conceptualized as important in the pathophysiology of TMD. However, while some TMD conditions manifest inflammation (e.g., rheumatoid arthritis or osteoarthritis), the majority of TMD cases does not appear to be associated with gross indications of inflammatory changes; the same applies to most more generalized pain conditions such as fibromyalgia [37–39]. This suggests that different receptor mechanisms may underlie the development of some chronic pain conditions involving deep musculoskeletal tissues such as TMD.

Several of the chemical mediators involved in peripheral nociceptive mechanisms (see 1.3.1) have been implicated in TMD. Inflammatory mediators such as neuropeptides, cytokines, prostaglandins, and 5-HT may play a role especially in those TMD conditions manifesting inflammation of the TMJ; for example, elevated levels of 5-HT, tumor necrosis factor alpha (TNF-α), and interleukin-1-beta (IL-1β) are a feature of these conditions [40,41]. The studies mentioned above with glutamate and its effects on nociceptive afferents, sensorimotor function, and pain that point to its possible role in peripheral mechanisms contributing to TMJ and myofascial pain, have led to the suggestion that changes in peripheral glutamate levels through cytosolic release from tissue damage, inflammation, or neurogenic release from nociceptive afferent activation may play an important role in chronic pain conditions such as TMD by modulating the sensitivity of deep craniofacial tissues through autocrine and/or paracrine regulation of ionotropic glutamate receptor mechanisms [14,17]. Glutamate itself does not induce inflammation in these tissues, but its tissue elevation can evoke peripheral sensitization and central sensitization as well as nociceptive jaw muscle reflex responses, which may contribute to typical features of TMD independent of signs of inflammation, that is, neuromuscular changes reflected in limitations in jaw movements, plus allodynia, hyperalgesia, pain spread and referral, and pain at rest. Furthermore, as the animal and human studies have revealed that peripheral effects of glutamate are sex dependent, sex differences in activation of peripheral glutamate receptors may conceivably be involved in the female predominance in TMD (and related conditions such as fibromyalgia).

1.5.3.2 Headaches. There are several types of headaches. Those such as migraines, cluster headaches, and other trigeminal autonomic cephalgias are sometimes referred to as neurovascular headaches [19,42]. *Migraines* come in attacks lasting up to 3 days, and patients often report nausea, vomiting, and increased sensitivity to sounds and light. Migraines with aura (classical migraine) or without aura (common migraine) manifest pain that is usually unilateral, moderate to severe in intensity, and with a pulsating quality that is aggravated by physical activity. The etiology and pathophysiology of migraines are not completely understood but appear to involve an interaction between neurovascular and myofascial nociceptive inputs into the CNS and modulation by descending influences from higher brain centers. In the case of the suspected peripheral mechanisms, both peripheral sensitization and neurogenic inflammation are thought to contribute to the pain and especially seem to involve 5-HTIB receptors on vessels and 5-HTID receptors on afferent endings in the meninges.

Cluster headache mainly occurs in men in series of attacks that are usually very painful and associated with autonomic reactions such as tears in the eye, blocked nose, and facial sweating. *Paroxysmal hemicrania* has many of the same characteristics as cluster headache but the pain attacks are more frequent and shorter and primarily occur in females. *Carotidynia* is a dull, aching pain near the upper portion of the carotid arteries, with referred pain to the face and head on the same side, and *temporal arteritis* is associated with a unilateral or bilateral headache principally with continuous or throbbing muscle pain in the temporal region. The extent to which peripheral mechanisms are involved in these conditions is unclear, but autonomic nervous system involvement and some predisposing factors have been identified [19].

Tension-type headaches are very common, with up to 80% of the population reported to experience this type of headache at least once in their life. The pain is described as a mild-to-moderate bilateral pressure or tightness in the frontal, temporal, parietal, and occipital regions and is not aggravated by physical activity. Peripheral sensitization of nociceptive afferent endings in temporal muscles may be involved, but CNS changes (e.g., central sensitization) likely also contribute [19,42].

1.6 SUMMARY

This chapter has noted the special emotional and psychological meaning and importance of the craniofacial region to the individual, and the various tissues and multiplicity of sensory functions manifested in this region. An overview is provided of the variety and complexity of the peripheral mechanisms underlying the activation and modulation of nociceptors, including the process of nociceptor or peripheral sensitization that may contribute to allodynia, hyperalgesia, pain spread, and spontaneous pain. Features of peripheral nociceptive mechanisms in specific craniofacial tissues are also outlined. It is also noted that the craniofacial region is the site of some of the most common pains in the body (e.g., toothaches, headaches, TMD), and the role that peripheral mechanisms may play in each of these and other craniofacial pain conditions is outlined.

ACKNOWLEDGMENT

Cited studies by the author have been supported by the National Institutes of Health grants DE04786 and 15420 and CIHR grant MOP 4918.

REFERENCES

1. Lipton, J.A., Ship, J.A., Larach-Robinson, D. (1997). Estimated prevalence and distribution of reported orofacial pain in the United States. *J Am Dent Assoc* 124:115–121.
2. LeResche, L., Drangsholt, M. (2008). Epidemiology of orofacial pain: prevalence, incidence, and risk factors. In: Sessle, B.J., Lavigne, G., Dubner, R., Lund, J.P. (eds.). *Orofacial Pain*, 2nd ed. Chicago, IL: Quintessence, pp. 13–18.
3. Dray, A. (2004). Future pharmacologic management of neuropathic pain. *J Orofac Pain* 18:381–385.
4. Gold, M.S. Molecular basis of receptors. (2005). In: Merskey, H., Loeser, J.D., Dubner, R. (eds.). *The Paths of Pain 1975–2005*. Seattle, WA: IASP Press, pp. 49–67.
5. Meyer, R.A., Ringkamp, M., Campbell, J.N., Raja, S.N. (2006). Peripheral mechanisms of cutaneous nociception. In: McMahon, S.B., Koltzenburg, M. (eds.). *Wall and Melzack's Textbook of Pain*, 5th ed. Amsterdam: Elsevier, pp. 3–34.
6. Woolf, C.J., Ma, Q. (2007). Nociceptors—noxious stimulus detectors. *Neuron* 55:353–364.
7. Hucho, T., Levine, J.D. (2007). Signaling pathways in sensitization: toward a nociceptor cell biology. *Neuron* 55:365–376.
8. Flor, H., Devor, M., Jensen, T.S. (2003). Phantom limb pain: causes and cures. In: Dostrovsky, J.O., Carr, D.B., Koltzenburg, M. (eds.). *Proceedings of the 10th World Congress on Pain, Progress in Pain Research and Management*, Vol. 24. Seattle, WA: IASP Press, pp. 767–790.
9. Woda, A., Salter, M.W. (2008). Mechanisms of neuropathic pain. In: Sessle, B.J., Lavigne, G., Dubner, R., Lund, J.P. (eds.). *Orofacial Pain*, 2nd ed. Chicago, IL: Quintessence, pp. 53–59.
10. Robinson, P.P., Boissonade, F.M., Loescher, A.R., Smith, K.G., Yates, J.M., Elcock, C., Bird, E.V., Davies, S.L., Smith, P.L., Vora, A.R. (2004). Peripheral mechanisms for the initiation of pain following trigeminal nerve injury. *J Orofac Pain* 18:287–292.
11. Sessle, B.J. (2005). Orofacial pain. In: Merskey, H., Loeser, J.D., Dubner, R. (eds.). *The Paths of Pain 1975–2005*. Seattle, WA: IASP Press, pp. 131–150.
12. Dubner, R., Sessle, B.J., Storey, A.T. (eds.) (1978). *The Neural Basis of Oral and Facial Function*. New York: Plenum Press.
13. Cooper, B. (2007). Nociceptors in the orofacial region: skin/mucosa. In: Schmidt, R.F., Willis, W.D. (eds.). *Encyclopedic Reference of Pain*. Heidelberg: Springer-Verlag, pp. 1422–1424.
14. Lam, D.K., Sessle, B.J., Cairns, B.E., Hu, J.W. (2005). Neural mechanisms of temporomandibular joint and masticatory muscle pain: a possible role for peripheral glutamate receptor mechanisms. *Pain Res Manage* 10:145–152.

15. Bakke, M., Hu, J.W., Sessle, B.J. (1998). Morphine application to peripheral tissues modulates nociceptive jaw reflex. *Neuroreport* 9:3315–3319.
16. Clemente, J.T., Parada, C.A., Veiga, M.C., Gear, R.W., Tambeli, C.H. (2004). Sexual dimorphism in the antinociception mediated by kappa opioid receptors in the rat temporomandibular joint. *Neurosci Lett* 372:250–255.
17. Cairns, B. (2007). Nociceptors in the orofacial region: TMJ and muscle. In: Schmidt, R.F., Willis, W.D. (eds.). *Encyclopedic Reference of Pain*. Heidelberg: Springer-Verlag, pp. 1424–1427.
18. Urtado, M.B., Gameiro, G.H., Tambeli, C.H., Fischer, L., Urtado, C.B., de Arruda Veiga, M.C. (2007). Involvement of peripheral TRPV1 in TMJ hyperalgesia induced by ethanol withdrawal. *Life Sci* 81:1622–1626.
19. Olesen, J., Goadsby, P., Ramadan, N., Tfelt-Hansen, P., Welch, K. (eds.) (2006). *The Headache*, 3rd ed. Philadelphia: Lippincott Williams & Wilkins.
20. Strassman, A.M., Levy, D. (2006). Response properties of dural nociceptors in relation to headache. *J Neurophysiol* 95:1298–1306.
21. Belmonte, C., Aracil, A., Acosta, M.C., Luna, C., Gallar, J. (2004). Nerves and sensations from the eye surface. *Ocul Surf* 2:248–253.
22. Hu, J.W. (2004). Tooth pulp. In: Miles, T.S., Nauntofte, B., Svensson, P. (eds.). *Clinical Oral Physiology*. Copenhagen: Quintessence, pp. 141–163.
23. Matthews, B., Sessle, B.J. (2008). Peripheral mechanisms of orofacial pain. In: Sessle, B.J., Lavigne, G., Dubner, R., Lund, J.P. (eds.). *Orofacial Pain*, 2nd ed. Chicago, IL: Quintessence, pp. 27–33.
24. Narhi, M.V.O. (2007). Nociceptors in the dental pulp. In: Schmidt, R.F., Willis, W.D. (eds.). *Encyclopedic Reference of Pain*. Heidelberg: Springer-Verlag, pp. 1418–1420.
25. Sessle, B.J. (2000). Acute and chronic craniofacial pain: brainstem mechanisms of nociceptive transmission and neuroplasticity, and their clinical correlates. *Crit Rev Oral Biol Med* 11:57–91.
26. Sessle, B.J., Lavigne, G., Dubner, R., Lund, J.P. (eds.) (2008). *Orofacial Pain*, 2nd ed. Chicago, IL: Quintessence.
27. Holland, G.R. (2008). Management of dental pain. In: Sessle, B.J., Lavigne, G., Dubner, R., Lund, J.P. (eds.). *Orofacial Pain*, 2nd ed. Chicago, IL: Quintessence, pp. 161–169.
28. Fricton, J.R., Schiffman, E.L. (2008). Management of masticatory myalgia and arthralgia. In: Sessle, B.J., Lavigne, G., Dubner, R., Lund, J.P. (eds.). *Orofacial Pain*, 2nd ed. Chicago, IL: Quintessence, pp. 179–185.
29. Young, E., Kajander, K.C., Rimell, F., Ho, B., Goldman, J. (2001). Substance P immunoreactive sensory axons as a subset of the total axonal population in the maxillary sinus of the rabbit: a characterization of normal and infected mucosa. *Am J Rhinol* 15:61–67.
30. Bennett, G.J. (2004). Neuropathic pain in the orofacial region: clinical and research challenges. *J Orofac Pain* 18:281–286.
31. Eliav, E., Max, M.B. (2008). Management of neuropathic pain. In: Sessle, B.J., Lavigne, G., Dubner, R., Lund, J.P. (eds.). *Orofacial Pain*, 2nd ed. Chicago, IL: Quintessence, pp. 195–202.
32. Fromm, G.H., Sessle, B.J. (1991). Summary and conclusions. In: Fromm, G.H., Sessle, B.J. (eds.). *Trigeminal: Current Concepts Regarding Pathogenesis and Treatment*. Stoneham, MA: Butterworths, pp. 205–219.

33. Sessle, B.J., Klineberg, I., Svensson, P.A. (2009). Neurophysiological perspective on rehabilitation with oral implants and their potential side effects. In: Jokstad, A. (ed.). *Osseointegration and Dental Implants*. Copenhagen: Blackwell Munksgaard (in press).

34. Ship, J.A., Grushka, M., Lipton, J.A., Mott, A.E., Sessle, B.J., Dionne, R. (1995). An update on burning mouth syndrome. *J Am Dent Assoc* 126:842–853.

35. Lauria, G., Majorana, A., Borgna, M., Lombardi, R., Penza, P., Padovani, A., Sapelli, P. (2005). Trigeminal small-fiber sensory neuropathy causes burning mouth syndrome. *Pain* 115:332–337.

36. Laskin, D., Greene, C.S., Hylander, W. (eds.) (2006). *TMDs. An Evidence-Based Approach to Diagnosis and Treatment*. Chicago, IL: Quintessence.

37. Henriksson, K.G. (2003). Fibromyalgia—from syndrome to disease. *J Rehabil Med* 41(Suppl.):89–94.

38. Stohler, C.S. (1995). Clinical perspectives on masticatory and related muscle disorders. In: Sessle, B.J., Bryant, P.S., Dionne, R.A. (eds.). *Temporomandibular Disorders and Related Pain Conditions. Progress in Pain Research and Management*, Vol. 4. Seattle, WA: IASP Press, pp. 3–29.

39. Zarb, G.A., Carlsson, G., Sessle, B.J., Mohl, N. (eds.) (1994). *Temporomandibular Joint and Masticatory Muscle Disorders*. Copenhagen: Munksgaard.

40. Kopp, S. (2001). Neuroendocrine, immune, and local responses related to temporomandibular disorders. *J Orofac Pain* 15:9–28.

41. Milam, S.B. (2006). TMJ osteoarthritis. In: Laskin, D., Greene, C.S., Hylander, W. (eds.). *TMDs. An Evidence-Based Approach to Diagnosis and Treatment*. Chicago, IL: Quintessence, pp: 105–123.

42. Okeson, J.P. (2008). Management of orofacial pain related to headache: principles and practices. In: Sessle, B.J., Lavigne, G., Dubner, R., Lund, J.P. (eds.). *Orofacial Pain*, 2nd ed. Chicago, IL: Quintessence, pp. 203–210.

43. Svensson, P., Sessle, B.J. (2004). Orofacial pain. In: Miles, T.S., Nauntofte, B., Svensson, P. (eds.). *Clinical Oral Physiology*. Copenhagen: Quintessence, pp. 93–139.

CHAPTER 2

Role of Peripheral Mechanisms in Spinal Pain Conditions

BRIAN E. CAIRNS[1] and PRADIT PRATEEPAVANICH[2]

[1]Faculty of Pharmaceutical Sciences, The University of British Columbia
[2]Department of Rehabilitation Medicine, Siriraj Hospital, Mahidol University

Content

Peripheral Receptor Targets for Analgesia: Novel Approaches to Pain Management, Edited by Brian E. Cairns

2.1 DIVERSITY OF SPINAL CORD INNERVATED TISSUES

The purpose of this chapter is to provide a description of peripheral pain transduction mechanisms and their role in several chronic pain conditions affecting spinal cord innervated areas of the body. This chapter is intended to provide both a general overview of the characteristics of nociceptors that innervate various tissues of the body as well as a clinical description of disorders with an overview of pathophysiology that emphasizes actual or suspected peripheral mechanisms in the affected tissues.

With the exception of the craniofacial region, the spinal cord innervates the entire body from the neck to the toes. Spinal cord sensory afferent fibers have their cell bodies in the dorsal root ganglion of the various spinal cord roots from the cervical to the sacral level. Spinal cord sensory afferent fibers are characterized physiologically by their conduction velocity into myelinated Aα- (muscle proprioceptors), Aβ- (low-threshold mechanoreceptors), and Aδ- (mechanoreceptors, thermoreceptors), and unmyelinated C-fibers (polymodal receptors) (Table 2.1). It is generally accepted that thinly myelinated Aδ- and unmyelinated C-fibers with nonspecialized endings are responsible for the transduction of noxious information from most spinal cord innervated tissues; however, more thickly myelinated fibers may also play a role in pain sensation, especially from the skin. The following sections review aspects of the afferent innervation of select organ systems by the spinal cord.

2.2 PERIPHERAL NOCICEPTIVE MECHANISMS IN SPINALLY INNERVATED TISSUES

2.2.1 Cutaneous Tissues

Peripheral nociceptive mechanisms in the skin are by far the best studied of any tissue in the body. The skin is innervated by fast-conducting, thickly

TABLE 2.1. Sensory Primary Afferent Subtypes and Their Function.

Fiber Type	Subtype	Function
A	Aα	Motor efferent fibers, spindle and golgi tendon organ afferent fibers, proprioception, stretch, reflex activity
	Aβ	Discriminative touch, pressure sensation (innocuous), joint rotation
	Aγ	Muscle spindle efferent fibers
	Aδ	Touch, temperature, pressure, and chemical (innocuous to noxious)
B		Preganglionic autonomic, vascular smooth muscle
C	Sympathetic	Postganglionic autonomic
	Sensory	Touch, temperature, pressure, and chemical (innocuous to noxious)

myelinated Aβ- (group II) and slowly conducting, thinly myelinated Aδ- (group III) and unmyelinated C-(group IV) fibers. Many of these fibers innervate the epidermis and terminate in nonspecialized endings. Cutaneous fibers that respond to stimuli that are potentially or actually tissue damaging (noxious stimuli), such as intense mechanical stimuli (pinch, pressure, indentation), algesic chemical, or elevated thermal (>45 °C) stimuli, are considered nociceptors (Figure 2.1a). Cutaneous afferent fibers that become responsive to noxious mechanical stimulation only after tissue inflammation or the application of algesic chemicals are known as "silent" nociceptors [1]. The vast majority of silent nociceptors are C-fibers, and it has been speculated that these fibers are normally chemoreceptive but can be sufficiently sensitized to respond to mechanical stimuli under conditions associated with tissue injury [1]. Cutaneous nociceptors project to the dorsal horn of the spinal cord. The major termination of cutaneous Aδ-fibers is lamina I, whereas cutaneous C-fibers project to both laminae I and II. In addition, cutaneous fibers also project to laminae III and IV of the spinal dorsal horn [1].

In addition to categorizing cutaneous nociceptors by conduction velocity, these fibers are usually categorized based on their response to different modalities of noxious stimuli. The two major classes of cutaneous nociceptors are Aδ mechanonociceptors and C polymodal nociceptors, although many other subcategories of cutaneous nociceptors have been described [1]. Other categories include Aδ mechano-heat nociceptors that tend to respond to higher temperatures than C polymodal fibers, Aδ/C cold nociceptors that respond to mechanical and intense cold, and C mechanonociceptors that respond to intense mechanical stimuli [1].

Mechanoreceptors are often categorized by their response to sustained mechanical stimulation [1]. Slowly adapting mechanoreceptors discharge while stimulus is maintained, while rapidly adapting mechanoreceptors discharge only at the initiation (and sometimes the termination) of the stimulus. Rapidly adapting mechanoreceptors are thought to code for the temporal component of stimulus application, while slowly adapting mechanoreceptors may signal information about intensity (such as displacement, velocity). The Aδ mechanonociceptors often exhibit slowly adapting responses to high-intensity mechanical stimuli while lacking a response to thermal stimuli, although some respond to thermal stimuli after sensitization by inflammation or algesic chemicals. In addition, a subpopulation of Aβ-fibers also appears to respond to noxious mechanical stimulation. Activation of Aβ-fibers in the skin by noxious stimuli may explain why the source of cutaneous pain, unlike pain from deeper tissues, is reasonably easy to discriminate [2].

C polymodal afferent fibers also respond to noxious mechanical stimuli. In addition, these nociceptors respond to noxious thermal (>45 °C) stimuli and cutaneous administration of algesic chemicals [1]. These nociceptors commonly express the transient receptor potential (TRP) receptors, such as the TRP vanilloid 1 (TRPV1) receptor that is responsive to capsaicin (Figure 2.1a). Many cutaneous nociceptors have other TRP receptors and receptors

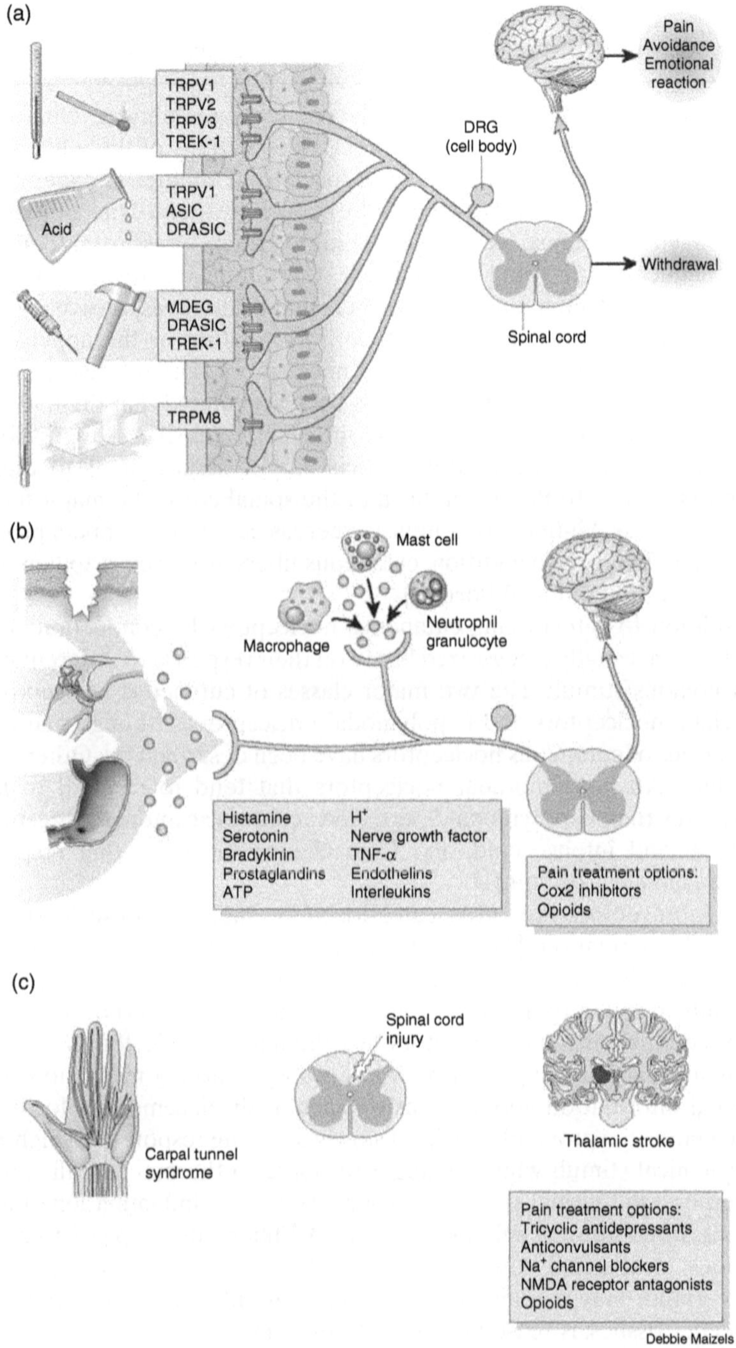

FIGURE 2.1. Pain can result from nociceptive, inflammatory, or neuropathic mechanisms that occur in the periphery. The transduction of noxious thermal (cold and heat), chemical, and mechanical stimuli occurs through the activation of specific receptors located on the nociceptor. Tissue inflammation leads to the release of a number of proinflammatory mediators that can excite and sensitize nociceptors. Neuropathic pain is often the result of an injury to a peripheral nerve but can also be produced by lesions in the central nervous system. Reprinted by permission from Macmillan Publishers: [NATURE NEUROSCIENCE] (Scholz, J., Woolf, CJ. (2002). Can we conquer pain? *Nat Neurosci* 5:1062–1067), copyright (2002).

such as the acid-sensing ion channels (ASICs), which allow them to respond to other algesic chemicals (menthol, mustard oil) and low pH [3].

2.2.2 Joints

A typical joint, such as the knee joint, is innervated by group II, group III, and a high proportion of group IV fibers. Group III and group IV fibers terminate as nonspecialized nerve endings in the capsule of the joint, or in joint-associated tissues such as adipose tissue, ligaments, menisci, and the periosteum [4]. Joint cartilage is not innervated. The majority of group III and group IV fibers responds to noxious mechanical and/or chemical stimuli applied to fibrous structures such as the joint capsule or ligaments and act as nociceptors. In noninjured joints, joint nociceptors are not activated by movement of the joint in the normal working range, but only respond to twisting the joint beyond its normal range of motion or intense pressure applied to the capsule [4,5]. During joint inflammation or after intra-articular injection of algesic chemicals such as bradykinin, prostaglandin (PG)E2, and PGE1, mechanonociceptors can become sensitized and respond to normal joint movements, while there may also be recruitment of silent nociceptors, which in the joint are primarily group IV fibers [6]. As in skeletal muscle, the majority of group III and IV fibers is also chemosensitive (Figure 2.1b).

2.2.3 Skeletal Muscle

Skeletal muscle is also innervated by large, myelinated fibers as well as group III (Aδ) and group IV (C) afferent fibers that have nonspecialized endings and can respond to noxious mechanical and/or chemical stimuli [7,8]. Anatomical and electrophysiological studies in animals suggest that in the skeletal muscle, many unmyelinated nerve fibers terminate near arterioles and venules, while many thinly myelinated nerve fibers terminate in the walls of small arteries, venules, and lymphatic segments [7]. These slowly conducting muscle afferent fibers project to lamina I and laminae IV/V of the spinal cord [9,10]. Slowly conducting fibers that innervate the skeletal muscle often have high mechanical thresholds and slowly adapting responses that are consistent with a role in mechanical nociception. These afferent fibers can also be excited by changes in interstitial osmolarity and pH as well as by increases in the interstitial concentrations of a number of compounds associated with tissue injury, such as potassium chloride (KCl), adenosine triphosphate (ATP), biogenic amine, and amino acid neurotransmitters, and algogenic substances such as bradykinin and various cytokines. Some slowly conducting muscle afferent fibers also respond to innocuous and noxious thermal stimuli [11,12]. At present, it is unclear whether there are silent nociceptors in the skeletal muscle. It is also apparent that in the muscle tissue, both Aδ- and C-fibers may serve as polymodal nociceptors.

2.2.4 The Viscera

The viscera are comprised of various organs of the body that are associated with painful conditions, such as those found in the cardiovascular system as well as the gastrointestinal and genitourinary tracts. In general, these organs are innervated by both thinly myelinated Aδ- and unmyelinated C-fibers that have their central terminations in the dorsal horn of the spinal cord. In many organs, visceral afferent fibers can be classified by their response to mechanical stimuli as intensity-encoding mechanoreceptors, high-threshold mechanoreceptors, or mechanically insensitive receptors [13,14]. Intensity-encoding mechanoreceptors have a low threshold but encode mechanical stimuli into the noxious range, and their activation has been suggested to be responsible for transition from nonpainful to painful visceral sensations. High-threshold mechanoreceptors, as their name implies, have a mechanical threshold in the noxious range. Mechanically insensitive receptors appear to be similar to the silent nociceptors described in the joint and skin in that they become mechanically responsive only under conditions associated with tissues damage such as inflammation or ischemia. Mechanically insensitive receptors are thought to be particularly important in visceral tissues where chemical sensation predominates, for example, in the heart where pain is related to ischemia or chemical stimuli and no noxious mechanical stimuli are known.

2.2.5 Heart

Sympathetic sensory afferent fibers with cell bodies in the dorsal root ganglion and projections to the upper thoracic spinal cord are thought to be the pathway by which nociceptive input from cardiac tissues is transmitted to the central nervous system [15]. These fibers form synaptic contacts in laminae I, V, VII, and X of the thoracic dorsal horn [15]. Thinly myelinated and unmyelinated parasympathetic afferent fibers with cell bodies in the nodose ganglion may also contribute to ischemic pain in this organ [16]. These fibers have nonspecialized endings that are branched and innervate the epicardium [15]. The heart also contains silent nociceptors that are activated by ischemia-related inflammation. Many unmyelinated sympathetic afferent fibers are excited by low pH, potassium, and adenosine and bradykinin, chemical stimuli associated with ischemic tissue damage [15,17].

2.2.6 Gastrointestinal Tract

The gastrointestinal tract is also innervated by slowly conducting, thinly myelinated and unmyelinated afferent fibers of the splanchnic and pelvic nerves that lack specialized endings and terminate in viscus muscle layers or in association with arteries and veins [13,18]. The majority of these fibers is mechanoreceptors and are activated by distension and contraction of the gastrointestinal smooth muscle [18]. Many of these fibers also encode mechanical distention into the noxious range and may be sensitized by either chemical or thermal stimuli, which suggests that these fibers serve as polymodal nociceptors [13,18]. These fibers can be sensitized by ischemia and by algesic substances such as bradykinin, ATP, capsaicin, and prostaglandins (Figure 2.1b) [19]. Bradykinin and prostaglandins interact in a potentiating way to modulate the sensitivity of spinal afferent endings, reducing the threshold for activation to cause hypersensitivity [13,18].

2.2.7 Bladder

The bladder is innervated by slowly conducting, thinly myelinated and unmyelinated afferent fibers of the splanchnic and pelvic nerves that are predominantly mechanoreceptive [20,21]. Although many of these fibers have low thresholds to mechanical stimulation, the vast majority of these fibers is also activated by the noxious distention of the bladder [20]. Bladder afferent fibers project to lamina I and laminae IV–V of the spinal cord dorsal horn [22]. It has been speculated that ATP release from the urothelium (bladder epithelium cells) acts on P2X3 receptors expressed on unmyelinated afferent fibers is necessary for normal triggering of reflex bladder activity as well as for the pain behavior resulting from bladder irritation [14,23]. ATP can be released from urothelium cells as a result of the activation of TRPV1 receptors present on the majority of afferents innervating the urinary tracts [14].

2.2.8 Uterus

The uterus appears to be innervated almost exclusively by C-fibers [24,25]. These fibers can be divided by their threshold response to mechanical distention of the uterus as low threshold, high threshold, or mechanically insensitive. Virtually all uterine fibers respond to bradykinin, and about 50% also respond to noxious thermal stimulation, which suggests that a large proportion of uterine afferent fibers in the hypogastric nerve are polymodal C-fibers. These afferent fibers differ from other visceral afferents in that they express TRPV1 but not P2X3 receptors [26]. Interestingly, it has been found that ~5–15% of afferent fibers that innervate the uterus appear to have collateral branches that innervate the colon [27]. If these fibers convey noxious information, this finding suggests that excitation of afferent endings in one organ could potentially alter afferent sensitivity in the other organ.

2.3 ROLE OF PERIPHERAL MECHANISMS IN SELECT PAIN CONDITIONS

2.3.1 Neuropathic Pain

Neuropathic pain occurs as a consequence of a lesion in the peripheral or central nervous system, although in many patients, the lesion and/or source of noxious input is not identified (Figure 2.2). This has resulted in the term "non-

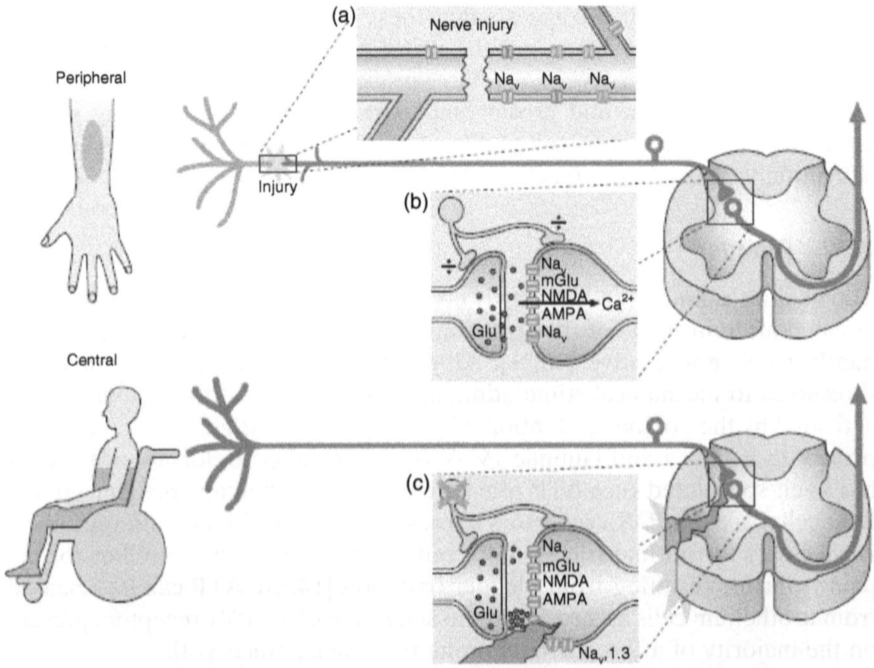

FIGURE 2.2. Both peripheral and central mechanisms can lead to the development of neuropathic pain conditions. A key change in this process is the development of central sensitization, which is mediated through an increase in glutamatergic synaptic activity. Reprinted by permission from Macmillan Publishers: [NATURE CLINICAL PRACTICE NEUROLOGY] (Finnerup, N.B., Jensen, T.S. (2006). Mechanisms of disease: mechanism-based classification of neuropathic pain—a critical analysis. *Nat Clin Pract Neurol* 2:107–115), copyright (2006).

nociceptive pain" being applied to pain symptoms associated with this group of conditions. Neuropathic pain usually produces not a single but a constellation of symptoms such as dysesthesia (spontaneous or evoked unpleasant sensations) or paroxysmal (intermittent, short-lasting, intense, stereotyped) pain and evidence of sensory, motor, and/or autonomic dysfunction in the pain area. These pain conditions are characterized by their resistance to treatment with conventional analgesics [28].

The diagnosis of neuropathic pain can be classified into one of three groups: possible, probable, or definite. Possible neuropathic pain requires both pain in a neuroanatomical area and a history of relevant disease or lesion in the nervous system. Probable neuropathic pain requires possible neuropathic pain criteria plus a decreased sensibility in the painful area. Definite neuropathic pain requires probable neuropathic pain criteria plus a documented nerve lesion. It is important to recognize that one mechanism can explain more than one symptom, but that one symptom may derive from many mechanisms.

In acute animal models of nerve injury, immune cells such as neutrophils, mast cells, and macrophages migrate to the site of injury and release a number of immune mediators. These compounds (cytokines, growth factors, inflammatory mediators, etc.) released in the vicinity of an acute nerve injury may act directly on nerve fibers to alter their activity or indirectly by influencing immune cells to result in pain [29,30]. They may also induce in phenotypic changes in the surviving nociceptors, for example, upregulation of tetrodotoxin-resistant sodium channels and the development of spontaneous afferent discharge. Over a period of months after the initial injury, dorsal root ganglion neurons are lost as resident immune cells in the dorsal root ganglion react to the remote nerve injury and act to destroy degenerating dorsal root ganglion neurons that have been axotomized [29,30]. In many animal models, the formation of sympathetic basketlike structures around the large dorsal root ganglion neurons has also been demonstrated, although their exact role in the development of pain remains a matter of debate. Consequences of a peripheral nerve injury on the central nervous system include the development of central sensitization and loss of inhibitory interneurons as a result of the ongoing afferent barrages, as well as the release of sensitizing agents (tumor necrosis factor alpha [TNF-α], cytokines), and changes in the expression of various receptors.

As mentioned, it is often not possible to identify the precipitating nerve lesion in patients with neuropathic pain. As a result, neuropathic pain is often categorized by the apparent underlying cause. For example, there are peripheral neuropathies for which the apparent cause is diabetes, viral infection (postherpetic neuralgia), or limb amputation (phantom limb pain), as well as central neuropathies are associated with strokes and spinal cord injuries [31]. Less common causes of peripheral neuropathies include complex regional pain syndromes (CRPSs), radiculopathies that occur as a result of dysfunction of spinal nerve roots as a result of nerve damage, and acquired immune deficiency syndrome, where about 2% develop neuropathic pain syndromes [32]. The following sections provide additional information about the more common causes of peripheral neuropathies.

2.3.2 Painful Diabetic Neuropathy

Diabetes mellitus is the most common cause of neuropathy, and neuropathic symptoms associated with this condition have been described for over 100 years [33,34]. Diabetic sensorimotor polyneuropathy is the most common form of diabetic neuropathies. Although sensory deficits from this condition can be demonstrated in the vast majority (~70%) of both type I and type II diabetics, only about 15–25% of diabetics have symptoms and only a small percentage will actually develop significant pain from these sensory changes [32,34,35]. Diabetic sensorimotor polyneuropathy is characterized by a slow progression of sensory deficits starting at the feet and spreading upwards to affect the legs and distal parts of the upper limbs over time. Symptoms can include numbness, burning foot pain, pins-and-needles sensations, and paroxysmal pains that are often more pronounced at night. It is thought that symptoms occur as a result of prolonged, hyperglycemia-induced epineural vascular damage, nerve fiber loss, and demyelination [33,34]. Slowing of nerve conduction due to demyelination can be demonstrated [33], and there is an apparent loss of small fiber (myelinated and unmyelinated) mechanonociceptors early in the process [33]. An increase in inflammatory reactions in the nerves has been demonstrated [33].

2.3.3 Postherpetic Neuralgia

Postherpetic neuralgia occurs as a result of pain developing or persisting after shingles, an acute reemergence of a herpes zoster infection [28,32]. It is estimated that somewhere between 7% and 27% of persons who have shingles can go on to develop postherpetic neuralgia [32]. Pain is typically neuropathic, with both brief episodes of sharp or lancinating pain lasting seconds, as well as more sustained and severe pain that can be either stimulus evoked or stimulus independent. Dynamic mechanical allodynia is one of the most common symptoms of this form of neuralgia [36]. The underlying cause of pain is thought to result from a combination of demyelination and ganglion neuron loss as a result of the herpes zoster infection. The lancinating nature of episodic pain in this condition has been suggested to result from ephaptic (axon to axon) transmission due to demyelination, although there is no evidence that this can occur *in vivo*. Shingles is also a significant cause of trigeminal neuralgia (see Chapter 1).

2.3.4 Phantom Limb Pain

Pain ascribed to an amputated limb is referred to as phantom limb pain and is differentiated from pain localized to the nerve stump. Its symptoms can include intense, burning pain, perceived cramping and tremor, and perceived swelling within the phantom limb [37]. There has been a suggestion of an association of this pain with somatosensory cortical reorganization, which occurs as a result of the loss of sensory input from the amputated limb, although this association is complex and is not predictive of the intensity of pain [37]. Phantom limb pain may occur during the first year after amputation in 53–85% of patients [32,37].

2.3.5 CRPSs I and II

CRPS comprises a group of neuropathic pain disorders associated with significant ongoing and stimulus-evoked pain, which often develop after a seemingly minor tissue trauma [38]. Normally, innocuous mechanical stimuli, such as clothing touching the affected area, may cause pain [39]. Some patients also become extremely sensitive to small changes in temperature [39]. Increased sweating and changes of skin, nail, and hair growth patterns are common in the affected area [39]. In addition, increased or decreased vascular tone within the affected area may make it either cold, blue, pale, and sweaty or hot, red, and dry [39,40]. There are two major subcategories of the disorder. CRPS I or reflex sympathetic dystrophy often occurs after injuries that are not clearly associated with an identifiable nerve injury (e.g., sprain or fracture) but results in immobilization, although central mechanisms such as stroke-related injury have also been identified in some patients [39,41]. Pain in CRPS I is disproportionate to the tissue injury and is not usually confined to tissues innervated by a single nerve. Ongoing pain in this disorder is often described as stinging or burning [38,39]. In a subgroup of CRPS patients, pain appears to be sympathetically maintained, as manipulations of the sympathetic nervous system (e.g., sympathetic blocks) attenuate pain [41]. In contrast, CRPS II or causalgia is usually associated with a definite nerve injury event, such as nerve damage during surgery or a crush injury [41]. Patients with CRPS II often report typical shooting or electrical pain symptoms similar to other neuropathic pain conditions and exhibit hypoesthesia with allodynia in the affected area [39].

The exact pathophysiology of CRPS has not been determined; however, there is evidence that both peripheral and central mechanisms contribute to the pain in this disorder. The best studied peripheral mechanism is the development of an interaction between the sympathetic and sensory nervous systems that occurs after nerve injury. In healthy animals, the sympathetic nervous system does not directly interact with the sensory nervous system. In animal nerve injury models, sprouting of sympathetic efferents into the dorsal root ganglion to form basket structures around the ganglion neuron has been observed, and dorsal root ganglion neurons become more responsive to norepinephrine [42]. In addition, experimental nerve injury causes sympathetic efferent fibers to wrap around the endings of sensory afferent fibers in the skin and may permit coupling between the sympathetic efferent sensory afferent nerve terminals [42]. Some cutaneous nociceptors appear to become responsive to norepinephrine under these conditions [41]. Anatomical changes are reasonably well correlated with changes in nocifensive behavior in the animal nerve injury models studied, which suggests that nerve injury results in a novel peripheral sympathetic–sensory interaction.

Local changes in sensitivity to sympathetic activation, as evidenced by changes in vascular function in the affected tissues, also occur in many CRPS patients. Further, blockade of sympathetic tone to an affected region may decrease edema, although neurogenic mechanisms that result in the release of vasoactive peptides such as calcitonin gene-related peptide (CGRP) or substance P, likely also contribute to this edema [43,44]. In a subset of CRPS patients, an association between sympathetic tone and ongoing pain intensity can be demonstrated [41]. In CRPS patients, the expression of α1-adrenoreceptors in the affected skin has been found to be increased [42], and a recent study suggests that mechanically insensitive C-fibers may be excited by norepinephrine in conditions of sympathetically maintained pain [45]. Nevertheless, it should be recognized that many CRPS patients do not exhibit characteristics of sympathetically maintained pain and that anti-inflammatory agents (e.g., nonsteroidal anti-inflammatory drugs [NSAIDs]) can be effective in treating CRPS-related pain, which suggest that other peripheral mechanisms, such as inflammation, also play a role in this pain disorder [40,42,44].

2.3.6 Arthritis

Osteoarthritis is characterized by joint pain, stiffness, and loss of mobility and commonly affects the hands, knees, hips, and spine [46]. Most individuals over the age of 65 have some evidence of osteoarthritis, and about 10% suffer pain as a result of this disorder [46,47]. Aging, traumatic injury, and, to some extent, genetic factors contribute to alterations in joint loading that result in damage to the cartilage [46,47]. This damage progresses to become chronic with remodeling changes to subchondral bone and low-level joint inflammation, although, unlike other inflammatory arthropathies, osteoarthritis lacks evidence of significant synovial inflammation or systemic manifestations of inflammation [46]. Nevertheless, it is likely that inflammatory mediators contribute to pain in the osteoarthritic joint, particularly in the later stages of the disease. It has also been proposed that loss of blood vessels in the joint over time produces ischemic pain in the joint and periarticular tissues [48]. In part, the age factor may be a reflection of the age-related loss of the chondrocyte capacity to remodel and repair joint cartilage [46]. There is also some evidence that joint afferent mechanosensation is augmented with age, which could also contribute to age-related increases in pain from this condition [47].

In contrast to osteoarthritis, rheumatoid arthritis is a chronic systemic inflammatory disease affecting approximately 0.5–1% of the adult general population [49]. Rheumatoid arthritis typically affects joints of the fingers, toes, and wrists initially and eventually leads to irreversible joint destruction of these and other joints [50]. The triggering event for the development of this condition is unknown [50]. The cause of this form of arthritis is usually attributed to an immune dysfunction, as the condition is characterized by antibody-induced invasion of the joint by T cells, and subsequent joint destruction [49–51]. In addition to the presence of a serological marker, rheumatoid factor, which does not actually appear to play a convincing role in the disease, ~50% of patients also have autoantibodies against collagen that do appear to contribute to arthritis and joint destruction [50]. It is thought that joint pain results from increased intra-articular pressure secondary to edema produce by the frank inflammation associated with this disorder. In the knee joints of rheumatoid arthritis sufferers, synovial fluid volume may be more than 10 times greater than healthy subjects, causing pressures within the knee joint to increase by 30 mmHg or more [12].

2.3.7 Fibromyalgia and Myofascial Pain Syndrome

Myofascial pain is one of the most common forms of chronic pain. For example, it has been estimated that at least 50% of the general population will experience back pain during their adult years [52], while around 85% of patients of specialized pain clinics report symptoms of chronic myofascial pain [53]. Perhaps, the most severe form of chronic myofascial pain occurs in fibromyalgia syndrome, which has a prevalence in the general population of about 2% [52]. The principal symptoms of fibromyalgia syndrome include chronic widespread pain with multiple tender points throughout the body as well as a propensity for increased muscle fatigue and weakness, often exacerbated by exercise [54]. Muscle pain in fibromyalgia fluctuates and is associated with generalized symptoms of increased sensitivity to several modalities of pain (mechanical, thermal), which can be manifested in multiple tissues (muscles, skin, etc.) [54–56].

Myofascial pain syndrome, a related disorder, differs from fibromyalgia in that the muscle pain is usually confined to discrete regions and is characterized by the presence of myofascial trigger points. Fibromyalgia syndrome can also be associated with the presence of myofascial trigger points, and thus, the two conditions are thought to be at least partially overlapping. Myofascial trigger points are regions of tissue (muscle or may be ligaments, periosteum, joints, skin, etc.) that are hyperirritable and, when palpated, cause the patients to report pain of a quality and referral pattern similar to that suffered on an ongoing basis due to their condition. In the muscle tissue, myofascial trigger points are often associated with "taut bands," which are described as areas of localized increased contraction within the muscle and exhibit increased electromyographic activity. In addition, myofascial trigger points appear to be regions of altered muscle function and may exhibit indications of ischemia or altered metabolic function, such as decreased pH and elevated cytokines (e.g., TNF-α, interleukin-6).

Muscle pain reported by myofascial pain syndrome sufferers is well localized. Even in fibromyalgia, sufferers do not complain of diffuse, generalized pain, but rather pain from specific, usually muscle, sources. The reasonably well-localized muscle pain in these conditions has led to the speculation that certain peripheral sites are important pain generators that initiate and may maintain pain in this condition [54]. Arendt-Nielsen and Henriksson have proposed that a majority of fibromyalgia patients fit into a "bottom-to-top model" where widespread pain occurs after a chronic but not localized muscle pain [56]. This proposal suggests that as more muscle sites become involved, there will be a tendency toward generalized pain sensitivity that is a hallmark of fibromyalgia. In other words, ongoing pain in the periphery is critical for the development and maintenance of the symptoms of many fibromyalgia syndrome patients. Nevertheless, it appears that a subgroup of fibromyalgia (FM) patients lack a peripheral locus for their pain.

Local muscle ischemia has been put forward as a mechanism for the development of myofascial trigger points. Hypoperfusion of the muscle can lead to the release of algogenic substances, which alters function and produces pain. The consequences of hypoperfusion are exacerbated under conditions of tonic exercise, making this an attractive hypothesis to explain some of the symptoms of both myofascial pain and fibromyalgia syndrome. In fibromyalgia, there is evidence of decreased blood flow in the trapezius muscle, a common source of muscle pain in this condition [54,55]. In addition, muscle exercise seems to have a more profound effect on muscle blood flow in fibromyalgia sufferers than healthy controls [54,55]. In active myofascial trigger points, it has been reported that pH is lowered and several vasoactive peptides (substance P, bradykinin, CGRP) and cytokines (interleukin-6, -8, and TNF-α) are elevated compared with normal muscle or nonactive trigger points [57,58]. Muscle tissue hypoxia due to hypoperfusion is an effective stimuli for the activation of muscle nociceptors [54,55]. Baseline blood flow in infraspinatus muscle (a shoulder blade muscle) of FM and controls was not different, but during static contractions, the majority of FM patients had poor or no increased blood flow compared with controls, who had increased blood flow [59]. It has been suggested that sympathetic dysfunction or loss of adrenergic beta receptors in muscle vascular beds may be responsible for this observation.

It is important to recognize that many of the symptoms associated with fibromyalgia syndrome indicate that a process of central nervous system sensitization is responsible. Although it has been proposed that tonic nociceptive input from the muscle is required to initiate and maintain central sensitization, other purely central mechanisms, such as a deficit in descending inhibitory mechanisms, have also been proposed [54,55]. The combination of central sensitization and decreased descending inhibition may lead to the more generalized pain complaints seen in fibromyalgia syndrome, even in the absence of peripheral nociceptive inputs [60]. In addition, central mechanisms involving abnormal stress response resulting in hyporeactivity to stress have been proposed to contribute to the development and maintenance of fibromyalgia syndrome [55,60].

2.3.8 Inflammatory Bowel Diseases and Irritable Bowel Syndrome

The highest prevalence of inflammatory bowel diseases, which encompass the two main conditions of Crohn's disease and ulcerative colitis, occurs in northern Europe and North America and have a prevalence of ~0.04% [61]. These conditions are characterized by relapsing abdominal pain, chronic diarrhea, weight loss, malaise, and fever [62–64]. Crohn's is characterized by the presence of discontinuous aphthous ulcers that may occur anywhere in the gastrointestinal tract, whereas in ulcerative colitis, inflammation is confined to the colon and is continuous [62,63].

The mechanisms that underlie the development of these conditions appear to be of peripheral origin and are multifactor. Environmental factors appear to play an important part in the development of inflammatory bowel disease, although they do not appear to be causative [62,65,66]. In Crohn's disease, which appears to be a condition of impaired immunologic tolerance, it is thought that enteric pathogens trigger an overshoot of the immune response or expose a defect in the ability of the immune system to downregulate after an acute insult, which leads to a chronic inflammatory response [62,66]. This inflammation is associated with the enhanced production of TNF-α and interleukin-12 p40 and overly aggressive acquired (T cell) immune responses to certain enteric bacteria [65,66]. These changes appear to occur in genetically susceptible hosts, as several mutated genes associated with the development of Crohn's disease appear to code for proteins that would be expected to modulate immune responsiveness [65,66]. For example, the *NOD2* gene, a cytosolic protein that recognizes a bacterial cell wall component, is associated with about 30% of European cases of Crohn's disease, and the *DLG5* gene, which encodes a scaffolding protein involved in the maintenance of epithelial integrity, also suggests a role for gene mutations in the development of Crohn's disease [64,65]. Ulcerative colitis is also associated with gene mutations, for example, the multidrug resistance gene (*MDR1*) encodes P-glycoprotein 170, a transporter that governs efflux of drugs and other compounds from cells [66].

In contrast, irritable bowel syndrome, with a prevalence of 10–20% in the general population, is a much more common condition that is not strongly associated with obvious pathophysiological change in the gastrointestinal mucosa [67]. This syndrome is characterized by abdominal pain with a change in bowel habits [68,69]. There is also evidence of visceral hypersensitivity (tenderness to palpation, ongoing pain, provoked pain, endoscopy, or balloon distension of colon) in these patients [68–70].

The initiating event in this syndrome remains obscure, although there is some evidence from animal studies that acute infection or low-grade inflammatory insult produces irritable bowel syndrome-like symptoms, and perhaps as many as 30% of patients report irritable bowel syndrome symptom initiation in association with a gastrointestinal infection [69]. Both peripheral and central mechanisms appear to play a role in the development of pain in irritable bowel syndrome. In addition to local symptoms of abdominal pain, irritable bowel syndrome patients exhibit increased sensitivity to remote noxious stimuli, and psychosocial factors (particularly stress) are associated with the development of this disorder, which suggest a role for central mechanisms [68,69]. However, it has been demonstrated that local anesthesia of the gastrointestinal tract of irritable bowel syndrome sufferers not only attenuates abdominal pain but also reverses symptoms of generalized pain hypersensitivity associated with this disorder, which suggests that tonic peripheral input is important in the maintenance of pain symptoms in this condition [68].

2.3.9 Dysmenorrhea

Primary dysmenorrhea is an example of a visceral condition for which a peripheral mechanism is reasonably well established. Primary dysmenorrhea is a condition of painful menstrual cramps without evidence of pathological change to the endometrium of the uterus [71,72]. The prevalence of this condition is reported around 50%, peaks in women 20–24 years of age, and decreases thereafter. Pain occurs just preceding or with the onset of menstruation and is described as fluctuating, spasmodic, and labor like. Pain is most intense in the first 24 hours, lasts 2–3 days, and may include backache, nausea, vomiting, and diarrhea. Approximately, two-thirds of dysmenorrhea sufferers report pain of moderate to severe intensity.

It is thought that the vast majority of primary dysmenorrheas results from an increase in the release of PGs, which increases uterine contractions and leads to a reduction in uterine blood flow, hypoxia, and pain [71,72]. This concept is reinforced by findings that most sufferers respond to NSAIDs, which block the production of PGs. NSAIDs reduce both pain and PG levels to or below those of women who do not have pain. Although many prostaglandins are produced by the endometrium, it appears that $PGF_{2\alpha}$, which is elevated in the endometrium and menstrual flow, may be the principal PG involved [71]. Indeed, menstrual cramp intensity has been shown to be proportional to $PGF_{2\alpha}$ content [71]. Nevertheless, a proportion of women have severe symptoms of dysmenorrhea that do not appear to be associated with increased PG levels, and it has been suggested that other compounds, such as prostacyclins or leukotrienes may be responsible for pain in these women [71,72].

2.4 SUMMARY

As reviewed above, pain in a number of common chronic painful conditions appears to result from specific peripheral nociceptive mechanisms. This suggests that pain in these conditions could be ameliorated by the use of locally acting analgesics that may minimize untoward side effects of similar systemically active agents. A current example of this approach is the treatment of arthritis by topical NSAIDs, such as diclofenac. Current research suggests that diclofenac is not only effective for arthritis-related pain when used topically, but that serious drug-related side effects associated with the use of this class of drug, such as exacerbation of hypertension, altered renal function, and gastrointestinal ulceration, are also markedly reduced when this agent is employed locally rather than systemically. On the other hand, local analgesic agents can also be particularly useful in helping to determine what component of ongoing pain in chronic pain sufferers is mediated through peripheral as opposed to central nervous system mechanisms. Thus, the development of a greater arsenal of peripherally acting analgesic agents will serve both to enhance the diagnosis of pain mechanisms and to improve their treatment in a number of challenging chronic pain conditions.

REFERENCES

1. Willis, W.D., Coggeshall, R.E. (1991). *Sensory Mechanisms of the Spinal Cord*. New York: Plenum Press.

2. Djouhri, L., Lawson, S.N. (2004). A-fiber nociceptive primary afferent neurons: a review of incidence and properties in relation to other afferent A-fiber neurons in mammals. *Brain Res Rev* 46:131–145.

3. Willis, W.D. (2007). The somatosensory system, with emphasis on structures important for pain. *Brain Res Rev* 55:297–313.

4. Schaible, H.-G. (2006). Articular nociceptors. In: Schmidt, R.F., Willis, W.D.J. (eds.). *Encyclopedic Reference of Pain*. Heidelberg: Springer-Verlag, pp. 124–127.

5. Schaible, H.G., Schmelz, M., Tegeder, I. (2006). Pathophysiology and treatment of pain in joint disease. *Adv Drug Deliv Rev* 58:323–342.

6. McDougall, J.J. (2006). Arthritis and pain. Neurogenic origin of joint pain. *Arthritis Res Ther* 8:220.

7. Haouzi, P., Chenuel, B., Huszczuk, A. (2004). Sensing vascular distension in skeletal muscle by slow conducting afferent fibers: neurophysiological basis and implication for respiratory control. *J Appl Physiol* 96:407–418.

8. Graven-Nielsen, T., Mense, S. (2001). The peripheral apparatus of muscle pain: evidence from animal and human studies. *Clin J Pain* 17:2–10.

9. Hoheisel, U., Lehmann-Willenbrock, E., Mense, S. (1989). Termination patterns of identified group II and III afferent fibres from deep tissues in the spinal cord of the cat. *Neuroscience* 28:495–507.

10. Panneton, W.M., Gan, Q., Juric, R. (2005). The central termination of sensory fibers from nerves to the gastrocnemius muscle of the rat. *Neuroscience* 134:175–187.

11. Mense, S., Meyer, H. (1988). Bradykinin-induced modulation of the response behaviour of different types of feline group III and IV muscle receptors. *J Physiol* 398:49–63.

12. Kumazawa, T., Mizumura, K. (1977). Thin-fibre receptors responding to mechanical, chemical, and thermal stimulation in the skeletal muscle of the dog. *J Physiol* 273:179–194.

13. Blackshaw, L.A., Gebhart, G.F. (2002). The pharmacology of gastrointestinal nociceptive pathways. *Curr Opin Pharmacol* 2:642–649.

14. Cervero, F., Laird, J.M. (2004). Understanding the signaling and transmission of visceral nociceptive events. *J Neurobiol* 61:45–54.

15. Foreman, R.D. (1999). Mechanisms of cardiac pain. *Annu Rev Physiol* 61:143–167.

16. Hisata, Y., Zeredo, J.L., Eishi, K., Toda, K. (2006). Cardiac nociceptors innervated by vagal afferents in rats. *Auton Neurosci* 126–127:174–178.

17. Wu, Z.Z., Pan, H.L. (2007). Role of TRPV1 and intracellular Ca2+ in excitation of cardiac sensory neurons by bradykinin. *Am J Physiol Regul Integr Comp Physiol* 293:R276–R283.

18. Grundy, D. (2002). Neuroanatomy of visceral nociception: vagal and splanchnic afferent. *Gut* 51:2–5.

19. Blackshaw, L.A., Brookes, S.J., Grundy, D., Schemann, M. (2007). Sensory transmission in the gastrointestinal tract. *Neurogastroenterol Motil* 19:1–19.

20. Sengupta, J.N., Gebhart, G.F. (1994). Mechanosensitive properties of pelvic nerve afferent fibers innervating the urinary bladder of the rat. *J Neurophysiol* 72: 2420–2430.

21. Xu, L., Gebhart, G.F. (2008). Characterization of mouse lumbar splanchnic and pelvic nerve urinary bladder mechanosensory afferents. *J Neurophysiol* 99: 244–253.

22. Wang, H.F., Shortland, P., Park, M.J., Grant, G. (1998). Retrograde and transganglionic transport of horseradish peroxidase-conjugated cholera toxin B subunit, wheatgerm agglutinin and isolectin B4 from *Griffonia simplicifolia* I in primary afferent neurons innervating the rat urinary bladder. *Neuroscience* 87:275–288.

23. Birder, L.A. (2005). More than just a barrier: urothelium as a drug target for urinary bladder pain. *Am J Physiol Renal Physiol* 289:F489–F495.

24. Sandner-Kiesling, A., Pan, H.L., Chen, S.R., James, R.L., DeHaven-Hudkins, D.L., Dewan, D.M., Eisenach, J.C. (2002). Effect of kappa opioid agonists on visceral nociception induced by uterine cervical distension in rats. *Pain* 96:13–22.

25. Liu, B., Eisenach, J.C., Tong, C. (2005). Chronic estrogen sensitizes a subset of mechanosensitive afferents innervating the uterine cervix. *J Neurophysiol* 93:2167–2173.

26. Tong, C., Conklin, D., Clyne, B.B., Stanislaus, J.D., Eisenach, J.C. (2006). Uterine cervical afferents in thoracolumbar dorsal root ganglia express transient receptor potential vanilloid type 1 channel and calcitonin gene-related peptide, but not P2X3 receptor and somatostatin. *Anesthesiology* 104:651–657.

27. Chaban, V., Christensen, A., Wakamatsu, M., McDonald, M., Rapkin, A., McDonald, J., Micevych, P. (2007). The same dorsal root ganglion neurons innervate uterus and colon in the rat. *Neuroreport* 18:209–212.

28. Wu, C.L., Raja, S.N. (2008). An update on the treatment of postherpetic neuralgia. *J Pain* 9:S19–S30.

29. Scholz, J., Woolf, C.J. (2007). The neuropathic pain triad: neurons, immune cells and glia. *Nat Neurosci* 10:1361–1368.

30. Thacker, M.A., Clark, A.K., Marchand, F., McMahon, S.B. (2007). Pathophysiology of peripheral neuropathic pain: immune cells and molecules. *Anesth Analg* 105:838–847.

31. Finnerup, N.B., Sindrup, S.H., Jensen, T.S. (2007). Chronic neuropathic pain: mechanisms, drug targets and measurement. *Fundam Clin Pharmacol* 21:129–136.

32. Sadosky, A., McDermott, A.M., Brandenburg, N.A., Strauss, M. (2008). A review of the epidemiology of painful diabetic peripheral neuropathy, postherpetic neuralgia, and less commonly studied neuropathic pain conditions. *Pain Pract* 8:45–56.

33. Said, G. (2007). Diabetic neuropathy—a review. *Nat Clin Pract Neurol* 3:331–340.

34. Tracy, J.A., Dyck, P.J. (2008). The spectrum of diabetic neuropathies. *Phys Med Rehabil Clin N Am* 19:1–26.

35. Boulton, A.J.M. (2007). Diabetic neuropathy: classification, measurement and treatment. *Curr Opin Endocrinol Diabetes Obes* 14:141–145.

36. Dworkin, R.H., Gnann, J.W.J., Oaklander, A.L., Raja, S.N., Schmader, K.E., Whitley, R.J. (2008). Diagnosis and assessment of pain associated with herpes zoster and postherpetic neuralgia. *J Pain* 9:S37–S44.

37. Acerra, N.E., Souvlis, T., Moseley, G.L. (2007). Stroke, complex regional pain syndrome and phantom limb pain: can commonalities direct future management? *J Rehabil Med* 39:109–114.

38. Stanton-Hicks, M. (2006). Complex regional pain syndrome: manifestations and the role of neurostimulation in its management. *J Pain Symptom Manage* 31: S20–S24.
39. Harden, R.N., Bruehl, S.P. (2006). Diagnosis of complex regional pain syndrome: signs, symptoms, and new empirically derived diagnostic criteria. *Clin J Pain* 22:415–419.
40. Sharma, A., Williams, K., Raja, S.N. (2006). Advances in treatment of complex regional pain syndrome: recent insights on a perplexing disease. *Curr Opin Anaesthesiol* 19:566–572.
41. Straub, R.H., Baerwald, C.G., Wahle, M., Jänig, W. (2005). Autonomic dysfunction in rheumatic diseases. *Rheum Dis Clin North Am* 31:61–75.
42. Gibbs, G.F., Drummond, P.D., Finch, P.M., Phillips, J.K. (2008). Unravelling the pathophysiology of complex regional pain syndrome: focus on sympathetically maintained pain. *Clin Exp Pharmacol Physiol* 35:717–724.
43. Birklein, F. (2005). Complex regional pain syndrome. *J Neurol* 252:131–138.
44. Jänig, W., Baron, R. (2004). Experimental approach to CRPS. *Pain* 108:3–7.
45. Jørum, E., Ørstavik, K., Schmidt, R., Namer, B., Carr, R.W., Kvarstein, G., Hilliges, M., Handwerker, H., Torebjörk, E., Schmelz, M. (2007). Catecholamine-induced excitation of nociceptors in sympathetically maintained pain. *Pain* 127:296–301.
46. Goldring, M.B., Goldring, S.R. (2007). Osteoarthritis. *J Cell Physiol* 213:626–634.
47. McDougall, J.J. (2006). Pain and OA. *J Musculoskelet Neuronal Interact* 6: 385–386.
48. Hancock, C.M., Riegger-Krugh, C. (2008). Modulation of pain in osteoarthritis: the role of nitric oxide. *Clin J Pain* 24:353–365.
49. Okroj, M., Heinegård, D., Holmdahl, R., Blom, A.M. (2007). Rheumatoid arthritis and the complement system. *Ann Med* 39:517–530.
50. Majithia, V., Geraci, S.A. (2007). Rheumatoid arthritis: diagnosis and management. *Am J Med* 120:936–939.
51. Klinkhoff, A. (2004). Biological agents for rheumatoid arthritis: targeting both physical function and structural damage. *Drugs* 64:1267–1283.
52. McBeth, J., Jones, K. (2007). Epidemiology of chronic musculoskeletal pain. *Best Pract Res Clin Rheumatol* 21:403–425.
53. Rooks, D.S. (2007). Fibromyalgia treatment update. *Curr Opin Rheumatol* 19:111–117.
54. Staud, R. (2007). Future perspectives: pathogenesis of chronic muscle pain. *Best Pract Res Clin Rheumatol* 21:581–596.
55. Staud, R. (2006). Biology and therapy of fibromyalgia: pain in fibromyalgia syndrome. *Arthritis Res Ther* 8:208.
56. Arendt-Nielsen, L., Henriksson, K.G. (2007). Pathophysiological mechanisms in chronic musculoskeletal pain (fibromyalgia): the role of central and peripheral sensitization and pain disinhibition. *Best Pract Res Clin Rheumatol* 21:465–480.
57. Shah, J.P., Danoff, J.V., Desai, M.J., Parikh, S., Nakamura, L.Y., Phillips, T.M., Gerber, L.H. (2008). Biochemicals associated with pain and inflammation are elevated in sites near to and remote from active myofascial trigger points. *Arch Phys Med Rehabil* 89:16–23.

58. Shah, J.P., Phillips, T.M., Danoff, J.V., Gerber, L.H. (2005). An in vivo microanalytical technique for measuring the local biochemical milieu of human skeletal muscle. *J Appl Physiol* 99:1977–1984.
59. Elvin, A., Siosteen, A.-K., Nilsson, A., Kosek, E. (2006). Decreased muscle blood flow in fibromyalgia patients during standardised muscle exercise: a contrast media enhanced colour Doppler study. *Eur J Pain* 10:137–144.
60. Price, D.D., Staud, R. (2005). Neurobiology of fibromyalgia syndrome. *J Rheumatol* 32:22–28.
61. Baumgart, D.C., Carding, S.R. (2007). Inflammatory bowel disease: cause and immunobiology. *Lancet* 369:1627–1640.
62. Panés, J., Gomollón, F., Taxonera, C., Hinojosa, J., Clofent, J., Nos, P. (2007). Crohn's disease: a review of current treatment with a focus on biologics. *Drugs* 67:2511–2537.
63. Thoreson, R., Cullen, J.J. (2007). Pathophysiology of inflammatory bowel disease: an overview. *Surg Clin North Am* 87:575–585.
64. Sands, B.E. (2007). Inflammatory bowel disease: past, present, and future. *J Gastroenterol* 42:16–25.
65. Scaldaferri, F., Fiocchi, C. (2007). Inflammatory bowel disease: progress and current concepts of etiopathogenesis. *J Dig Dis* 8:171–178.
66. Sartor, R.B. (2006). Mechanisms of disease: pathogenesis of Crohn's disease and ulcerative colitis. *Nat Clin Pract Gastroenterol Hepatol* 3:390–407.
67. Videlock, E.J., Chang, L. (2007). Irritable bowel syndrome: current approach to symptoms, evaluation, and treatment. *Gastroenterol Clin North Am* 36:665–685.
68. Price, D.D., Zhou, Q., Moshiree, B., Robinson, M.E., Nicholas Verne, G. (2006). Peripheral and central contributions to hyperalgesia in irritable bowel syndrome. *J Pain* 7:529–535.
69. Schwetz, I., Bradesi, S., Mayer, E.A. (2004). The pathophysiology of irritable bowel syndrome. *Minerva Med* 95:419–426.
70. Gebhart, G.F. (2000). Visceral pain—peripheral sensitisation. *Gut* 47:iv54–iv55.
71. Dawood, M.Y. (2006). Primary dysmenorrhea: advances in pathogenesis and management. *Obstet Gynecol* 108:428–441.
72. French, L. (2005). Dysmenorrhea. *Am Fam Physician* 71:285–291.

PART II

SPECIFIC RECEPTOR TARGETS FOR PERIPHERAL ANALGESICS

CHAPTER 3

Voltage-Gated Sodium Channels in Peripheral Nociceptive Neurons as Targets for the Treatment of Pain

THEODORE R. CUMMINS

Department of Pharmacology and Toxicology, Stark Neurosciences Research Institute, Indiana University School of Medicine

Content

Peripheral Receptor Targets for Analgesia: Novel Approaches to Pain Management, Edited by Brian E. Cairns

3.1 INTRODUCTION

Voltage-gated sodium channels are a crucial component of action potential electrogenesis in the majority of mammalian electrically excitable cells, including peripheral nociceptive sensory neurons involved in the transduction and transmission of noxious stimuli [1]. These channels are specialized transmembrane proteins that form a highly selective pathway for sodium to flow from one side of the cytoplasmic membrane to the other, and as the name implies, the flow of sodium through these proteins is controlled, or gated, by the voltage difference across the cytoplasmic membrane. Changes in voltage-sensitive sodium channel properties and voltage-gated sodium currents can clearly contribute to alterations in the generation and propagation of action potentials. While under normal conditions nociceptive sensory neurons are typically quiescent [2], peripheral sensory neurons can become hyperexcitable after nerve injury [3–7] or in response to inflammation [2,8]. This hyperexcitability can contribute to pain, and based on this and other lines of evidence, voltage-gated sodium channels are acknowledged as possible targets for analgesics. Indeed, drugs that inhibit sodium channel activity are used as local anesthetics (LAs) to block pain sensations and in the treatment of inflammatory and neuropathic pain [9–11]. However, sodium channel therapeutics are often associated with undesirable cardiac and central nervous system (CNS) side effects as the available drugs target sodium channels in multiple tissues or have nonspecific actions on additional ion channels and proteins [12,13]. Furthermore, for many individuals with chronic or neuropathic pain, the currently available treatments are not effective [14]. Better and more specific pharmacological agents and therapeutic strategies are needed to treat pain. Advances in our understanding of the molecular biology and pharmacology of voltage-gated sodium channels and the role different voltage-gated sodium channels play in normal and abnormal nociceptor excitability have provided significant insight into how better analgesics that target voltage-gated sodium channels can be developed. This chapter focuses on the role of peripheral neuronal voltage-gated sodium channels in pain and highlights what is known about their pharmacology, genetics, structure, and function.

3.2 FUNCTION OF VOLTAGE-GATED SODIUM CHANNELS

Voltage-gated sodium channels generate ionic currents that are gated in a complex fashion by changes in the electrical potential across the cytoplasmic membrane. A typical voltage-gated sodium channel is ~30 times more permeable to sodium than potassium [15], and as the sodium ion concentration is typically ~10 times higher outside the cell than inside, the sodium currents conducted by these channels flow into the cell under most physiological conditions. Voltage-gated sodium channels are closed at negative membrane potentials, and therefore, at typical resting membrane potentials in neurons (e.g.,

–65 mV), the vast majority of sodium channels is in a nonconducting, closed state (Figure 3.1a). Depolarizations of the membrane potential (which can be induced by excitatory neurotransmitters or, in the case of nociceptive neurons, noxious stimuli) induces the activation of sodium channels, resulting in conducting (open) channels. The large inward sodium gradient results in sodium ions flowing into the cell (Figure 3.1b), and this inward sodium current can cause a further depolarization of the cell membrane potential. This of course can result in more sodium channels opening, and thus, sodium channel activity is considered regenerative. The regenerative sodium channel activity underlies the all-or-none phenomenon known as the action potential whose mechanism was so elegantly dissected by Hodgkin and Huxley [16–20]. Crucial to the termination of the action potential is a second gating process, referred to as inactivation. Inactivation occurs within one to several milliseconds and is often referred to as fast inactivation to distinguish it from a distinct process termed

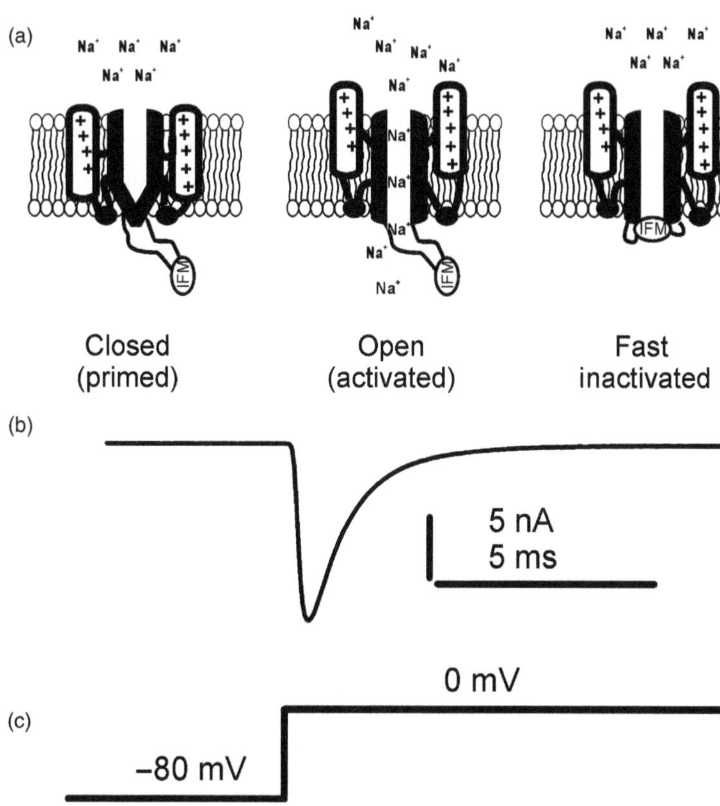

FIGURE 3.1. (a) Cartoon depicting close, open, and fast-inactivated gating confirmations for voltage-gated sodium channels. (b) Voltage clamp recording showing typical voltage-gated sodium currents. The downward deflection reflects the inward movement of sodium ions in response to a depolarizing voltage pulse (c) from a holding potential of –80 mV.

slow inactivation, which occurs during prolonged depolarizations lasting on the order of seconds. Inactivation (either fast or slow) also results in nonconducting channels, and channels must return to negative membrane potentials before they can recover from inactivation (also referred to as repriming). Fast inactivation stops the flow of sodium ions into the cell interior. This, coupled with the activation of potassium channels allowing positively activated potassium ions to flow out of the cell, helps terminate the action potential and allows the repolarization of the membrane potential. The time course for recovery from inactivation can help determine the rate at which excitable cells can generate repetitive action potentials.

Hodgkin and Huxley initially proposed that sodium channels contained three independent charged activation "particles" that responded to changes in membrane potential and determined the activation properties of voltage-gated sodium channels. In the absence of ionic currents, extremely small "gating" currents can be recorded from sodium channels, and a large body of data indicates that these gating currents correspond to the movement of the charged regions of the channel that sense transmembrane potential and are crucial to the activation process [21,22]. Inactivation was initially proposed to be a voltage-dependent process that was completely independent of activation; however, there is now solid evidence demonstrating that inactivation is coupled to activation and derives at least some of its voltage dependence from activation [23]. Sodium channels can inactivate from both open and closed states. Closed-state inactivation, which may actually reflect inactivation of partially activated channels [24], is slower than open-channel inactivation and likely also plays a role in modulating the relative excitability of neurons and muscle. Many of the clinically useful sodium channel blockers enhance the stability of the inactivated state (see below) and increase the proportion of channels that undergo closed-state-inactivation.

For many years, voltage-gated sodium channels were considered to have one basic function, generating the regenerative upstroke of the action potential. The recognition that sodium channels can exhibit complex gating behaviors and that some neurons express more than one type of sodium current has led to the conclusion that sodium channels play a more complicated role in regulating neuronal excitability. This complexity is especially true for peripheral sensory neurons. Although CNS neurons seem to express relatively homogeneous currents exhibiting rapid activation, rapid inactivation, and uniform high sensitivity (IC_{50} ~10nM) to the puffer fish toxin tetrodotoxin (TTX), dorsal root ganglia (DRG) neurons obviously express more complex currents (Figure 3.2) that contain both rapidly inactivating TTX-sensitive components and slowly inactivating TTX-resistant (IC_{50} ≥50µm) components [25,26]. It was proposed that the slower TTX-resistant currents might serve to prolong the duration of the action potential, possibly modulating neurotransmitter release at the nerve terminals. More recently, it has been shown that sensory neurons actually express two distinct types of TTX-resistant currents: both slow-inactivating and persistent TTX-resistant currents [27,28]. Persistent sodium

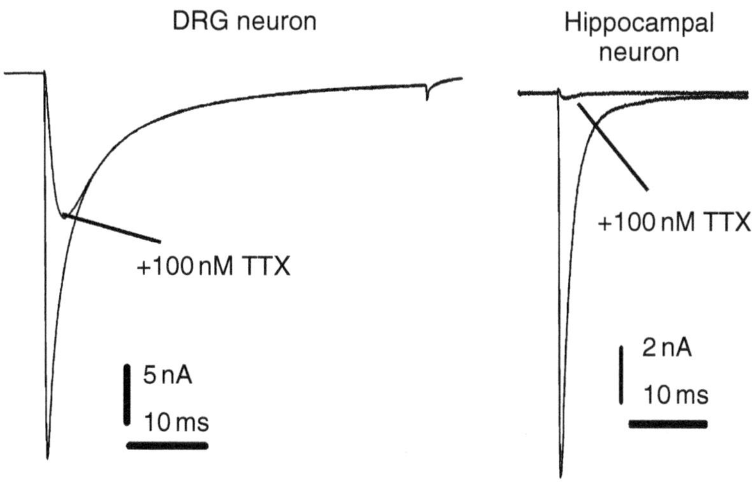

FIGURE 3.2. Comparison of sodium currents recorded from a small-diameter DRG sensory neuron and a hippocampal CA1 neuron. Sodium currents were elicited with step depolarizations from a holding potential of –100 to –10 mV. Tetrodotoxin (TTX) blocks all of the current in the hippocampal neurons but only the fast-inactivating component of the current in the DRG sensory neuron.

currents, sodium currents that persist for prolonged periods during depolarizations, are also often referred to as "noninactivating" sodium current components and can be either TTX sensitive or TTX resistant. Persistent sodium currents have been identified in CNS neurons [29] and in peripheral sensory neurons [30–32] and can have significant influences on the threshold for the generation of the action potential. Resurgent sodium currents are even more unusual and complex types of sodium current that can modulate the excitability of neurons. Resurgent currents were first discovered in cerebellar Purkinje neurons [33] but are also observed in ~40% of medium- and large-diameter DRG sensory neurons [34]. Resurgent currents are atypical currents that are observed during repolarization of the membrane following strong depolarizations. This is surprising because typical sodium currents inactivate during strong depolarizations and, as they close before recovering from inactivation, do not reopen during repolarization. In cerebellar Purkinje neurons, resurgent currents are thought to arise from a distinct inactivation mechanism [35] and play a crucial role in generating bursts of multiple action potentials [36]. The complex gating associated with voltage-gated sodium channels arises, at least in part, from their complex structure.

3.3 STRUCTURE OF VOLTAGE-GATED SODIUM CHANNELS

Biochemical analyses were used to determine that voltage-gated sodium channels are large transmembrane protein complexes. The main functional subunit is the α-subunit, which is an integral membrane protein of ~260kD, that by itself can selectively conduct sodium ions in a voltage-gated manner [37]. As the α-subunit can function by itself, the α-subunits are often referred to as sodium channels, and throughout the rest of this chapter, α-subunit and sodium channel are often used interchangeably. However, typically, the α-subunit is associated with one to two β-subunits [38]. These β-subunits are smaller transmembrane proteins (~30–40kD), and some of them are attached to the α-subunit by a disulfide bond. The first voltage-gated sodium channel α-subunit to be sequenced was from the electric eel [39]. The same group subsequently cloned two different sodium channels from rat brain with similar overall structures [40]. From the amino acid sequences, they deduced that sodium channels had 24 membrane-spanning segments arranged in four repeated homology units often referred to as domains I–IV (Figure 3.3). The fourth transmembrane segment, often referred to as S4, of each domain contains four to seven positively charged amino acid residues that are largely acknowledged as the basis of the gating currents and the voltage-sensors of voltage-gated sodium channels [21,41]. The linker between the S5 and S6 segments, which is on the extracellular side of the channel, actually dips into the plane of the membrane and helps form the external half of the channel pore, including the selectivity filter for sodium ions (referred to as the P-loops). The intracellular half of the pore is thought to be formed by the portion of the S6 segments that is closer to the cytoplasmic face of the channel. Although a high-resolution crystal structure has not been determined for voltage-gated sodium channels, crystal structures have been determined for voltage-gated potassium channels, and the major details relating to the pore and activation structures are believed to be similar. In particular, the crystal structure of the $K_v1.2$ potassium channel [42,43] shows that the S5, S6, and P-loops indeed form the core of the channel pore and that the S1–S4 regions form a relatively independent voltage-sensor structure that is coupled to the pore structure by the S4–S5 linker of each subunit (or domain in the case of voltage-gated sodium channels). Potassium

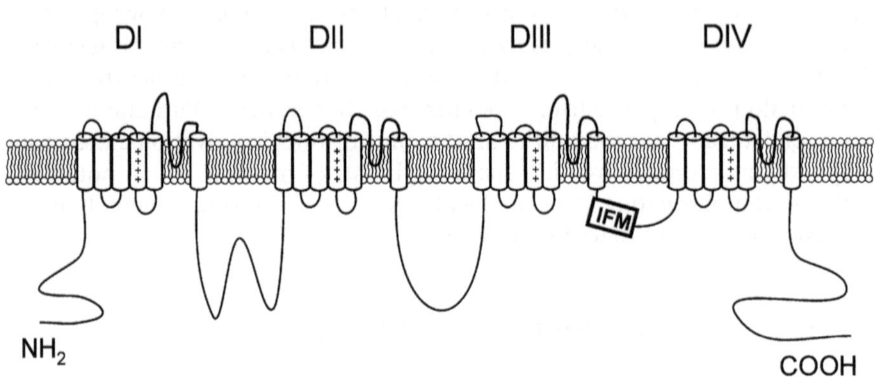

FIGURE 3.3. Linear diagram of a typical voltage-gated sodium channel showing the overall secondary structure.

channels that inactivate can do so by a "ball-and-chain" mechanism involving the C-terminus [44]. In contrast, fast inactivation of voltage-gated sodium channels is believed to operate by a "hinged-lid" mechanism, with the intracellular linker between domains III and IV (the III–IV linker) somehow occluding the conduction pathway during depolarizations [45]. A triplet of amino acid residues in the III–IV linker (isoleucine, phenylalanine, and methionine, or IFM) has been shown to be especially important for fast inactivation, as has the voltage sensor of domain IV [23,46]. It is not entirely clear how the IFM motif interacts with the channel pore, although some studies have implicated the S4–S5 linkers of domains III and IV [47,48]. The precise mechanisms for the development of persistent currents, resurgent currents, and slow inactivation are less clear, although some intriguing hypotheses have been proposed.

3.4 MOLECULAR GENETICS OF VOLTAGE-GATED SODIUM CHANNELS

As mentioned above, the sequences of the first two mammalian voltage-gated sodium channel α-subunits to be determined were published by Noda and colleagues in 1986 [40]. These channels, initially referred to as "brain sodium channels I and II," are now referred to as $Na_v1.1$ and $Na_v1.2$ and were the first mammalian voltage-gated channels to be cloned. Over the next 12 years, before the first draft of the human genome sequence was completed, seven additional voltage-gated sodium channel α-subunits were cloned. All mammals seem to have nine voltage-gated sodium channels ($Na_v1.1$–1.9) generated by distinct genes [49]. Compared with other types of ion channels, the voltage-gated sodium channels are highly conserved. Overall, they exhibit ~80% similarity at the amino acid level, with identity ranging from ~86% between $Na_v1.1$ and $Na_v1.2$ to ~45% between $Na_v1.9$ and each of the other isoforms. Based on the high degree of similarity, it is unlikely that there is another member of the Na_v1 family in humans waiting to be discovered. A tenth gene with some homology to the Na_v1 voltage-gated sodium channels (~40% identity at the amino acid level) has also been identified. However, this channel, referred to as Na_x under the standardized nomenclature, is not believed to belong to the Na_v1 family [50]. The amino acid sequence of Na_x differs from the Na_v1 sequences in key regions that are very highly conserved among the Na_v1 family, such as the pore loops, the S4 voltage-sensors, and the III–IV linker that forms the inactivation gate. Furthermore, several lines of evidence indicate that Na_x is a sodium-gated, not voltage-gated, channel [51,52]. Although Na_x is expressed in many neurons, including nociceptive neurons, the role of Na_x in neuronal excitability is not known, and because Na_x has not been functionally expressed or isolated, virtually nothing is known about the pharmacology of Na_x. It is not known if Na_x could be a target for pain therapeutics, and Na_x will therefore not be considered in the rest of this chapter.

Although the Na_v1 channels are highly conserved, over the last 20 years, research has shown that the different Na_v1 α-subunits have distinctive properties and physiological roles [53,54]. Each of the nine isoforms has specific developmental, tissue, and cellular distributions [55,56]. Although there is overlap in the functional properties and channel distributions, and in some instances, it does appear that loss of a particular isoform can be partially compensated for by increased expression of other isoforms, data from knockout animals and human loss-of-function mutations clearly indicate that this compensation is generally incomplete. Indeed, homozygous knockouts of several of the voltage-gated sodium channels are lethal. Interestingly, seven of the isoforms exhibit significant expression in peripheral sensory neurons [54,55,57,58]. Several of these are thought to play crucial roles in nociception and are likely to be excellent targets for the development of novel therapeutics. In the sections below, what is known about the role(s) of each Na_v1 isoform in physiology is described, with an emphasis on those isoforms that are believed to be especially important in peripheral analgesia. It is important to note that individual neurons—nociceptive neurons in particular—typically express multiple voltage-gated sodium channel genes. Although it is not entirely clear what the importance of this is, it is thought that different isoforms can differentially contribute to excitability, that they are subject to different forms of modulation, and that some may have distinct cellular localizations.

3.4.1 $Na_v1.1$

$Na_v1.1$ is a TTX-sensitive voltage-gated sodium channel (VGSC) that is widely expressed in nervous tissues, including both CNS neurons and peripheral nervous system (PNS) neurons. In CNS neurons, $Na_v1.1$ immunoreactivity is predominantly localized in cell bodies. In expression systems, $Na_v1.1$ produces fast-activating and fast-inactivating sodium currents that are likely to contribute in a major way to the upstroke of action potentials in neurons [59,60]. Interestingly, a large number of $Na_v1.1$ mutations, both gain of function and loss of function, have been identified in patients with inherited epilepsies [61]. $Na_v1.1$ mutations have been identified in patients with migraine [62]; however, it is not clear if these mutations impact the excitability of trigeminal neurons or if the migraine might be due to alterations in CNS neuronal excitability. *In situ* hybridization studies indicate that $Na_v1.1$ mRNA is expressed at fairly high levels in peripheral sensory neurons, with the highest levels in large-diameter sensory neurons, medium expression in medium-diameter neurons, and low-expression levels in small-diameter neurons [57]. Although this expression pattern suggests a limited role in nociceptive neurons, characterization of $Na_v1.1$ current properties and the role of $Na_v1.1$ current in sensory neurons are lacking. In part, this is because $Na_v1.1$ is one of the more difficult sodium channel isoforms to work with, and in part, it is because there are no data implicating $Na_v1.1$ in pain mechanisms. Patients with $Na_v1.1$ mutations that cause epilepsy are not reported to have altered nociception or any other alterations in peripheral sensory functions. It is not believed that $Na_v1.1$ channels play a special role in nociception and pain. Homozygous $Na_v1.1$ knockout mice die at postnatal day 15 [63] following ataxia, seizures, and general deficits in CNS function. Heterozygous mice with haploinsufficiency of $Na_v1.1$ also develop seizures and exhibit a specific loss of sodium currents in neurons that secrete gamma-aminobutyric acid (GABAergic neurons). $Na_v1.1$ has also been found in some cardiac muscle cells [64]. Overall, these results suggest that drugs that specifically target $Na_v1.1$ are likely to be associated with severe CNS side effects and, possibly, some cardiac side effects as well. In addition, because $Na_v1.1$-specific inhibitors are predicted to reduce the activity of GABAergic neurons in the spinal cord, such compounds might even increase pain sensations. $Na_v1.1$ is not believed to be a valid target for the development of novel analgesics.

3.4.2 $Na_v1.2$

$Na_v1.2$ is also not believed to be a good target for analgesics. $Na_v1.2$ is ~90% identical to $Na_v1.1$ and generates fast-activating, fast-inactivating TTX-sensitive sodium currents [65]. $Na_v1.2$ is predominantly expressed in CNS neurons; however, in contrast to $Na_v1.1$, $Na_v1.2$ immunoreactivity is more pronounced in unmyelinated axons than in cell bodies [66,67]. The expression of $Na_v1.2$ is thought to be negligible in peripheral neurons [57]. The restricted CNS expression pattern of $Na_v1.2$ and the fact that knockout of $Na_v1.2$ in mice is perinatally lethal [68] indicate that drugs that specifically target $Na_v1.2$ are also likely to induce significant CNS side effects with no impact on the activity of nociceptive neurons.

3.4.3 $Na_v1.3$

Although $Na_v1.3$ has high homology (~90%) with $Na_v1.1$ and $Na_v1.2$ channels, and also generates fast-activating, fast-inactivating TTX-sensitive currents in neurons [69], $Na_v1.3$ has been proposed as a potential target for analgesics. However, the role of $Na_v1.3$ channels in nociception and pain is controversial. In animal models, $Na_v1.3$ is expressed in developing neurons, but its expression is significantly downregulated as neurons mature [70]. Intriguingly, $Na_v1.3$ expression (as judged by both mRNA levels and protein immunostaining) is significantly increased following axotomy [71,72] and inflammation [73] in rats. Based on these findings, it was hypothesized that the reexpression of $Na_v1.3$ channels, under conditions associated with pain, might contribute to increased excitability of DRG neurons, and therefore, $Na_v1.3$ could play a role in nociceptor hyperexcitability. The increased expression of $Na_v1.3$ in axotomized neurons is correlated with the observation that TTX-sensitive currents in axotomized DRG neurons recover from inactivation much faster than TTX-sensitive currents in uninjured DRG neurons [32]. Increases in recovery from inactivation rates could lead to increased firing frequencies. $Na_v1.3$ channels are also able to generate relatively large ramp currents in response to slow ramp depolarizations [69] and, under some conditions, prominent persistent (or noninactivating) currents [74,75], which could reduce the threshold for action potential initiation and neuronal excitability. Therefore, based on the characteristics of the currents generated by $Na_v1.3$ channels, the reexpression of $Na_v1.3$ is predicted to increase neuronal excitability. However, functional $Na_v1.3$ currents have not been identified in adult sensory neurons. Isoform-specific blockers of $Na_v1.3$ channels are not available, and therefore, it is difficult to determine if $Na_v1.3$ channels contribute to the neuronal hyperexcitability in DRG sensory neurons following nerve injury and/or inflammation using a pharmacological approach.

The role $Na_v1.3$ channels in neuronal hyperexcitability and pain behaviors has been investigated using strategies that knock down $Na_v1.3$ expression, including using antisense oligodeoxynucleotides [76–78] and $Na_v1.3$ null mutant transgenic mice [79]. Intrathecally administered $Na_v1.3$ antisense was shown to reduce hyperexcitability of dorsal horn neurons and to attenuate pain-related behaviors following spinal cord injury as well as chronic constriction injury (CCI) of the peripheral nerve [76,77]. However, using a different $Na_v1.3$ antisense construct, Lindia et al. reported that the reduction of $Na_v1.3$ did not impact the allodynia associated with the spared nerve injury (SNI) model in rats [78]. Furthermore, acute, inflammatory, and neuropathic pain behavior was normal in $Na_v1.3$ knockout transgenic mice [79]. It is not entirely clear what accounts for the differences in these studies. $Na_v1.3$-specific blockers would certainly help determine the role that $Na_v1.3$ channels play in inflammatory and neuropathic pain. Until this has been established, the potential usefulness of $Na_v1.3$-specific blockers (or modulators) as analgesics remains unclear.

3.4.4 $Na_v1.4$

$Na_v1.4$ is clearly not a good target for analgesics as $Na_v1.4$ is almost exclusively expressed in the skeletal muscle [80]. Although $Na_v1.4$ currents are also fast activating, fast inactivating, and TTX sensitive, at the amino acid level, $Na_v1.4$ is only ~62% identical to $Na_v1.1$–$Na_v1.3$ and the other TTX-sensitive channels. $Na_v1.4$ is sometimes referred to as a short sodium channel because the loop between domains I and II is about 200 amino acids shorter than it is in most of the other voltage-gated sodium channels. The only other short sodium channel is $Na_v1.9$. In the "long" channels, the loop between domains I and II contains multiple phosphorylation sites; however, the precise number and kinases associated with these sites differs between the different long isoforms. $Na_v1.4$ is the only sodium channel expressed in mature innervated skeletal muscle, and this channel generates the upstroke of the action potential in the skeletal muscle. The lack of loops I–II phosphorylation sites may reflect that $Na_v1.4$ is subject to less posttranslational modulation than the other isoforms.

3.4.5 $Na_v1.5$

In the adult, $Na_v1.5$ is predominantly expressed in the cardiac muscle [81]. $Na_v1.5$ is also expressed in immature and denervated skeletal muscle [82,83], and $Na_v1.5$ message and current are detectable, at least at low levels, in neonatal DRG tissue and DRG neurons [84]. $Na_v1.5$ message is detectable in some adult DRG neurons, but expression is considered to be very low under most conditions. This channel, often referred to as the cardiac sodium channel, produces unique currents, with voltage dependencies of activation and steady-state inactivation that are hyperpolarized when compared with those of most of the other sodium channels, as well as an intermediate (IC_{50} ~1–2 μM) sensitivity to TTX. Despite the observation that $Na_v1.5$ likely underlies the "third" TTX-resistant current that has been observed in some sensory neurons [84,85], no data have been reported that indicate $Na_v1.5$ channels play a role in pain sensations or influence the excitability of peripheral sensory neurons. As $Na_v1.5$ is the predominant channel expressed in the cardiac muscle, drugs that exert pronounced effects on $Na_v1.5$ activity are likely to be associated with undesirable side effects and narrow therapeutic windows if systemically administered.

3.4.6 $Na_v1.6$

$Na_v1.6$ is another fast-activating, fast-inactivating, TTX-sensitive voltage-gated sodium channel that is widely expressed in the CNS and PNS. Like $Na_v1.1$, $Na_v1.6$ expression has also been detected in the transverse tubules of cardiac ventricular myocytes [64]. $Na_v1.6$ differs from $Na_v1.1$ in its expression pattern; $Na_v1.6$ is the predominant voltage-gated sodium channel in the nodes of ranvier in both PNS and CNS myelinated neurons [86,87]. Transgenic mice that lack functional $Na_v1.6$ channels die during the third postnatal week when myelination of axons occurs [88], and it is likely that this is due to an inability of other voltage-gated sodium channels to compensate for $Na_v1.6$ at the nodes of ranvier. *In situ* hybridization evidence suggests that in the DRG, $Na_v1.6$ is heavily expressed in medium- and large-diameter DRG neurons and only lightly expressed in small-diameter neurons [57]. Immunocytochemical evidence does indicate that $Na_v1.6$ is expressed in unmyelinated peripheral axons [89], but it is not clear if $Na_v1.6$ channels make a significant contribution to conduction in these axons. $Na_v1.6$ channels, like $Na_v1.4$ channels, exhibit very fast recovery from inactivation [90], indicating that neurons and axons expressing $Na_v1.6$ channels should be able to sustain high firing frequencies. Indeed, sodium currents in large-diameter DRG neurons, which can fire at relatively high frequencies [91,92], exhibit rapid recovery from inactivation that is similar to that of $Na_v1.6$ [93]. It should be noted, however, that recovery from inactivation of $Na_v1.6$ can be modulated by fibroblast growth factor homologous factors [94], indicating that firing frequency might be regulated by modulating $Na_v1.6$. $Na_v1.6$ current density is modulated by calmodulin [95] and p38 mitogen-activated protein kinases [96], which could also regulate the excitability of neurons.

Another unique property of $Na_v1.6$ is that $Na_v1.6$ channels are able to produce the specialized resurgent currents, described earlier, that can be observed in cerebellar Purkinje neurons [33] and in some medium- and large-diameter DRG neurons [34]. Although resurgent currents in Purkinje neurons are thought to be predominantly carried by $Na_v1.6$ channels, they are not recorded from all neuronal subtypes that express $Na_v1.6$ channels [97,98]. Cummins et al. demonstrated that resurgent currents are present in ~40% of large-diameter DRG neurons from control mice but are not expressed in DRG neurons isolated from $Na_v1.6$ null mice, and demonstrated that recombinant $Na_v1.6$ channels can produce resurgent currents in cultured DRG neurons [34]. These data indicate that $Na_v1.1$, $Na_v1.7$, $Na_v1.8$, and $Na_v1.9$ currents do not produce resurgent currents in DRG neurons. Resurgent currents contribute to rapid, burst firing in cerebellar Purkinje neurons [36]. However, it is not clear what the impact of resurgent currents generated by $Na_v1.6$ is in sensory neuronal excitability and what role, if any, $Na_v1.6$ might play in nociception and pain sensations. As $Na_v1.6$ is crucial to axonal conduction in myelinated fibers, drugs that specifically target $Na_v1.6$ channels could be associated with pronounced adverse side effects.

3.4.7 $Na_v1.7$

Multiple lines of evidence demonstrate that $Na_v1.7$ is an excellent target for analgesics. First, $Na_v1.7$, previously referred to as PN1, hNE9, and NaS, is almost exclusively expressed in the PNS and is highly expressed in small-diameter and nociceptive neurons. Second, the properties of $Na_v1.7$ currents are distinct in several ways from those of other voltage-gated sodium channels, and these differences may allow $Na_v1.7$ to play an important role in fine-tuning the excitability of nociceptors. Third, gain-of-function mutations have been identified as underlying two distinct inherited chronic pain syndromes in humans, demonstrating that alterations in $Na_v1.7$ activity can cause severe pain. Finally, human mutations that cause loss of function of $Na_v1.7$ indicate that $Na_v1.7$ plays an absolutely crucial, and perhaps selective, role in pain sensations (although, as is discussed below, transgenic animal studies suggest a more complex role for $Na_v1.7$). In the next few paragraphs, the evidence supporting the assertion that $Na_v1.7$ is possibly an ideal target for the development of novel analgesics is examined in detail.

Although early functional studies suggested that TTX-sensitive sodium channels in the peripheral nerve are similar in several ways to those in central neurons and the skeletal muscle, biochemical analyses [99] indicated that sodium channels in the peripheral nerve have distinct molecular properties. Although it was not initially clear whether this was due to tissue-specific post-translational modifications or genetic differences, *in situ* hybridization studies provided evidence that novel sodium channel mRNAs were expressed in peripheral neurons [70]. Within the next decade, several groups independently cloned what is now referred to as $Na_v1.7$. Interestingly, $Na_v1.7$ was cloned from a variety of tissues. A novel TTX-sensitive voltage-gated sodium channel was cloned in 1995 from a human medullary thyroid carcinoma cell line [100]. Because this transcript was not found in the brain, heart, or kidney, they proposed that this sodium channel, which they called hNE, was exclusively expressed in neuroendocrine cells. A nearly identical sodium channel, called NaS, was cloned around the same time from rabbit Schwann cells [101]. For several years, Mandel's group had been studying a unique sodium channel expressed in PC12 cells and peripheral neurons [102], which they referred to as PN1. In 1997, they [102] and another group [103] published the full-length sequence for PN1 from rats. Based on sequence homology, it was concluded that PN1 was the ortholog of hNE and NaS. Based on Northern blot, Western blot, and immunohistochemistry analyses, Toledo-Aral et al. concluded that PN1 (referred to as $Na_v1.7$ from here on) was predominantly expressed in peripheral neurons and might be preferentially targeted to the nerve endings of peripheral neurons. They did not find evidence for expression in Schwann cells or central neurons. They did, however, find that $Na_v1.7$ was expressed in superior cervical ganglion (sympathetic) neurons in addition to DRG (sensory) neurons. Many subsequent studies have examined the expression pattern of $Na_v1.7$, although sometimes with conflicting results. In general, the consensus is that $Na_v1.7$ is predominantly expressed in peripheral neurons, both sympathetic and sensory, with expression also sometimes detectable in adrenal and thyroid tissues [55,57,103]. Although these early studies indicated that $Na_v1.7$ was expressed at significant levels in small-, medium-, and large-diameter sensory neurons, more recent studies strongly suggest that $Na_v1.7$ is more abundant in C-fiber than A-fibers [104] and has greater expression in nociceptive compared with non-nociceptive sensory neurons [105]. The predominant expression of $Na_v1.7$ in peripheral neurons, and possible preferential expression in nociceptive neurons, led to the proposal that $Na_v1.7$ might be a valid target for analgesics. Interestingly, the expression of $Na_v1.7$ in DRG neurons is upregulated in animal models of painful diabetic neuropathy [106] and chronic inflammation [107,108].

Functionally, $Na_v1.7$ currents are similar in several respects to other TTX-sensitive channels, although important differences have been identified. $Na_v1.7$ currents exhibit rapid activation and rapid inactivation from the open configuration [100], similar to $Na_v1.1$–$Na_v1.4$ and $Na_v1.6$. However, in contrast to $Na_v1.4$ and $Na_v1.6$, which exhibit rapid recovery from fast inactivation, $Na_v1.7$ channels exhibit substantially slower recovery from fast inactivation [90,109]. Thus, neurons expressing only $Na_v1.7$ channels should not be capable of firing at high frequencies, while neurons expressing $Na_v1.6$ channels would. This is grossly consistent with the expression patterns of $Na_v1.7$ and $Na_v1.6$ as maximal firing rate of DRG C-fibers is significantly lower than that of A-fibers [110]. Overall, the biophysical properties of sodium currents generated by cloned human $Na_v1.7$ channels closely resemble those of the predominant TTX-sensitive current expressed in small-diameter DRG sensory neurons [109]. $Na_v1.7$ currents can take five times longer than $Na_v1.4$ or $Na_v1.6$ currents to inactivate at negative membrane potentials (membrane potentials close to the resting membrane potential of neurons), where channels are likely to inactivate directly from resting or closed states. This slower rate of closed-state inactivation is thought to contribute to the propensity of $Na_v1.7$ channels to generate relatively large currents during slow ramp depolarizations (currents often referred to as ramp currents) compared with $Na_v1.4$ and $Na_v1.6$ channels [90,109]. Based on their biophysical properties, $Na_v1.7$ channels are thought to be important in setting the threshold for the generation of action potentials in small-diameter nociceptive neurons.

The confirmation that $Na_v1.7$ is an important contributor to pain sensations in humans has come from the study of inherited painful neuropathies. Single point mutations in $Na_v1.7$ have been identified as underlying two distinct autosomal dominant, chronic burning pain syndromes in humans: inherited erythromelalgia (IE) and paroxysmal extreme pain disorder (PEPD) [111]. Studies of these painful syndromes, and the functional consequences of the mutations that cause them, have provided compelling evidence that changes in the gating properties of $Na_v1.7$ can result in dramatically increased pain sensations. At least nine distinct point mutations in *SCN9A*, the gene that encodes $Na_v1.7$, have been identified in patients with IE [112–117]. These mutations, which primarily cause severe burning sensations in a patient's hands and feet, all cause significant hyperpolarizing shifts in the voltage dependence of activation [115–120]. Eight of the nine IE mutations that have been characterized to date also produce larger ramp currents and slow the rate at which the channels deactivate (or return to the closed state from the open state). DRG neurons transfected with recombinant $Na_v1.7$ containing one of the IE mutations exhibit lower thresholds for firing action potentials and fire at higher-than-normal frequencies in response to suprathreshold stimulation [115,117,121], demonstrating that the IE mutations can indeed increase the excitability of sensory neurons. The majority of the IE mutations is located at or near parts of the channel that are associated with activation gating (Figure 3.4).

Fertleman et al. identified eight distinct $Na_v1.7$ missense mutations in different PEPD families that are distinct from the IE mutations [122]. The PEPD mutations, which cause severe burning sensations in rectal, ocular, and submandibular regions, are predominantly located in regions of the sodium channel that are associated with inactivation gating (Figure 3.4). The effects of the mutations on $Na_v1.7$ current properties are distinct from those seen with IE mutations. The PEPD mutations cause depolarizing shifts in voltage dependence of steady-state inactivation and slow the rate of fast inactivation, leading to persistent currents [122,123]. Thus, while IE mutations predominantly enhance activation, PEPD mutations impair inactivation [111]. These studies not only demonstrate that alterations in $Na_v1.7$ currents are sufficient to cause severe chronic pain in humans, but they also indicate that alterations of dif-

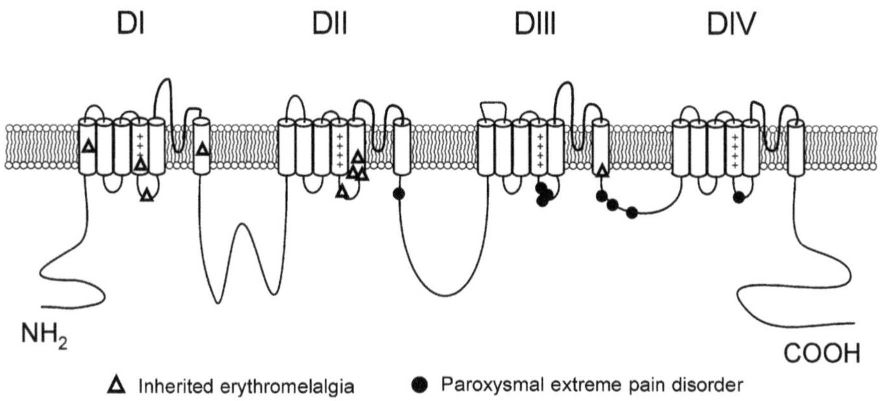

FIGURE 3.4. Linear diagram of $Na_v1.7$ showing locations of single point mutations indicated in the painful neuropathies inherited erythromelalgia (unfilled triangles) and paroxymsal extreme pain disorder (filled circles).

ferent properties of $Na_v1.7$ may determine the phenotype of the pain associated with the mutations. Interestingly, while PEPD patients often respond well to treatment with carbamazepine, IE patients reportedly do not [122,124].

Studies of individuals with complete insensitivity to pain or congenital indifference to pain (CIP) provided the strongest evidence that $Na_v1.7$ plays a crucial role in our ability to perceive pain [125–127]. Genetic analysis of families determined that the pain insensitivity was congenital and could be mapped as an autosomal-recessive trait linked to *SCN9A*. Distinct homozygous nonsense mutations were identified in each of the affected individuals, with different mutations identified in the unrelated families with CIP studied from several different countries. These truncating mutations have been either shown to or predicted to result in a complete loss of functional $Na_v1.7$ currents. Family members who were heterozygous for the *SCN9A* mutations, and therefore should have one functional *SCN9A* allele, reportedly exhibited normal pain phenotypes. The individuals who exhibited an inability to experience pain otherwise appeared normal based on neurological examinations. The only noted exceptions to this selective effect on pain were deficits in olfaction in some patients [126] and awkward gait in others [125]; these exceptions have not been noted in all individuals with CIP. This predominantly selective effect on pain sensations was surprising, as $Na_v1.7$ is expressed in sympathetic neurons as well as small-diameter sensory neurons. Indeed, in order to assess autonomic function, Goldberg et al. tested sweating, tear formation, blood pressure regulation, and temperature regulation and reported these were normal in patients with CIP [126]. This led to the proposal that $Na_v1.7$ might truly be an ideal target for the development of novel analgesics.

Although the human data are very compelling, there are still some concerns and questions regarding $Na_v1.7$ as an analgesic target. Transgenic mice that have a global knockout of $Na_v1.7$ die just after birth [128]. This could be due to the loss of $Na_v1.7$ in sympathetic neurons; however, it is not clear why humans are able to tolerate the loss of $Na_v1.7$ throughout the body. Nociceptor-specific deletion of $Na_v1.7$ in mice did show that $Na_v1.7$ plays a major role in inflammatory and acute pain, but neuropathic pain behavior was not reduced in these mice [129], suggesting that $Na_v1.7$ may not be important in the production of neuropathic pain. It is not yet clear if humans who lack $Na_v1.7$ have a complete inability to develop all types of neuropathic pain; it remains to be determined if patients with CIP still might eventually develop specific pain disorders, such as painful diabetic neuropathy or cancer-related pain.

In summary, multiple lines of evidence, including gain-of-function mutations that cause severe pain and loss-of-function mutations that apparently cause a relatively selective and complete loss of pain sensations, indicate that $Na_v1.7$ might be an ideal target for novel analgesics. However, $Na_v1.7$ expression in sympathetic neurons and possibly neuroendocrine tissues, may have some impact on the usefulness of $Na_v1.7$-specific inhibitors in treating pain.

3.4.8 $Na_v1.8$

As mentioned above, peripheral sensory neurons are rather unusual in that they often express TTX-resistant voltage-gated sodium currents in addition to the TTX-sensitive sodium currents found in most neurons [25]. TTX-resistant sodium currents are primarily observed in small-diameter sensory neurons [26,130–132]. In 1996, Akopian and colleagues [133] cloned $Na_v1.8$ (which they referred to as SNS at that time) and demonstrated that this isoform produced currents that were highly resistant to TTX and that were similar to the classic TTX-resistant sodium currents recorded in DRG neurons. In 1999, they used $Na_v1.8$ null transgenic mice to show that $Na_v1.8$ was the predominant TTX-resistant sodium channel in sensory neurons [134]. Since then, substantial data have been accumulated implicating $Na_v1.8$- and $Na_v1.8$-like TTX-resistant currents channels in nociception. Although it is now known that there are two distinct TTX-resistant sodium channel isoforms expressed at high levels in DRG neurons ($Na_v1.8$ and $Na_v1.9$), the majority of studies have focused on currents conducted by $Na_v1.8$ channels. $Na_v1.8$ channels exhibit unique patterns of expression, biophysical properties, and second messenger modifications compared with TTX-sensitive channels.

The expression pattern of $Na_v1.8$ has been examined by a number of different groups. In their initial description, Akopian et al. reported that $Na_v1.8$ was virtually exclusively expressed in peripheral sensory ganglia, with no expression detected in CNS tissue, sympathetic ganglia, or muscle tissues [134]. Interestingly, $Na_v1.8$ expression was not detected in the sciatic nerve. Benn et al. [135] used immunocytochemistry to examine the developmental expression pattern of $Na_v1.8$ and to identify which neuronal subpopulations in the DRG expressed $Na_v1.8$. They found that $Na_v1.8$ expression increased substantially with age; in adults, approximately 50% of DRG neurons express $Na_v1.8$ immunoreactivity. $Na_v1.8$ was found mainly in small-diameter neurons;

however, some medium-diameter neurons also expressed $Na_v1.8$. In a very difficult study, it was demonstrated that the majority of DRG neurons that responded to noxious stimuli *in vivo* exhibited pronounced $Na_v1.8$ immunoreactivity in their cell bodies, whereas muscle afferents and low-threshold mechanoreceptor afferents exhibited negligible staining [136]. These data suggest that $Na_v1.8$ could be an excellent target for analgesics.

While it can be difficult to distinguish between the currents produced by the different neuronal TTX-sensitive channels, the currents produced by $Na_v1.8$ channels are distinctive. $Na_v1.8$ currents and the predominant TTX-resistant currents observed in peripheral sensory neurons display substantially slower rates of activation and fast inactivation than TTX-sensitive currents (see Figure 3.2). Conversely, recovery from fast inactivation can be significantly faster for $Na_v1.8$ currents. These results indicate that the inactivated state of $Na_v1.8$ is destabilized compared with TTX-sensitive currents. Consistent with this destabilization, the voltage dependence of steady-state fast inactivation is typically 30–40 mV more depolarized for $Na_v1.8$ currents than for TTX-sensitive currents [32,133]. The voltage dependence of activation also tends to be more depolarized for $Na_v1.8$ currents. These differences in functional properties have important implications for the influence of $Na_v1.8$ on sensory neuronal excitability. The slower rate of inactivation suggests that $Na_v1.8$ channels should contribute to broader action potentials; indeed, small-diameter sensory neurons typically have action potentials that are broader than those of other types of neurons. The depolarized voltage dependence of inactivation should make neurons that express $Na_v1.8$ less susceptible to depolarization block; this could be important for the continued activation of nociceptive nerve terminals subjected to chronic depolarization as a result of tissue damage. By comparing DRG neurons isolated from control mice and $Na_v1.8$ knockout mice, Renganathan et al. showed that $Na_v1.8$ is a major contributor to the upstroke of action potentials and to continuous firing activity during sustained depolarizations in small-diameter peripheral sensory neurons (Figure 3.5) [137]. However, because of the depolarized voltage dependence of activation, $Na_v1.8$ channels are likely to be activated after TTX-sensitive currents in response to depolarizing inputs, and thus, in contrast to $Na_v1.7$, $Na_v1.8$ is not likely to determine the threshold for the generation of action potentials in peripheral sensory neurons [121,138]. However, the amplitude and activity of $Na_v1.8$ currents in DRG neurons are increased by inflammatory mediators, and these changes are likely to contribute to increased excitability of sensory neurons [139–141]. A number of different molecules have been implicated in modulating $Na_v1.8$ currents, including calmodulin [142], protein kinase A [143], and p38 mitogen-activated protein kinase [144]. Drugs that specifically target the second messenger-induced modulation of $Na_v1.8$ could be effective analgesics.

Behavioral studies also support the notion that $Na_v1.8$ plays an important role in nociception. Mice lacking functional $Na_v1.8$ channels display decreases in behavioral responses to noxious thermal and mechanical stimulus as well

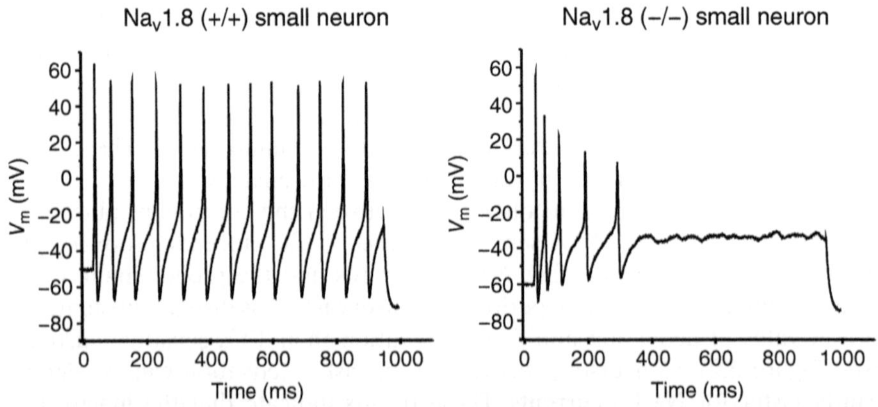

FIGURE 3.5. (a) $Na_v1.8$ (+/+) neurons show robust and sustained repetitive firing in response to injecting depolarizing stimuli of 150pA (b). $Na_v1.8$ (–/–) neurons failed to sustain high-frequency firing in response to the same stimuli. Reprinted with permission from Renganathan, M., Cummins, T.R., Waxman, S.G. (2001). Contribution of Na(v)1.8 sodium channels to action potential electrogenesis in DRG neurons. *J Neurophysiol* 86:629–640 [137].

as exhibiting delayed inflammatory hyperalgesia [134]. Decreasing $Na_v1.8$ mRNA levels using antisense oligodeoxynucleotides was also effective at reducing pain behaviors associated with peripheral inflammation [145,146]. These results help confirm that $Na_v1.8$ is important in normal pain function and that $Na_v1.8$ plays a role in inflammatory pain. In contrast, the contribution of $Na_v1.8$ currents to neuropathic pain conditions remains somewhat controversial. Several studies demonstrated that $Na_v1.8$ mRNA, protein, and current are substantially decreased in axotomized DRG neurons [32,147,148]. This could suggest that $Na_v1.8$ may not be involved in pain associated with nerve injury. However, knockdown of $Na_v1.8$ by intrathecal administration of specific antisense oligodeoxynucleotides was antiallodynic and antihyperalgesic in rats with pain caused by spinal nerve ligation [149]. This knockdown is rapidly reversible, suggesting that $Na_v1.8$ channels play an important role in the maintenance of neuropathic pain. Roza et al. reported that spontaneous activity in damaged sensory axons was greatly reduced in $Na_v1.8$ knockout mice compared with wild type [150], and Joshi et al. reported that $Na_v1.8$ antisense could reduce pain behaviors associated with chronic constrictive nerve injury (although they also found that this was not effective at reducing pain behaviors associated with vincristine chemotherapy or with skin incisions) [146]. Finally, Dong et al. showed that small interfering RNAs that knockdown $Na_v1.8$ could reverse mechanical allodynia caused by CCI in rats [151]. In contrast, other studies on $Na_v1.8$ knockout mice have concluded that $Na_v1.8$ does not play any role in neuropathic pain [129,152]. It is not entirely clear what accounts for the different observations regarding the role of $Na_v1.8$ in neuropathic pain mechanisms. Interestingly, $Na_v1.8$ channels also appear to be important for the hyperexcitability caused by $Na_v1.7$ erythromelalgia mutations in DRG neurons. Rush et al. showed that an $Na_v1.7$ erythromelalgia mutation that increases the excitability of DRG neurons, which express $Na_v1.8$ channels, decreases the excitability of sympathetic ganglion neurons, which lack $Na_v1.8$ channels, unless the sympathetic neurons are also transfected with $Na_v1.8$ [121]. The relatively depolarized voltage dependence of inactivation of $Na_v1.8$ channels are thought to be important determinants of the neuropathic pain induced by the erythromelalgia mutations. A selective $Na_v1.8$ inhibitor is likely to be useful in treating inflammatory pain and should help identify the role(s) of $Na_v1.8$ in human neuropathic pain.

It is predicted that it should be easier to develop analgesic compounds that specifically target $Na_v1.8$ than $Na_v1.7$. $Na_v1.8$ exhibits much less homology to the other voltage-gated sodium channels than does $Na_v1.7$; while >75% of the amino acids are identical between $Na_v1.2$ and $Na_v1.7$, only ~53% are identical between $Na_v1.2$ and $Na_v1.8$. A large proportion of the differences in $Na_v1.8$ are in the long intracellular loops, and this could contribute to the substantial differences in second messenger modulation that are observed between $Na_v1.8$ and other neuronal voltage-gated sodium channels. Although there are fewer differences in the transmembrane segments and in the pore region, there are some important differences that have already been identified as contributing to important pharmacological differences. It is predicted that increased knowledge of the structure–function relationships of $Na_v1.8$ will aid the rational development of $Na_v1.8$-specific blockers. As will be discussed below, several peptidic compounds that exhibit some selectivity to $Na_v1.8$ have been described, and a small molecule, selective inhibitor of $Na_v1.8$, has shown analgesic activity in animal models of pain, indicating that it is indeed feasible to selectively target $Na_v1.8$.

3.4.9 $Na_v1.9$

The role of $Na_v1.9$, a second neuronal TTX-resistant channel previously referred to as NaN and SNS2, in pain is not as clear as that of $Na_v1.8$. Within the peripheral sensory ganglia, $Na_v1.9$ is preferentially expressed in small-diameter neurons [28,58,153] and may be predominantly associated with nociceptive neurons [154,155]. This suggests a role in nociception. However, other studies have indicated that $Na_v1.9$ is also expressed in enteric neurons [156], leading to the suggestion that $Na_v1.9$ plays a role in regulating gastrointestinal function. If so, then analgesic drugs that target $Na_v1.9$ might induce gastrointestinal side effects. Although $Na_v1.9$ was originally cloned in 1998, it has proven extremely difficult to study in heterologous expression systems [157]. The initial studies attempting to identify the functional properties of $Na_v1.9$ did not agree on what type of current $Na_v1.9$ generated. Akopian et al. proposed that $Na_v1.9$ might not produce functional sodium currents [134]. Tate et al. proposed that $Na_v1.9$ produced a fast-inactivating current that resembled the currents generated by cardiac $Na_v1.5$ channel [153]. Cummins et al. isolated a TTX-resistant current in DRG neurons from $Na_v1.8$ null mice that activated at potentials close to resting membrane potential (–60 to –70 mV) but, in contrast to all other voltage-gated sodium channel currents, exhibited extremely slow inactivation [27]. It was proposed that this "persistent" TTX-resistant current (Figure 3.6) was generated by $Na_v1.9$ and was likely to play a role in setting resting membrane potential as well as contributing to subthreshold electrogenesis in small DRG neurons [27,158]. Electrophysiological studies on DRG neurons from $Na_v1.9$ knockout mice [159,160] confirmed that $Na_v1.9$ does indeed generate the persistent TTX-resistant current. Interestingly, it was also proposed [161] that $Na_v1.9$ produced current in CNS neurons that is activated by brain-derived neurotrophic factor (BDNF), a current that is inhibited by nanomolar concentrations of the neurotoxin saxitoxin (STX). However, this work has not been replicated in either CNS neurons or in PNS neurons and is considered unlikely as the native $Na_v1.9$ current in DRG neurons is insensitive to submicromolar concentrations of STX [159,162]. Several studies have indicated that $Na_v1.9$ persistent TTX-resistant current is subject to other types of modulation [163–168], including by inflammatory mediators such as prostaglandin E_2 (PGE_2). It has therefore been proposed that modulation of $Na_v1.9$ could substantially impact firing thresholds in nociceptive neurons. Modulation of $Na_v1.9$ can be both acute and chronic. Inflammation induces an upregulation of $Na_v1.9$ mRNA after 7 days and, conversely, axotomy causes a downregulation [58,153], possibly indicating a role for $Na_v1.9$ in sensory neuronal hyperexcitability associated with inflam-

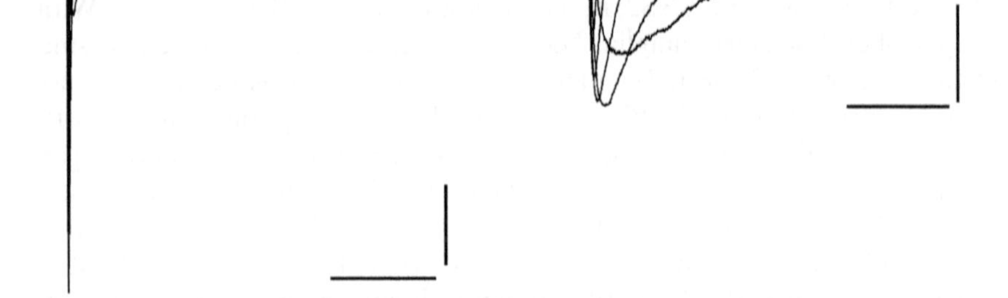

FIGURE 3.6. (a) Voltage-clamp recordings of total sodium currents recorded from the small dorsal root ganglion (DRG) neuron shows both fast-inactivating and persistent sodium current components. (b) Persistent TTX-resistant sodium currents recorded from another small DRG neuron. Horizontal calibration: 10 ms, vertical calibration: 5 nA. Reprinted with permission from Herzog, R.I., Cummins, T.R., Waxman, S.G. (2001). Persistent TTX-resistant Na+ current affects resting potential and response to depolarization in simulated spinal sensory neurons. *J Neurophysiol* 86:1351–1364 [158].

matory pain but not nerve injury-induced pain. Indeed, transgenic mice that lack functional $Na_v1.9$ showed a reduced hypersensitivity to inflammatory hyperalgesia induced by formalin, carrageenan, complete Freund's adjuvant (CFA), and PGE_2 [159] and a reduced sensitivity to specific inflammatory mediators such as bradykinin, serotonin, and ATP [160]. In contrast, such mice do not show altered pain behavior in nerve injury models of neuropathic pain [160]. $Na_v1.9$ is likely to be an important contributor to inflammatory pain, but may not be crucial to neuropathic pain associated with nerve injury. Because transgenic mice lacking functional $Na_v1.9$ are grossly indistinguishable from wild-type mice, exhibit normal eating behaviors, weight gain, and blood chemistry, and are fertile [159,160], drugs that specifically target $Na_v1.9$ could effectively treat pain caused by inflammation with minimal side effects. As $Na_v1.9$ exhibits significant differences at the amino acid level from other voltage-gated sodium channels, including $Na_v1.8$, it seems likely that $Na_v1.9$-specific modulators can be developed.

Of the nine different voltage-gated sodium channel α-subunits, seven are expressed predominantly in neurons (Table 3.1). Interestingly, many small-diameter DRG neurons, which are likely to be nociceptors, express $Na_v1.8$,

TABLE 3.1. Voltage-Gated Sodium Channel α-Subunits.

Isoform	Other Common Names	Predominant Expression	Functional Properties	TTX Sensitivity
$Na_v1.1$	Type I	CNS, PNS	Fast activation, fast inactivation	High
$Na_v1.2$	Type II	CNS	Fast activation, fast inactivation	High
$Na_v1.3$	Type III	CNS, PNS	Fast activation, fast inactivation	High
$Na_v1.4$	Skm1, μ1	Skeletal muscle	Fast activation, fast inactivation	High
$Na_v1.5$	Skm2, H1	Cardiac muscle, uninervated skeletal muscle	Fast activation, fast inactivation	Intermediate
$Na_v1.6$	Na6, PN4, Scn8a	CNS, PNS	Fast activation, fast inactivation, resurgent currents	High
$Na_v1.7$	hNE, PN1, NaS	PNS	Fast activation, fast inactivation, slow recovery from inactivation	High
$Na_v1.8$	SNS, PN3	DRG	Slow inactivation	Low
$Na_v1.9$	NaN, SNS2	PNS	Slow activation, persistent currents	Low

CNS, central nervous system; PNS, peripheral nervous system.

$Na_v1.9$, and TTX-sensitive current that might be largely generated by $Na_v1.7$. Based on the available evidence, $Na_v1.7$, $Na_v1.8$, and $Na_v1.9$ are likely to be the best targets for novel analgesics.

3.4.10 β-Subunits

Four different β-subunits have been identified (β1, β2, β3, and β4) [169–172]. Although initial studies using recombinant subunits expressed in *Xenopus* oocytes indicated that β-subunits substantially modulate the kinetic properties of the sodium currents conducted by α-subunits, this effect on gating is not as pronounced in mammalian cells [69,173,174]. The β-subunits are likely to play an important role in the stabilization of the α-subunits in the membrane and/or localization of the α-subunits to specific membrane domains [169]. The β4-subunit, in combination with the activity of a yet to be identified kinase, seems to be involved in the generation of resurgent sodium currents [175,176], at least in cerebellar Purkinje neurons. Several other accessory proteins, such as calmodulin [95] or annexin II [177], have also been identified as complexing with sodium channels and as modulators of sodium currents and therefore may also be considered as sodium channel accessory subunits. It has been proposed that accessory subunits, including β-subunits, might be important in modulating pain sensations. For example, sodium currents and sodium channel expression in peripheral sensory neurons are altered in mice lacking β2-subunits [178]. These mice showed attenuated inflammatory pain behaviors. Conversely, β2 expression is upregulated in the DRG of rats that exhibit neuropathic pain behaviors after SNI [179]. In the CCI rat model of neuropathic pain, β3 is upregulated in DRG neurons [180]. It is intriguing to think that drugs that disrupt the interaction between specific sodium channel α- and β-subunits might have analgesic activity; however, agents that target the interaction between α- and β-subunits have not been identified.

3.5 SODIUM CHANNEL PHARMACOLOGY

Sodium channels are sensitive to modulation by a variety of pharmacological agents [181,182]. A good deal of research has been conducted on these important compounds, and we have extensive knowledge about many drugs and toxins that interact with sodium channels. Sodium currents and channels, as outlined above, are clearly appealing targets for analgesics. Even if changes in sodium channel properties or expression are not directly responsible for increased pain, sodium channels in the PNS and/or the CNS are involved in the neuronal activity necessary for pain sensations.

A number of different drugs that interact with sodium channels, such as LAs, tricyclic compounds, and anticonvulsants, have been used to treat pain [12,183–185]. The clinically relevant sodium channel modulators (e.g., lidocaine and carbamazepine) seem to all interact with channel residues in the inner portion of the S6 segments of domains I, III, and IV [185–188] and, in general, result in inhibition, at least acutely, of voltage-gated sodium currents. Although a few of the drugs produce a simple "tonic" block of the sodium currents, similar in some respects to that obtained with classic channel-blocking toxins such as TTX, most of the clinically relevant modulators also exhibit pronounced "use dependence." As the name implies, use dependence refers to the increased block that is observed when sodium channels are rapidly and repeatedly activated. Use dependence (also referred to as "phasic" block) is likely to be important in limiting the activity of cells exhibiting fast firing rates, such as the neurons involved in seizure activity or, possibly, hyperactive nociceptive neurons [189]. The use-dependent phenomenon is postulated to arise from the state-dependent binding of the drugs to the sodium channels. In a simple gating scheme, voltage-gated sodium channels have four distinct states: open, closed, fast inactivated, and slow inactivated. A drug that displays state-dependent binding exhibits a higher binding affinity for one or two of these states. The majority of the clinically useful drugs that target sodium channels is believed to have a higher affinity for the open and/or one of the inactivated states than for the closed state. As channels that are depolarized are more likely to open and become inactivated, the inhibition caused by these drugs can also be considered voltage dependent (although this may be indirect). It is important to note that aberrant neuronal activity is not only associated with high-frequency action potential firing, but is also often associated with depolarized membrane potentials in excitable cells. The voltage-dependent inhibition of sodium channels is therefore likely to be important in the mechanism of action for many of the drugs that target voltage-gated sodium channels in chronically depolarized neurons [190].

Although anticonvulsants, anti-arrhythmic drugs, LAs, and even tricyclic compounds that interact with voltage-gated sodium channels are believed to bind at an overlapping site in the intracellular part of the pore, the potency, rate of onset, rate of offset, and other properties can exhibit important differences. For example, bupivacaine and lidocaine are both effective LAs, but bupivacine has a slower dissociate rate. This likely contributes to its higher cardiotoxicity compared with lidocaine. While lidocaine can dissociate from cardiac sodium channels between cardiac action potentials, bupivacaine might not and thus inhibits contraction of cardiac myocytes to a greater extent. Differences in the sensitivity of sodium channel α-subunits to some drugs have been reported. Mexiletine, an analog of lidocaine that can be given orally, has been reported to have a 10-fold higher affinity for inactivated $Na_v1.5$ channels than for inactivated $Na_v1.2$ channels [191]. Differences have also been reported for the sensitivity of TTX-resistant and TTX-sensitive currents in sensory neurons to sodium channel inhibitors [192,193]. However, overall, the differences in the drug sensitivity of the various sodium channel subtypes are not believed to be large. Therefore, the drugs in clinical use that target voltage-gated sodium channels typically can inhibit cardiac, CNS, and PNS sodium channels, and as a result typically have relatively narrow therapeutic windows.

The region of the S6 segments that contributes to the binding of LAs and other clinically relevant sodium channel inhibitors is generally highly conserved among the different isoforms, and therefore, it is not clear if drugs targeting this region of the sodium channels that have higher isoform selectivity can be developed.

Lidocaine is one of the most widely used LAs and can be used for treating neuropathic pain (although success can be limited) as well as to provide localized anesthesia and relief from acute pain sensations. Lidocaine is widely believed to preferentially bind to fast-inactivated channels, although this remains somewhat controversial as some studies indicate preferential binding to activated states [194] and others to slow-inactivated states [195]. The analgesic activity of lidocaine, like that of other LAs, is generally fully reversible. Lidocaine is effective at inhibiting sensory neuronal sodium channels [192,196,197], evoked and spontaneous peripheral nerve activity in experimental systems [198,199], and pain in animal models [200]. Lidocaine has proven very versatile and can be delivered in a variety of ways. The lidocaine patch (5%) is one of the more effective treatments for postherpetic neuropathic pain, reducing both allodynic pain and ongoing pain [201]. Lidocaine patches might also be effective at treating painful diabetic neuropathy [202] and painful idiopathic distal polyneuropathy [203]. Serious side effects have not been associated with the lidocaine patch, with the primary reported adverse effect being mild skin irritation at the site of the patch [204]. Lidocaine has also been given systemically to treat neuropathic pain [9,205]. In a study with 31 subjects, intravenous lidocaine was significantly more effective than placebo at reducing pain intensity, and the pain relief persisted for several hours after lidocaine infusion was stopped [205]. Interestingly, although lidocaine can inhibit cardiac sodium channels [206], cardiotoxicity is usually only a problem with very high dosages. CNS toxicity can be more problematic with systemic lidocaine, and adverse effects include lightheadedness, drowsiness, headaches, and other CNS toxicity symptoms associated with LAs. In some studies, systemic lidocaine has failed to provide substantial pain relief [207]. Mexilitine, an orally active analog of lidocaine used for treating ventricular arrhythmias, has shown some efficacy in animal studies for treating pain [208,209]. Although mexilitine can reduce pain associated with diabetic neuropathy [210], it is not considered as effective as other treatment options [211]. There are many different LAs that target voltage-gated sodium channels. These can differ in terms of rate of onset, cardiotoxicity, CNS toxicity, degree of protein binding, and lipid solubility. Despite the extensive usefulness of LAs for treating acute pain, with the possible exception of lidocaine, LAs have had limited use in treating neuropathic pain.

Anticonvulsants, such as phenytoin and carbamezapine that block voltage-gated sodium channels, can be useful for treating pain [212]. Carbamazepine has been very effective in treating patients with PEPD (which as previously described is often caused by mutations in $Na_v1.7$) [124]. Anticonvulsants are use-dependent blockers of sodium channels and are thought to preferentially interact with inactivated channels at either the same site as LAs or an overlapping site [185,213]. Anticonvulsants inhibit both TTX-sensitive and TTX-resistant neuronal sodium channels, although differences in the pharmacodynamics have been observed [193,214]. Phenytoin and carbamezapine have both been used to treat trigeminal neuralgia, but the use of phenytoin has been limited due to its poor side-effect profile; carbamazepine is also considered useful in treating migraine. Carbamazepine does not seem to be very effective for treating painful diabetic neuropathy or other types of neuropathic pain [212,215]. Oxcarbazepine, an analog of carbamazepine with reduced liver metabolism [216], has been shown to reduce allodynia and hyperalgesia in animal models of neuropathic pain [217]. Clinical studies suggest that oxcarbazepine may be effective at treating several types of neuropathic pain [218], including pain associated with multiple sclerosis [219] and painful diabetic neuropathy [220–222]. Lamotrigine is another anticonvulsant whose activity is due, at least in part, to inhibition of voltage-gated sodium channels [212,223], which has been investigated as an analgesic. Lamotrigine has been reported to be effective at treating HIV-associated neuropathy, trigeminal neuralgia, and diabetic neuropathy [212]. However, in a large placebo-controlled study on pain associated with diabetic neuropathy, lamotrigine was reported to be inconsistently effective at reducing pain [224]. Lacosamide is a relatively new compound that was not only developed originally as an anticonvulsant [225,226] but has also been shown to be effective at reducing chronic pain [227–229]. An important mechanism of action of lacosamide appears to be a block of voltage-gated sodium channels [226,230,231]. Interestingly, lacosamide does not appear to interact with the fast-inactivation state of sodium channels but rather seems to specifically enhance slow inactivation. This effect can take seconds to develop, as opposed to millisecond timescales for the actions of lidocaine and carbamazepine. As a result, neurons that are abnormally depolarized for prolonged durations might be more susceptible to block by lacosamide than neurons with normal resting membrane potentials, and thus, lacosamide may represent an example of a sodium channel blocker that preferentially targets abnormal electrical activity in neurons in a distinct manner compared with other drugs that target voltage-gated sodium channels. Phase II clinical trials suggest that lacosamide is effective at treating painful diabetic peripheral neuropathy and indicated that lacosamide was well tolerated, with a good safety profile [232]. It is interesting to note that, currently, the most commonly used anticonvulsants for treating pain are gabapentin and pregabalin, which are not thought to be potent inhibitors of voltage-gated sodium channels.

Tricyclic antidepressants have been successfully used for several decades to treat pain and can be considered as a first-line treatment for some types of neuropathic pain, such as postherpetic neuralgia [233–235]. Tricyclic antidepressants are potent inhibitors of reuptake of the monoamines serotonin and norepinephrine, and this is clearly an important part of their antidepressant activity and may contribute to their analgesic activity. However, tricyclic antidepressants can also inhibit receptors, such as N-methyl-d-aspartic acid (NMDA) receptors, and ion channels, including calcium channels and sodium channels. It has been proposed that the sodium channel blocking activity might be especially important for the analgesic efficacy of tricyclics. Amitriptyline is the most commonly used antidepressant for neuropathic pain and is able to inhibit voltage-dependent sodium channels at concentrations that are therapeutically effective for treating neuropathic pain [236–238]. Amitriptyline shows higher affinity for inactivated sodium channels, exhibits use-dependent binding, and interacts with the LA binding site of sodium channels [192,237]. Amitriptyline does not appear to be isoform selective as skeletal muscle ($Na_v1.4$) and cardiac ($Na_v1.5$) sodium channels can be blocked in addition to neuronal isoforms [237,239]. A study comparing the analgesic effects of intrathecal administration of nine tricyclic antidepressants and three LAs in rats determined that although all of the compounds had analgesic activity, amitriptyline was the most potent and provided the longest duration of spinal anesthesia [240]. Imipramine, desipramine, nortriptyline, and maprotiline have also been shown to preferentially block inactivated sensory neuronal sodium channels at concentrations near therapeutic plasma concentrations [238]. It is interesting to note that selective serotonin reuptake inhibitors, which are not that effective at treating neuropathic pain [241], are not effective blockers of sodium channels at therapeutic concentrations [238], supporting the hypothesis that sodium channel blockade is important for the effectiveness of tricyclic antidepressants against neuropathic pain. It is important to note that, although two-thirds of neuropathic pain patients receive some degree of pain relief with tricyclic antidepressants, approximately one in five patients consider the side effects to be unacceptable. It is unclear if tricyclic compounds that are selective for sodium channels can be identified.

As described in the last section, while there are many drugs currently available targeting sodium channels that are clinically useful as analgesics, they often do not provide adequate relief, especially for neuropathic pain and, because they are generally not very specific, typically have narrow therapeutic windows. There is a preponderance of evidence demonstrating that sodium channel activity and specific sodium channel isoforms play important roles in peripheral mechanisms of nociception and in neuropathic pain, and therefore, considerable effort has been devoted to identifying and developing novel agents that target sodium channels. In the next few paragraphs, several different strategies that have been used to identify novel analgesics that target sodium channels are described.

It has been proposed that broad spectrum sodium channel blockers with enhanced potency might be useful for treating neuropathic pain. Drugs that can inhibit TTX-resistant and TTX-sensitive channels in the PNS as well as CNS sodium channels might target pain activity at multiple levels. Many novel compounds that are state-dependent, broad-spectrum sodium channel blockers have been recently identified [242–245]. Several of these are more potent than available sodium channels blockers and indeed appear to be effective at decreasing neuropathic pain sensations [243,246]. Of course, a significant disadvantage of the sodium channel blockers currently in use for treating pain is that they are often associated with CNS side effects, such as dizziness or sedation. It is hoped that novel sodium channel blockers with higher potency that do not alter the activity of other channels or proteins will have reduced side effects. PPPA (2-[4-(4-chloro-2-fluorophenoxy)phenyl]-pyrimidine-4-carboxamide) is a compound that reportedly exhibits 1000-fold greater potency for sodium channels compared with carbamazepine and lamotrigine [245]. PPPA shows greater affinity for inactivated channels than for resting channels and significant use-dependent block and effectively reduced pain behaviors in animal models of inflammatory and neuropathic pain at doses that had negligible effects on motor performance [245]. However, it is not known if PPPA will ultimately prove useful in the clinic. Another strategy to limit CNS side effects is to identify sodium channel blockers that do not penetrate the blood-brain barrier. Theoretically, such compounds could inhibit sodium channels in peripheral neurons but would have much lower CNS side effects because they would not reach CNS neurons. Cyclopentane dicarboxamide (CDA54) is a sodium channel blocker that exhibited a 33-fold lower concentration in the brain than plasma concentrations when given orally to rats [247]. CDA54 preferentially blocked inactivated sodium channels and was effective in two different animal neuropathic pain models. Importantly, although CDA54 blocks $Na_v1.2$, $Na_v1.5$, $Na_v1.7$, and $Na_v1.8$ channels at roughly the same range of concentrations *in vitro*, CDA54 did indeed show significantly lower CNS side effects than mexilitine.

Another clever strategy for specifically targeting sodium channels in nociceptive sensory neurons was described by Binshtok et al. [248]. In this study, nociceptive sensory neurons were specifically targeted by combining the application of a membrane-impermeant lidocaine derivative (QX-314) with capsaicin, the active component of hot peppers. Capsaicin is a selective agonist for the transient receptor potential vanilloid 1 (TRPV1) channel, which is a sensor for noxious heat that is predominantly expressed on nociceptive sensory neurons. The pore of TRPV1 is large enough to allow small charged molecules such as QX-314 to pass through it, and therefore, extracellularly applied QX-314 is able to traverse activated TRPV1 channels to the interior of nociceptive neurons, where QX-314 can readily access the LA binding site on the sensory neuronal sodium channels and inhibit nociceptor excitability. Because motor neurons and other non-nociceptive neurons do not express TRPV1 channels, QX-314 does not alter the activity of these other neurons. In rats, capsaicin injected with QX-314 into the hind paw, or near the sciatic nerve, was able to significantly decrease pain sensitivity without apparent motor or tactile deficits. While this approach specifically targets nociceptive neurons, it is not clear how useful it will ultimately be clinically. Capsaicin by itself can produce intense burning pain sensations, as it excites nociceptive neurons via activation of TRPV1 receptors. Furthermore, although QX-314 does not inhibit neuronal sodium channels when applied externally, it can inhibit cardiac sodium channels, and therefore, cardiotoxicity may be a potential concern.

Yet another strategy to specifically target pain sensations is to use drugs that specifically target voltage-gated sodium channel isoforms predominantly expressed in nociceptive neurons, such as Nav1.7, Nav1.8, and Nav1.9. An example of this is A-803467, a small molecule that was discovered in an extensive screen for blockers of $Na_v1.8$ [249]. A-803467 blocks recombinant $Na_v1.8$ channels with ~100-fold higher selectivity over recombinant $Na_v1.2$, $Na_v1.3$, $Na_v1.5$, and $Na_v1.7$ channels [249]. This is the first small molecule to be described with selectivity for $Na_v1.8$ over cardiac and TTX-sensitive neuronal channels. It should be noted that A-803467 activity against $Na_v1.9$ currents was not determined. A-803467 blocked both spontaneous and evoked action potentials in sensory neurons and, although A-803467 was found to be extensively bound to plasma proteins (98.7%) in rats, analgesic activity was observed in a number of different animal pain models at free plasma concentrations ~200–300 nM. A-803467 showed significant activity against several inflammatory and neuropathic models of pain, but it was not very effective against skin incision models of postoperative pain, a chemotherapy-induced pain model and visceral pain model. This raises the possibility that $Na_v1.8$ activity is not important in all types of pain. Importantly, A-803467 did not adversely impact spontaneous exploratory behavior or motor coordination of rats, supporting the proposal that this drug is selective for $Na_v1.8$ channels. Like many drugs with analgesic activity that target sodium channels, A-803467 showed higher affinity for inactivated $Na_v1.8$ channels than for resting $Na_v1.8$ channels. However, it did not show significant use-dependent block, possibly suggesting that A-803467 might not bind to the LA binding site of $Na_v1.8$. Although A-803467 may not be useful in humans for treating pain because of pharmacokinetic properties, the discovery of A-803467 provides proof of principle that it is feasible to develop small-molecule inhibitors of $Na_v1.8$ that have the potential to become very useful analgesics [249].

A promising source of isoform-specific blockers of sensory neuronal voltage-gated sodium channels are biological toxins. Biological toxins can be highly potent blockers or modulators of sodium channel activity and are being investigated as potential compounds on which to base novel therapeutics for treating neuropathic pain. There is a large amount of diversity in the types of toxins that target voltage-gated sodium channels. As many as seven distinct toxin binding sites have been identified on sodium channel α-subunits [182].

Biological toxins such as TTX, a guanidine toxin isolated from puffer fish, can block voltage-gated sodium currents with a high degree of selectivity over ionic currents. TTX and another guanidine toxin, STX, which is also highly selective for sodium channels, are small water-soluble toxins that block six of the nine sodium channel isoforms at nanomolar concentrations ($Na_v1.1$–$Na_v1.4$, $Na_v1.6$, and $Na_v1.7$). The cardiac channel, $Na_v1.5$, is ~50-fold less sensitive to

TTX and STX. $Na_v1.8$ and $Na_v1.9$ are almost completely resistant to these toxins. The residues that are involved in the binding of these toxins have been extensively investigated and the binding site has been designated as toxin binding site 1. TTX and STX bind within the outer portion of the channel pore [250]. A single residue in the pore loop of domain I dictates the resistance of $Na_v1.5$, $Na_v1.8$, and $Na_v1.9$ channels to TTX and STX [162,251–254]. TTX can inhibit ectopic activity in animal models of neuropathic pain [255,256] and has been used in limited clinical trials for treating pain, such as severe cancer pain [257]. Neosaxitoxin, an analog of STX, is also being investigated as an analgesic in humans [258]. However, as TTX and neosaxitoxin can block all CNS neuronal sodium channels, there is significant concern about systemic toxicity [259,260]. Interestingly, a TTX analog that appears selective for $Na_v1.6$ has recently been reported [261], indicating that it may be feasible to develop other isoform-selective small-molecule pore blockers that target toxin site 1.

Another group of molecules that selectively target sodium channels and bind at site 1 are the μ-conotoxins (e.g., GIIIA), which are large peptide toxins of ~22 amino acids isolated from the venom of marine cone snails [262–264]. In contrast to TTX, GIIIA potently inhibits rat $Na_v1.4$ channels but has ~20-fold lower affinity for neuronal TTX-sensitive channels [263,265], and this isoform specificity is due to specific amino acid residues at the outer edge of the channel pore [262]. Two groups reported that MrVIb, another peptide toxin from marine cone snails that is composed of 31 amino acids, has substantial analgesic activity in animal models of pain [4,266]. MrVIb is interesting because it is somewhat selective for $Na_v1.8$ (which again is almost exclusively expressed in peripheral sensory neurons) compared with neuronal TTX-sensitive channels, the cardiac channel and $Na_v1.9$. However, MrVIb only shows ~10-fold higher affinity for $Na_v1.8$ compared with $Na_v1.5$ and $Na_v1.7$ [266], and thus, the therapeutic window may still be small. MrVIb was able to reduce pain in rats in an incisional pain model [4] and a nerve injury model of neuropathic pain [266]. Analogs of MrVIb that are more selective for $Na_v1.8$, if they can be developed, should effectively decrease chronic pain with better therapeutic indices than the nonselective sodium channel inhibitors currently available. It is interesting to note that another conotoxin that binds in the pore of N-type calcium channels (sometimes referred to as zinconotide and marketed under the name Prialt) is clinically efficacious in the treatment of neuropathic pain [267] and has been U.S. Food and Drug Administration (FDA) approved for the treatment of some types of severe chronic pain. This demonstrates that large peptidic channel blockers can be useful clinically as analgesics.

Several other toxin binding sites have been identified on sodium channels [182]. It is important to note that many of these toxins (e.g., batrachotoxin) are gating modifiers that generally do not inhibit or block sodium currents but actually promote activation. Therefore, some biological toxins are not likely to be good candidates for blocking neuronal activity associated with pain but rather are likely to be proalgesic. Interestingly, veratridine and batrachotoxin, which promote sodium channel activity, bind to residues in the S6 segments [188] that overlaps the LA binding site. These are classified as site 2 toxins.

A number of different peptidic toxins isolated from spiders have been shown to inhibit voltage-gated sodium currents [268–270]. Some of these spider toxins also exhibit interesting isoform specificities. ProTx-II, a 30 amino-acid-long peptide with three disulfide bonds, is ~50-fold more selective for $Na_v1.7$ channels over $Na_v1.5$ channels [270,271]. Although Smith et al. proposed that ProTx-II might bind at a novel site, Sokolov et al. [272] proposed that it interacts with the voltage sensor of domain II. The tarantula toxins Huwentoxin-I and Huwentoxin-IV have virtually no effect on muscle sodium channels ($Na_v1.4$ and $Na_v1.5$) but are potent inhibitor of neuronal TTX-sensitive channels, especially $Na_v1.7$ [273,274]. Xiao et al. showed that exchanging just two amino acid residues between the IIS3–S4 linker of $Na_v1.4$ and $Na_v1.7$ results in a near complete switch in the sensitivity of these channels to Huwentoxin-I and Huwentoxin-IV [274]. This and other recent evidences demonstrate that these tarantula toxins bind at or near neurotoxin site 4 [274]. Thus, these spider toxins behave functionally as pure current inhibitors but are actually voltage-gating modifiers that block channel activity by locking the voltage sensor of domain II in the closed configuration [272,274]. This research indicates that the voltage sensors are viable targets for the development of sodium channel inhibitors and analgesics. Large peptide toxins are likely to interact with numerous residues on voltage-gated sodium channels, and this increases the potential for isoform specificity. As many of these peptidic toxins are charged, they are also unlikely to cross the blood-brain barrier, which could be an advantage for their use as peripheral analgesics. Huwentoxin-I has been shown to have analgesic activity in the rat formalin pain model [275]. While it is not yet clear at this time if biological toxins that target voltage-gated sodium channels can be developed into effective analgesics that can be used clinically, the toxin binding sites that have been identified are located in different regions of the sodium channels, and studies on biological toxins are helping to identify target sites for the development of novel pain therapeutics.

Other genetic approaches to targeting specific sodium channel isoforms are also being pursued. Oligonucleotide antisense and small interfering RNA-mediated knockdown of $Na_v1.8$ have shown promise in animal models of neuropathic pain [149,151,276]. Viral delivery of short hairpin RNAs for selective knockdown of $Na_v1.7$ and $Na_v1.8$ sodium channels also seems promising for treating pain [277,278]. The promoter region of $Na_v1.7$ has been identified [279], and it is likely that this knowledge will also open up new avenues for suppressing the electrical activity of nociceptive neurons.

3.6 SUMMARY

Although peripheral neuronal voltage-gated sodium channels are clearly appealing targets for treating pain, the drugs that are currently available for targeting sodium channels are not ideal. Our understanding of the genetics, molecular biology, pharmacology, and biophysical properties of voltage-gated sodium channels has progressed at a rapid pace. Two peripheral neuronal sodium channels, $Na_v1.7$ and $Na_v1.8$, have been shown to play crucial roles in pain mechanisms, and $Na_v1.9$ could also have an important role in inflammatory pain mechanisms. Although novel therapeutics that target sodium channel activity in CNS neurons involved in pain might be difficult to develop, drugs that specifically target peripheral neuronal sodium channels are feasible and have great potential as analgesics for treating peripheral neuropathic pain.

REFERENCES

1. Catterall, W.A. (2000). From ionic currents to molecular mechanisms: the structure and function of voltage-gated sodium channels. *Neuron* 26:13–25.
2. Djouhri, L., Dawbarn, D., Robertson, A., Newton, R., Lawson, S.N. (2001). Time course and nerve growth factor dependence of inflammation-induced alterations in electrophysiological membrane properties in nociceptive primary afferent neurons. *J Neurosci* 21:8722–8733.
3. Wall, P.D., Gutnick, M. (1974). Ongoing activity in peripheral nerves: the physiology and pharmacology of impulses originating from a neuroma. *Exp Neurol* 43:580–593.
4. Bulaj, G., Zhang, M.M., Green, B.R., Fiedler, B., Layer, R.T., Wei, S., Nielsen, J.S., Low, S.J., Klein, B.D., Wagstaff, J.D., Chicoine, L., Harty, T.P., Terlau, H., Yoshikami, D., Olivera, B.M. (2006). Synthetic muO-conotoxin MrVIB blocks TTX-resistant sodium channel NaV1.8 and has a long-lasting analgesic activity. *Biochemistry* 45:7404–7414.
5. Zhang, J.M., Donnelly, D.F., Song, X.J., Lamotte, R.H. (1997). Axotomy increases the excitability of dorsal root ganglion cells with unmyelinated axons. *J Neurophysiol* 78:2790–2794.
6. Zhang, J.M., Song, X.J., LaMotte, R.H. (1997). An in vitro study of ectopic discharge generation and adrenergic sensitivity in the intact, nerve-injured rat dorsal root ganglion. *Pain* 72:51–57.
7. Kim, Y.I., Na, H.S., Kim, S.H., Han, H.C., Yoon, Y.W., Sung, B., Nam, H.J., Shin, S.L., Hong, S.K. (1998). Cell type-specific changes of the membrane properties of peripherally-axotomized dorsal root ganglion neurons in a rat model of neuropathic pain. *Neuroscience* 86:301–309.
8. Xu, G.Y., Zhao, Z.Q. (2001). Change in excitability and phenotype of substance P and its receptor in cat Abeta sensory neurons following peripheral inflammation. *Brain Res* 923:112–119.
9. Mao, J., Chen, L.L. (2000). Systemic lidocaine for neuropathic pain relief. *Pain* 87:7–17.
10. Massey, G.V., Pedigo, S., Dunn, N.L., Grossman, N.J., Russell, E.C. (2002). Continuous lidocaine infusion for the relief of refractory malignant pain in a terminally ill pediatric cancer patient. *J Pediatr Hematol Oncol* 24:566–568.
11. Strichartz, G.R., Zhou, Z., Sinnott, C., Khodorova, A. (2002). Therapeutic concentrations of local anaesthetics unveil the potential role of sodium channels in

neuropathic pain. *Novartis Found Symp* 241:189–201; discussion 202–185, 226–132.

12. Gold, M.S. (2008). Na(+) channel blockers for the treatment of pain: context is everything, almost. *Exp Neurol* 210:1–6.
13. Cummins, T.R., Rush, A.M. (2007). Voltage-gated sodium channel blockers for the treatment of neuropathic pain. *Expert Rev Neurother* 7:1597–1612.
14. Namaka, M., Gramlich, C.R., Ruhlen, D., Melanson, M., Sutton, I., Major, J. (2004). A treatment algorithm for neuropathic pain. *Clin Ther* 26:951–979.
15. Favre, I., Moczydlowski, E., Schild, L. (1996). On the structural basis for ionic selectivity among Na+, K+, and Ca2+ in the voltage-gated sodium channel. *Biophys J* 71:3110–3125.
16. Hodgkin, A.L., Huxley, A.F. (1952). A quantitative description of membrane current and its application to conduction and excitation in nerve. *J Physiol* 117:500–544.
17. Hodgkin, A.L., Huxley, A.F. (1952). The dual effect of membrane potential on sodium conductance in the giant axon of Loligo. *J Physiol* 116:497–506.
18. Hodgkin, A.L., Huxley, A.F. (1952). The components of membrane conductance in the giant axon of Loligo. *J Physiol* 116:473–496.
19. Hodgkin, A.L., Huxley, A.F. (1952). Currents carried by sodium and potassium ions through the membrane of the giant axon of Loligo. *J Physiol* 116:449–472.
20. Hodgkin, A.L., Huxley, A.F. (1952). Movement of sodium and potassium ions during nervous activity. *Cold Spring Harb Symp Quant Biol* 17:43–52.
21. Stuhmer, W., Conti, F., Suzuki, H., Wang, X.D., Noda, M., Yahagi, N., Kubo, H., Numa, S. (1989). Structural parts involved in activation and inactivation of the sodium channel. *Nature* 339:597–603.
22. Sigworth, F.J. (1994). Voltage gating of ion channels. *Q Rev Biophys* 27:1–40.
23. Chahine, M., George, A.L., Jr., Zhou, M., Ji, S., Sun, W., Barchi, R.L., Horn, R. (1994). Sodium channel mutations in paramyotonia congenita uncouple inactivation from activation. *Neuron* 12:281–294.
24. Armstrong, C.M. (2006). Na channel inactivation from open and closed states. *Proc Natl Acad Sci U S A* 103:17991–17996.
25. Kostyuk, P.G., Veselovsky, N.S., Tsyndrenko, A.Y. (1981). Ionic currents in the somatic membrane of rat dorsal root ganglion neurons—I. Sodium currents. *Neuroscience* 6:2423–2430.
26. Roy, M.L., Narahashi, T. (1992). Differential properties of tetrodotoxin-sensitive and tetrodotoxin-resistant sodium channels in rat dorsal root ganglion neurons. *J Neurosci* 12:2104–2111.
27. Cummins, T.R., Dib-Hajj, S.D., Black, J.A., Akopian, A.N., Wood, J.N., Waxman, S.G. (1999). A novel persistent tetrodotoxin-resistant sodium current in SNS-null and wild-type small primary sensory neurons. *J Neurosci* 19:RC43.
28. Dib-Hajj, S.D., Tyrrell, L., Cummins, T.R., Black, J.A., Wood, P.M., Waxman, S.G. (1999). Two tetrodotoxin-resistant sodium channels in human dorsal root ganglion neurons. *FEBS Lett* 462:117–120.
29. Crill, W.E. (1996). Persistent sodium current in mammalian central neurons. *Annu Rev Physiol* 58:349–362.

30. Baker, M.D., Bostock, H. (1997). Low-threshold, persistent sodium current in rat large dorsal root ganglion neurons in culture. *J Neurophysiol* 77:1503–1513.

31. Kiernan, M.C., Baker, M.D., Bostock, H. (2003). Characteristics of late Na(+) current in adult rat small sensory neurons. *Neuroscience* 119:653–660.

32. Cummins, T.R., Waxman, S.G. (1997). Downregulation of tetrodotoxin-resistant sodium currents and upregulation of a rapidly repriming tetrodotoxin-sensitive sodium current in small spinal sensory neurons after nerve injury. *J Neurosci* 17:3503–3514.

33. Raman, I.M., Bean, B.P. (1997). Resurgent sodium current and action potential formation in dissociated cerebellar Purkinje neurons. *J Neurosci* 17:4517–4526.

34. Cummins, T.R., Dib-Hajj, S.D., Herzog, R.I., Waxman, S.G. (2005). Nav1.6 channels generate resurgent sodium currents in spinal sensory neurons. *FEBS Lett* 579:2166–2170.

35. Raman, I.M., Bean, B.P. (2001). Inactivation and recovery of sodium currents in cerebellar Purkinje neurons: evidence for two mechanisms. *Biophys J* 80:729–737.

36. Khaliq, Z.M., Gouwens, N.W., Raman, I.M. (2003). The contribution of resurgent sodium current to high-frequency firing in Purkinje neurons: an experimental and modeling study. *J Neurosci* 23:4899–4912.

37. Noda, M., Ikeda, T., Suzuki, H., Takeshima, H., Takahashi, T., Kuno, M., Numa, S. (1986). Expression of functional sodium channels from cloned cDNA. *Nature* 322:826–828.

38. Isom, L.L., De Jongh, K.S., Catterall, W.A. (1994). Auxiliary subunits of voltage-gated ion channels. *Neuron* 12:1183–1194.

39. Noda, M., Shimizu, S., Tanabe, T., Takai, T., Kayano, T., Ikeda, T., Takahashi, H., Nakayama, H., Kanaoka, Y., Minamino, N., et al. (1984). Primary structure of *Electrophorus electricus* sodium channel deduced from cDNA sequence. *Nature* 312:121–127.

40. Noda, M., Ikeda, T., Kayano, T., Suzuki, H., Takeshima, H., Kurasaki, M., Takahashi, H., Numa, S. (1986). Existence of distinct sodium channel messenger RNAs in rat brain. *Nature* 320:188–192.

41. Bezanilla, F. (2000). The voltage sensor in voltage-dependent ion channels. *Physiol Rev* 80:555–592.

42. Long, S.B., Campbell, E.B., Mackinnon, R. (2005). Crystal structure of a mammalian voltage-dependent Shaker family K+ channel. *Science* 309:897–903.

43. Long, S.B., Campbell, E.B., Mackinnon, R. (2005). Voltage sensor of Kv1.2: structural basis of electromechanical coupling. *Science* 309:903–908.

44. Hoshi, T., Zagotta, W.N., Aldrich, R.W. (1990). Biophysical and molecular mechanisms of Shaker potassium channel inactivation. *Science* 250:533–538.

45. West, J.W., Patton, D.E., Scheuer, T., Wang, Y., Goldin, A.L., Catterall, W.A. (1992). A cluster of hydrophobic amino acid residues required for fast Na(+)-channel inactivation. *Proc Natl Acad Sci U S A* 89:10910–10914.

46. Chanda, B., Asamoah, O.K., Bezanilla, F. (2004). Coupling interactions between voltage sensors of the sodium channel as revealed by site-specific measurements. *J Gen Physiol* 123:217–230.

47. Lerche, H., Peter, W., Fleischhauer, R., Pika-Hartlaub, U., Malina, T., Mitrovic, N., Lehmann-Horn, F. (1997). Role in fast inactivation of the IV/S4-S5 loop of the human muscle Na+ channel probed by cysteine mutagenesis. *J Physiol* 505(Pt 2):345–352.
48. Smith, M.R., Goldin, A.L. (1997). Interaction between the sodium channel inactivation linker and domain III S4–S5. *Biophys J* 73:1885–1895.
49. Goldin, A.L., Barchi, R.L., Caldwell, J.H., Hofmann, F., Howe, J.R., Hunter, J.C., Kallen, R.G., Mandel, G., Meisler, M.H., Netter, Y.B., Noda, M., Tamkun, M.M., Waxman, S.G., Wood, J.N., Catterall, W.A. (2000). Nomenclature of voltage-gated sodium channels. *Neuron* 28:365–368.
50. Catterall, W.A., Goldin, A.L., Waxman, S.G. (2005). International Union of Pharmacology. XLVII. Nomenclature and structure-function relationships of voltage-gated sodium channels. *Pharmacol Rev* 57:397–409.
51. Akopian, A.N., Souslova, V., Sivilotti, L., Wood, J.N. (1997). Structure and distribution of a broadly expressed atypical sodium channel. *FEBS Lett* 400:183–187.
52. Hiyama, T.Y., Watanabe, E., Ono, K., Inenaga, K., Tamkun, M.M., Yoshida, S., Noda, M. (2002). Na(x) channel involved in CNS sodium-level sensing. *Nat Neurosci* 5:511–512.
53. Goldin, A.L. (2001). Resurgence of sodium channel research. *Annu Rev Physiol* 63:871–894.
54. Rush, A.M., Cummins, T.R., Waxman, S.G. (2007). Multiple sodium channels and their roles in electrogenesis within dorsal root ganglion neurons. *J Physiol* 579:1–14.
55. Felts, P.A., Yokoyama, S., Dib-Hajj, S., Black, J.A., Waxman, S.G. (1997). Sodium channel alpha-subunit mRNAs I, II, III, NaG, Na6 and hNE (PN1): different expression patterns in developing rat nervous system. *Brain Res Mol Brain Res* 45:71–82.
56. Trimmer, J.S., Rhodes, K.J. (2004). Localization of voltage-gated ion channels in mammalian brain. *Annu Rev Physiol* 66:477–519.
57. Black, J.A., Dib-Hajj, S., McNabola, K., Jeste, S., Rizzo, M.A., Kocsis, J.D., Waxman, S.G. (1996). Spinal sensory neurons express multiple sodium channel alpha-subunit mRNAs. *Brain Res Mol Brain Res* 43:117–131.
58. Dib-Hajj, S.D., Tyrrell, L., Black, J.A., Waxman, S.G. (1998). NaN, a novel voltage-gated Na channel, is expressed preferentially in peripheral sensory neurons and down-regulated after axotomy. *Proc Natl Acad Sci U S A* 95:8963–8968.
59. Smith, R.D., Goldin, A.L. (1998). Functional analysis of the rat I sodium channel in xenopus oocytes. *J Neurosci* 18:811–820.
60. Lossin, C., Wang, D.W., Rhodes, T.H., Vanoye, C.G., George, A.L., Jr. (2002). Molecular basis of an inherited epilepsy. *Neuron* 34:877–884.
61. George, A.L., Jr. (2005). Inherited disorders of voltage-gated sodium channels. *J Clin Invest* 115:1990–1999.
62. Dichgans, M., Freilinger, T., Eckstein, G., Babini, E., Lorenz-Depiereux, B., Biskup, S., Ferrari, M.D., Herzog, J., van den Maagdenberg, A.M., Pusch, M., Strom, T.M. (2005). Mutation in the neuronal voltage-gated sodium channel SCN1A in familial hemiplegic migraine. *Lancet* 366:371–377.
63. Yu, F.H., Mantegazza, M., Westenbroek, R.E., Robbins, C.A., Kalume, F., Burton, K.A., Spain, W.J., McKnight, G.S., Scheuer, T., Catterall, W.A. (2006). Reduced

sodium current in GABAergic interneurons in a mouse model of severe myoclonic epilepsy in infancy. *Nat Neurosci* 9:1142–1149.

64. Maier, S.K., Westenbroek, R.E., McCormick, K.A., Curtis, R., Scheuer, T., Catterall, W.A. (2004). Distinct subcellular localization of different sodium channel alpha and beta subunits in single ventricular myocytes from mouse heart. *Circulation* 109:1421–1427.
65. Rush, A.M., Dib-Hajj, S.D., Waxman, S.G. (2005). Electrophysiological properties of two axonal sodium channels, Nav1.2 and Nav1.6, expressed in mouse spinal sensory neurones. *J Physiol* 564:803–815.
66. Westenbroek, R.E., Merrick, D.K., Catterall, W.A. (1989). Differential subcellular localization of the RI and RII Na+ channel subtypes in central neurons. *Neuron* 3:695–704.
67. Kaplan, M.R., Cho, M.H., Ullian, E.M., Isom, L.L., Levinson, S.R., Barres, B.A. (2001). Differential control of clustering of the sodium channels Na(v)1.2 and Na(v)1.6 at developing CNS nodes of Ranvier. *Neuron* 30:105–119.
68. Planells-Cases, R., Caprini, M., Zhang, J., Rockenstein, E.M., Rivera, R.R., Murre, C., Masliah, E., Montal, M. (2000). Neuronal death and perinatal lethality in voltage-gated sodium channel alpha(II)-deficient mice. *Biophys J* 78:2878–2891.
69. Cummins, T.R., Aglieco, F., Renganathan, M., Herzog, R.I., Dib-Hajj, S.D., Waxman, S.G. (2001). Nav1.3 sodium channels: rapid repriming and slow closed-state inactivation display quantitative differences after expression in a mammalian cell line and in spinal sensory neurons. *J Neurosci* 21:5952–5961.
70. Beckh, S., Noda, M., Lubbert, H., Numa, S. (1989). Differential regulation of three sodium channel messenger RNAs in the rat central nervous system during development. *EMBO J* 8:3611–3616.
71. Waxman, S.G., Kocsis, J.D., Black, J.A. (1994). Type III sodium channel mRNA is expressed in embryonic but not adult spinal sensory neurons, and is reexpressed following axotomy. *J Neurophysiol* 72:466–470.
72. Kim, C.H., Oh, Y., Chung, J.M., Chung, K. (2002). Changes in three subtypes of tetrodotoxin sensitive sodium channel expression in the axotomized dorsal root ganglion in the rat. *Neurosci Lett* 323:125–128.
73. Black, J.A., Cummins, T.R., Plumpton, C., Chen, Y.H., Hormuzdiar, W., Clare, J.J., Waxman, S.G. (1999). Upregulation of a silent sodium channel after peripheral, but not central, nerve injury in DRG neurons. *J Neurophysiol* 82:2776–2785.
74. Chen, Y.H., Dale, T.J., Romanos, M.A., Whitaker, W.R., Xie, X.M., Clare, J.J. (2000). Cloning, distribution and functional analysis of the type III sodium channel from human brain. *Eur J Neurosci* 12:4281–4289.
75. Lampert, A., Hains, B.C., Waxman, S.G. (2006). Upregulation of persistent and ramp sodium current in dorsal horn neurons after spinal cord injury. *Exp Brain Res* 174:660–666.
76. Hains, B.C., Klein, J.P., Saab, C.Y., Craner, M.J., Black, J.A., Waxman, S.G. (2003). Upregulation of sodium channel Nav1.3 and functional involvement in neuronal hyperexcitability associated with central neuropathic pain after spinal cord injury. *J Neurosci* 23:8881–8892.
77. Hains, B.C., Saab, C.Y., Klein, J.P., Craner, M.J., Waxman, S.G. (2004). Altered sodium channel expression in second-order spinal sensory neurons contributes to pain after peripheral nerve injury. *J Neurosci* 24:4832–4839.

78. Lindia, J.A., Kohler, M.G., Martin, W.J., Abbadie, C. (2005). Relationship between sodium channel NaV1.3 expression and neuropathic pain behavior in rats. *Pain* 117:145–153.

79. Nassar, M.A., Baker, M.D., Levato, A., Ingram, R., Mallucci, G., McMahon, S.B., Wood, J.N. (2006). Nerve injury induces robust allodynia and ectopic discharges in Nav1.3 null mutant mice. *Mol Pain* 2:33.

80. Trimmer, J.S., Cooperman, S.S., Tomiko, S.A., Zhou, J.Y., Crean, S.M., Boyle, M.B., Kallen, R.G., Sheng, Z.H., Barchi, R.L., Sigworth, F.J., et al. (1989). Primary structure and functional expression of a mammalian skeletal muscle sodium channel. *Neuron* 3:33–49.

81. Rogart, R.B., Cribbs, L.L., Muglia, L.K., Kephart, D.D., Kaiser, M.W. (1989). Molecular cloning of a putative tetrodotoxin-resistant rat heart Na+ channel isoform. *Proc Natl Acad Sci U S A* 86:8170–8174.

82. Rogart, R.B., Regan, L.J. (1985). Two subtypes of sodium channel with tetrodotoxin sensitivity and insensitivity detected in denervated mammalian skeletal muscle. *Brain Res* 329:314–318.

83. White, M.M., Chen, L.Q., Kleinfield, R., Kallen, R.G., Barchi, R.L. (1991). SkM2, a Na+ channel cDNA clone from denervated skeletal muscle, encodes a tetrodotoxin-insensitive Na+ channel. *Mol Pharmacol* 39:604–608.

84. Renganathan, M., Dib-Hajj, S., Waxman, S.G. (2002). Na(v)1.5 underlies the "third TTX-R sodium current" in rat small DRG neurons. *Brain Res Mol Brain Res* 106:70–82.

85. Rush, A.M., Brau, M.E., Elliott, A.A., Elliott, J.R. (1998). Electrophysiological properties of sodium current subtypes in small cells from adult rat dorsal root ganglia. *J Physiol* 511(Pt 3):771–789.

86. Caldwell, J.H., Schaller, K.L., Lasher, R.S., Peles, E., Levinson, S.R. (2000). Sodium channel Na(v)1.6 is localized at nodes of ranvier, dendrites, and synapses. *Proc Natl Acad Sci U S A* 97:5616–5620.

87. Krzemien, D.M., Schaller, K.L., Levinson, S.R., Caldwell, J.H. (2000). Immunolocalization of sodium channel isoform NaCh6 in the nervous system. *J Comp Neurol* 420:70–83.

88. Garcia, K.D., Sprunger, L.K., Meisler, M.H., Beam, K.G. (1998). The sodium channel Scn8a is the major contributor to the postnatal developmental increase of sodium current density in spinal motoneurons. *J Neurosci* 18:5234–5239.

89. Black, J.A., Renganathan, M., Waxman, S.G. (2002). Sodium channel Na(v)1.6 is expressed along nonmyelinated axons and it contributes to conduction. *Brain Res Mol Brain Res* 105:19–28.

90. Herzog, R.I., Cummins, T.R., Ghassemi, F., Dib-Hajj, S.D., Waxman, S.G. (2003). Distinct repriming and closed-state inactivation kinetics of Nav1.6 and Nav1.7 sodium channels in mouse spinal sensory neurons. *J Physiol* 551:741–750.

91. Harper, A.A., Lawson, S.N. (1985). Electrical properties of rat dorsal root ganglion neurones with different peripheral nerve conduction velocities. *J Physiol* 359:47–63.

92. Lee, K.H., Chung, K., Chung, J.M., Coggeshall, R.E. (1986). Correlation of cell body size, axon size, and signal conduction velocity for individually labelled dorsal root ganglion cells in the cat. *J Comp Neurol* 243:335–346.

93. Everill, B., Cummins, T.R., Waxman, S.G., Kocsis, J.D. (2001). Sodium currents of large (Abeta-type) adult cutaneous afferent dorsal root ganglion neurons display

rapid recovery from inactivation before and after axotomy. *Neuroscience* 106:161–169.

94. Rush, A.M., Wittmack, E.K., Tyrrell, L., Black, J.A., Dib-Hajj, S.D., Waxman, S.G. (2006). Differential modulation of sodium channel Na(v)1.6 by two members of the fibroblast growth factor homologous factor 2 subfamily. *Eur J Neurosci* 23:2551–2562.
95. Herzog, R.I., Liu, C., Waxman, S.G., Cummins, T.R. (2003). Calmodulin binds to the C terminus of sodium channels Nav1.4 and Nav1.6 and differentially modulates their functional properties. *J Neurosci* 23:8261–8270.
96. Wittmack, E.K., Rush, A.M., Hudmon, A., Waxman, S.G., Dib-Hajj, S.D. (2005). Voltage-gated sodium channel Nav1.6 is modulated by p38 mitogen-activated protein kinase. *J Neurosci* 25:6621–6630.
97. Raman, I.M., Sprunger, L.K., Meisler, M.H., Bean, B.P. (1997). Altered subthreshold sodium currents and disrupted firing patterns in Purkinje neurons of Scn8a mutant mice. *Neuron* 19:881–891.
98. Pan, F., Beam, K.G. (1999). The absence of resurgent sodium current in mouse spinal neurons. *Brain Res* 849:162–168.
99. Wollner, D.A., Catterall, W.A. (1985). Antigenic differences among the voltage-sensitive sodium channels in the peripheral and central nervous systems and skeletal muscle. *Brain Res* 331:145–149.
100. Klugbauer, N., Lacinova, L., Flockerzi, V., Hofmann, F. (1995). Structure and functional expression of a new member of the tetrodotoxin-sensitive voltage-activated sodium channel family from human neuroendocrine cells. *EMBO J* 14: 1084–1090.
101. Belcher, S.M., Zerillo, C.A., Levenson, R., Ritchie, J.M., Howe, J.R. (1995). Cloning of a sodium channel alpha subunit from rabbit Schwann cells. *Proc Natl Acad Sci U S A* 92:11034–11038.
102. Toledo-Aral, J.J., Moss, B.L., He, Z.J., Koszowski, A.G., Whisenand, T., Levinson, S.R., Wolf, J.J., Silos-Santiago, I., Halegoua, S., Mandel, G. (1997). Identification of PN1, a predominant voltage-dependent sodium channel expressed principally in peripheral neurons. *Proc Natl Acad Sci U S A* 94:1527–1532.
103. Sangameswaran, L., Fish, L.M., Koch, B.D., Rabert, D.K., Delgado, S.G., Ilnicka, M., Jakeman, L.B., Novakovic, S., Wong, K., Sze, P., Tzoumaka, E., Stewart, G.R., Herman, R.C., Chan, H., Eglen, R.M., Hunter, J.C. (1997). A novel tetrodotoxin-sensitive, voltage-gated sodium channel expressed in rat and human dorsal root ganglia. *J Biol Chem* 272:14805–14809.
104. Fukuoka, T., Kobayashi, K., Yamanaka, H., Obata, K., Dai, Y., Noguchi, K. (2008). Comparative study of the distribution of the alpha-subunits of voltage-gated sodium channels in normal and axotomized rat dorsal root ganglion neurons. *J Comp Neurol* 510:188–206.
105. Djouhri, L., Newton, R., Levinson, S.R., Berry, C.M., Carruthers, B., Lawson, S.N. (2003). Sensory and electrophysiological properties of guinea-pig sensory neurones expressing Nav 1.7 (PN1) Na+ channel alpha subunit protein. *J Physiol* 546:565–576.
106. Hong, S., Morrow, T.J., Paulson, P.E., Isom, L.L., Wiley, J.W. (2004). Early painful diabetic neuropathy is associated with differential changes in tetrodotoxin-sensitive and -resistant sodium channels in dorsal root ganglion neurons in the rat. *J Biol Chem* 279:29341–29350.

107. Black, J.A., Liu, S., Tanaka, M., Cummins, T.R., Waxman, S.G. (2004). Changes in the expression of tetrodotoxin-sensitive sodium channels within dorsal root ganglia neurons in inflammatory pain. *Pain* 108:237–247.

108. Tanaka, M., Cummins, T.R., Ishikawa, K., Dib-Hajj, S.D., Black, J.A., Waxman, S.G. (1998). SNS Na+ channel expression increases in dorsal root ganglion neurons in the carrageenan inflammatory pain model. *Neuroreport* 9:967–972.

109. Cummins, T.R., Howe, J.R., Waxman, S.G. (1998). Slow closed-state inactivation: a novel mechanism underlying ramp currents in cells expressing the hNE/PN1 sodium channel. *J Neurosci* 18:9607–9619.

110. Waddell, P.J., Lawson, S.N. (1990). Electrophysiological properties of subpopulations of rat dorsal root ganglion neurons in vitro. *Neuroscience* 36:811–822.

111. Dib-Hajj, S.D., Cummins, T.R., Black, J.A., Waxman, S.G. (2007). From genes to pain: Na v 1.7 and human pain disorders. *Trends Neurosci* 30:555–563.

112. Drenth, J.P., te Morsche, R.H., Guillet, G., Taieb, A., Kirby, R.L., Jansen, J.B. (2005). SCN9A mutations define primary erythermalgia as a neuropathic disorder of voltage gated sodium channels. *J Invest Dermatol* 124:1333–1338.

113. Michiels, J.J., te Morsche, R.H., Jansen, J.B., Drenth, J.P. (2005). Autosomal dominant erythermalgia associated with a novel mutation in the voltage-gated sodium channel alpha subunit Nav1.7. *Arch Neurol* 62:1587–1590.

114. Yang, Y., Wang, Y., Li, S., Xu, Z., Li, H., Ma, L., Fan, J., Bu, D., Liu, B., Fan, Z., Wu, G., Jin, J., Ding, B., Zhu, X., Shen, Y. (2004). Mutations in SCN9A, encoding a sodium channel alpha subunit, in patients with primary erythermalgia. *J Med Genet* 41:171–174.

115. Dib-Hajj, S.D., Rush, A.M., Cummins, T.R., Hisama, F.M., Novella, S., Tyrrell, L., Marshall, L., Waxman, S.G. (2005). Gain-of-function mutation in Nav1.7 in familial erythromelalgia induces bursting of sensory neurons. *Brain* 128:1847–1854.

116. Han, C., Lampert, A., Rush, A.M., Dib-Hajj, S.D., Wang, X., Yang, Y., Waxman, S.G. (2007). Temperature dependence of erythromelalgia mutation L858F in sodium channel Nav1.7. *Mol Pain* 3:3.

117. Harty, T.P., Dib-Hajj, S.D., Tyrrell, L., Blackman, R., Hisama, F.M., Rose, J.B., Waxman, S.G. (2006). Na(V)1.7 mutant A863P in erythromelalgia: effects of altered activation and steady-state inactivation on excitability of nociceptive dorsal root ganglion neurons. *J Neurosci* 26:12566–12575.

118. Choi, J.S., Dib-Hajj, S.D., Waxman, S.G. (2006). Inherited erythermalgia: limb pain from an S4 charge-neutral Na channelopathy. *Neurology* 67:1563–1567.

119. Cummins, T.R., Dib-Hajj, S.D., Waxman, S.G. (2004). Electrophysiological properties of mutant Nav1.7 sodium channels in a painful inherited neuropathy. *J Neurosci* 24:8232–8236.

120. Sheets, P.L., Jackson, J.O., 2nd, Waxman, S.G., Dib-Hajj, S.D., Cummins, T.R. (2007). A Nav1.7 channel mutation associated with hereditary erythromelalgia contributes to neuronal hyperexcitability and displays reduced lidocaine sensitivity. *J Physiol* 581:1019–1031.

121. Rush, A.M., Dib-Hajj, S.D., Liu, S., Cummins, T.R., Black, J.A., Waxman, S.G. (2006). A single sodium channel mutation produces hyper- or hypoexcitability in different types of neurons. *Proc Natl Acad Sci U S A* 103:8245–8250.

122. Fertleman, C.R., Baker, M.D., Parker, K.A., Moffatt, S., Elmslie, F.V., Abrahamsen, B., Ostman, J., Klugbauer, N., Wood, J.N., Gardiner, R.M., Rees, M. (2006). SCN9A

mutations in paroxysmal extreme pain disorder: allelic variants underlie distinct channel defects and phenotypes. *Neuron* 52:767–774.

123. Jarecki, B.W., Sheets, P.L., Jackson Ii, J.O., Cummins, T.R. (2008). Paroxysmal extreme pain disorder mutations within the D3/S4-S5 linker of Nav1.7 cause moderate destabilization of fast-inactivation. *J Physiol* 586:4137–4153.

124. Fertleman, C.R., Ferrie, C.D., Aicardi, J., Bednarek, N.A., Eeg-Olofsson, O., Elmslie, F.V., Griesemer, D.A., Goutieres, F., Kirkpatrick, M., Malmros, I.N., Pollitzer, M., Rossiter, M., Roulet-Perez, E., Schubert, R., Smith, V.V., Testard, H., Wong, V., Stephenson, J.B. (2007). Paroxysmal extreme pain disorder (previously familial rectal pain syndrome). *Neurology* 69:586–595.

125. Cox, J.J., Reimann, F., Nicholas, A.K., Thornton, G., Roberts, E., Springell, K., Karbani, G., Jafri, H., Mannan, J., Raashid, Y., Al-Gazali, L., Hamamy, H., Valente, E.M., Gorman, S., Williams, R., McHale, D.P., Wood, J.N., Gribble, F.M., Woods, C.G. (2006). An SCN9A channelopathy causes congenital inability to experience pain. *Nature* 444:894–898.

126. Goldberg, Y.P., MacFarlane, J., MacDonald, M.L., Thompson, J., Dube, M.P., Mattice, M., Fraser, R., Young, C., Hossain, S., Pape, T., Payne, B., Radomski, C., Donaldson, G., Ives, E., Cox, J., Younghusband, H.B., Green, R., Duff, A., Boltshauser, E., Grinspan, G.A., Dimon, J.H., Sibley, B.G., Andria, G., Toscano, E., Kerdraon, J., Bowsher, D., Pimstone, S.N., Samuels, M.E., Sherrington, R., Hayden, M.R. (2007). Loss-of-function mutations in the Nav1.7 gene underlie congenital indifference to pain in multiple human populations. *Clin Genet* 71:311–319.

127. Ahmad, S., Dahllund, L., Eriksson, A.B., Hellgren, D., Karlsson, U., Lund, P.E., Meijer, I.A., Meury, L., Mills, T., Moody, A., Morinville, A., Morten, J., O'Donnell, D., Raynoschek, C., Salter, H., Rouleau, G.A., Krupp, J.J. (2007). A stop codon mutation in SCN9A causes lack of pain sensation. *Hum Mol Genet* 16:2114–2121.

128. Nassar, M.A., Stirling, L.C., Forlani, G., Baker, M.D., Matthews, E.A., Dickenson, A.H., Wood, J.N. (2004). Nociceptor-specific gene deletion reveals a major role for Nav1.7 (PN1) in acute and inflammatory pain. *Proc Natl Acad Sci U S A* 101:12706–12711.

129. Nassar, M.A., Levato, A., Stirling, L.C., Wood, J.N. (2005). Neuropathic pain develops normally in mice lacking both Nav1.7 and Nav1.8. *Mol Pain* 1:24.

130. Caffrey, J.M., Eng, D.L., Black, J.A., Waxman, S.G., Kocsis, J.D. (1992). Three types of sodium channels in adult rat dorsal root ganglion neurons. *Brain Res* 592:283–297.

131. Elliott, A.A., Elliott, J.R. (1993). Characterization of TTX-sensitive and TTX-resistant sodium currents in small cells from adult rat dorsal root ganglia. *J Physiol* 463:39–56.

132. Arbuckle, J.B., Docherty, R.J. (1995). Expression of tetrodotoxin-resistant sodium channels in capsaicin-sensitive dorsal root ganglion neurons of adult rats. *Neurosci Lett* 185:70–73.

133. Akopian, A.N., Sivilotti, L., Wood, J.N. (1996). A tetrodotoxin-resistant voltage-gated sodium channel expressed by sensory neurons. *Nature* 379:257–262.

134. Akopian, A.N., Souslova, V., England, S., Okuse, K., Ogata, N., Ure, J., Smith, A., Kerr, B.J., McMahon, S.B., Boyce, S., Hill, R., Stanfa, L.C., Dickenson, A.H., Wood, J.N. (1999). The tetrodotoxin-resistant sodium channel SNS has a specialized function in pain pathways. *Nat Neurosci* 2:541–548.

135. Benn, S.C., Costigan, M., Tate, S., Fitzgerald, M., Woolf, C.J. (2001). Developmental expression of the TTX-resistant voltage-gated sodium channels Nav1.8 (SNS) and Nav1.9 (SNS2) in primary sensory neurons. *J Neurosci* 21:6077–6085.

136. Djouhri, L., Fang, X., Okuse, K., Wood, J.N., Berry, C.M., Lawson, S.N. (2003). The TTX-resistant sodium channel Nav1.8 (SNS/PN3): expression and correlation with membrane properties in rat nociceptive primary afferent neurons. *J Physiol* 550(Pt 3):739–752.

137. Renganathan, M., Cummins, T.R., Waxman, S.G. (2001). Contribution of Na(v)1.8 sodium channels to action potential electrogenesis in DRG neurons. *J Neurophysiol* 86:629–640.

138. Zimmermann, K., Leffler, A., Babes, A., Cendan, C.M., Carr, R.W., Kobayashi, J., Nau, C., Wood, J.N., Reeh, P.W. (2007). Sensory neuron sodium channel Nav1.8 is essential for pain at low temperatures. *Nature* 447:855–858.

139. Gold, M.S., Reichling, D.B., Shuster, M.J., Levine, J.D. (1996). Hyperalgesic agents increase a tetrodotoxin-resistant Na+ current in nociceptors. *Proc Natl Acad Sci U S A* 93:1108–1112.

140. Zhang, Y.H., Vasko, M.R., Nicol, G.D. (2002). Ceramide, a putative second messenger for nerve growth factor, modulates the TTX-resistant Na(+) current and delayed rectifier K(+) current in rat sensory neurons. *J Physiol* 544:385–402.

141. Cardenas, C.G., Del Mar, L.P., Cooper, B.Y., Scroggs, R.S. (1997). 5HT4 receptors couple positively to tetrodotoxin-insensitive sodium channels in a subpopulation of capsaicin-sensitive rat sensory neurons. *J Neurosci* 17:7181–7189.

142. Choi, J.S., Hudmon, A., Waxman, S.G., Dib-Hajj, S.D. (2006). Calmodulin regulates current density and frequency-dependent inhibition of sodium channel Nav1.8 in DRG neurons. *J Neurophysiol* 96:97–108.

143. Fitzgerald, E.M., Okuse, K., Wood, J.N., Dolphin, A.C., Moss, S.J. (1999). cAMP-dependent phosphorylation of the tetrodotoxin-resistant voltage-dependent sodium channel SNS. *J Physiol* 516(Pt 2):433–446.

144. Hudmon, A., Choi, J.S., Tyrrell, L., Black, J.A., Rush, A.M., Waxman, S.G., Dib-Hajj, S.D. (2008). Phosphorylation of sodium channel Na(v)1.8 by p38 mitogen-activated protein kinase increases current density in dorsal root ganglion neurons. *J Neurosci* 28:3190–3201.

145. Khasar, S.G., Gold, M.S., Levine, J.D. (1998). A tetrodotoxin-resistant sodium current mediates inflammatory pain in the rat. *Neurosci Lett* 256:17–20.

146. Joshi, S.K., Mikusa, J.P., Hernandez, G., Baker, S., Shieh, C.C., Neelands, T., Zhang, X.F., Niforatos, W., Kage, K., Han, P., Krafte, D., Faltynek, C., Sullivan, J.P., Jarvis, M.F., Honore, P. (2006). Involvement of the TTX-resistant sodium channel Nav 1.8 in inflammatory and neuropathic, but not post-operative, pain states. *Pain* 123:75–82.

147. Dib-Hajj, S., Black, J.A., Felts, P., Waxman, S.G. (1996). Down-regulation of transcripts for Na channel alpha-SNS in spinal sensory neurons following axotomy. *Proc Natl Acad Sci U S A* 93:14950–14954.

148. Decosterd, I., Ji, R.R., Abdi, S., Tate, S., Woolf, C.J. (2002). The pattern of expression of the voltage-gated sodium channels Na(v)1.8 and Na(v)1.9 does not change in uninjured primary sensory neurons in experimental neuropathic pain models. *Pain* 96:269–277.

149. Lai, J., Gold, M.S., Kim, C.S., Bian, D., Ossipov, M.H., Hunter, J.C., Porreca, F. (2002). Inhibition of neuropathic pain by decreased expression of the tetrodotoxin-resistant sodium channel, NaV1.8. *Pain* 95:143–152.
150. Roza, C., Laird, J.M., Souslova, V., Wood, J.N., Cervero, F. (2003). The tetrodotoxin-resistant Na+ channel Nav1.8 is essential for the expression of spontaneous activity in damaged sensory axons of mice. *J Physiol* 550:921–926.
151. Dong, X.W., Goregoaker, S., Engler, H., Zhou, X., Mark, L., Crona, J., Terry, R., Hunter, J., Priestley, T. (2007). Small interfering RNA-mediated selective knockdown of Na(V)1.8 tetrodotoxin-resistant sodium channel reverses mechanical allodynia in neuropathic rats. *Neuroscience* 146:812–821.
152. Kerr, B.J., Souslova, V., McMahon, S.B., Wood, J.N. (2001). A role for the TTX-resistant sodium channel Nav 1.8 in NGF-induced hyperalgesia, but not neuropathic pain. *Neuroreport* 12:3077–3080.
153. Tate, S., Benn, S., Hick, C., Trezise, D., John, V., Mannion, R.J., Costigan, M., Plumpton, C., Grose, D., Gladwell, Z., Kendall, G., Dale, K., Bountra, C., Woolf, C.J. (1998). Two sodium channels contribute to the TTX-R sodium current in primary sensory neurons. *Nat Neurosci* 1:653–655.
154. Fang, X., Djouhri, L., Black, J.A., Dib-Hajj, S.D., Waxman, S.G., Lawson, S.N. (2002). The presence and role of the tetrodotoxin-resistant sodium channel Na(v)1.9 (NaN) in nociceptive primary afferent neurons. *J Neurosci* 22: 7425–7433.
155. Fang, X., Djouhri, L., McMullan, S., Berry, C., Waxman, S.G., Okuse, K., Lawson, S.N. (2006). Intense isolectin-B4 binding in rat dorsal root ganglion neurons distinguishes C-fiber nociceptors with broad action potentials and high Nav1.9 expression. *J Neurosci* 26:7281–7292.
156. Rugiero, F., Mistry, M., Sage, D., Black, J.A., Waxman, S.G., Crest, M., Clerc, N., Delmas, P., Gola, M. (2003). Selective expression of a persistent tetrodotoxin-resistant Na+ current and NaV1.9 subunit in myenteric sensory neurons. *J Neurosci* 23:2715–2725.
157. Dib-Hajj, S., Black, J.A., Cummins, T.R., Waxman, S.G. (2002). NaN/Nav1.9: a sodium channel with unique properties. *Trends Neurosci* 25:253–259.
158. Herzog, R.I., Cummins, T.R., Waxman, S.G. (2001). Persistent TTX-resistant Na+ current affects resting potential and response to depolarization in simulated spinal sensory neurons. *J Neurophysiol* 86:1351–1364.
159. Priest, B.T., Murphy, B.A., Lindia, J.A., Diaz, C., Abbadie, C., Ritter, A.M., Liberator, P., Iyer, L.M., Kash, S.F., Kohler, M.G., Kaczorowski, G.J., MacIntyre, D.E., Martin, W.J. (2005). Contribution of the tetrodotoxin-resistant voltage-gated sodium channel NaV1.9 to sensory transmission and nociceptive behavior. *Proc Natl Acad Sci U S A* 102:9382–9387.
160. Amaya, F., Wang, H., Costigan, M., Allchorne, A.J., Hatcher, J.P., Egerton, J., Stean, T., Morisset, V., Grose, D., Gunthorpe, M.J., Chessell, I.P., Tate, S., Green, P.J., Woolf, C.J. (2006). The voltage-gated sodium channel Na(v)1.9 is an effector of peripheral inflammatory pain hypersensitivity. *J Neurosci* 26:12852–12860.
161. Blum, R., Kafitz, K.W., Konnerth, A. (2002). Neurotrophin-evoked depolarization requires the sodium channel Na(V)1.9. *Nature* 419:687–693.
162. Leffler, A., Herzog, R.I., Dib-Hajj, S.D., Waxman, S.G., Cummins, T.R. (2005). Pharmacological properties of neuronal TTX-resistant sodium channels and the role of a critical serine pore residue. *Pflugers Arch* 451:454–463.

163. Cummins, T.R., Black, J.A., Dib-Hajj, S.D., Waxman, S.G. (2000). Glial-derived neurotrophic factor upregulates expression of functional SNS and NaN sodium channels and their currents in axotomized dorsal root ganglion neurons. *J Neurosci* 20:8754–8761.

164. Coste, B., Osorio, N., Padilla, F., Crest, M., Delmas, P. (2004). Gating and modulation of presumptive NaV1.9 channels in enteric and spinal sensory neurons. *Mol Cell Neurosci* 26:123–134.

165. Maingret, F., Coste, B., Padilla, F., Clerc, N., Crest, M., Korogod, S.M., Delmas, P. (2008). Inflammatory mediators increase Nav1.9 current and excitability in nociceptors through a coincident detection mechanism. *J Gen Physiol* 131:211–225.

166. Rush, A.M., Craner, M.J., Kageyama, T., Dib-Hajj, S.D., Waxman, S.G., Ranscht, B. (2005). Contactin regulates the current density and axonal expression of tetrodotoxin-resistant but not tetrodotoxin-sensitive sodium channels in DRG neurons. *Eur J Neurosci* 22:39–49.

167. Rush, A.M., Waxman, S.G. (2004). PGE2 increases the tetrodotoxin-resistant Nav1.9 sodium current in mouse DRG neurons via G-proteins. *Brain Res* 1023:264–271.

168. Ostman, J.A., Nassar, M.A., Wood, J.N., Baker, M.D. (2008). GTP up-regulated persistent Na+ current and enhanced nociceptor excitability require NaV1.9. *J Physiol* 586:1077–1087.

169. Isom, L.L. (2001). Sodium channel beta subunits: anything but auxiliary. *Neuroscientist* 7:42–54.

170. Isom, L.L., De Jongh, K.S., Patton, D.E., Reber, B.F., Offord, J., Charbonneau, H., Walsh, K., Goldin, A.L., Catterall, W.A. (1992). Primary structure and functional expression of the beta 1 subunit of the rat brain sodium channel. *Science* 256: 839–842.

171. Shah, B.S., Stevens, E.B., Gonzalez, M.I., Bramwell, S., Pinnock, R.D., Lee, K., Dixon, A.K. (2000). Beta3, a novel auxiliary subunit for the voltage-gated sodium channel, is expressed preferentially in sensory neurons and is upregulated in the chronic constriction injury model of neuropathic pain. *Eur J Neurosci* 12: 3985–3990.

172. Yu, F.H., Westenbroek, R.E., Silos-Santiago, I., McCormick, K.A., Lawson, D., Ge, P., Ferriera, H., Lilly, J., DiStefano, P.S., Catterall, W.A., Scheuer, T., Curtis, R. (2003). Sodium channel beta4, a new disulfide-linked auxiliary subunit with similarity to beta2. *J Neurosci* 23:7577–7585.

173. Chen, C., Westenbroek, R.E., Xu, X., Edwards, C.A., Sorenson, D.R., Chen, Y., McEwen, D.P., O'Malley, H.A., Bharucha, V., Meadows, L.S., Knudsen, G.A., Vilaythong, A., Noebels, J.L., Saunders, T.L., Scheuer, T., Shrager, P., Catterall, W.A., Isom, L.L. (2004). Mice lacking sodium channel beta1 subunits display defects in neuronal excitability, sodium channel expression, and nodal architecture. *J Neurosci* 24:4030–4042.

174. Meadows, L.S., Chen, Y.H., Powell, A.J., Clare, J.J., Ragsdale, D.S. (2002). Functional modulation of human brain Nav1.3 sodium channels, expressed in mammalian cells, by auxiliary beta 1, beta 2 and beta 3 subunits. *Neuroscience* 114:745–753.

175. Grieco, T.M., Afshari, F.S., Raman, I.M. (2002). A role for phosphorylation in the maintenance of resurgent sodium current in cerebellar Purkinje neurons. *J Neurosci* 22:3100–3107.

176. Grieco, T.M., Malhotra, J.D., Chen, C., Isom, L.L., Raman, I.M. (2005). Open-channel block by the cytoplasmic tail of sodium channel beta4 as a mechanism for resurgent sodium current. *Neuron* 45:233–244.
177. Okuse, K., Malik-Hall, M., Baker, M.D., Poon, W.Y., Kong, H., Chao, M.V., Wood, J.N. (2002). Annexin II light chain regulates sensory neuron-specific sodium channel expression. *Nature* 417:653–656.
178. Lopez-Santiago, L.F., Pertin, M., Morisod, X., Chen, C., Hong, S., Wiley, J., Decosterd, I., Isom, L.L. (2006). Sodium channel beta2 subunits regulate tetrodotoxin-sensitive sodium channels in small dorsal root ganglion neurons and modulate the response to pain. *J Neurosci* 26:7984–7994.
179. Pertin, M., Ji, R.R., Berta, T., Powell, A.J., Karchewski, L., Tate, S.N., Isom, L.L., Woolf, C.J., Gilliard, N., Spahn, D.R., Decosterd, I. (2005). Upregulation of the voltage-gated sodium channel beta2 subunit in neuropathic pain models: characterization of expression in injured and non-injured primary sensory neurons. *J Neurosci* 25:10970–10980.
180. Shah, B.S., Gonzalez, M.I., Bramwell, S., Pinnock, R.D., Lee, K., Dixon, A.K. (2001). Beta3, a novel auxiliary subunit for the voltage-gated sodium channel is upregulated in sensory neurones following streptozocin induced diabetic neuropathy in rat. *Neurosci Lett* 309:1–4.
181. Catterall, W.A. (2002). Molecular mechanisms of gating and drug block of sodium channels. *Novartis Found Symp* 241:206–218; discussion 218–232.
182. Cestele, S., Catterall, W.A. (2000). Molecular mechanisms of neurotoxin action on voltage-gated sodium channels. *Biochimie* 82:883–892.
183. Ragsdale, D.S., Avoli, M. (1998). Sodium channels as molecular targets for antiepileptic drugs. *Brain Res Brain Res Rev* 26:16–28.
184. Clare, J.J., Tate, S.N., Nobbs, M., Romanos, M.A. (2000). Voltage-gated sodium channels as therapeutic targets. *Drug Discov Today* 5:506–520.
185. Ragsdale, D.S., McPhee, J.C., Scheuer, T., Catterall, W.A. (1996). Common molecular determinants of local anesthetic, antiarrhythmic, and anticonvulsant block of voltage-gated Na+ channels. *Proc Natl Acad Sci U S A* 93:9270–9275.
186. Yarov-Yarovoy, V., McPhee, J.C., Idsvoog, D., Pate, C., Scheuer, T., Catterall, W.A. (2002). Role of amino acid residues in transmembrane segments IS6 and IIS6 of the Na+ channel alpha subunit in voltage-dependent gating and drug block. *J Biol Chem* 277:35393–35401.
187. Yarov-Yarovoy, V., Brown, J., Sharp, E.M., Clare, J.J., Scheuer, T., Catterall, W.A. (2001). Molecular determinants of voltage-dependent gating and binding of pore-blocking drugs in transmembrane segment IIIS6 of the Na(+) channel alpha subunit. *J Biol Chem* 276:20–27.
188. Nau, C., Wang, G.K. (2004). Interactions of local anesthetics with voltage-gated Na+ channels. *J Membr Biol* 201:1–8.
189. Sills, G.J., Brodie, M.J. (2001). Update on the mechanisms of action of antiepileptic drugs. *Epileptic Disord* 3:165–172.
190. Ritter, A.M., Ritchie, C., Martin, W.J. (2007). Relationship between the firing frequency of injured peripheral neurons and inhibition of firing by sodium channel blockers. *J Pain* 8:287–295.
191. Kawagoe, H., Yamaoka, K., Kinoshita, E., Fujimoto, Y., Maejima, H., Yuki, T., Seyama, I. (2002). Molecular basis for exaggerated sensitivity to mexiletine in the cardiac isoform of the fast Na channel. *FEBS Lett* 513:235–241.

192. Leffler, A., Reiprich, A., Mohapatra, D.P., Nau, C. (2007). Use-dependent block by lidocaine but not amitriptyline is more pronounced in tetrodotoxin (TTX)-resistant Nav1.8 than in TTX-sensitive Na+ channels. *J Pharmacol Exp Ther* 320:354–364.

193. Rush, A.M., Elliott, J.R. (1997). Phenytoin and carbamazepine: differential inhibition of sodium currents in small cells from adult rat dorsal root ganglia. *Neurosci Lett* 226:95–98.

194. Vedantham, V., Cannon, S.C. (1999). The position of the fast-inactivation gate during lidocaine block of voltage-gated Na+ channels. *J Gen Physiol* 113:7–16.

195. Balser, J.R., Nuss, H.B., Romashko, D.N., Marban, E., Tomaselli, G.F. (1996). Functional consequences of lidocaine binding to slow-inactivated sodium channels. *J Gen Physiol* 107:643–658.

196. Scholz, A., Vogel, W. (2000). Tetrodotoxin-resistant action potentials in dorsal root ganglion neurons are blocked by local anesthetics. *Pain* 89:47–52.

197. Brau, M.E., Dreimann, M., Olschewski, A., Vogel, W., Hempelmann, G. (2001). Effect of drugs used for neuropathic pain management on tetrodotoxin-resistant Na(+) currents in rat sensory neurons. *Anesthesiology* 94:137–144.

198. Persaud, N., Strichartz, G.R. (2002). Micromolar lidocaine selectively blocks propagating ectopic impulses at a distance from their site of origin. *Pain* 99:333–340.

199. Chabal, C., Russell, L.C., Burchiel, K.J. (1989). The effect of intravenous lidocaine, tocainide, and mexiletine on spontaneously active fibers originating in rat sciatic neuromas. *Pain* 38:333–338.

200. Smith, L.J., Shih, A., Miletic, G., Miletic, V. (2002). Continual systemic infusion of lidocaine provides analgesia in an animal model of neuropathic pain. *Pain* 97: 267–273.

201. Meier, T., Wasner, G., Faust, M., Kuntzer, T., Ochsner, F., Hueppe, M., Bogousslavsky, J., Baron, R. (2003). Efficacy of lidocaine patch 5% in the treatment of focal peripheral neuropathic pain syndromes: a randomized, double-blind, placebo-controlled study. *Pain* 106:151–158.

202. Barbano, R.L., Herrmann, D.N., Hart-Gouleau, S., Pennella-Vaughan, J., Lodewick, P.A., Dworkin, R.H. (2004). Effectiveness, tolerability, and impact on quality of life of the 5% lidocaine patch in diabetic polyneuropathy. *Arch Neurol* 61: 914–918.

203. Herrmann, D.N., Barbano, R.L., Hart-Gouleau, S., Pennella-Vaughan, J., Dworkin, R.H. (2005). An open-label study of the lidocaine patch 5% in painful idiopathic sensory polyneuropathy. *Pain Med* 6:379–384.

204. Gammaitoni, A.R., Alvarez, N.A., Galer, B.S. (2003). Safety and tolerability of the lidocaine patch 5%, a targeted peripheral analgesic: a review of the literature. *J Clin Pharmacol* 43:111–117.

205. Tremont-Lukats, I.W., Hutson, P.R., Backonja, M.M. (2006). A randomized, double-masked, placebo-controlled pilot trial of extended IV lidocaine infusion for relief of ongoing neuropathic pain. *Clin J Pain* 22:266–271.

206. Bean, B.P., Cohen, C.J., Tsien, R.W. (1983). Lidocaine block of cardiac sodium channels. *J Gen Physiol* 81:613–642.

207. Gottrup, H., Bach, F.W., Juhl, G., Jensen, T.S. (2006). Differential effect of ketamine and lidocaine on spontaneous and mechanical evoked pain in patients with nerve injury pain. *Anesthesiology* 104:527–536.

208. Tzeng, J.I., Cheng, K.I., Huang, K.L., Chen, Y.W., Chu, K.S., Chu, C.C., Wang, J.J. (2007). The cutaneous analgesic effect of class I antiarrhythmic drugs. *Anesth Analg* 104:955–958.
209. Erichsen, H.K., Hao, J.X., Xu, X.J., Blackburn-Munro, G. (2003). A comparison of the antinociceptive effects of voltage-activated Na+ channel blockers in two rat models of neuropathic pain. *Eur J Pharmacol* 458:275–282.
210. Oskarsson, P., Ljunggren, J.G., Lins, P.E. (1997). Efficacy and safety of mexiletine in the treatment of painful diabetic neuropathy. The Mexiletine Study Group. *Diabetes Care* 20:1594–1597.
211. Adriaensen, H., Plaghki, L., Mathieu, C., Joffroy, A., Vissers, K. (2005). Critical review of oral drug treatments for diabetic neuropathic pain-clinical outcomes based on efficacy and safety data from placebo-controlled and direct comparative studies. *Diabetes Metab Res Rev* 21:231–240.
212. Eisenberg, E., River, Y., Shifrin, A., Krivoy, N. (2007). Antiepileptic drugs in the treatment of neuropathic pain. *Drugs* 67:1265–1289.
213. Lipkind, G.M., Fozzard, H.A. (2005). Molecular modeling of local anesthetic drug binding by voltage-gated sodium channels. *Mol Pharmacol* 68:1611–1622.
214. Cardenas, C.A., Cardenas, C.G., de Armendi, A.J., Scroggs, R.S. (2006). Carbamazepine interacts with a slow inactivation state of NaV1.8-like sodium channels. *Neurosci Lett* 408:129–134.
215. Wiffen, P.J., McQuay, H.J., Moore, R.A. (2005). Carbamazepine for acute and chronic pain. *Cochrane Database Syst Rev* 3:CD005451.
216. Beydoun, A., Kutluay, E. (2002). Oxcarbazepine. *Expert Opin Pharmacother* 3:59–71.
217. Jang, Y., Kim, E.S., Park, S.S., Lee, J., Moon, D.E. (2005). The suppressive effects of oxcarbazepine on mechanical and cold allodynia in a rat model of neuropathic pain. *Anesth Analg* 101:800–806.
218. Magenta, P., Arghetti, S., Di Palma, F., Jann, S., Sterlicchio, M., Bianconi, C., Galimberti, V., Osio, M., Siciliano, G., Cavallotti, G., Sterzi, R. (2005). Oxcarbazepine is effective and safe in the treatment of neuropathic pain: pooled analysis of seven clinical studies. *Neurol Sci* 26:218–226.
219. Solaro, C., Restivo, D., Mancardi, G.L., Tanganelli, P. (2007). Oxcarbazepine for treating paroxysmal painful symptoms in multiple sclerosis: a pilot study. *Neurol Sci* 28:156–158.
220. Beydoun, A., Shaibani, A., Hopwood, M., Wan, Y. (2006). Oxcarbazepine in painful diabetic neuropathy: results of a dose-ranging study. *Acta Neurol Scand* 113: 395–404.
221. Dogra, S., Beydoun, S., Mazzola, J., Hopwood, M., Wan, Y. (2005). Oxcarbazepine in painful diabetic neuropathy: a randomized, placebo-controlled study. *Eur J Pain* 9:543–554.
222. Grosskopf, J., Mazzola, J., Wan, Y., Hopwood, M. (2006). A randomized, placebo-controlled study of oxcarbazepine in painful diabetic neuropathy. *Acta Neurol Scand* 114:177–180.
223. Cheung, H., Kamp, D., Harris, E. (1992). An in vitro investigation of the action of lamotrigine on neuronal voltage-activated sodium channels. *Epilepsy Res* 13: 107–112.
224. Vinik, A.I., Tuchman, M., Safirstein, B., Corder, C., Kirby, L., Wilks, K., Quessy, S., Blum, D., Grainger, J., White, J., Silver, M. (2007). Lamotrigine for treatment of

pain associated with diabetic neuropathy: results of two randomized, double-blind, placebo-controlled studies. *Pain* 128:169–179.

225. Stohr, T., Kupferberg, H.J., Stables, J.P., Choi, D., Harris, R.H., Kohn, H., Walton, N., White, H.S. (2007). Lacosamide, a novel anti-convulsant drug, shows efficacy with a wide safety margin in rodent models for epilepsy. *Epilepsy Res* 74: 147–154.
226. Beyreuther, B.K., Freitag, J., Heers, C., Krebsfanger, N., Scharfenecker, U., Stohr, T. (2007). Lacosamide: a review of preclinical properties. *CNS Drug Rev* 13:21–42.
227. Beyreuther, B., Callizot, N., Stohr, T. (2006). Antinociceptive efficacy of lacosamide in a rat model for painful diabetic neuropathy. *Eur J Pharmacol* 539:64–70.
228. Beyreuther, B.K., Callizot, N., Brot, M.D., Feldman, R., Bain, S.C., Stohr, T. (2007). Antinociceptive efficacy of lacosamide in rat models for tumor- and chemotherapy-induced cancer pain. *Eur J Pharmacol* 565:98–104.
229. Hao, J.X., Stohr, T., Selve, N., Wiesenfeld-Hallin, Z., Xu, X.J. (2006). Lacosamide, a new anti-epileptic, alleviates neuropathic pain-like behaviors in rat models of spinal cord or trigeminal nerve injury. *Eur J Pharmacol* 553:135–140.
230. Errington, A.C., Stohr, T., Heers, C., Lees, G. (2008). The investigational anticonvulsant lacosamide selectively enhances slow inactivation of voltage-gated sodium channels. *Mol Pharmacol* 73:157–169.
231. Sheets, P.L., Heers, C., Stoehr, T., Cummins, T.R. (2008). Differential block of sensory neuronal voltage-gated sodium channels by lacosamide [(2R)-2-(acetylamino)-N-benzyl-3-methoxypropanamide], lidocaine, and carbamazepine. *J Pharmacol Exp Ther* 326:89–99.
232. Rauck, R.L., Shaibani, A., Biton, V., Simpson, J., Koch, B. (2007). Lacosamide in painful diabetic peripheral neuropathy: a phase 2 double-blind placebo-controlled study. *Clin J Pain* 23:150–158.
233. Kishore-Kumar, R., Max, M.B., Schafer, S.C., Gaughan, A.M., Smoller, B., Gracely, R.H., Dubner, R. (1990). Desipramine relieves postherpetic neuralgia. *Clin Pharmacol Ther* 47:305–312.
234. Max, M.B., Schafer, S.C., Culnane, M., Smoller, B., Dubner, R., Gracely, R.H. (1988). Amitriptyline, but not lorazepam, relieves postherpetic neuralgia. *Neurology* 38:1427–1432.
235. Watson, C.P., Evans, R.J., Reed, K., Merskey, H., Goldsmith, L., Warsh, J. (1982). Amitriptyline versus placebo in postherpetic neuralgia. *Neurology* 32:671–673.
236. Song, J.H., Ham, S.S., Shin, Y.K., Lee, C.S. (2000). Amitriptyline modulation of Na(+) channels in rat dorsal root ganglion neurons. *Eur J Pharmacol* 401: 297–305.
237. Wang, G.K., Russell, C., Wang, S.Y. (2004). State-dependent block of voltage-gated Na+ channels by amitriptyline via the local anesthetic receptor and its implication for neuropathic pain. *Pain* 110:166–174.
238. Dick, I.E., Brochu, R.M., Purohit, Y., Kaczorowski, G.J., Martin, W.J., Priest, B.T. (2007). Sodium channel blockade may contribute to the analgesic efficacy of antidepressants. *J Pain* 8:315–324.
239. Nau, C., Seaver, M., Wang, S.Y., Wang, G.K. (2000). Block of human heart hH1 sodium channels by amitriptyline. *J Pharmacol Exp Ther* 292:1015–1023.

240. Chen, Y.W., Huang, K.L., Liu, S.Y., Tzeng, J.I., Chu, K.S., Lin, M.T., Wang, J.J. (2004). Intrathecal tri-cyclic antidepressants produce spinal anesthesia. *Pain* 112:106–112.

241. Sindrup, S.H., Otto, M., Finnerup, N.B., Jensen, T.S. (2005). Antidepressants in the treatment of neuropathic pain. *Basic Clin Pharmacol Toxicol* 96:399–409.

242. Ilyin, V.I., Hodges, D.D., Whittemore, E.R., Carter, R.B., Cai, S.X., Woodward, R.M. (2005). V102862 (Co 102862): a potent, broad-spectrum state-dependent blocker of mammalian voltage-gated sodium channels. *Br J Pharmacol* 144: 801–812.

243. Ilyin, V.I., Pomonis, J.D., Whiteside, G.T., Harrison, J.E., Pearson, M.S., Mark, L., Turchin, P.I., Gottshall, S., Carter, R.B., Nguyen, P., Hogenkamp, D.J., Olanrewaju, S., Benjamin, E., Woodward, R.M. (2006). Pharmacology of 2-[4-(4-chloro-2-fluorophenoxy)phenyl]-pyrimidine-4-carboxamide: a potent, broad-spectrum state-dependent sodium channel blocker for treating pain states. *J Pharmacol Exp Ther* 318:1083–1093.

244. Ko, S.H., Jochnowitz, N., Lenkowski, P.W., Batts, T.W., Davis, G.C., Martin, W.J., Brown, M.L., Patel, M.K. (2006). Reversal of neuropathic pain by alpha-hydroxyphenylamide: a novel sodium channel antagonist. *Neuropharmacology* 50: 865–873.

245. Jones, P.J., Wang, Y., Smith, M.D., Hargus, N.J., Eidam, H.S., White, H.S., Kapur, J., Brown, M.L., Patel, M.K. (2007). Hydroxyamide analogs of propofol exhibit state-dependent block of sodium channels in hippocampal neurons: implications for anticonvulsant activity. *J Pharmacol Exp Ther* 320:828–836.

246. Stummann, T.C., Salvati, P., Fariello, R.G., Faravelli, L. (2005). The anti-nociceptive agent ralfinamide inhibits tetrodotoxin-resistant and tetrodotoxin-sensitive Na+ currents in dorsal root ganglion neurons. *Eur J Pharmacol* 510:197–208.

247. Brochu, R.M., Dick, I.E., Tarpley, J.W., McGowan, E., Gunner, D., Herrington, J., Shao, P.P., Ok, D., Li, C., Parsons, W.H., Stump, G.L., Regan, C.P., Lynch, J.J., Jr., Lyons, K.A., McManus, O.B., Clark, S., Ali, Z., Kaczorowski, G.J., Martin, W.J., Priest, B.T. (2006). Block of peripheral nerve sodium channels selectively inhibits features of neuropathic pain in rats. *Mol Pharmacol* 69:823–832.

248. Binshtok, A.M., Bean, B.P., Woolf, C.J. (2007). Inhibition of nociceptors by TRPV1-mediated entry of impermeant sodium channel blockers. *Nature* 449:607–610.

249. Jarvis, M.F., Honore, P., Shieh, C.C., Chapman, M., Joshi, S., Zhang, X.F., Kort, M., Carroll, W., Marron, B., Atkinson, R., Thomas, J., Liu, D., Krambis, M., Liu, Y., McGaraughty, S., Chu, K., Roeloffs, R., Zhong, C., Mikusa, J.P., Hernandez, G., Gauvin, D., Wade, C., Zhu, C., Pai, M., Scanio, M., Shi, L., Drizin, I., Gregg, R., Matulenko, M., Hakeem, A., Gross, M., Johnson, M., Marsh, K., Wagoner, P.K., Sullivan, J.P., Faltynek, C.R., Krafte, D.S. (2007). A-803467, a potent and selective Nav1.8 sodium channel blocker, attenuates neuropathic and inflammatory pain in the rat. *Proc Natl Acad Sci U S A* 104:8520–8525.

250. Lipkind, G.M., Fozzard, H.A. (1994). A structural model of the tetrodotoxin and saxitoxin binding site of the Na+ channel. *Biophys J* 66:1–13.

251. Satin, J., Kyle, J.W., Chen, M., Bell, P., Cribbs, L.L., Fozzard, H.A., Rogart, R.B. (1992). A mutant of TTX-resistant cardiac sodium channels with TTX-sensitive properties. *Science* 256:1202–1205.

252. Sivilotti, L., Okuse, K., Akopian, A.N., Moss, S., Wood, J.N. (1997). A single serine residue confers tetrodotoxin insensitivity on the rat sensory-neuron-specific sodium channel SNS. *FEBS Lett* 409:49–52.

253. Backx, P.H., Yue, D.T., Lawrence, J.H., Marban, E., Tomaselli, G.F. (1992). Molecular localization of an ion-binding site within the pore of mammalian sodium channels. *Science* 257:248–251.

254. Heinemann, S.H., Terlau, H., Imoto, K. (1992). Molecular basis for pharmacological differences between brain and cardiac sodium channels. *Pflugers Arch* 422:90–92.

255. Marcil, J., Walczak, J.S., Guindon, J., Ngoc, A.H., Lu, S., Beaulieu, P. (2006). Antinociceptive effects of tetrodotoxin (TTX) in rodents. *Br J Anaesth* 96:761–768.

256. Omana-Zapata, I., Khabbaz, M.A., Hunter, J.C., Clarke, D.E., Bley, K.R. (1997). Tetrodotoxin inhibits neuropathic ectopic activity in neuromas, dorsal root ganglia and dorsal horn neurons. *Pain* 72:41–49.

257. Hagen, N.A., du Souich, P., Lapointe, B., Ong-Lam, M., Dubuc, B., Walde, D., Love, R., Ngoc, A.H. (2008). Tetrodotoxin for moderate to severe cancer pain: a randomized, double blind, parallel design multicenter study. *J Pain Symptom Manage* 35:420–429.

258. Rodriguez-Navarro, A.J., Lagos, N., Lagos, M., Braghetto, I., Csendes, A., Hamilton, J., Figueroa, C., Truan, D., Garcia, C., Rojas, A., Iglesias, V., Brunet, L., Alvarez, F. (2007). Neosaxitoxin as a local anesthetic: preliminary observations from a first human trial. *Anesthesiology* 106:339–345.

259. Kohane, D.S., Smith, S.E., Louis, D.N., Colombo, G., Ghoroghchian, P., Hunfeld, N.G., Berde, C.B., Langer, R. (2003). Prolonged duration local anesthesia from tetrodotoxin-enhanced local anesthetic microspheres. *Pain* 104:415–421.

260. Kohane, D.S., Yieh, J., Lu, N.T., Langer, R., Strichartz, G.R., Berde, C.B. (1998). A re-examination of tetrodotoxin for prolonged duration local anesthesia. *Anesthesiology* 89:119–131.

261. Rosker, C., Lohberger, B., Hofer, D., Steinecker, B., Quasthoff, S., Schreibmayer, W. (2007). The TTX metabolite 4,9-anhydro-TTX is a highly specific blocker of the Na(v1.6) voltage-dependent sodium channel. *Am J Physiol Cell Physiol* 293:C783–C789.

262. Cummins, T.R., Aglieco, F., Dib-Hajj, S.D. (2002). Critical molecular determinants of voltage-gated sodium channel sensitivity to mu-conotoxins GIIIA/B. *Mol Pharmacol* 61:1192–1201.

263. Cruz, L.J., Kupryszewski, G., LeCheminant, G.W., Gray, W.R., Olivera, B.M., Rivier, J. (1989). Mu-conotoxin GIIIA, a peptide ligand for muscle sodium channels: chemical synthesis, radiolabeling, and receptor characterization. *Biochemistry* 28:3437–3442.

264. Terlau, H., Olivera, B.M. (2004). Conus venoms: a rich source of novel ion channel-targeted peptides. *Physiol Rev* 84:41–68.

265. Cruz, L.J., Gray, W.R., Olivera, B.M., Zeikus, R.D., Kerr, L., Yoshikami, D., Moczydlowski, E. (1985). *Conus geographus* toxins that discriminate between neuronal and muscle sodium channels. *J Biol Chem* 260:9280–9288.

266. Ekberg, J., Jayamanne, A., Vaughan, C.W., Aslan, S., Thomas, L., Mould, J., Drinkwater, R., Baker, M.D., Abrahamsen, B., Wood, J.N., Adams, D.J., Christie,

M.J., Lewis, R.J. (2006). MuO-conotoxin MrVIB selectively blocks Nav1.8 sensory neuron specific sodium channels and chronic pain behavior without motor deficits. *Proc Natl Acad Sci U S A* 103:17030–17035.

267. Jain, K.K. (2000). An evaluation of intrathecal ziconotide for the treatment of chronic pain. *Expert Opin Investig Drugs* 9:2403–2410.

268. Liang, S. (2004). An overview of peptide toxins from the venom of the Chinese bird spider *Selenocosmia huwena* Wang [=*Ornithoctonus huwena* (Wang)]. *Toxicon* 43:575–585.

269. Blumenthal, K.M., Seibert, A.L. (2003). Voltage-gated sodium channel toxins: poisons, probes, and future promise. *Cell Biochem Biophys* 38:215–238.

270. Middleton, R.E., Warren, V.A., Kraus, R.L., Hwang, J.C., Liu, C.J., Dai, G., Brochu, R.M., Kohler, M.G., Gao, Y.D., Garsky, V.M., Bogusky, M.J., Mehl, J.T., Cohen, C.J., Smith, M.M. (2002). Two tarantula peptides inhibit activation of multiple sodium channels. *Biochemistry* 41:14734–14747.

271. Smith, J.J., Cummins, T.R., Alphy, S., Blumenthal, K.M. (2007). Molecular interactions of the gating modifier toxin ProTx-II with NaV 1.5: implied existence of a novel toxin binding site coupled to activation. *J Biol Chem* 282:12687–12697.

272. Sokolov, S., Kraus, R.L., Scheuer, T., Catterall, W.A. (2008). Inhibition of sodium channel gating by trapping the domain II voltage sensor with protoxin II. *Mol Pharmacol* 73:1020–1028.

273. Peng, K., Shu, Q., Liu, Z., Liang, S. (2002). Function and solution structure of huwentoxin-IV, a potent neuronal tetrodotoxin (TTX)-sensitive sodium channel antagonist from Chinese bird spider *Selenocosmia huwena*. *J Biol Chem* 277:47564–47571.

274. Xiao, Y., Bingham, J.P., Zhu, W., Moczydlowski, E., Liang, S., Cummins, T.R. (2008). Tarantula huwentoxin-IV inhibits neuronal sodium channels by binding to receptor site 4 and trapping the domain II voltage sensor in the closed configuration. *J Biol Chem* 283:27300–27313.

275. Chen, J.Q., Zhang, Y.Q., Dai, J., Luo, Z.M., Liang, S.P. (2005). Antinociceptive effects of intrathecally administered huwentoxin-I, a selective N-type calcium channel blocker, in the formalin test in conscious rats. *Toxicon* 45:15–20.

276. Gold, M.S., Weinreich, D., Kim, C.S., Wang, R., Treanor, J., Porreca, F., Lai, J. (2003). Redistribution of Na(V)1.8 in uninjured axons enables neuropathic pain. *J Neurosci* 23:158–166.

277. Yeomans, D.C., Levinson, S.R., Peters, M.C., Koszowski, A.G., Tzabazis, A.Z., Gilly, W.F., Wilson, S.P. (2005). Decrease in inflammatory hyperalgesia by herpes vector-mediated knockdown of Nav1.7 sodium channels in primary afferents. *Hum Gene Ther* 16:271–277.

278. Mikami, M., Yang, J. (2005). Short hairpin RNA-mediated selective knockdown of NaV1.8 tetrodotoxin-resistant voltage-gated sodium channel in dorsal root ganglion neurons. *Anesthesiology* 103:828–836.

279. Diss, J.K., Calissano, M., Gascoyne, D., Djamgoz, M.B., Latchman, D.S. (2008). Identification and characterization of the promoter region of the Nav1.7 voltage-gated sodium channel gene (SCN9A). *Mol Cell Neurosci* 37:537–547.

CHAPTER 4

Potassium Channels

DAISUKE NISHIZAWA,[1] TORU KOBAYASHI,[1,2] and KAZUTAKA IKEDA[1]

[1]Division of Psychobiology, Tokyo Institute of Psychiatry
[2]Department of Molecular Neuropathology, Brain Research Institute, Niigata University

Content

4.1 OVERVIEW OF POTASSIUM CHANNELS

The potassium channel family is the largest of all known ion channel families. Since the initial cDNA cloning of genomic and complementary DNA of a voltage-dependent potassium channel gene on the basis of electrophysiological analysis of "Shaker" mutants in *Drosophila melanogaster* [1], approximately 90 potassium channel members have been identified according to the HUGO Gene Nomenclature Committee (HGNC) Database (Department of Biology, University College London, London, U.K.) (http://www.genenames.org) [2]. The HGNC Database stores the approved human gene names and symbols (short-form abbreviations). Each gene name that encodes each potas-

Peripheral Receptor Targets for Analgesia: Novel Approaches to Pain Management, Edited by Brian E. Cairns

sium channel in these four groups was also named by the International Union of Pharmacology (IUPHAR) committee [3]. To date, members of the potassium channel family have been divided into four groups, including voltage-gated (K_V), calcium-activated (K_{Ca}), inward-rectifying (K_{ir}), and two-pore domain (K_{2P}) potassium channels, based on their structure and functional properties. Figure 4.1 illustrates the phylogenetic tree of the potassium channel family. The phylogeny was reconstructed using Molecular Evolutionary Genetics Analysis (MEGA) v.4.0.1 [4] from the human reference sequences (RefSeqs) that are available in the National Center for Biotechnology Information (NCBI) Database, which are linked to the HGNC Database. As shown in Figure 4.1, the members in the K_V, K_{Ca}, K_{ir}, and K_{2P} groups and their homologous genes are largely clustered together in the tree.

The K_V channel subfamily contains the largest number of subunits among all potassium channel subfamilies and is the most diverse, both structurally and functionally, of all voltage-gated ion channels [5]. The K_V subfamily comprises 12 groups (K_V1–K_V12) and each group contains several subunits, resulting in a total of at least 40 K_V subunits [6]. The basic architectural modules of these members of potassium channel subunits are common to other voltage-gated cation channel subunits, such as voltage-gated Na^+ and Ca^{2+} channel subunits. K_V channel is composed of four α-subunits. Each α-subunit contains six transmembrane (TM) domains (S1–S6) and a pore-forming loop between S5 and S6, with cytoplasmic N- and C-terminal domains. The S4 region, with its multiple positive charges, serves as a voltage sensor that enables ion conduction in response to changes in cell membrane voltage [7]. Additionally, some K_V channels include an auxiliary β-subunit that is a cytoplasmic protein. K_V channel subunits are distributed in the brain, spinal cord, heart, retina, skeletal muscle, smooth muscle, kidney, pancreas, and many other organs. These K_V channels play an important role in maintaining and regulating membrane potential and modulating electrical excitability in various cell types, including neurons and muscles [6].

The K_{ir} channel subfamily is the second largest potassium channel subfamily. In contrast to the outward rectification exhibited in delayed rectifying K_V channels, currents through K_{ir} channels flow more readily in an inward rather than an outward direction [8,9]. Since the early cDNA cloning that encoded $K_{ir}1.1$ and $K_{ir}2.1$ channel subunits [8,10], the K_{ir} channel subfamily has been classified into seven groups based on their structure, function, and channel regulation [11]. The basic structure of the channel subunits contains two TM domains (S1–S2) and the pore-forming loop (H5) located between S1 and S2. The functional channels exist as homo- or heterotetramers. K_{ir} channel subunits are also widely distributed in the brain, heart, retina, skeletal muscle, testis, kidney, pancreas, and other organs. These K_{ir} channels play an important role in maintaining resting membrane potential, repolarizing cardiac action potential, and modulating cell excitability [12].

The K_{Ca} channel subfamily is the smallest among the four potassium channel subfamilies (Figure 4.1). The basic structure of K_{Ca} subunits is similar to that

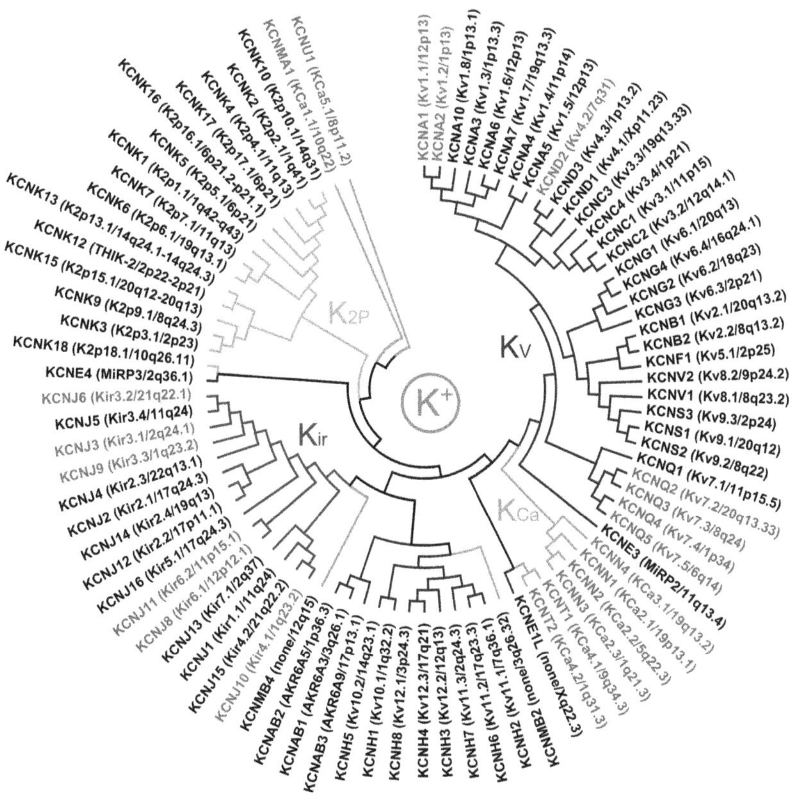

FIGURE 4.1. The potassium channel family phylogenetic tree reconstructed from human reference sequences (RefSeqs) for potassium channel subunits available in the NCBI Database, by the maximum parsimony method with bootstrap replications set at 1000 using MEGA. Only the amino acid sequences for potassium channel genes and their homologs that are linked to and collected in the HGNC Database are used. The tree was constructed from the aligned sequences from the ClustalW algorithm using MEGA. The HGNC gene name was allotted to each potassium channel subunit, as well as the IUPHAR name (or a representative alias) and its chromosomal localization in parentheses. The potassium channel subunits that have been suggested to be involved in analgesia or pain in previous studies are highlighted in color. Red characters represent subunits whose involvement in analgesia or pain is suggested for each specific subunit in the subgroups of the same color, whereas pink characters represent subunits whose involvement in analgesia or pain is suggested, but not for each specific subunit in the subgroups of the same color. See color insert.

of K_V subunits. K_{Ca} subunits are members of the 6TM family of potassium channels. The K_{Ca} channel subfamily is further divided into three subgroups [13] based on ion conductance: small conductance (SK; $K_{Ca}2.1$, $K_{Ca}2.2$), intermediate conductance (IK; $K_{Ca}3.1$), and big conductance (BK; $K_{Ca}1.1$, $K_{Ca}4.1$–4.2, $K_{Ca}5.1$). The BK channel subunits possess an additional TM domain in the

N-terminus (S0) and two regulator of conductance (RCK for K^+) domains in the cytosolic C-terminus [14]. The SK and BK channels have extra domains in the C-terminus—calmodulin-binding domain (CaMBD) and "calcium bowl," respectively—that are associated with regulation by Ca^{2+} or interaction with Ca^{2+} [14,15]. The SK and IK channels are activated by cytoplasmic Ca^{2+} concentrations, whereas BK channels are additionally voltage sensitive because of their S4 regions serving as voltage sensors [13,14]. K_{Ca} channels have ubiquitous distribution, such as in the brain, heart, skeletal muscle, smooth muscle, testis, kidney, pancreas, and other organs. The channels are involved in neuronal afterhyperpolarization [16].

The K_{2P} channel subfamily is hypothesized to underlie background or leak currents that set resting potential. The unique structure of this channel subunit contains two pore domains and 4TM domains and forms functional dimers. They are divided into six groups that are uniquely termed TIWK, TREK (TRAAK), TASK, TALK, THIK, and TRESK, based on their structural and functional properties [11]. K_{2P} channel subunits are also widely distributed in the brain, heart, lung, small intestine, placenta, kidney, liver, pancreas, and other organs. The physiological functions of some of these channels have been shown to be involved in cell volume regulation and sensing external basolateral pH changes associated with HCO_3^- transport, although their roles remain largely unresolved [17].

Because potassium channels are a diverse family, many of their roles in analgesia (antinociception) are poorly understood, especially with regard to K_{2P} channels [15]. Furthermore, only a limited number of studies have investigated the involvement of peripheral potassium channels in analgesia. The several potassium channel subunits presented in Figure 4.1 have been suggested to be involved in analgesia or pain. Although many subunits have not been examined specifically, the K_{ir} channels $K_{ir}3.x$ (G protein-activated K_{ir} [GIRK], K_G) or $K_{ir}6.x$ (K_{ATP}), K_{Ca} channels, and some of the K_V channels appear to be potent molecules involved in analgesia (Figure 4.1). In the following two sections, $K_{ir}3$ channels, probably the most potent molecules involved in analgesia, are particularly detailed. In the following section, the characteristics of other potassium channel subunits and their involvement in analgesia are reviewed, and the possibility of utilizing these channels as therapeutic targets for analgesia is discussed.

4.2 INVOLVEMENT OF GIRK CHANNELS IN ANALGESIA

$K_{ir}3$ channels are GIRK (K_G) channels. GIRK channels are expressed in many tissues, including the pancreas, small intestine, testis, skeletal and smooth muscles [18], heart [19], spinal cord [20,21], and various regions of the central nervous system (CNS) with different subunit compositions [22–24]. Four GIRK subunits (GIRK1–GIRK4; $K_{ir}3.1$–$K_{ir}3.4$) have been identified in mammals. Neuronal GIRK channels function predominantly as heteromultimers composed of GIRK1 and either GIRK2 or GIRK3 [25]. $K_{ir}3$ channels are gated by activation of several $G_{i/o}$ protein-coupled receptors, such as M_2-muscarinic [26], D_2- and D_4-dopaminergic [27], α_2-adrenergic [28], metabotropic glutamate [29], somatostatin [30], CB_1-cannabinoid [31,32], nociceptin/orphanin FQ [33], adenosine A_1 [34], and opioid receptors [35]. GIRK channel activation causes membrane hyperpolarization and thus leads to inhibitory regulation of neuronal excitability. Activation of GIRK channels that are expressed with opioid receptors in the spinal cord blocks nociceptive transmission, resulting in opioid-induced analgesia. The involvement of GIRK channels in analgesia has been shown *in vivo* using *weaver* mutant mice [36,37] that have a nonsynonymous point mutation in the pore-forming region of the $K_{ir}3.2$ subunit [38], with loss of K^+ selectivity [39,40] and various aberrant changes in cerebellar granule cells [41], nerve cell loss in areas of the mesencephalic dopamine cell system, including substantia nigra [42], significantly lower analgesia compared with wild-type mice [36], and lack of activating effects of ethanol [43]. GIRK channels play a key role in analgesia induced by opioids [36,44]. Studies using $K_{ir}3$ knockout mice have further elucidated the role of GIRK channels in analgesia. Mice lacking GIRK channels display decreased analgesia in response to activation of opioid or other $G_{i/o}$ protein-coupled receptors compared with wild-type mice [20,21,45–47]. GIRK channel modulators are able to affect the physiology or behaviors of these mice. For example, the selective serotonin reuptake inhibitor (SSRI) fluoxetine inhibits *weaver* channels, and chronic fluoxetine treatment markedly alleviated the motor disturbances of *weaver* mice and substantially suppressed abnormal neuronal cell death in *weaver* mouse cerebellum and pontine nuclei [48].

Another recent study revealed the genomic region responsible for genetic mediation of analgesia induced by multiple drug classes using quantitative trait locus mapping in 872 (C57BL/6 × 129P3) F2 mice [49]. A region on distal chromosome 1, including the *Girk3* (*Kcnj9*) gene, has shown significant linkage to variability in the analgesic effects of opioid (morphine), α_2-adrenergic (clonidine), and cannabinoid (WIN55,212-2) drugs on thermal nociception. Furthermore, the *Girk3* gene of 129P3 mice, compared with C57BL/6 mice, has been shown to be differentially expressed in the midbrain periaqueductal gray (PAG), a brain region implicated in analgesia [49]. The results support the hypothesis that GIRK channels are involved in analgesia mediated by several $G_{i/o}$ protein-coupled receptors.

GIRK channels are modulated by various activating and inhibiting compounds [50]. Figure 4.2 illustrates a schematic representation of GIRK activators and inhibitors from several different studies. GIRK channels have been shown to be inhibited by a wide variety of pharmacological ligands/agents with varying degrees of potency and efficacy, such as antidepressants (e.g., fluoxetine, paroxetine, imipramine, desipramine, amitriptyline, nortriptyline, clomipramine, and maprotiline [51–54]), antipsychotics (e.g., thioridazine, clozapine, pimozide, and haloperidol [53,55,56]), anesthetics (e.g., halothane, isoflurane, enflurane, F3 [1-chloro-1,2,2-trifluorocyclobutane]

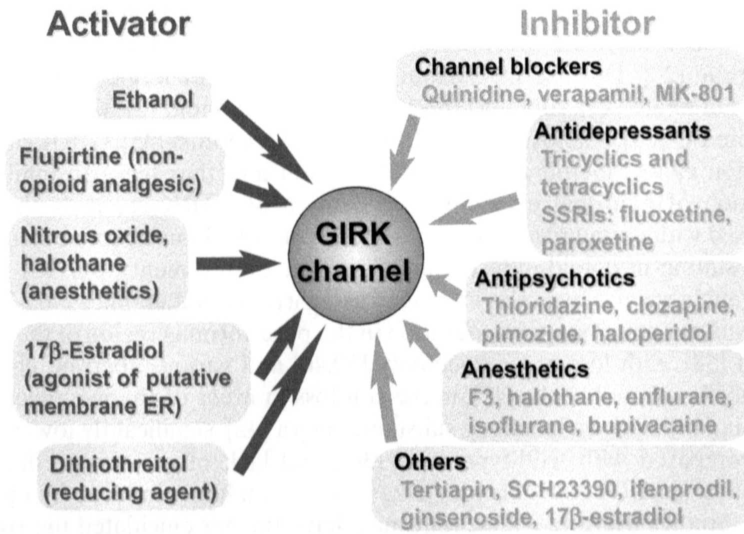

FIGURE 4.2. Various modulators of GIRK channels. Blue and red arrows show the activating and inhibiting effect on GIRK channels, respectively. See color insert.

and the structurally related nonimmobilizer F6 [1,2-dichlorohexafluorocyclobutane], and bupivacaine [57–59]), and other compounds such as quinidine, verapamil, MK-801 ([+]-5-methyl-10,11-dihydro-5H-dibenzo[a,d]cyclohepten-5,10-iminehydrogen maleate; dizocilpine), tertiapin, SCH23390 (R-[+]-7-chloro-8-hydroxy-3-methyl-1-phenyl-2,3,4,5-tetrahydro-1H-3-benzazepine hydrochloride), ginsenoside, and ifenprodil [50]. The most well-known $K_{ir}3$ activator is ethanol [43,60]. Some anesthetics, such as nitrous oxide and halothane (at high concentrations), also activate GIRK channels [57,58]. The nonopioid analgesic flupirtine was reported to activate GIRK channels [61], and 17β-estradiol and dithiothreitol (DTT) were found to activate GIRK channels [62,63]. Recently, another GIRK activator was identified through screening various chemical compounds using an *in vitro Xenopus* oocyte expression system [64]. Although the roles of these substances in peripheral analgesia remain to be clarified, selective GIRK activators could be candidate therapeutic agents for analgesia and may benefit many patients with chronic pain that is poorly managed by current therapies.

4.3 GIRK CHANNELS FOR PERIPHERAL ANALGESIA

To date, few studies have focused on the role of GIRK channels in peripheral analgesia. However, Khodorova et al. have shown that endothelin-1 (ET-1), which is synthesized by keratinocytes in normal skin and is locally released after cutaneous injury, produced analgesia through endothelin-B (ET_B) receptors and triggered pain through local endothelin-A (ET_A) nociceptors. ET_B receptor activation has been shown to induce the release of β-endorphin from keratinocytes, in which the colocalization of ET_B receptors with β-endorphin has been confirmed in rat plantar hind paw epidermis adjacent to nociceptive sensory terminals, and to result in the activation of GIRK channels linked to opioid receptors on nociceptors [65]. μ- and δ-opioid receptors have been shown using GIRK2 knockout mice to significantly contribute to attenuation of ET-1-induced pain, and activation of channels with GIRK2 subunit was shown to be crucial to ET-1-mediated analgesia [65]. The results of this study indicated the existence of an intrinsic feedback mechanism that controls peripheral pain through the action of β-endorphin secreted in the skin [66] and highlighted the possibility that peripheral GIRK channels and ET_B receptors may be important and useful targets for the treatment of pain.

4.4 OTHER PERIPHERAL POTASSIUM CHANNEL TARGETS FOR ANALGESIA

4.4.1 K_{ir} Channels

To date, many studies have suggested the involvement of other K_{ir} channel subunits in addition to GIRK subunits in analgesia or pain. $K_{ir}6.x$ (K_{ATP}) channels, among the K_{ir} channels, have been suggested to be important channel targets for central and peripheral analgesia, although K_{ATP} channels in pancreatic β-cells are well known to link glucose metabolism to insulin release [67]. Functional K_{ATP} channels are composed of four $K_{ir}6$ subunits and four sulfonylurea receptors (SUR1, SUR2A, or SUR2B, depending on the tissue) that regulate the opening and closing of $K_{ir}6$ channels [67]. The four $K_{ir}6$ subunits form a channel pore that is surrounded by four sulfonylurea receptors. The activity of K_{ATP} channels is regulated not only by intracellular adenosine triphosphate (ATP) concentration but also by G protein βγ-subunits through activation of several G protein-coupled receptors (GPCRs), such as α_2-adrenergic, somatostatin, adenosine, and opioid receptors [68]. Accordingly, activation of these receptors by their agonists is antagonized by K_{ATP} channel blockers in tests of analgesia.

Ocaña and Baeyens showed that intracerebroventricular (i.c.v.) pretreatment with the K_{ATP} channel blockers gliquidone, glipizide, glibenclamide, and tolbutamide (antidiabetic sulfonylureas) antagonized morphine-induced analgesia in the tail-flick test in mice, whereas these blockers did not antagonize the analgesic effect induced by U-50,488H (trans-[±]-3,4-dichloro-*N*-methyl-*N*-[2(1-pirrolidynyl)cyclohexyl]benzeneacetamide methanesulfonate salt), a κ-opioid receptor agonist [69]. The spinally mediated analgesic effect of intrathecally (i.t.) injected morphine is also antagonized by i.t. glibenclamide administration in different rat models of pain [70]. Moreover, the analgesia induced by epidural administration of morphine in a tail-flick test in rats was potentiated by epidural administration of the K_{ATP} channel openers nicorandil and levcromakalim, and this potentiation was abolished by glibenclamide [71]. Rodrigues and Duarte have shown that glibenclamide and tolbutamide injected subcutaneously (s.c.) into the rat hind paw antagonized the peripheral antinociception induced by morphine administered s.c. into the hind paw of hyperalgesic rats [72]. These results suggest that K_{ATP} channels are involved in morphine-induced analgesia through μ- and δ-opioid receptors, possibly at supraspinal, spinal, and peripheral levels.

K_{ATP} channels have been shown to be involved in analgesia induced by other GPCR agonists. For example, i.c.v. or i.t. glibenclamide administration antagonized the antinociception induced by the α_2-adrenoceptor agonists clonidine (i.c.v. and i.t.) and tizanidine (i.c.v.) [73,74], suggesting that K_{ATP} channel blockers antagonize both supraspinal and spinal antinociception induced by α_2-adrenoceptor agonists. Similarly, the antinociception induced by i.c.v. administration of the adenosine A_1 receptor agonist R-PIA ([-]-N6-[2-phenylisopropyl]-adenosine), the muscarinic receptor agonist pilocarpine, and several 5-HT_{1A} receptor agonists was antagonized by gliquidone in the tail-flick and hot-plate tests in mice [73,75,76].

Furthermore, several studies have suggested the involvement of K_{ATP} channels in the analgesic effects induced by nonsteroidal anti-inflammatory drugs (NSAIDs) [77], activation of the nitric oxide (NO)/cyclic guanosine monophosphate (cGMP) pathway by sodium nitroprusside or dibutyryl cGMP [78], tricyclic antidepressants such as amitriptyline and clomipramine [79], H_1-antihistamines [80], and the antiepileptic gabapentin [81].

In addition, the involvement of $K_{ir}4.1$ in pain was suggested in a recent study in which specific silencing of Kir4.1 using RNA interference in the rat trigeminal ganglion led to spontaneous and evoked facial painlike behavior in freely moving rats [82].

In summary, K_{ATP} channels may be involved in analgesic effects induced not only by the mediation of GPCRs but also by many other drugs at supraspinal, spinal, and even peripheral levels [77,78].

4.4.2 K_V Channels

Several studies have demonstrated the involvement of K_V channels in central or peripheral analgesia. Galeotti et al. showed that i.c.v. administration of an antisense oligodeoxyribonucleotide (aODN) for the $K_V1.1$ gene inhibited the antinociceptive effects of morphine, the gamma-aminobutyric acid B ($GABA_B$) receptor agonist baclofen, clonidine, and the α_2-adrenoceptor agonist guanabenz in the mouse hot-plate test [83,84], suggesting the involvement of the $K_V1.1$ subunits in central analgesia mediated by opioid, $GABA_B$, and α_2-adrenergic receptors. The involvement of the $K_V1.1$ subunits in central opioid analgesia has been further corroborated by evidence indicating that morphine-induced antinociception in $K_V1.1$ null mutant mice is blunted [85]. Additionally, i.c.v. injection of the aODN for the $K_V1.1$ subunits dose-dependently inhibited clomipramine- and amitriptyline-induced antinociception in the mouse hot-plate test, suggesting the involvement of the $K_V1.1$ subunits in tricyclic antidepressant-induced analgesia [83,86]. In addition to the K_V1.1 subunits, Finnegan et al. examined the effect of μ-opioid receptor stimulation on the inhibitory and excitatory synaptic inputs to basolateral amygdala (BLA) neurons that are projected to the central nucleus of the amygdala (CeA) and considered to be important for opioid analgesia. These researchers found that two K_V channel blockers of dendrotoxin-K (K_V1.1) and tityustoxin-Kα (K_V1.2) attenuated the inhibitory effect of the μ-opioid receptor agonist D-Ala^2,*N*-Me-Phe^4,Gly^5-ol-enkephalin (DAMGO) on miniature inhibitory postsynaptic currents (mIPSCs) [87].

With regard to K_V channel subunits other than K_V1, forms of pain hypersensitivity that are dependent on extracellular signal-regulated kinases (ERKs, which mediate central sensitization during inflammatory pain in spinal cord dorsal horn neurons) were absent in K_V4.2 knockout mice compared with wild-type littermates [88]. This result suggests that the K_V4.2 channel subunit is a downstream target of ERK in the spinal cord and plays a crucial role in pain plasticity. Furthermore, the neuronal K_V7 channel opener retigabine (K_V7.2–7.5, also known as KCNQ2-5 subunits) significantly attenuated mechanical hypersensitivity in response to pinprick stimulation of an injured hind paw in the rat chronic constriction injury model and spared nerve models of neuropathic pain [89]. Retigabine also inhibited carrageenan-induced hyperalgesia in a rat model of chronic pain, an effect that was reversed by the KCNQ channel blocker XE991 (10,10-bis[4-pyridinylmethyl]-9[10H]-anthracenone) [90]. These two studies indicated that K_V7 channels may play a key role in nociceptive sensory systems. In addition, retigabine suppressed capsaicin-induced licking as an index of visceral pain behavior and prolonged the latency to first lick in mice [91], providing evidence that activation of K_V7 channels also plays an inhibitory role in the visceral pain pathway.

In summary, K_V1.1, K_V1.2, K_V4.2, and K_V7 (K_V7.2–7.5) channel subunits have been shown to be involved in antinociception in several pain models and could be potential analgesic targets.

4.4.3 K_{Ca} Channels

K_{Ca} channels have also been shown to be involved in analgesia. The SK channel blocker apamin (i.t.) completely blocked [2-D-penicillamine, 5-D-penicillamine]-enkephalin (DPDPE)-induced antinociception in mouse tail-flick tests, suggesting the involvement of the SK channel in the analgesia mediated by the δ-opioid receptor [92]. Apamin (i.t.) also antagonized the antinociception induced by i.t. administration of the cannabinoids Δ^9-THC (tetrahydrocannabinol), Δ^8-THC, and CP 55,940 ([−]-cis-3-[2-hydroxy-4(1,1-dimethylheptyl)phenyl]-trans-4-[3-hydroxypropyl]cyclohexanol) in mouse tail-flick tests, although apamin (i.c.v.) failed to block the antinociceptive effects of these cannabinoids (i.c.v.), suggesting the involvement of the SK channel in the analgesia mediated by cannabinoid receptors at the spinal level but not at the supraspinal level [93]. Furthermore, several reports have suggested the involvement of SK channels in the analgesic effects induced by the administration of i.c.v. tricyclic antidepressants [79], i.c.v. H_1-antihistamines (e.g., pyrilamine, diphenhydramine, and promethazine) [80], and i.t. gabapentin [81].

Yamazumi et al. demonstrated that antinociception induced by i.t. clonidine or bethanechol, a muscarinic receptor agonist, in rat tail-flick tests was partially antagonized by i.t. administration of the BK channel blocker charybdotoxin [74], suggesting the involvement of the BK channel in analgesia mediated by the α_2-adrenoceptor and muscarinic receptor. Additionally, the involvement of BK channels in the analgesic effects induced by i.t. gabapentin has also been demonstrated [81].

Although little is known about the involvement of IK channels in analgesia or pain, the IK ($K_{Ca}3.1$) channel inhibitor clotrimazole prevented the antinociceptive effects of the peroxisome proliferator-activated receptor-α (PPAR-α) agonists GW7647 (2-[4-(2-[1-cyclohexanebutyl-3-cyclohexylureido]ethyl) phenylthio]-2-methylpropionic acid) and palmitoylethanolamide (PEA) in the formalin test in mice, suggesting that IK channels mediate PPAR-α antinociception [94].

In summary, K_{Ca} channels, especially SK and BK channels, appear to play a role in the analgesic effects mediated by some GPCRs at the spinal level, as well as those mediated by several types of drugs at the supraspinal or spinal levels.

4.4.4 K_{2P} Channels

Only a limited number of studies have investigated the involvement of K_{2P} channels in analgesia, although these channels are widely expressed in central and peripheral tissues, including dorsal root ganglia [95]. Interestingly, K_{2P} channels are sensitive to some types of volatile general anesthetics. TRESK ($K_{2P}18.1$) is activated by clinical concentrations of isoflurane, halothane, sevoflurane, and desflurane [96]. TREK-1 ($K_{2P}2.1$) and TREK-2 ($K_{2P}10.1$) are also opened by chloroform, diethyl ether, halothane, and isoflurane [97,98]. TASK-1 ($K_{2P}3.1$) is activated by halothane and isoflurane, and TASK-2 ($K_{2P}5.1$) is activated by halothane, isoflurane, and chloroform [97]. Indeed, TASK-1 and TASK-3 ($K_{2P}9.1$) knockout mice are less sensitive to the anesthetic effects of halothane and isoflurane than their wild-type littermates [99,100], and TASK-1 knockout mice display increased sensitivity to thermal nociception and reduced analgesic effects of s.c. administration of the cannabinoid agonist WIN55212-2 in the hot-plate test [99]. TREK-1 ($K_{2P}2.1$) knockout mice are resistant to anesthesia induced by volatile anesthetics and more sensitive to painful heat sensations near the threshold between anoxious warmth and painful heat [101,102]. TRAAK ($K_{2P}4.1$) is structurally and functionally similar to TREK and is insensitive to volatile anesthetics. In contrast, halothane inhibits TWIK, THIK, and TALK [97]. These studies indicate that activation of some K_{2P} channels by inhalational anesthetics might be involved in some of the mechanisms of general anesthesia and pain relief. Although further studies will be

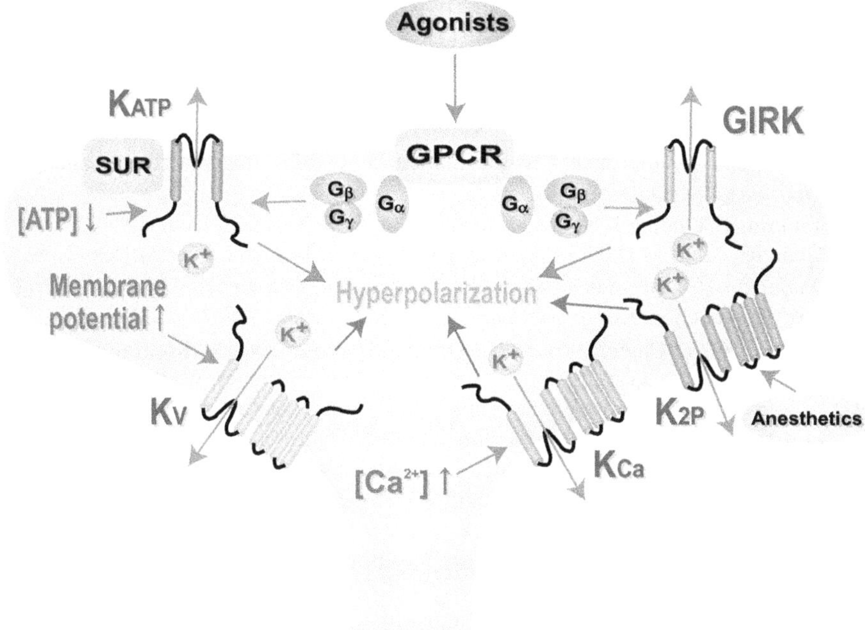

FIGURE 4.3. Schematic illustration of peripheral endogenous analgesia, focusing on major potassium channels, induced by hyperpolarization of membrane potential in the nerve terminus of the peripheral sensory neuron. GPCR, G protein-coupled receptor; SUR, sulfonylurea receptor. See color insert.

needed, K_{2P} channel activators may also be candidates as potent therapeutic analgesics.

4.5 CONCLUDING REMARKS

Figure 4.3 shows a schematic illustration of the peripheral endogenous analgesia mediated by the major potassium channels. GIRK channels and K_{ATP} channels appear to play the most important role in central and peripheral analgesia. However, increasing evidence suggests the involvement of other subunits in analgesia or pain. Far more potassium channel subunits may contribute to the mechanisms of analgesia or pain transduction than the currently known channels. The development of therapeutic drugs targeting such potassium channels may lead to effective pain treatment in the future.

REFERENCES

1. Papazian, D.M., Schwarz, T.L., Tempel, B.L., Jan, Y.N., Jan, L.Y. (1987). Cloning of genomic and complementary DNA from Shaker, a putative potassium channel gene from *Drosophila*. *Science* 237:749–753.

2. Eyre, T.A, Ducluzeau, F., Sneddon, T.P., Povey, S., Bruford, E.A., Lush, M.J. (2006). The HUGO Gene Nomenclature Database, 2006 updates. *Nucleic Acids Res* 34(Database issue):D319–D321.
3. Catterall, W.A., Chandy, K.G., Clapham, D.E., Gutman, G.A., Hofmann, F., Harmar, A.J., Abernethy, D.R., Spedding, M. (2003). International Union of Pharmacology: approaches to the nomenclature of voltage-gated ion channels. *Pharmacol Rev* 55:573–574.
4. Tamura, K., Dudley, J., Nei, M., Kumar, S. (2007). MEGA4: Molecular Evolutionary Genetics Analysis (MEGA) software version 4.0. *Mol Biol Evol* 24:1596–1599.
5. Anderson, P.A, Greenberg, R.M. (2001). Phylogeny of ion channels: clues to structure and function. *Comp Biochem Physiol B Biochem Mol Biol* 129:17–28.
6. Gutman, G.A., Chandy, K.G., Grissmer, S., Lazdunski, M., McKinnon, D., Pardo, L.A., Robertson, G.A., Rudy, B., Sanguinetti, M.C., Stühmer, W., Wang, X. (2005). International Union of Pharmacology. LIII. Nomenclature and molecular relationships of voltage-gated potassium channels. *Pharmacol Rev* 57:473–508.
7. Yellen, G. (2002). The voltage-gated potassium channels and their relatives. *Nature* 419:35–42.
8. Kubo, Y., Reuveny, E., Slesinger, P.A., Jan, Y.N., Jan, L.Y. (1993). Primary structure and functional expression of a rat G-protein-coupled muscarinic potassium channel. *Nature* 364:802–806.
9. Reimann, F., Ashcroft, F.M. (1999). Inwardly rectifying potassium channels. *Curr Opin Cell Biol* 11:503–508.
10. Ho, K., Nichols, C.G., Lederer, W.J., Lytton, J., Vassilev, P.M., Kanazirska, M.V., Hebert, S.C. (1993). Cloning and expression of an inwardly rectifying ATP-regulated potassium channel. *Nature* 362:31–38.
11. Alexander, S.P.H., Mathie, A., Peters, J.A. (2008). Guide to Receptors and Channels (GRAC), 3rd edition. *Br J Pharmacol* 153(Suppl. 2):S1–S209.
12. Kubo, Y., Adelman, J.P., Clapham, D.E., Jan, L.Y., Karschin, A., Kurachi, Y., Lazdunski, M., Nichols, C.G., Seino, S., Vandenberg, C.A. (2005). International Union of Pharmacology. LIV. Nomenclature and molecular relationships of inwardly rectifying potassium channels. *Pharmacol Rev* 57:509–526.
13. Vergara, C., Latorre, R., Marrion, N.V., Adelman, J.P. (1998). Calcium-activated potassium channels. *Curr Opin Neurobiol* 8:321–329.
14. Roosild, T.P., Lê, K.T., Choe, S. (2004). Cytoplasmic gatekeepers of K^+-channel flux: a structural perspective. *Trends Biochem Sci* 29:39–45.
15. Ocaña, M., Cendán, C.M., Cobos, E.J., Entrena, J.M., Baeyens, J.M. (2004). Potassium channels and pain: present realities and future opportunities. *Eur J Pharmacol* 500:203–219.
16. Wei, A.D., Gutman, G.A., Aldrich, R., Chandy, K.G., Grissmer, S., Wulff, H. (2005). International Union of Pharmacology. LII. Nomenclature and molecular relationships of calcium-activated potassium channels. *Pharmacol Rev* 57:463–472.
17. Goldstein, S.A., Bayliss, D.A., Kim, D., Lesage, F., Plant, L.D., Rajan, S. (2005). International Union of Pharmacology. LV. Nomenclature and molecular relationships of two-P potassium channels. *Pharmacol Rev* 57:527–540.
18. Vaughn, J., Wolford, J.K., Prochazka, M., Permana, P.A. (2000). Genomic structure and expression of human *KCNJ9* (*Kir3.3/GIRK3*). *Biochem Biophys Res Commun* 274:302–309.

19. Corey, S., Clapham, D.E. (1998). Identification of native atrial G-protein-regulated inwardly rectifying K^+ (GIRK4) channel homomultimers. *J Biol Chem* 273:27499–27504.
20. Marker, C.L., Stoffel, M., Wickman, K. (2004). Spinal G-protein-gated K^+ channels formed by GIRK1 and GIRK2 subunits modulate thermal nociception and contribute to morphine analgesia. *J Neurosci* 24:2806–2812.
21. Marker, C.L., Lujan, R., Loh, H.H., Wickman, K. (2005). Spinal G-protein-gated potassium channels contribute in a dose-dependent manner to the analgesic effect of μ- and δ- but not κ-opioids. *J Neurosci* 25:3551–3559.
22. Jelacic, T.M., Kennedy, M.E., Wickman, K., Clapham, D.E. (2000). Functional and biochemical evidence for G-protein-gated inwardly rectifying K^+ (GIRK) channels composed of GIRK2 and GIRK3. *J Biol Chem* 275:36211–36216.
23. Kobayashi, T., Ikeda, K., Ichikawa, T., Abe, S., Togashi, S., Kumanishi, T. (1995). Molecular cloning of a mouse G-protein-activated K^+ channel (mGIRK1) and distinct distributions of three GIRK (GIRK1, 2 and 3) mRNAs in mouse brain. *Biochem Biophys Res Commun* 208:1166–1173.
24. Wickman, K., Karschin, C., Karschin, A., Picciotto, M.R., Clapham, D.E. (2000). Brain localization and behavioral impact of the G-protein-gated K^+ channel subunit GIRK4. *J Neurosci* 20:5608–5615.
25. Kofuji, P., Davidson, N., Lester, H.A. (1995). Evidence that neuronal G-protein-gated inwardly rectifying K^+ channels are activated by Gβγ subunits and function as heteromultimers. *Proc Natl Acad Sci U S A* 92:6542–6546.
26. Fernandez-Fernandez, J.M., Wanaverbecq, N., Halley, P., Caulfield, M.P., Brown, D.A. (1999). Selective activation of heterologously expressed G protein-gated K^+ channels by M_2 muscarinic receptors in rat sympathetic neurones. *J Physiol* 515(Pt 3):631–637.
27. Pillai, G., Brown, N.A., McAllister, G., Milligan, G., Seabrook, G.R. (1998). Human D_2 and D_4 dopamine receptors couple through βγ G-protein subunits to inwardly rectifying K^+ channels (GIRK1) in a *Xenopus* oocyte expression system: selective antagonism by L-741,626 and L-745,870 respectively. *Neuropharmacology* 37:983–987.
28. Bünemann, M., Bücheler, M.M., Philipp, M., Lohse, M.J., Hein, L. (2001). Activation and deactivation kinetics of α_{2A}- and α_{2C}-adrenergic receptor-activated G protein-activated inwardly rectifying K^+ channel currents. *J Biol Chem* 276:47512–47517.
29. Saugstad, J.A., Segerson, T.P., Westbrook, G.L. (1996). Metabotropic glutamate receptors activate G-protein-coupled inwardly rectifying potassium channels in *Xenopus* oocytes. *J Neurosci* 16:5979–5985.
30. Kreienkamp, H.J., Hönck, H.H., Richter, D. (1997). Coupling of rat somatostatin receptor subtypes to a G-protein gated inwardly rectifying potassium channel (GIRK1). *FEBS Lett* 419:92–94.
31. Ho, B.Y., Uezono, Y., Takada, S., Takase, I., Izumi, F. (1999). Coupling of the expressed cannabinoid CB1 and CB2 receptors to phospholipase C and G protein-coupled inwardly rectifying K^+ channels. *Receptors Channels* 6:363–374.
32. McAllister, S.D., Griffin, G., Satin, L.S., Abood, M.E. (1999). Cannabinoid receptors can activate and inhibit G protein-coupled inwardly rectifying potassium channels in a *Xenopus* oocyte expression system. *J Pharmacol Exp Ther* 291:618–626.

33. Ikeda, K., Kobayashi, K., Kobayashi, T., Ichikawa, T., Kumanishi, T., Kishida, H., Yano, R., Manabe, T. (1997). Functional coupling of the nociceptin/orphanin FQ receptor with the G-protein-activated K^+ (GIRK) channel. *Brain Res Mol Brain Res* 45:117–126.

34. Kobayashi, T., Ikeda, K., Kumanishi, T. (2002). Functional characterization of an endogenous *Xenopus* oocyte adenosine receptor. *Br J Pharmacol* 135:313–322.

35. Ikeda, K., Kobayashi, T., Ichikawa, T., Usui, H., Kumanishi, T. (1995). Functional couplings of the δ- and the κ-opioid receptors with the G-protein-activated K^+ channel. *Biochem Biophys Res Commun* 208:302–308.

36. Ikeda, K., Kobayashi, T., Kumanishi, T., Niki, H., Yano, R. (2000). Involvement of G-protein-activated inwardly rectifying K (GIRK) channels in opioid-induced analgesia. *Neurosci Res* 38:113–116.

37. Ikeda, K., Yoshii, M., Sora, I., Kobayashi, T. (2003). Opioid receptor coupling to GIRK channels: in vitro studies using a *Xenopus* oocyte expression system and in vivo studies on *weaver* mutant mice. *Methods Mol Med* 84:53–64.

38. Patil, N., Cox, D.R., Bhat, D., Faham, M., Myers, R.M., Peterson, A.S. (1995). A potassium channel mutation in weaver mice implicates membrane excitability in granule cell differentiation. *Nat Genet* 11:126–129.

39. Navarro, B., Kennedy, M.E., Velimirovic, B., Bhat, D., Peterson, A.S., Clapham, D.E. (1996). Nonselective and $G_{\beta\gamma}$-insensitive weaver K^+ channels. *Science* 272: 1950–1953.

40. Tong, Y., Wei, J., Zhang, S., Strong, J.A., Dlouhy, S.R., Hodes, M.E., Ghetti, B., Yu, L. (1996). The weaver mutation changes the ion selectivity of the affected inwardly rectifying potassium channel GIRK2. *FEBS Lett* 390:63–68.

41. Rakic, P., Sidman, R.L. (1973). Weaver mutant mouse cerebellum: defective neuronal migration secondary to abnormality of Bergmann glia. *Proc Natl Acad Sci U S A* 70:240–244.

42. Triarhou, L.C., Norton, J., Ghetti, B. (1988). Mesencephalic dopamine cell deficit involves areas A8, A9 and A10 in weaver mutant mice. *Exp Brain Res* 70:256–265.

43. Kobayashi, T., Ikeda, K., Kojima, H., Niki, H., Yano, R., Yoshioka, T., Kumanishi, T. (1999). Ethanol opens G-protein-activated inwardly rectifying K^+ channels. *Nat Neurosci* 2:1091–1097.

44. Ikeda, K., Kobayashi, T., Kumanishi, T., Yano, R., Sora, I., Niki, H. (2002). Molecular mechanisms of analgesia induced by opioids and ethanol: is the GIRK channel one of the keys? *Neurosci Res* 44:121–131.

45. Blednov, Y.A., Stoffel, M., Alva, H., Harris, R.A. (2003). A pervasive mechanism for analgesia: activation of GIRK2 channels. *Proc Natl Acad Sci U S A* 100:277–282.

46. Marker, C.L., Cintora, S.C., Roman, M.I., Stoffel, M., Wickman, K. (2002). Hyperalgesia and blunted morphine analgesia in G protein-gated potassium channel subunit knockout mice. *Neuroreport* 13:2509–2513.

47. Mitrovic, I., Margeta-Mitrovic, M., Bader, S., Stoffel, M., Jan, L.Y., Basbaum, A.I. (2003). Contribution of GIRK2-mediated postsynaptic signaling to opiate and α_2-adrenergic analgesia and analgesic sex differences. *Proc Natl Acad Sci U S A* 100:271–276.

48. Takahashi, T., Kobayashi, T., Ozaki, M., Takamatsu, Y., Ogai, Y., Ohta, M., Yamamoto, H., Ikeda, K. (2006). G protein-activated inwardly rectifying K^+ channel inhibition and rescue of *weaver* mouse motor functions by antidepressants. *Neurosci Res* 54:104–111.
49. Smith, S.B., Marker, C.L., Perry, C., Liao, G., Sotocinal, S.G., Austin, J.S., Melmed, K., Clark, J.D., Peltz, G., Wickman, K., Mogil, J.S. (2008). Quantitative trait locus and computational mapping identifies *Kcnj9* (GIRK3) as a candidate gene affecting analgesia from multiple drug classes. *Pharmacogenet Genomics* 18:231–241.
50. Kobayashi, T., Ikeda, K. (2006). G protein-activated inwardly rectifying potassium channels as potential therapeutic targets. *Curr Pharm Des* 12:4513–4523.
51. Kobayashi, T., Washiyama, K., Ikeda, K. (2003). Inhibition of G protein-activated inwardly rectifying K^+ channels by fluoxetine (Prozac). *Br J Pharmacol* 138: 1119–1128.
52. Kobayashi, T., Washiyama, K., Ikeda, K. (2004). Inhibition of G protein-activated inwardly rectifying K^+ channels by various antidepressant drugs. *Neuropsychopharmacology* 29:1841–1851.
53. Kobayashi, T., Washiyama, K., Ikeda, K. (2004). Modulators of G protein-activated inwardly rectifying K^+ channels: potentially therapeutic agents for addictive drug users. *Ann N Y Acad Sci* 1025:590–594.
54. Kobayashi, T., Washiyama, K., Ikeda, K. (2006). Inhibition of G protein-activated inwardly rectifying K^+ channels by the antidepressant paroxetine. *J Pharmacol Sci* 102:278–287.
55. Kobayashi, T., Ikeda, K., Kumanishi, T. (1998). Effects of clozapine on the δ- and κ-opioid receptors and the G-protein-activated K^+ (GIRK) channel expressed in *Xenopus* oocytes. *Br J Pharmacol* 123:421–426.
56. Kobayashi, T., Ikeda, K., Kumanishi, T. (2000). Inhibition by various antipsychotic drugs of the G-protein-activated inwardly rectifying K^+ (GIRK) channels expressed in *Xenopus* oocytes. *Br J Pharmacol* 129:1716–1722.
57. Yamakura, T., Lewohl, J.M., Harris, R.A. (2001). Differential effects of general anesthetics on G protein-coupled inwardly rectifying and other potassium channels. *Anesthesiology* 95:144–153.
58. Weigl, L.G., Schreibmayer, W. (2001). G protein-gated inwardly rectifying potassium channels are targets for volatile anesthetics. *Mol Pharmacol* 60:282–289.
59. Zhou, W., Arrabit, C., Choe, S., Slesinger, P.A. (2001). Mechanism underlying bupivacaine inhibition of G protein-gated inwardly rectifying K^+ channels. *Proc Natl Acad Sci U S A* 98:6482–6487.
60. Lewohl, J.M., Wilson, W.R., Mayfield, R.D., Brozowski, S.J., Morrisett, R.A., Harris, R.A. (1999). G-protein-coupled inwardly rectifying potassium channels are targets of alcohol action. *Nat Neurosci* 2:1084–1090.
61. Jakob, R., Krieglstein, J. (1997). Influence of flupirtine on a G-protein coupled inwardly rectifying potassium current in hippocampal neurones. *Br J Pharmacol* 122:1333–1338.
62. Kelly, M.J., Rønnekleiv, O.K., Ibrahim, N., Lagrange, A.H., Wagner, E.J. (2002). Estrogen modulation of K^+ channel activity in hypothalamic neurons involved in the control of the reproductive axis. *Steroids* 67:447–456.
63. Zeidner, G., Sadja, R., Reuveny, E. (2001). Redox-dependent gating of G protein-coupled inwardly rectifying K^+ channels. *J Biol Chem* 276:35564–35570.

64. Nishizawa, D., Gajya, N., Ikeda, K. (forthcoming). Identification of selective agonists and antagonists to G protein-activated inwardly rectifying potassium channels: candidate medicines for drug dependence and pain. *Ann N Y Acad Sci* (in press).
65. Khodorova, A., Navarro, B., Jouaville, L.S., Murphy, J.E., Rice, F.L., Mazurkiewicz, J.E., Long-Woodward, D., Stoffel, M., Strichartz, G.R., Yukhananov, R., Davar, G. (2003). Endothelin-B receptor activation triggers an endogenous analgesic cascade at sites of peripheral injury. *Nat Med* 9:1055–1061.
66. Zanello, S.B., Jackson, D.M., Holick, M.F. (1999). An immunocytochemical approach to the study of β-endorphin production in human keratinocytes using confocal microscopy. *Ann N Y Acad Sci* 885:85–99.
67. Campbell, J.D., Sansom, M.S., Ashcroft, F.M. (2003). Potassium channel regulation. *EMBO Rep* 4:1038–1042.
68. Wada, Y., Yamashita, T., Imai, K., Miura, R., Takao, K., Nishi, M., Takeshima, H., Asano, T., Morishita, R., Nishizawa, K., Kokubun, S., Nukada, T. (2000). A region of the sulfonylurea receptor critical for a modulation of ATP-sensitive K^+ channels by G-protein βγ-subunits. *EMBO J* 19:4915–4925.
69. Ocaña, M., Baeyens, J.M. (1993). Differential effects of K^+ channel blockers on antinociception induced by α_2-adrenoceptor, $GABA_B$ and κ-opioid receptor agonists. *Br J Pharmacol* 110:1049–1054.
70. Kang, Y., Zhang, C., Qiao, J. (1997). Involvement of endogenous opioids and ATP-sensitive potassium channels in the mediation of carbachol-induced antinociception at the spinal level: a behavioral study in rats. *Brain Res* 761:342–346.
71. Asano, T., Dohi, S., Iida, H. (2000). Antinociceptive action of epidural K^+_{ATP} channel openers via interaction with morphine and an α_2-adrenergic agonist in rats. *Anesth Analg* 90:1146–1151.
72. Rodrigues, A.R., Duarte, I.D. (2000). The peripheral antinociceptive effect induced by morphine is associated with ATP-sensitive K^+ channels. *Br J Pharmacol* 129:110–114.
73. Raffa, R.B., Martinez, R.P. (1995). The "glibenclamide-shift" of centrally-acting antinociceptive agents in mice. *Brain Res* 677:277–282.
74. Yamazumi, I., Okuda, T., Koga, Y. (2001). Involvement of potassium channels in spinal antinociceptions induced by fentanyl, clonidine and bethanechol in rats. *Jpn J Pharmacol* 87:268–276.
75. Ocaña, M., Baeyens, J.M. (1994). Role of ATP-sensitive K^+ channels in antinociception induced by R-PIA, an adenosine A1 receptor agonist. *Naunyn Schmiedebergs Arch Pharmacol* 350:57–62.
76. Robles, L.I., Barrios, M., Del Pozo, E., Dordal, A., Baeyens, J.M. (1996). Effects of K^+ channel blockers and openers on antinociception induced by agonists of $5\text{-}HT_{1A}$ receptors. *Eur J Pharmacol* 295:181–188.
77. Ortiz, M.I., Torres-López, J.E., Castañeda-Hernández, G., Rosas, R., Vidal-Cantú, G.C., Granados-Soto, V. (2002). Pharmacological evidence for the activation of K^+ channels by diclofenac. *Eur J Pharmacol* 438:85–91.
78. Alves, D.P., Soares, A.C., Francischi, J.N., Castro, M.S., Perez, A.C., Duarte, I.D. (2004). Additive antinociceptive effect of the combination of diazoxide, an activator of ATP-sensitive K^+ channels, and sodium nitroprusside and dibutyryl-cGMP. *Eur J Pharmacol* 489:59–65.

79. Galeotti, N., Ghelardini, C., Bartolini, A. (2001). Involvement of potassium channels in amitriptyline and clomipramine analgesia. *Neuropharmacology* 40:75–84.

80. Galeotti, N., Ghelardini, C., Bartolini, A. (1999). The role of potassium channels in antihistamine analgesia. *Neuropharmacology* 38:1893–1901.

81. Mixcoatl-Zecuatl, T., Medina-Santillán, R., Reyes-García, G., Vidal-Cantú, G.C., Granados-Soto, V. (2004). Effect of K^+ channel modulators on the antiallodynic effect of gabapentin. *Eur J Pharmacol* 484:201–208.

82. Vit, J.P., Ohara, P.T., Bhargava, A., Kelley, K., Jasmin, L. (2008). Silencing the Kir4.1 potassium channel subunit in satellite glial cells of the rat trigeminal ganglion results in pain-like behavior in the absence of nerve injury. *J Neurosci* 28:4161–4171.

83. Galeotti, N., Ghelardini, C., Papucci, L., Capaccioli, S., Quattrone, A., Bartolini, A. (1997). An antisense oligonucleotide on the mouse Shaker-like potassium channel Kv1.1 gene prevents antinociception induced by morphine and baclofen. *J Pharmacol Exp Ther* 281:941–949.

84. Galeotti, N., Ghelardini, C., Vinci, M.C., Bartolini, A. (1999). Role of potassium channels in the antinociception induced by agonists of α_2-adrenoceptors. *Br J Pharmacol* 126:1214–1220.

85. Clark, J.D., Tempel, B.L. (1998). Hyperalgesia in mice lacking the Kv1.1 potassium channel gene. *Neurosci Lett* 251:121–124.

86. Galeotti, N., Ghelardini, C., Capaccioli, S., Quattrone, A., Nicolin, A., Bartolini, A. (1997). Blockade of clomipramine and amitriptyline analgesia by an antisense oligonucleotide to mKv1.1, a mouse Shaker-like K^+ channel. *Eur J Pharmacol* 330:15–25.

87. Finnegan, T.F., Chen, S.R., Pan, H.L. (2006). μ Opioid receptor activation inhibits GABAergic inputs to basolateral amygdala neurons through Kv1.1/1.2 channels. *J Neurophysiol* 95:2032–2041.

88. Hu, H.J., Carrasquillo, Y., Karim, F., Jung, W.E., Nerbonne, J.M., Schwarz, T.L., Gereau, R.W., 4th. (2006). The Kv4.2 potassium channel subunit is required for pain plasticity. *Neuron* 50:89–100.

89. Blackburn-Munro, G., Jensen, B.S. (2003). The anticonvulsant retigabine attenuates nociceptive behaviours in rat models of persistent and neuropathic pain. *Eur J Pharmacol* 460:109–116.

90. Passmore, G.M., Selyanko, A.A., Mistry, M., Al-Qatari, M., Marsh, S.J., Matthews, E.A., Dickenson, A.H., Brown, T.A., Burbidge, S.A., Main, M., Brown, D.A. (2003). KCNQ/M currents in sensory neurons: significance for pain therapy. *J Neurosci* 23:7227–7236.

91. Hirano, K., Kuratani, K., Fujiyoshi, M., Tashiro, N., Hayashi, E., Kinoshita, M. (2007). Kv7.2-7.5 voltage-gated potassium channel (KCNQ2-5) opener, retigabine, reduces capsaicin-induced visceral pain in mice. *Neurosci Lett* 413:159–162.

92. Welch, S.P., Dunlow, L.D. (1993). Antinociceptive activity of intrathecally administered potassium channel openers and opioid agonists: a common mechanism of action? *J Pharmacol Exp Ther* 267:390–399.

93. Welch, S.P., Thomas, C., Patrick, G.S. (1995). Modulation of cannabinoid-induced antinociception after intracerebroventricular versus intrathecal administration to

mice: possible mechanisms for interaction with morphine. *J Pharmacol Exp Ther* 272:310–321.

94. LoVerme, J., Russo, R., La Rana, G., Fu, J., Farthing, J., Mattace-Raso, G., Meli, R., Hohmann, A., Calignano, A., Piomelli, D. (2006). Rapid broad-spectrum analgesia through activation of peroxisome proliferator-activated receptor-α. *J Pharmacol Exp Ther* 319:1051–1061.
95. Medhurst, A.D., Rennie, G., Chapman, C.G., Meadows, H., Duckworth, M.D., Kelsell, R.E., Gloger, I.I., Pangalos, M.N. (2001). Distribution analysis of human two pore domain potassium channels in tissues of the central nervous system and periphery. *Mol Brain Res* 86:101–114.
96. Liu, C., Au, J.D., Zou, H.L., Cotton, J.F., Yost, C.S. (2004). Potent activation of the human tandem pore domain K channel TRESK with clinical concentrations of volatile anesthetics. *Anesth Analg* 99:1715–1722.
97. Patel, A.J., Honoré, E. (2001). Properties and modulation of mammalian 2P domain K^+ channels. *Trends Neurosci* 24:339–346.
98. Patel, A.J., Honoré, E., Lesage, F., Fink, M., Romey, G., Lazdunski, M. (1999). Inhalational anesthetics activate two-pore-domain background K^+ channels. *Nat Neurosci* 2:422–426.
99. Linden, A.M., Aller, M.I., Leppä, E., Vekovischeva, O., Aitta-Aho, T., Veale, E.L., Mathie, A., Rosenberg, P., Wisden, W., Korpi, E.R. (2006). The in vivo contributions of TASK-1-containing channels to the actions of inhalation anesthetics, the α_2 adrenergic sedative dexmedetomidine, and cannabinoid agonists. *J Pharmacol Exp Ther* 317:615–626.
100. Linden, A.M., Sandu, C., Aller, M.I., Vekovischeva, O.Y., Rosenberg, P.H., Wisden, W., Korpi, E.R. (2007). TASK-3 knockout mice exhibit exaggerated nocturnal activity, impairments in cognitive functions, and reduced sensitivity to inhalation anesthetics. *J Pharmacol Exp Ther* 323:924–934.
101. Alloui, A., Zimmermann, K., Mamet, J., Duprat, F., Noël, J., Chemin, J., Guy, N., Blondeau, N., Voilley, N., Rubat-Coudert, C., Borsotto, M., Romey, G., Heurteaux, C., Reeh, P., Eschalier, A., Lazdunski, M. (2006). TREK-1, a K^+ channel involved in polymodal pain perception. *EMBO J* 25:2368–2376.
102. Honoré, E. (2007). The neuronal background K_{2P} channels: focus on TREK1. *Nat Rev Neurosci* 8:251–261.

CHAPTER 5

Voltage-Gated Calcium Channels as Targets for the Treatment of Chronic Pain

JOSEPH G. McGIVERN

Amgen Inc.

Content

5.1 OVERVIEW

Multiple subtypes of voltage-gated Ca^{2+} channels exist, but several lines of evidence suggest that it is primarily the N-type and T-type Ca^{2+} channels that play important roles in the process of nociception, especially under conditions of chronic pain. The powerful analgesic effects of intrathecal ziconotide in humans provide the most convincing evidence for the validation of the N-type Ca^{2+} channel as an analgesic target. Compared with other analgesic drugs, ziconotide has a unique molecular mechanism of action that involves potent and selective block of N-type channels. These channels are found in presynaptic nerve terminals, where they govern the Ca^{2+} influx that is required to trigger neurotransmitter release. The efficacy of ziconotide likely results from

Peripheral Receptor Targets for Analgesia: Novel Approaches to Pain Management, Edited by Brian E. Cairns

its ability to interrupt pain signaling by reducing the release of pronociceptive neurotransmitters in the spinal cord, but it is fair to say that its precise analgesic mechanism has not been proven. In contrast, the involvement of T-type channels in sensory processing is an emerging story. T-type Ca^{2+} channels are found mainly in postsynaptic dendrites, where they contribute to the integration of synaptic inputs, and in neuronal cell bodies, where they regulate membrane excitability and action potential firing patterns. No potent and selective blockers of T-type channels are available for testing in pharmacology experiments, and so, it is only recently that they have begun to receive attention as potential targets for treating pain. Currently, the strongest evidence for their validation as analgesic targets comes from antisense oligonucleotide experiments and gene knockout approaches in animals. It will be exciting to learn if selective blockers of T-type Ca^{2+} channels will prove to be efficacious and safe analgesic drugs in patients.

5.2 INTRODUCTION

Ca^{2+} is a ubiquitous signaling element that activates a wide range of physiological processes in virtually all cell types, including neurons [1]. Under normal resting conditions, the cytoplasmic concentration of Ca^{2+} in neurons is maintained within a very narrow range (10–100nM), but it can increase rapidly during neuronal activity as a result of Ca^{2+} influx from the extracellular space or Ca^{2+} release from intracellular stores. Ca^{2+} usually enters neurons through ion channels, which are highly specialized transport proteins found in the plasma membrane. The passage of positively charged ions across the neuronal cell membrane can exert a depolarizing influence on the membrane, which in turn may lead to the activation of voltage-gated ion channels, including Na^+ and K^+ channels. Thus, Ca^{2+} entering a neuron can directly modulate membrane excitability and promote potential generation and propagation. In addition, Ca^{2+} can function as a second messenger that triggers a multitude of downstream signaling processes by binding to and activating effector proteins, such as Ca^{2+}-gated ion channels, enzymes, and other Ca^{2+}-sensing proteins, for example, calmodulin. Of particular note, increased cytoplasmic Ca^{2+} in presynaptic nerve terminals can evoke the release of neurotransmitters. Consistent with the neurophysiological roles of Ca^{2+}, dysregulation of Ca^{2+} signaling in neurons can lead to unusual electrical activity, abnormal neurotransmission, and even altered gene transcription in certain pathological states.

5.3 VOLTAGE-GATED CALCIUM CHANNEL STRUCTURE AND DIVERSITY

Ca^{2+} channels form a large diverse family, whose members can be classified broadly as either voltage-gated, that is, activated by changes in membrane potential [2], or ligand-gated, that is, activated by the binding of a chemical substance, such as a neurotransmitter [3]. Voltage-gated Ca^{2+} channels are widely expressed in peripheral and central neurons. Multiple subtypes exist, and these can be categorized on the basis of their molecular, structural, and functional characteristics (Table 5.1). Most voltage-gated Ca^{2+} channels appear to be multi-subunit protein complexes that contain a large (>2000 amino acids) pore-forming α_1-subunit in association with smaller auxiliary $\alpha_2\delta$-, β-, and, in some cases, γ-subunits [4,5]. Extensive structural diversity among Ca^{2+} channels arises from the large number of possible combinations of pore-forming and auxiliary subunits. Ten membrane-spanning α_1-subunits (termed $Ca_V1.1$–1.4, $Ca_V2.1$–2.3, and $Ca_V3.1$–3.3) have been identified, and these are believed to underlie all native Ca^{2+} currents. In addition, four $\alpha_2\delta$-subunits, four β-subunits, and eight γ-subunits have been identified. These auxiliary subunits are either cytosolic (β) or membrane-spanning ($\alpha_2\delta$ and γ) proteins that serve to fine-tune the biophysical properties of the channel and modulate its trafficking to the membrane. Although the genes that encode the Ca^{2+} channel subunits are the primary source of the molecular diversity within the family, alternative splicing of messenger RNA (mRNA) transcripts enhances this diversity significantly. Splice variants often display unique biophysical properties and can be expressed in a tissue-specific way, suggesting that cells can tailor their ion channel expression to match the physiological functions that they need to perform. All known voltage-gated Ca^{2+} channels are activated by membrane depolarization, although the various subtypes often operate over distinct ranges of membrane potential. For instance, Ca^{2+} channels can be described either as high-voltage activated (HVA), that is, L-, N-, P/Q-, and R-types, or as low-voltage activated (LVA), that is, T-type.

The α_1-subunit is the most important subunit of a voltage-gated Ca^{2+} channel as it forms the ion permeation pathway and defines the majority of the channel's biophysical properties [4,5]. It also contains the binding sites for most pharmacological agents, including channel blockers and activators. The α_1-subunit is a membrane-spanning protein with intracellular N- and C-termini. It comprises four homologous domains (DI through DIV) that are connected sequentially by intracellular loops. Each domain is analogous to one α-subunit of the prototypic tetrameric delayed rectifier subtypes of K^+ channel, that is, the *Shaker*-, *Shab*-, *Shaw*-, and *Shal*-related families. Within each domain, there are six transmembrane α-helical segments (S1 through S6) that are connected in series by short extracellular and intracellular loops. These α-helices not only serve to anchor the α_1-subunit in the membrane but also contain many of the structural elements that determine the channel's functional properties. For instance, the S5 and S6 α-helices are believed to line the pore of the channel, whereas the S4 α-helices appear to function as the channel's voltage sensor. The S4 α-helices can move in response to changes in the transmembrane electric field and, as they are coupled to S5 and S6, their movement can induce conformational changes in the structure of the channel causing the pore to open. Some of the loops that connect the α-helices also contribute to the

TABLE 5.1. Summary of Ca^{2+} Channel Diversity, Expression, and Pharmacology.

α_1-Subunit	Classification	Associated Auxiliary Subunits	Expression	Pharmacology (Blockers)
$Ca_v1.1$ (α_{1S})	L-type (HVA)	$\alpha_2\delta$, β, and γ	Skeletal muscle cells	Dihydropyridines, e.g., nitrendipine Phenylalkylamines, e.g., verapamil Benzothiazepines, e.g., diltiazem Divalent cations, e.g., Cd^{2+}
$Ca_v1.2$ (α_{1C})			Cardiac myocytes, neurons, endocrine cells	
$Ca_v1.3$ (α_{1D})			Neurons, cardiac myocytes, pancreatic β-cells	
$Ca_v1.4$ (α_{1F})			Retinal cells	
$Ca_v2.1$ (α_{1A})	P/Q-type (HVA)	$\alpha_2\delta$ and β	Neurons, pancreatic β-cells	ω-conotoxin MVIIC ω-agatoxin IVA Gabapentin/ pregabalin?
$Ca_v2.2$ (α_{1B})	N-type (HVA)		Neurons, pancreatic β-cells	ω-conotoxins, e.g., ω-MVIIA, ω-GVIA, ω-CVID Gabapentin/ pregabalin?
$Ca_v2.3$ (α_{1E})	R-type (HVA)		Neurons, endocrine cells	SNX-482 (from tarantula venom)
$Ca_v3.1$ (α_{1G})	T-type (LVA)	?	Neurons, cardiac myocytes, smooth muscle cells, endocrine cells	Ethosuximide Zonisamide Mibefradil Divalent cations, e.g., Ni^{2+}
$Ca_v3.2$ (α_{1H})			Cardiac myocytes, kidney cells, neurons, smooth muscle cells, endocrine cells	
$Ca_v3.3$ (α_{1I})			Neurons	

channel's properties. Unlike the loops that connect the other α-helices, the extracellular loops that connect S5 and S6 in each domain actually reenter (but do not traverse) the cell membrane. These so-called pore loops (P-loops) are believed to control the ionic selectivity and permeation characteristics of the channel. They do this by cooperating to form a putative ringlike structure within the lumen of the pore. This structure is believed to comprise four negatively charged amino acids (one contributed per P-loop) [6]. In HVA Ca^{2+} channels, each P-loop contributes a glutamate (E) residue, leading to the formation of an EEEE motif, whereas in LVA Ca^{2+} channels, the E residues from the third and fourth P-loops are replaced with aspartate (D) residues to form an EEDD motif. These motifs serve to bind and release Ca^{2+} during the permeation process. Finally, the inactivation of voltage-gated Ca^{2+} channels is believed to proceed via a hinged-lid mechanism, with the inactivation gate formed by the relatively long intracellular loop that connects DI and DII. Interestingly, the DI–DII loop is also important for the interaction between the α_1- and β-subunits, which provides a mechanism to explain how β-subunits can alter Ca^{2+} channel gating [7].

The Ca^{2+} channel α_1-subunit requires the lipid environment of the plasma membrane to maintain a native functional structure. Due to technical challenges, it is very difficult to obtain large quantities of membrane proteins, such as the pore-forming subunits of most ion channels, for crystallization purposes. Thus, there have been no reports so far describing the three-dimensional structure of a Ca^{2+} channel α_1-subunit. However, the tertiary structure of the Ca^{2+} channel α_1-subunit is presumed to be generally similar to the structure of other voltage-gated ion channels such as the tetrameric K^+ channel $K_V1.2$, which has been crystallized in its open state [8,9]. Thus, a functional Ca^{2+} channel likely involves a circular arrangement of the four domains, with the ion-conducting pathway located in the center. Also, the exact spatial arrangement of the α_1-, $\alpha_2\delta$-, β-, and γ-subunits within the channel complex remains unclear, even though protein–protein interaction domains have been identified in some Ca^{2+} channel subunits.

For the purposes of this chapter, the voltage-gated Ca^{2+} channels that are most relevant to the process of nociception are the N-type and T-type channels [10,11]. It has been suggested that the P-type [12,13] and R-type Ca^{2+} channels [14,15] also play roles in pain processing under certain circumstances, but at this time, the data are considered to be inadequate for validation of these channels as analgesic targets in humans.

5.4 N-TYPE CALCIUM CHANNEL

The N-type Ca^{2+} channel belongs to the HVA class of channels (Table 5.1) and is characterized by a slow inactivation process and sensitivity to inhibition by ω-conotoxins that have been isolated from the venoms of various marine cone snails. The N-type channel is expressed almost exclusively in neurons and is found throughout the peripheral and central nervous systems. It exists as a protein complex containing the $Ca_V2.2$ (α_{1B}) subtype of α_1-subunit in association with $\alpha_2\delta$- and β-subunits. Immunohistochemical studies with specific antibodies [16] and autoradiographic studies with selective peptides [17] have revealed that the N-type channel is expressed at high density in presynaptic nerve terminals, where it tends to be associated with intracellular proteins that are involved in exocytotic neurotransmitter release [18]. In the dorsal horn of the spinal cord, the N-type channel is colocalized with substance P and displays its highest expression in the superficial laminae where the afferent fibers of primary sensory neurons terminate [19].

Peripheral nerve injury can induce changes in the expression of multiple ion channel genes [20]. These changes are often associated with increased membrane excitability of both primary and secondary sensory neurons and with development of behavioral signs of pain in animals. For instance, $Ca_V2.2$ immunoreactivity is increased in the dorsal horn of the spinal cord, particularly in lamina II, following loose ligation of the sciatic nerve, and this is correlated with the development of mechanical and cold allodynia [21]. Upregulation of $Ca_V2.2$ at the level of the spinal cord may explain the increased potency of N-type channel blockers in reducing membrane responses of dorsal horn neurons to electrical, mechanical, and thermal stimuli following spinal nerve ligation (SNL) in rats [12]. However, depending on the specific neuron tested and the nerve injury paradigm, N-type Ca^{2+} currents at the level of the dorsal root ganglia (DRG) neuronal soma may be either increased [22] or reduced in amplitude [23]. Unfortunately, it is difficult to determine using electrophysiological methods how the expression of functional N-type Ca^{2+} channels might have changed at the level of the presynaptic nerve terminals in the spinal cord.

The $Ca_V2.2$ subunit is subject to alternative splicing. Of particular relevance to nociceptive processing in primary sensory neurons, there are two equal length versions of exon 37, namely 37a and 37b, which yield Ca^{2+} channel α_1-subunit proteins that differ by 14 amino acids in the C-terminus [24]. These exon variants appear to be expressed in a mutually exclusive manner in neuronal tissue. Although exon 37b is the most widely expressed variant in the nervous system, exon 37a appears to be highly enriched in capsaicin-responsive, $Na_V1.8$-containing neurons of rat DRG. It is unclear if this splice variant is also present in human N-type Ca^{2+} channels. When compared with capsaicin-insensitive neurons, it appears that larger Ca^{2+} currents can be recorded in capsaicin-responsive neurons, which presumably express exon 37a. This mechanism may permit greater Ca^{2+} influx during action potentials and lead to increased neurotransmitter release from these neurons. It is conceivable that this mechanism could facilitate the transmission of painful sensory information and possibly increase the analgesic potency of N-type channel blockers. Exon 37a appears to be required for acute thermal and mechanical nociception and for the development of thermal and mechanical hyperalgesia following tissue and nerve injury in animals [25]. Interestingly, the expression of mRNA sequences containing exon 37a appears to be downregulated by

~50% following nerve injury, suggesting that sensory neurons might be able to tailor the expression of N-type Ca^{2+} channel variants according to the specific type of painful information they need to transmit. It is tempting to speculate that Ca^{2+} channel blockers that selectively target exon 37a-containing channels might be able to provide analgesia with an excellent safety profile. However, this particular approach is considered unlikely to succeed because exon 37 is located at the C-terminus where few, if any, Ca^{2+} channel blockers bind. Nevertheless, the existence of other nociceptor-specific splice variants may provide opportunities for the discovery of selective N-type Ca^{2+} channel blockers that could be used to elucidate the influence of Ca^{2+} channel variants on the process of nociception and to pave the way potentially for the identification of novel analgesic drugs [26].

Lending support to the notion that N-type channels are critical components of nociceptive signaling, $Ca_V2.2$ knockout mice are resistant to the development of chronic pain-associated behavioral phenomena, such as allodynia and hyperalgesia [27,28]. There is also an abundance of preclinical and clinical pharmacological evidence supporting a role of N-type Ca^{2+} channels in pain signal processing. The most valuable data come from studies that have been conducted with ω-conotoxins, for example, ω-MVIIA, ω-GVIA, and ω-CVID, which are selective peptide blockers of N-type Ca^{2+} channels [29]. Ziconotide (SNX-111) is a synthetic version of ω-MVIIA that is found in the venom of the species *Conus magus*. Ziconotide comprises 25 amino acids, six of which are cysteine residues that are linked in pairs by three disulfide bonds [30]. The pharmacology of ziconotide has been reviewed recently [31]. Briefly, radioligand-binding experiments have revealed that ziconotide binds rapidly, reversibly, and with high affinity (1–18 pM) to N-type Ca^{2+} channels [32–35]. Voltage-clamp experiments have revealed that it is a potent and selective inhibitor of N-type Ca^{2+} currents in cells that express either native or recombinant channels [36–39]. The molecular mechanism of action of ziconotide (and the other ω-conotoxins) appears to involve inhibition of Ca^{2+} flux by direct occlusion of the channel's pore.

Consistent with the critical role of N-type Ca^{2+} channels in controlling synaptic transmission, ziconotide and other ω-conotoxins inhibit depolarization-evoked release of neurotransmitters and neuromodulators *in vitro* [25,40–43]. Electrophysiology experiments have demonstrated that ω-conotoxins can also reduce excitatory neurotransmission in spinal cord slices *in vitro* [44] and inhibit formalin-induced windup in the spinal cord *in vivo* [12]. Windup is an electrophysiological phenomenon whereby dorsal horn neurons display facilitated responses following high intensity C-fiber discharging. It is dependent on the activation of the *N*-methyl-D-aspartate subtype of glutamate receptor and is believed to be a correlate of the central sensitization that is associated with hypersensitivity to pain in many chronic pain conditions.

Ziconotide can induce long-lasting inhibition of behavioral responses in multiple animal models of persistent and chronic pain (Table 5.2). In general, ziconotide tends to be more potent than morphine, and its efficacy is not

TABLE 5.2. Antinociceptive and Analgesic Effects of Ca^{2+} Channel Blockers.

Drug	Animal Models	Human Conditions Treated
Ziconotide	Hot plate (52.5 °C) [45,46,48] Paw pressure [48] Tail immersion (50 °C water) [48] Formalin (phases 1 and 2) [45–48] Carrageenan (heat hyperalgesia) [49] CFA (heat hyperalgesia) [43] Paw incision [53] SNL (L5/L6) (mechanical allodynia) [47,50,51] Sciatic nerve CCI (heat hyperalgesia) [52] Partial sciatic nerve injury (heat hyperalgesia) [52]	Intractable severe pain due to cancer or AIDS [54] Intractable nonmalignant severe chronic pain [55] Intractable severe chronic pain [56] Postoperative pain [57] Intractable deafferentation pain [58] General neuropathic pain [59,60]
Gabapentin/ pregabalin	Formalin (phase 2) [77] Carrageenan (heat hyperalgesia) [77] Sciatic nerve CCI (cold allodynia) [78,80] Infraorbital nerve CCI (mechanical allodynia) [79] SNL (L5/L6) (tactile allodynia) [78,80] Streptozotocin-induced peripheral neuropathy (mechanical allodynia) [80]	Postherpetic neuralgia [65,71] Diabetic neuropathy [66,72–74] Trigeminal neuralgia [67,75] Neuropathic pain due to spinal cord injury [68] Cancer pain [69] Intermittent claudication due to lumbar spinal stenosis [70] Fibromyalgia [76]
Ethosuximide	Thermal nociception [152] Formalin (phases 1 and 2) [133] Carrageenan (heat hyperalgesia) [133] Sciatic nerve CCI (cold allodynia) [133] SNL (L5/L6) (tactile allodynia) [133] Paclitaxel- or vincristine-induced peripheral neuropathy (cold allodynia, mechanical allodynia and mechanical hyperalgesia.) [135]	Migraine pain [136]
Zonisamide	Formalin test (phase 2) [140] Sciatic nerve CCI (heat hyperalgesia) [141] Streptozotocin-induced peripheral neuropathy (mechanical allodynia) [140]	Migraine pain [142] Poststroke pain [143]
Mibefradil	Formalin (phases 1 and 2) [151] SNL (L5/L6) (tactile allodynia and heat hyperalgesia) [134]	No longer used clinically

limited by the development of tolerance. Spinally administered ziconotide (bolus or continuous infusion) inhibits behavioral responses in both the early and late phases of the formalin model [45–48], which is consistent with the *in vivo* electrophysiology findings mentioned earlier. Ziconotide is particularly efficacious in models of inflammatory and neuropathic pain. It prevents and reverses thermal hyperalgesia caused by injection of carrageenan [49] or complete Freund's adjuvant (CFA) [43] into the knee or paw. In addition, ziconotide reverses mechanical allodynia and thermal hyperalgesia following SNL [47,50,51] or chronic constriction injury (CCI) of the sciatic nerve [52]. Ziconotide also displays efficacy in a paw incision model that involves tissue injury [53].

By far, the most compelling evidence for a critical role of N-type Ca^{2+} channels in pain signal processing comes from the powerful analgesic effects of ziconotide (Prialt®, Elan Corporation, plc, Dublin, Ireland) in humans (Table 5.2). Due to its large size and hydrophilic nature, ziconotide cannot easily cross the blood-brain barrier. Therefore, due to the spinal localization of the Ca^{2+} channel target, it is necessary to administer ziconotide intrathecally using an implanted pump in order to provide effective analgesia to patients. The intrathecal route of delivery increases the probability that ziconotide will reach its site of action rapidly and also reduces the rate of clearance by metabolism and excretion. Intrathecal infusion of ziconotide is an approved approach in many countries for the treatment of severe chronic pain that is refractory to treatment with opioid drugs, such as morphine. The approval of this approach followed the completion of three large placebo-controlled phase 3 clinical trials, as well as several smaller open-label trials, that demonstrated prolonged analgesic efficacy and good safety of the drug in more than 600 patients [54–60]. These patients were experiencing pain that could be categorized in a number of ways, for example, due to nerve injury, cancer, AIDS, or major surgery. The use of an implanted continuous infusion device allows the dose of ziconotide to be controlled by the patient in order to achieve an acceptable balance of efficacy and side effects. Ziconotide infusion-induced analgesia is usually dose dependent, and many patients achieve moderate-to-complete pain relief. However, despite the use of an intrathecal infusion pump, the local concentration of ziconotide near the central nerve terminals of the primary sensory neurons is difficult to predict and control. The most common side effects that were observed during the clinical trials included postural hypotension, sedation, dizziness, nystagmus, and nausea. The side effects of ziconotide are also dose dependent, but their severity can be reduced by lowering the dose of drug.

In summary, owing to the potent analgesic effects of ziconotide in patients, the N-type Ca^{2+} channel is considered to be a validated analgesic target in humans. Nevertheless, there remains a significant opportunity to identify N-type Ca^{2+} channel blocking agents that offer the potential for improved safety, tolerability, and ease of use. For instance, it is not feasible for every patient with intractable severe chronic pain to accept an intrathecal infusion pump, so a more conveniently administered drug could greatly enlarge the pool of treatable patients. Even if it were possible to achieve spinally mediated analgesia with a parenterally administered N-type Ca^{2+} channel blocking peptide, rapid enzymatic degradation of the drug would be expected to reduce its stability in plasma and shorten its half-life. Although certain modifications to such a peptide could help to slow its elimination and increase its bioavailability [61], it seems more likely that a small molecule agent will overcome the dosing limitations of ziconotide. Several pharmaceutical and biotechnology companies are pursuing this approach and at least one experimental drug (NMED-160, also known as MK-6721) had advanced to phase 2 clinical testing [62,63]. However, although this molecule appeared to be safe and well tolerated, its development was terminated due to undisclosed issues with its pharmaceutical characteristics.

5.5 CALCIUM CHANNEL AUXILIARY SUBUNITS

With the notable exception of the so-called Ca^{2+} channel $\alpha_2\delta$ ligands, all known Ca^{2+} channel modulators exert their effects by binding to the α_1-subunit. The Ca^{2+} channel $\alpha_2\delta$ ligands are a group of analgesic and antiepileptic drugs, including gabapentin (Neurontin®, Pfizer Inc., New York, NY) and pregabalin (Lyrica®, Pfizer Inc.) [64]. Both drugs are analgesic in patients with a variety of chronic neuropathic pain syndromes (Table 5.2). Gabapentin has demonstrated clinical efficacy in the treatment of postherpetic neuralgia [65], diabetic peripheral neuropathy [66], trigeminal neuralgia [67], neuropathic pain due to spinal cord injury [68], cancer-related neuropathic pain [69], and intermittent claudication due to lumbar spinal stenosis [70]. It is approved in the United States for the treatment of postherpetic neuralgia and throughout Europe for the treatment of peripheral neuropathic pain. Worldwide, it is often prescribed off-label for the management of general neuropathic pain syndromes. Gabapentin dosing must often be titrated to high levels in search of adequate pain control, and even though it is a safe drug, pain relief is often suboptimal. Pregabalin is a newer $\alpha_2\delta$ ligand that has improved potency and superior bioavailability compared with gabapentin. In a variety of clinical situations, pregabalin is effective against pain associated with postherpetic neuralgia [71], diabetic peripheral neuropathy [72–74], trigeminal neuralgia [75], and fibromyalgia [76]. Pregabalin has been approved in many countries for the treatment of diabetic peripheral neuropathy and postherpetic neuralgia.

Gabapentin and pregabalin are antinociceptive in various animal models of inflammatory and neuropathic pain (Table 5.2) [77–80]. They share a common molecular mechanism of action that involves high-affinity binding (13–38 nM) to the $\alpha_2\delta_1$-subunit of HVA Ca^{2+} channels [81–83]. Under certain conditions, drug binding to the $\alpha_2\delta_1$-subunit may lead to inhibition of presynaptic Ca^{2+} currents [84–89] and to reduced neurotransmitter release [90]. The $\alpha_2\delta_1$-subunit appears to be essential for the analgesic actions of the Ca^{2+} channel $\alpha_2\delta$ ligands. A significant reduction in the binding of [^{3}H]-pregabalin in the brain and spinal cord is associated with a loss of the drug's analgesic efficacy in $\alpha_2\delta_1$ mutant mice [82]. Conversely, a variety of methods, including *in situ* hybridization, reverse transcriptase-polymerase chain reaction, Western blotting, and [^{3}H]-pregabalin binding, have revealed that peripheral nerve injury induces upregulation of the $\alpha_2\delta_1$-subunit in primary sensory neurons and in the dorsal horn of the spinal cord [91–94]. The upregulation of $\alpha_2\delta_1$ is associated with increased gabapentin sensitivity following SNL- and streptozotocin-induced peripheral neuropathy [80]. In transgenic mice that have been engineered to overexpress the $\alpha_2\delta_1$-subunit, the electrophysiological responses of dorsal horn neurons to mechanical and thermal stimulation are facilitated, as are some pain-related animal behaviors [95]. Furthermore, the HVA Ca^{2+} current in sensory neurons from these transgenic mice is increased in amplitude and is sensitive to inhibition by gabapentin (IC_{50} 2 μM), which is unlike the current in neurons taken from wild-type mice. In summary, the analgesic mechanism of action of the Ca^{2+} channel $\alpha_2\delta$ ligands remains incompletely understood, but it may involve decreased pronociceptive synaptic transmission in the brain and superficial layers of the dorsal horn in the spinal cord [90,96–98].

5.6 T-TYPE CALCIUM CHANNELS

The family of T-type Ca^{2+} channels belongs to the LVA class and is characterized by a rapid inactivation process. Three Ca^{2+} channel α_1-subunits, that is, α_{1G}, α_{1H}, and α_{1I} (or $Ca_V3.1$–3.3, respectively) produce T-type-like currents when expressed in mammalian cells and *Xenopus laevis* oocytes (Table 5.1) [99–101]. The three Ca_V3 subtypes can be distinguished on the basis of their biophysical and pharmacological properties. For instance, $Ca_V3.1$ and $Ca_V3.2$ both have faster activation and inactivation kinetics than $Ca_V3.3$, but can be distinguished from each other on the basis of the higher sensitivity of $Ca_V3.2$ to block by Ni^{2+} [102]. Even though auxiliary subunits can modulate the functional properties of the Ca_V3 subunits in mammalian expression systems, it remains unclear if native T-type channels exist as multi-subunit protein complexes [103–105].

T-type Ca^{2+} currents have been recorded from many cell types, including peripheral neurons [106,107] and central (spinal cord and brain) neurons [108,109]. Activation of neuronal T-type channels can lead to complex effects on neuronal membrane excitability and action potential firing patterns. The unique biophysical properties of T-type Ca^{2+} channels underlie their contributions to neurophysiology, particularly the switch between phasic and tonic firing modes in primary sensory and thalamic neurons [110,111]. T-type channels are activated by small membrane depolarizations, and under voltage-clamp conditions, they inactivate rapidly and give rise to transient Ca^{2+} currents. Due to their negative voltage dependence of inactivation, the majority of T-type channels is unavailable for opening at membrane potentials that are more depolarized than −70 mV, which is close to the resting membrane potential of a typical neuron. When a neuron is resting or in a depolarized state and the T-type channels are inactivated, it is more likely to respond to excitatory inputs by firing a series of regularly spaced single action potentials. In order for T-type Ca^{2+} channels to become available for opening, their inactivation must be removed by membrane hyperpolarization, which is often accomplished in neurons by the activation of K^+ or Cl^- channels, perhaps as a result of inhibitory synaptic input. When the T-type channels are opened by subsequent membrane depolarization, the resulting Ca^{2+} influx can generate a low-threshold Ca^{2+} spike (LTS). The LTS is a prolonged membrane depolarization that can facilitate the activation of higher-threshold voltage-gated ion channels, such as Na^+ and K^+ channels. Under these conditions, the neuron is more likely to respond to excitation with a high-frequency burst of action potentials. Burst firing usually terminates as a consequence of T-type channel inactivation along with activation of voltage-gated and Ca^{2+}-gated K^+ channels. The subsequent flow of repolarizing current through these channels may cause the neuronal membrane to hyperpolarize, thereby allowing the T-type channels to recover from inactivation and become available again for opening. In the neuronal circuits that exist in the thalamus, activity in reciprocally connected excitatory (relay nuclei) and inhibitory (reticular nucleus) neurons can promote the development of electrical oscillations. The presence of burst firing and oscillatory behavior in neuronal circuits can alter the input–output relationships on sensory pathways, including the pain pathway.

Most neurons express multiple Ca^{2+} channels [112], but the distribution of the various subtypes throughout the neuronal membrane is often nonoverlapping. Unlike the N-type Ca^{2+} channel, which is found primarily on presynaptic nerve terminals, T-type Ca^{2+} channels are expressed preferentially on dendrites and cell bodies, where they are postulated to play important roles in the integration of synaptic inputs as well as the regulation of membrane excitability and action potential firing patterns. *In situ* hybridization and immunohistochemical approaches have shown that $Ca_V3.1$ is the predominant subtype in the brain, although $Ca_V3.2$ and $Ca_V3.3$ are also expressed there [113,114]. Along the pain pathway, $Ca_V3.1$ is found in neurons of the spinal cord and the thalamic relay nuclei, whereas $Ca_V3.2$ is expressed by a subset of primary sensory neurons in the DRG and in neurons of the thalamic reticular nucleus. The $Ca_V3.3$ subunit appears to be localized almost exclusively in neurons, including those of the thalamic reticular nucleus. Unfortunately, very little is known at this time about the expression or the roles of T-type Ca^{2+} channel splice variants in the pain pathway [26]. Consistent with the distribution of $Ca_V3.1$, $Ca_V3.2$, and $Ca_V3.3$ mRNA and protein, T-type Ca^{2+} currents have been recorded from neurons of the DRG and spinal cord as well as from neurons of the thalamic relay and reticular nuclei [106–109]. Of relevance to sensory information processing, T-type Ca^{2+} channels are also expressed in the receptive fields of peripheral sensory neurons, where they may play a role in initiating the process of nociception [115]. When injected into peripheral receptive fields *in vivo*, reducing agents such as the endogenous amino acid L-cysteine can induce thermal hyperalgesia and mechanical sensitivity. Interestingly, T-type Ca^{2+} channels in DRG neurons are subject to tonic block by Zn^{2+}, which appears to bind to extracellular histidine residues of the channel [116]. Reducing agents and Zn^{2+} chelators can remove the bound Zn^{2+} and increase the amplitude of $Ca_V3.2$-mediated currents, which appears to be the major subtype underlying T-type currents in DRG neurons [117]. This action appears to sensitize nociceptors and to lower their threshold for activation.

The amplitude of T-type Ca^{2+} currents in primary sensory neurons may be altered in conditions associated with nerve injury [22,118–121]. However, the magnitude and direction of effect appear to be variable, perhaps reflecting differences in the severity of the nerve injury and/or the specific neurons examined. For instance, it has been suggested that the amplitude of T-type Ca^{2+} currents in nodose ganglion neurons is increased following transection of the vagus nerve, and that the resulting enhancement in Ca^{2+} influx could contribute to increased activity of Ca^{2+}-gated Cl^- channels along with depolarizing after-potentials. In contrast, other reports suggest that T-type Ca^{2+} currents in DRG neurons can be reduced in amplitude or eliminated following sciatic nerve transection or ligation. Paradoxically, reduced Ca^{2+} influx could lead to less activation of Ca^{2+}-gated K^+ channels, along with action potential prolongation and increased neuronal membrane excitability [121]. The changes in the expression of T-type Ca^{2+} channels in the neuronal soma would be expected to impact the overall excitability and action potential firing properties of the neuron. However, due to technical challenges it is difficult to elucidate what might be happening to the number of channels at other neuronal sites, such as the peripheral receptive fields and dendrites. Consequently, these studies have shed little light on the possible effects of nerve injury on the contribution of T-type Ca^{2+} channels to pain signal initiation and synaptic integration along the pain pathway.

Studies using subtype-specific antisense oligonucleotides and gene knockout approaches have revealed that the $Ca_V3.2$ channel is a major contributor to the process of nociception under normal (acute pain) and nerve injury (chronic pain) conditions [122,123]. Intrathecally administered anti-$Ca_V3.2$ antisense oligonucleotides caused a reduction in the expression of $Ca_V3.2$ mRNA and protein, as well as a large reduction in the amplitude of fast, Ni^{2+}-sensitive T-type ($Ca_V3.2$-like) currents in small- and medium-sized DRG neurons. In normal rats, anti-$Ca_V3.2$ antisense oligonucleotides exerted long-lasting (up to 4 days) antinociceptive effects, as evidenced by reduced vocalization responses to pressure applied to the paw. When compared with untreated or missense-treated animals, animals that had been treated with anti-$Ca_V3.2$ antisense oligonucleotides exhibited less tactile allodynia and mechanical hyperalgesia in the CCI model of neuropathic pain. The antinociceptive effects of anti-$Ca_V3.2$ antisense oligonucleotides in tests of acute pain are consistent with the results from behavioral studies using $Ca_V3.2$ knockout mice [124]. However, the $Ca_V3.2$ knockout mice developed behavioral signs of neuropathic pain in the SNL model, possibly suggesting that compensatory changes in the expression of other ion channels might have occurred in the pain pathway. Overall, the available evidence suggests that $Ca_V3.2$ channels normally perform pronociceptive functions at the level of the DRG and that $Ca_V3.2$-selective blockers might be able to exert antinociceptive effects *in vivo*. In contrast, $Ca_V3.1$ knockout mice displayed hyperalgesic responses in a model of visceral pain [125]. Interestingly, this hyperalgesia appears to be associated with reduced burst firing in thalamocortical relay neurons. Consistent with these observations, infusion of mibefradil (a nonselective T-type Ca^{2+} channel blocker) into the thalamus enhanced pain responses in wild-type mice. This suggests that $Ca_V3.1$ channels normally perform antinociceptive functions at the level of the thalamus. The mechanism that has been proposed to explain the hyperalgesic consequences of $Ca_V3.1$ channel inhibition (whether pharmacological or genetic) involves, in the first instance, a switch in the action potential firing behavior of thalamic relay neurons from a phasic (burst firing) mode to a tonic mode. The reduced burst firing in neurons of the thalamic relay nuclei appears to lead to a reduction in oscillatory behavior in thalamic circuits, with facilitated passage of nociceptive signals to the sensory cortex. Interestingly, thalamocortical dysrhythmias have been reported in patients with neurogenic pain, and these may lead to alterations in sensory gating processes such that the patient experiences persistent pain [126]. However, it remains a matter of speculation whether pain-associated thalamocortical dysrhythmias are the result of T-type Ca^{2+} channel mutations (*channelopathies*) or if they arise through some other mechanism.

Pharmacological evidence supporting a role for T-type Ca^{2+} channels in pain processing is limited by the poor availability of potent and selective blockers. Although T-type channels are blocked by a variety of antiepileptic, antihypertensive, anesthetic, and antipsychotic drugs, none of these agents are highly selective [127]. Animal studies with the antiepileptic drugs ethosuximide (Zarontin®, Pfizer Inc.) and zonisamide (Zonegran®, Eisai Inc., Woodcliff Lake, NJ) as well as the antihypertensive agent mibefradil have begun to lay the foundation of a pharmacological rationale for the involvement of these channels in nociception (Table 5.2). Ethosuximide is a nonselective and not very potent (7 μM–24 mM) blocker of T-type Ca^{2+} channels. It inhibits currents through the three T-type channel subtypes expressed in HEK-293 cells, apparently in a state-dependent manner [128]. Ethosuximide also inhibits native currents in primary sensory neurons [129] and thalamic neurons [130], although there is at least one report that it also interacts with persistent Na^+ channels and Ca^{2+}-gated K^+ channels [131]. Consistent with a role of T-type Ca^{2+} channels in spinal processing of nociceptive information, ethosuximide inhibits electrophysiological responses of dorsal horn neurons to electrical, mechanical, and thermal stimuli and reduces the phenomenon of windup [132]. Ethosuximide is efficacious in several behavioral models of pain [133–135]. For instance, it reduces tactile allodynia and thermal hyperalgesia in SNL rats and inhibits the mechanical and cold allodynia that result from chemotherapy agent-induced peripheral neuropathy in rats. Although ethosuximide does not appear to have been tested in patients with neuropathic pain, there is one anecdotal report that it could provide complete pain relief in a small number of patients who suffer from migraine [136]. Like ethosuximide, zonisamide is a nonselective blocker of T-type Ca^{2+} channels (50–500 μM) [137–139]. It reduces licking and biting behaviors in mice following formalin injection into the paw [140] and also exhibits antihyperalgesic and antiallodynic effects in nerve-injured rats and mice [141]. The antinociceptive effects of zonisamide may involve both central and peripheral mechanisms. Importantly, zonisamide has been used successfully as an analgesic drug in patients with migraine and poststroke pain [142,143]. Finally, even though mibefradil was withdrawn from the market due to drug–drug interactions, it remains in widespread use as a research tool to explore the role of T-type Ca^{2+} channels in various physiological processes. It is a moderately potent T-type channel blocker (0.1–5 μM) [144–149] and has been shown to have efficacy in several animal models of pain [134,150,151].

In summary, multiple lines of evidence support a role of T-type Ca^{2+} channels in nociception. The antinociceptive effect of anti-$Ca_V3.2$ antisense oligonucleotides currently represents the most solid evidence in support of a role of T-type Ca^{2+} channels in nociception. The results from the knockout mice suggest that blockers of the $Ca_V3.2$ subtype of T-type channels might exert antinociceptive effects at the level of the DRG and possibly the spinal cord, whereas blockers of the $Ca_V3.1$ subtype might exert pronociceptive effects at the level of the thalamus. However, direct pharmacological evidence for a role of T-type Ca^{2+} channels in nociception remains rather weak due to the nonselective nature of the available tools; these agents not only block T-type Ca^{2+} channel nonselectively but also block several subtypes of voltage-gated Na^+ channels, which represent a class of pain-related targets in their own right. A significant opportunity exists to discover and develop novel agents that could block T-type channels selectively. However, it appears that most efforts to find potent and selective T-type channel blocking agents remain at an early stage, and so the clinical validation of T-type channels as analgesic targets is not expected for several more years.

5.7 CONCLUSION

Chronic pain represents a major unmet medical need. Consequently, a significant amount of basic research is being conducted to understand the molecular and cellular mechanisms that underlie the development and maintenance of chronic pain. As a result of these efforts, many voltage-gated and ligand-gated ion channels have been demonstrated to be important in controlling neuronal activity at various points along the pain pathway. Beyond such basic research, significant investment is being made by pharmaceutical and biotechnology companies to discover pharmacological agents that modulate the function of the many proteins (including ion channels) that are involved in the process of nociception. The hope is that these agents could be developed as novel analgesic drugs with improved efficacy and safety profiles compared with existing therapies. Among the family of voltage-gated Ca^{2+} channels, the evidence outlined in this chapter illustrates that N-type and T-type channels are key players in nociception. Even though both subtypes conduct Ca^{2+} into neurons, their unique biophysical properties and subcellular distributions allow each one to exert distinct effects on neuronal function. The N-type channel is intricately involved in synaptic transmission in the dorsal horn of the spinal cord and has been validated convincingly as a pain target by the potent analgesic effects of ziconotide. However, tremendous efforts are being made now to improve on ziconotide, and it is likely to be only a matter of time before an orally active small molecule drug becomes available. On the other hand, the role of T-type channels in the processing of painful information is an emerging story that is relatively underdeveloped at this time. This small family of Ca^{2+} channels is involved in controlling neuronal membrane excitability and in integrating synaptic inputs in peripheral, spinal, and brain neurons. These channels have been implicated in pain processing primarily as a result of experiments in animals where gene expression has been manipulated. Although a few T-type Ca^{2+} channel blockers have shown analgesic efficacy in patients, these agents fail to discriminate between different channel subtypes, and so satisfactory clinical validation of this family of targets remains to be demonstrated. In conclusion, clear opportunities remain to discover and develop potent and selective blockers and N-type and T-type Ca^{2+} channels for potential use as novel analgesic drugs.

REFERENCES

1. Berridge, M.J. (1998). Neuronal calcium signaling. *Neuron* 21(1):13–26.
2. McGivern, J.G., Worley, J.F. (2007). Ion channels: voltage gated. In: Triggle, D.J., Taylor, J.B. (eds.). *Comprehensive Medicinal Chemistry II*, Vol. 2. Elsevier: Oxford, pp. 827–875.
3. Briggs, C.A., Gopalakrishnan, M. (2007). Ion channels: ligand gated. In: Triggle, D.J., Taylor, J.B. (eds.). *Comprehensive Medicinal Chemistry II*, Vol. 2. Elsevier: Oxford, pp. 877–918.
4. Catterall, W.A., Striessnig, J., Snutch, T.P., Perez-Reyes, E. (2003). International Union of Pharmacology. XL. Compendium of voltage-gated ion channels: calcium channels. *Pharmacol Rev* 55(4):579–581.
5. Ertel, E.A., Campbell, K.P., Harpold, M.M., Hofmann, F., Mori, Y., Perez-Reyes, E., Schwartz, A., Snutch, T.P., Tanabe, T., Birnbaumer, L., Tsien, R.W., Catterall, W.A. (2000). Nomenclature of voltage-gated calcium channels. *Neuron* 25(3):533–535.
6. Sather, W.A., McCleskey, E.W. (2003). Permeation and selectivity in calcium channels. *Annu Rev Physiol* 65:133–159.

7. Richards, M.W., Butcher, A.J., Dolphin, A.C. (2004). Ca2+ channel beta-subunits: structural insights AID our understanding. *Trends Pharmacol Sci* 25(12): 626–632.
8. Long, S.B., Campbell, E.B., Mackinnon, R. (2005). Crystal structure of a mammalian voltage-dependent Shaker family K+ channel. *Science* 309(5736): 897–903.
9. Long, S.B., Campbell, E.B., Mackinnon, R. (2005). Voltage sensor of Kv1.2: structural basis of electromechanical coupling. *Science* 309(5736):903–908.
10. McGivern, J.G., McDonough, S.I. (2004). Voltage-gated calcium channels as targets for the treatment of chronic pain. *Curr Drug Targets CNS Neurol Disord* 3(6): 457–478.
11. McGivern, J.G. (2006). Targeting N-type and T-type calcium channels for the treatment of pain. *Drug Discov Today* 11(5–6):245–253.
12. Matthews, E.A., Dickenson, A.H. (2001). Effects of spinally delivered N- and P-type voltage-dependent calcium channel antagonists on dorsal horn neuronal responses in a rat model of neuropathy. *Pain* 92(1–2):235–246.
13. Luvisetto, S., Marinelli, S., Panasiti, M.S., D'Amato, F.R., Fletcher, C.F., Pavone, F., Pietrobon, D. (2006). Pain sensitivity in mice lacking the Ca(v)2.1alpha1 subunit of P/Q-type Ca2+ channels. *Neuroscience* 142(3):823–832.
14. Matthews, E.A., Bee, L.A., Stephens, G.J., Dickenson, A.H. (2007). The Cav2.3 calcium channel antagonist SNX-482 reduces dorsal horn neuronal responses in a rat model of chronic neuropathic pain. *Eur J Neurosci* 25(12):3561–3569.
15. Fang, Z., Park, C.K., Li, H.Y., Kim, H.Y., Park, S.H., Jung, S.J., Kim, J.S., Monteil, A., Oh, S.B., Miller, R.J. (2007). Molecular basis of Ca(v)2.3 calcium channels in rat nociceptive neurons. *J Biol Chem* 282(7):4757–4764.
16. Westenbroek, R.E., Hell, J.W., Warner, C., Dubel, S.J., Snutch, T.P., Catterall, W.A. (1992). Biochemical properties and subcellular distribution of an N-type calcium channel alpha 1 subunit. *Neuron* 9(6):1099–1115.
17. Takemura, M., Kiyama, H., Fukui, H., Tohyama, M., Wada, H. (1989). Distribution of the omega-conotoxin receptor in rat brain. An autoradiographic mapping. *Neuroscience* 32(2):405–416.
18. Zamponi, G.W. (2003). Regulation of presynaptic calcium channels by synaptic proteins. *J Pharmacol Sci* 92(2):79–83.
19. Westenbroek, R.E., Hoskins, L., Catterall, W.A. (1998). Localization of Ca2+ channel subtypes on rat spinal motor neurons, interneurons, and nerve terminals. *J Neurosci* 18(16):6319–6330.
20. Abdulla, F.A., Moran, T.D., Balasubramanyan, S., Smith, P.A. (2003). Effects and consequences of nerve injury on the electrical properties of sensory neurons. *Can J Physiol Pharmacol* 81(7):663–682.
21. Cizkova, D., Marsala, J., Lukacova, N., Marsala, M., Jergova, S., Orendacova, J., Yaksh, T.L. (2002). Localization of N-type Ca2+ channels in the rat spinal cord following chronic constrictive nerve injury. *Exp Brain Res* 147(4):456–463.
22. Lancaster, E., Oh, E.J., Gover, T., Weinreich, D. (2002). Calcium and calcium-activated currents in vagotomized rat primary vagal afferent neurons. *J Physiol* 540(Pt 2):543–556.
23. Baccei, M.L., Kocsis, J.D. (2000). Voltage-gated calcium currents in axotomized adult rat cutaneous afferent neurons. *J Neurophysiol* 83(4):2227–2238.

24. Bell, T.J., Thaler, C., Castiglioni, A.J., Helton, T.D., Lipscombe, D. (2004). Cell-specific alternative splicing increases calcium channel current density in the pain pathway. *Neuron* 41(1):127–138.

25. Altier, C., Dale, C.S., Kisilevsky, A.E., Chapman, K., Castiglioni, A.J., Matthews, E.A., Evans, R.M., Dickenson, A.H., Lipscombe, D., Vergnolle, N., Zamponi, G.W. (2007). Differential role of N-type calcium channel splice isoforms in pain. *J Neurosci* 27(24):6363–6373.

26. Swayne, L.A., Bourinet, E. (2008). Voltage-gated calcium channels in chronic pain: emerging role of alternative splicing. *Pflugers Arch* 456(3):459–466.

27. Saegusa, H., Kurihara, T., Zong, S., Kazuno, A., Matsuda, Y., Nonaka, T., Han, W., Toriyama, H., Tanabe, T. (2001). Suppression of inflammatory and neuropathic pain symptoms in mice lacking the N-type Ca2+ channel. *EMBO J* 20(10): 2349–2356.

28. Kim, C., Jun, K., Lee, T., Kim, S.S., McEnery, M.W., Chin, H., Kim, H.L., Park, J.M., Kim, D.K., Jung, S.J., Kim, J., Shin, H.S. (2001). Altered nociceptive response in mice deficient in the alpha(1B) subunit of the voltage-dependent calcium channel. *Mol Cell Neurosci* 18(2):235–245.

29. Schroeder, C.I., Doering, C.J., Zamponi, G.W., Lewis, R.J. (2006). N-type calcium channel blockers: novel therapeutics for the treatment of pain. *Med Chem* 2(5):535–543.

30. Chung, D., Gaur, S., Bell, J.R., Ramachandran, J., Nadasdi, L. (1995). Determination of disulfide bridge pattern in omega-conopeptides. *Int J Pept Protein Res* 46(3–4):320–325.

31. McGivern, J.G. (2007). Ziconotide: a review of its pharmacology and use in the treatment of pain. *Neuropsychiatr Dis Treat* 3(1):69–85.

32. Stoehr, S.J., Dooley, D.J. (1993). Characteristics of [125I]omega-conotoxin MVIIA binding to rat neocortical membranes. *Neurosci Lett* 161(1):113–116.

33. Kristipati, R., Nadasdi, L., Tarczy-Hornoch, K., Lau, K., Miljanich, G.P., Ramachandran, J., Bell, J.R. (1994). Characterization of the binding of omega-conopeptides to different classes of non-L-type neuronal calcium channels. *Mol Cell Neurosci* 5(3):219–228.

34. Nielsen, K.J., Adams, D., Thomas, L., Bond, T., Alewood, P.F., Craik, D.J., Lewis, R.J. (1999). Structure-activity relationships of omega-conotoxins MVIIA, MVIIC and 14 loop splice hybrids at N and P/Q-type calcium channels. *J Mol Biol* 289(5):1405–1421.

35. Lewis, R.J., Nielsen, K.J., Craik, D.J., Loughnan, M.L., Adams, D.A., Sharpe, I.A., Luchian, T., Adams, D.J., Bond, T., Thomas, L., Jones, A., Matheson, J.L., Drinkwater, R., Andrews, P.R., Alewood, P.F. (2000). Novel omega-conotoxins from *Conus catus* discriminate among neuronal calcium channel subtypes. *J Biol Chem* 275(45):35335–35344.

36. Fox, J.A. (1995). Irreversible and reversible blockade of IMR32 calcium channel currents by synthetic MVIIA and iodinated MVIIC omega-conopeptides. *Pflugers Arch* 429(6):873–875.

37. Sanger, G.J., Ellis, E.S., Harries, M.H., Tilford, N.S., Wardle, K.A., Benham, C.D. (2000). Rank-order inhibition by omega-conotoxins in human and animal autonomic nerve preparations. *Eur J Pharmacol* 388(1):89–95.

38. Wen, L., Yang, S., Qiao, H., Liu, Z., Zhou, W., Zhang, Y., Huang, P. (2005). SO-3, a new O-superfamily conopeptide derived from *Conus striatus*, selectively inhibits N-type calcium currents in cultured hippocampal neurons. *Br J Pharmacol* 145(6): 728–739.

39. Bleakman, D., Bowman, D., Bath, C.P., Brust, P.F., Johnson, E.C., Deal, C.R., Miller, R.J., Ellis, S.B., Harpold, M.M., Hans, M., Grantham, C.J. (1995). Characteristics of a human N-type calcium channel expressed in HEK293 cells. *Neuropharmacology* 34(7):753–765.

40. Gaur, S., Newcomb, R., Rivnay, B., Bell, J.R., Yamashiro, D., Ramachandran, J., Miljanich, G.P. (1994). Calcium channel antagonist peptides define several components of transmitter release in the hippocampus. *Neuropharmacology* 33(10): 1211–1219.

41. Newcomb, R., Palma, A., Fox, J., Gaur, S., Lau, K., Chung, D., Cong, R., Bell, J.R., Horne, B., Nadasdi, L., Ramachandran, J. (1995). SNX-325, a novel calcium antagonist from the spider *Segestria florentina*. *Biochemistry* 34(26):8341–8347.

42. Wang, Y.X., Bezprozvannaya, S., Bowersox, S.S., Nadasdi, L., Miljanich, G., Mezo, G., Silva, D., Tarczy-Hornoch, K., Luther, R.R. (1998). Peripheral versus central potencies of N-type voltage-sensitive calcium channel blockers. *Naunyn Schmiedebergs Arch Pharmacol* 357(2):159–168.

43. Smith, M.T., Cabot, P.J., Ross, F.B., Robertson, A.D., Lewis, R.J. (2002). The novel N-type calcium channel blocker, AM336, produces potent dose-dependent antinociception after intrathecal dosing in rats and inhibits substance P release in rat spinal cord slices. *Pain* 96(1–2):119–127.

44. Motin, L., Adams, D.J. (2008). Omega-conotoxin inhibition of excitatory synaptic transmission evoked by dorsal root stimulation in rat superficial dorsal horn. *Neuropharmacology* 55(5):860–864.

45. Malmberg, A.B., Yaksh, T.L. (1994). Voltage-sensitive calcium channels in spinal nociceptive processing: blockade of N- and P-type channels inhibits formalin-induced nociception. *J Neurosci* 14(8):4882–4890.

46. Malmberg, A.B., Yaksh, T.L. (1995). Effect of continuous intrathecal infusion of omega-conopeptides, N-type calcium-channel blockers, on behavior and antinociception in the formalin and hot-plate tests in rats. *Pain* 60(1):83–90.

47. Bowersox, S.S., Gadbois, T., Singh, T., Pettus, M., Wang, Y.X., Luther, R.R. (1996). Selective N-type neuronal voltage-sensitive calcium channel blocker, SNX-111, produces spinal antinociception in rat models of acute, persistent and neuropathic pain. *J Pharmacol Exp Ther* 279(3):1243–1249.

48. Wang, Y.X., Gao, D., Pettus, M., Phillips, C., Bowersox, S.S. (2000). Interactions of intrathecally administered ziconotide, a selective blocker of neuronal N-type voltage-sensitive calcium channels, with morphine on nociception in rats. *Pain* 84(2–3):271–281.

49. Sluka, K.A. (1998). Blockade of N- and P/Q-type calcium channels reduces the secondary heat hyperalgesia induced by acute inflammation. *J Pharmacol Exp Ther* 287(1):232–237.

50. Chaplan, S.R., Pogrel, J.W., Yaksh, T.L. (1994). Role of voltage-dependent calcium channel subtypes in experimental tactile allodynia. *J Pharmacol Exp Ther* 269(3):1117–1123.

51. Scott, D.A., Wright, C.E., Angus, J.A. (2002). Actions of intrathecal omega-conotoxins CVID, GVIA, MVIIA, and morphine in acute and neuropathic pain in the rat. *Eur J Pharmacol* 451(3):279–286.

52. Yamamoto, T., Sakashita, Y. (1998). Differential effects of intrathecally administered N- and P-type voltage-sensitive calcium channel blockers upon two models of experimental mononeuropathy in the rat. *Brain Res* 794(2):329–332.

53. Wang, Y.X., Pettus, M., Gao, D., Phillips, C., Scott Bowersox, S. (2000). Effects of intrathecal administration of ziconotide, a selective neuronal N-type calcium channel blocker, on mechanical allodynia and heat hyperalgesia in a rat model of postoperative pain. *Pain* 84(2–3):151–158.

54. Staats, P.S., Yearwood, T., Charapata, S.G., Presley, R.W., Wallace, M.S., Byas-Smith, M., Fisher, R., Bryce, D.A., Mangieri, E.A., Luther, R.R., Mayo, M., McGuire, D., Ellis, D. (2004). Intrathecal ziconotide in the treatment of refractory pain in patients with cancer or AIDS: a randomized controlled trial. *JAMA* 291(1):63–70.

55. Wallace, M.S., Charapata, S.G., Fisher, R., Byas-Smith, M., Staats, P.S., Mayo, M., McGuire, D., Ellis, D. (2006). Intrathecal ziconotide in the treatment of chronic nonmalignant pain: a randomized, double-blind, placebo-controlled clinical trial. *Neuromodulation* 9(2):75–86.

56. Rauck, R.L., Wallace, M.S., Leong, M.S., Minehart, M., Webster, L.R., Charapata, S.G., Abraham, J.E., Buffington, D.E., Ellis, D., Kartzinel, R. (2006). A randomized, double-blind, placebo-controlled study of intrathecal ziconotide in adults with severe chronic pain. *J Pain Symptom Manage* 31(5):393–406.

57. Atanassoff, P.G., Hartmannsgruber, M.W., Thrasher, J., Wermeling, D., Longton, W., Gaeta, R., Singh, T., Mayo, M., McGuire, D., Luther, R.R. (2000). Ziconotide, a new N-type calcium channel blocker, administered intrathecally for acute postoperative pain. *Reg Anesth Pain Med* 25(3):274–278.

58. Brose, W.G., Gutlove, D.P., Luther, R.R., Bowersox, S.S., McGuire, D. (1997). Use of intrathecal SNX-111, a novel, N-type, voltage-sensitive, calcium channel blocker, in the management of intractable brachial plexus avulsion pain. *Clin J Pain* 13(3):256–259.

59. Wermeling, D., Drass, M., Ellis, D., Mayo, M., McGuire, D., O'Connell, D., Hale, V., Chao, S. (2003). Pharmacokinetics and pharmacodynamics of intrathecal ziconotide in chronic pain patients. *J Clin Pharmacol* 43(6):624–636.

60. Wermeling, D.P., Berger, J.R. (2006). Ziconotide infusion for severe chronic pain: case series of patients with neuropathic pain. *Pharmacotherapy* 26(3):395–402.

61. Fuertges, F., Abuchowski, A. (1990). The clinical efficacy of poly(ethylene glycol)-modified proteins. *J Control Release* 11(1–3):139–148.

62. Snutch, T.P. (2004). N-type channels, small organic molecules and pain. Spring Pain Research Conference. Grand Cayman, BWI, April 24–May 1.

63. Snutch, T.P., Feng, Z.P., Belardetti, F., Vanderah, T., Zamponi, G.W., Porreca, F. (2003). Novel N-type calcium channel blockers efficacious in animal models of chronic pain. 226th American Chemical Society National Meeting. New York, September 7–11.

64. Maneuf, Y.P., Luo, Z.D., Lee, K. (2006). Alpha2delta and the mechanism of action of gabapentin in the treatment of pain. *Semin Cell Dev Biol* 17(5):565–570.

65. Curran, M.P., Wagstaff, A.J. (2003). Gabapentin: in postherpetic neuralgia. *CNS Drugs* 17(13):975–982.

66. Morello, C.M., Leckband, S.G., Stoner, C.P., Moorhouse, D.F., Sahagian, G.A. (1999). Randomized double-blind study comparing the efficacy of gabapentin with amitriptyline on diabetic peripheral neuropathy pain. *Arch Intern Med* 159(16): 1931–1937.

67. Cheshire, W.P., Jr. (2002). Defining the role for gabapentin in the treatment of trigeminal neuralgia: a retrospective study. *J Pain* 3(2):137–142.

68. Levendoglu, F., Ogun, C.O., Ozerbil, O., Ogun, T.C., Ugurlu, H. (2004). Gabapentin is a first line drug for the treatment of neuropathic pain in spinal cord injury. *Spine* 29(7):743–751.

69. Caraceni, A., Zecca, E., Bonezzi, C., Arcuri, E., Yaya Tur, R., Maltoni, M., Visentin, M., Gorni, G., Martini, C., Tirelli, W., Barbieri, M., De Conno, F. (2004). Gabapentin for neuropathic cancer pain: a randomized controlled trial from the Gabapentin Cancer Pain Study Group. *J Clin Oncol* 22(14):2909–2917.

70. Yaksi, A., Ozgonenel, L., Ozgonenel, B. (2007). The efficiency of gabapentin therapy in patients with lumbar spinal stenosis. *Spine* 32(9):939–942.

71. Dworkin, R.H., Corbin, A.E., Young, J.P., Jr., Sharma, U., LaMoreaux, L., Bockbrader, H., Garofalo, E.A., Poole, R.M. (2003). Pregabalin for the treatment of postherpetic neuralgia: a randomized, placebo-controlled trial. *Neurology* 60(8):1274–1283.

72. Lesser, H., Sharma, U., LaMoreaux, L., Poole, R.M. (2004). Pregabalin relieves symptoms of painful diabetic neuropathy: a randomized controlled trial. *Neurology* 63(11):2104–2110.

73. Rosenstock, J., Tuchman, M., LaMoreaux, L., Sharma, U. (2004). Pregabalin for the treatment of painful diabetic peripheral neuropathy: a double-blind, placebo-controlled trial. *Pain* 110(3):628–638.

74. Richter, R.W., Portenoy, R., Sharma, U., Lamoreaux, L., Bockbrader, H., Knapp, L.E. (2005). Relief of painful diabetic peripheral neuropathy with pregabalin: a randomized, placebo-controlled trial. *J Pain* 6(4):253–260.

75. Obermann, M., Yoon, M.S., Sensen, K., Maschke, M., Diener, H.C., Katsarava, Z. (2008). Efficacy of pregabalin in the treatment of trigeminal neuralgia. *Cephalalgia* 28(2):174–181.

76. Crofford, L.J., Rowbotham, M.C., Mease, P.J., Russell, I.J., Dworkin, R.H., Corbin, A.E., Young, J.P., Jr., LaMoreaux, L.K., Martin, S.A., Sharma, U. (2005). Pregabalin for the treatment of fibromyalgia syndrome: results of a randomized, double-blind, placebo-controlled trial. *Arthritis Rheum* 52(4):1264–1273.

77. Field, M.J., Oles, R.J., Lewis, A.S., McCleary, S., Hughes, J., Singh, L. (1997). Gabapentin (neurontin) and S-(+)-3-isobutylgaba represent a novel class of selective antihyperalgesic agents. *Br J Pharmacol* 121(8):1513–1522.

78. Hunter, J.C., Gogas, K.R., Hedley, L.R., Jacobson, L.O., Kassotakis, L., Thompson, J., Fontana, D.J. (1997). The effect of novel anti-epileptic drugs in rat experimental models of acute and chronic pain. *Eur J Pharmacol* 324(2–3):153–160.

79. Christensen, D., Gautron, M., Guilbaud, G., Kayser, V. (2001). Effect of gabapentin and lamotrigine on mechanical allodynia-like behaviour in a rat model of trigeminal neuropathic pain. *Pain* 93(2):147–153.

80. Luo, Z.D., Calcutt, N.A., Higuera, E.S., Valder, C.R., Song, Y.H., Svensson, C.I., Myers, R.R. (2002). Injury type-specific calcium channel alpha 2 delta-1 subunit up-regulation in rat neuropathic pain models correlates with antiallodynic effects of gabapentin. *J Pharmacol Exp Ther* 303(3):1199–1205.

81. Suman-Chauhan, N., Webdale, L., Hill, D.R., Woodruff, G.N. (1993). Characterisation of [3H]gabapentin binding to a novel site in rat brain: homogenate binding studies. *Eur J Pharmacol* 244(3):293–301.

82. Field, M.J., Cox, P.J., Stott, E., Melrose, H., Offord, J., Su, T.Z., Bramwell, S., Corradini, L., England, S., Winks, J., Kinloch, R.A., Hendrich, J., Dolphin, A.C., Webb, T., Williams, D. (2006). Identification of the alpha2-delta-1 subunit of voltage-dependent calcium channels as a molecular target for pain mediating the analgesic actions of pregabalin. *Proc Natl Acad Sci U S A* 103(46):17537–17542.

83. Gee, N.S., Brown, J.P., Dissanayake, V.U., Offord, J., Thurlow, R., Woodruff, G.N. (1996). The novel anticonvulsant drug, gabapentin (Neurontin), binds to the alpha2delta subunit of a calcium channel. *J Biol Chem* 271(10):5768–5776.

84. McClelland, D., Evans, R.M., Barkworth, L., Martin, D.J., Scott, R.H. (2004). A study comparing the actions of gabapentin and pregabalin on the electrophysiological properties of cultured DRG neurones from neonatal rats. *BMC Pharmacol* 4(1):14.

85. Stefani, A., Spadoni, F., Bernardi, G. (1998). Gabapentin inhibits calcium currents in isolated rat brain neurons. *Neuropharmacology* 37(1):83–91.

86. Stefani, A., Spadoni, F., Giacomini, P., Lavaroni, F., Bernardi, G. (2001). The effects of gabapentin on different ligand- and voltage-gated currents in isolated cortical neurons. *Epilepsy Res* 43(3):239–248.

87. Alden, K.J., Garcia, J. (2001). Differential effect of gabapentin on neuronal and muscle calcium currents. *J Pharmacol Exp Ther* 297(2):727–735.

88. Martin, D.J., McClelland, D., Herd, M.B., Sutton, K.G., Hall, M.D., Lee, K., Pinnock, R.D., Scott, R.H. (2002). Gabapentin-mediated inhibition of voltage-activated Ca2+ channel currents in cultured sensory neurones is dependent on culture conditions and channel subunit expression. *Neuropharmacology* 42(3):353–366.

89. Sutton, K.G., Martin, D.J., Pinnock, R.D., Lee, K., Scott, R.H. (2002). Gabapentin inhibits high-threshold calcium channel currents in cultured rat dorsal root ganglion neurones. *Br J Pharmacol* 135(1):257–265.

90. Maneuf, Y.P., Blake, R., Andrews, N.A., McKnight, A.T. (2004). Reduction by gabapentin of K+-evoked release of [3H]-glutamate from the caudal trigeminal nucleus of the streptozotocin-treated rat. *Br J Pharmacol* 141(4):574–579.

91. Newton, R.A., Bingham, S., Case, P.C., Sanger, G.J., Lawson, S.N. (2001). Dorsal root ganglion neurons show increased expression of the calcium channel alpha2delta-1 subunit following partial sciatic nerve injury. *Brain Res Mol Brain Res* 95(1–2):1–8.

92. Abe, M., Kurihara, T., Han, W., Shinomiya, K., Tanabe, T. (2002). Changes in expression of voltage-dependent ion channel subunits in dorsal root ganglia of rats with radicular injury and pain. *Spine* 27(14):1517–1524.

93. Melrose, H.L., Kinloch, R.A., Cox, P.J., Field, M.J., Collins, D., Williams, D. (2007). [3H] pregabalin binding is increased in ipsilateral dorsal horn following chronic constriction injury. *Neurosci Lett* 417(2):187–192.

94. Luo, Z.D., Chaplan, S.R., Higuera, E.S., Sorkin, L.S., Stauderman, K.A., Williams, M.E., Yaksh, T.L. (2001). Upregulation of dorsal root ganglion (alpha)2(delta) calcium channel subunit and its correlation with allodynia in spinal nerve-injured rats. *J Neurosci* 21(6):1868–1875.

95. Li, C.Y., Zhang, X.L., Matthews, E.A., Li, K.W., Kurwa, A., Boroujerdi, A., Gross, J., Gold, M.S., Dickenson, A.H., Feng, G., Luo, Z.D. (2006). Calcium channel alpha2delta1 subunit mediates spinal hyperexcitability in pain modulation. *Pain* 125(1–2):20–34.

96. Fehrenbacher, J.C., Taylor, C.P., Vasko, M.R. (2003). Pregabalin and gabapentin reduce release of substance P and CGRP from rat spinal tissues only after inflammation or activation of protein kinase C. *Pain* 105(1–2):133–141.

97. Bayer, K., Ahmadi, S., Zeilhofer, H.U. (2004). Gabapentin may inhibit synaptic transmission in the mouse spinal cord dorsal horn through a preferential block of P/Q-type Ca2+ channels. *Neuropharmacology* 46(5):743–749.

98. Coderre, T.J., Kumar, N., Lefebvre, C.D., Yu, J.S. (2005). Evidence that gabapentin reduces neuropathic pain by inhibiting the spinal release of glutamate. *J Neurochem* 94(4):1131–1139.

99. Cribbs, L.L., Lee, J.H., Yang, J., Satin, J., Zhang, Y., Daud, A., Barclay, J., Williamson, M.P., Fox, M., Rees, M., Perez-Reyes, E. (1998). Cloning and characterization of alpha1H from human heart, a member of the T-type Ca2+ channel gene family. *Circ Res* 83(1):103–109.

100. Lee, J.H., Daud, A.N., Cribbs, L.L., Lacerda, A.E., Pereverzev, A., Klockner, U., Schneider, T., Perez-Reyes, E. (1999). Cloning and expression of a novel member of the low voltage-activated T-type calcium channel family. *J Neurosci* 19(6): 1912–1921.

101. Perez-Reyes, E., Cribbs, L.L., Daud, A., Lacerda, A.E., Barclay, J., Williamson, M.P., Fox, M., Rees, M., Lee, J.H. (1998). Molecular characterization of a neuronal low-voltage-activated T-type calcium channel. *Nature* 391(6670):896–900.

102. Lee, J.H., Gomora, J.C., Cribbs, L.L., Perez-Reyes, E. (1999). Nickel block of three cloned T-type calcium channels: low concentrations selectively block alpha1H. *Biophys J* 77(6):3034–3042.

103. Gao, B., Sekido, Y., Maximov, A., Saad, M., Forgacs, E., Latif, F., Wei, M.H., Lerman, M., Lee, J.H., Perez-Reyes, E., Bezprozvanny, I., Minna, J.D. (2000). Functional properties of a new voltage-dependent calcium channel alpha(2)delta auxiliary subunit gene (CACNA2D2). *J Biol Chem* 275(16):12237–12242.

104. Klugbauer, N., Dai, S., Specht, V., Lacinova, L., Marais, E., Bohn, G., Hofmann, F. (2000). A family of gamma-like calcium channel subunits. *FEBS Lett* 470(2):189–197.

105. Leuranguer, V., Bourinet, E., Lory, P., Nargeot, J. (1998). Antisense depletion of beta-subunits fails to affect T-type calcium channels properties in a neuroblastoma cell line. *Neuropharmacology* 37(6):701–708.

106. Scroggs, R.S., Fox, A.P. (1992). Calcium current variation between acutely isolated adult rat dorsal root ganglion neurons of different size. *J Physiol* 445:639–658.

107. Scroggs, R.S., Fox, A.P. (1992). Multiple Ca2+ currents elicited by action potential waveforms in acutely isolated adult rat dorsal root ganglion neurons. *J Neurosci* 12(5):1789–1801.

108. Coulter, D.A., Huguenard, J.R., Prince, D.A. (1989). Calcium currents in rat thalamocortical relay neurones: kinetic properties of the transient, low-threshold current. *J Physiol* 414:587–604.

109. Huguenard, J.R., Prince, D.A. (1992). A novel T-type current underlies prolonged Ca(2+)-dependent burst firing in GABAergic neurons of rat thalamic reticular nucleus. *J Neurosci* 12(10):3804–3817.

110. White, G., Lovinger, D.M., Weight, F.F. (1989). Transient low-threshold Ca2+ current triggers burst firing through an afterdepolarizing potential in an adult mammalian neuron. *Proc Natl Acad Sci U S A* 86(17):6802–6806.

111. Suzuki, S., Rogawski, M.A. (1989). T-type calcium channels mediate the transition between tonic and phasic firing in thalamic neurons. *Proc Natl Acad Sci U S A* 86(18):7228–7232.

112. Miller, R.J. (1987). Multiple calcium channels and neuronal function. *Science* 235(4784):46–52.

113. Kase, M., Kakimoto, S., Sakuma, S., Houtani, T., Ohishi, H., Ueyama, T., Sugimoto, T. (1999). Distribution of neurons expressing alpha 1G subunit mRNA of T-type voltage-dependent calcium channel in adult rat central nervous system. *Neurosci Lett* 268(2):77–80.

114. Talley, E.M., Cribbs, L.L., Lee, J.H., Daud, A., Perez-Reyes, E., Bayliss, D.A. (1999). Differential distribution of three members of a gene family encoding low voltage-activated (T-type) calcium channels. *J Neurosci* 19(6):1895–1911.

115. Todorovic, S.M., Jevtovic-Todorovic, V., Meyenburg, A., Mennerick, S., Perez-Reyes, E., Romano, C., Olney, J.W., Zorumski, C.F. (2001). Redox modulation of T-type calcium channels in rat peripheral nociceptors. *Neuron* 31(1):75–85.

116. Nelson, M.T., Woo, J., Kang, H.W., Vitko, I., Barrett, P.Q., Perez-Reyes, E., Lee, J.H., Shin, H.S., Todorovic, S.M. (2007). Reducing agents sensitize C-type nociceptors by relieving high-affinity zinc inhibition of T-type calcium channels. *J Neurosci* 27(31):8250–8260.

117. Lambert, R.C., McKenna, F., Maulet, Y., Talley, E.M., Bayliss, D.A., Cribbs, L.L., Lee, J.H., Perez-Reyes, E., Feltz, A. (1998). Low-voltage-activated Ca2+ currents are generated by members of the CavT subunit family (alpha1G/H) in rat primary sensory neurons. *J Neurosci* 18(21):8605–8613.

118. Abdulla, F.A., Smith, P.A. (2001). Axotomy- and autotomy-induced changes in Ca2+ and K+ channel currents of rat dorsal root ganglion neurons. *J Neurophysiol* 85(2):644–658.

119. Hogan, Q.H., McCallum, J.B., Sarantopoulos, C., Aason, M., Mynlieff, M., Kwok, W.M., Bosnjak, Z.J. (2000). Painful neuropathy decreases membrane calcium current in mammalian primary afferent neurons. *Pain* 86(1–2):43–53.

120. McCallum, J.B., Kwok, W.M., Mynlieff, M., Bosnjak, Z.J., Hogan, Q.H. (2003). Loss of T-type calcium current in sensory neurons of rats with neuropathic pain. *Anesthesiology* 98(1):209–216.

121. McCallum, J.B., Kwok, W.M., Sapunar, D., Fuchs, A., Hogan, Q.H. (2006). Painful peripheral nerve injury decreases calcium current in axotomized sensory neurons. *Anesthesiology* 105(1):160–168.

122. Wen, X.J., Li, Z.J., Chen, Z.X., Fang, Z.Y., Yang, C.X., Li, H., Zeng, Y.M. (2006). Intrathecal administration of Cav3.2 and Cav3.3 antisense oligonucleotide

reverses tactile allodynia and thermal hyperalgesia in rats following chronic compression of dorsal root of ganglion. *Acta Pharmacol Sin* 27(12):1547–1552.

123. Bourinet, E., Alloui, A., Monteil, A., Barrere, C., Couette, B., Poirot, O., Pages, A., McRory, J., Snutch, T.P., Eschalier, A., Nargeot, J. (2005). Silencing of the Cav3.2 T-type calcium channel gene in sensory neurons demonstrates its major role in nociception. *EMBO J* 24(2):315–324.

124. Choi, S., Na, H.S., Kim, J., Lee, J., Lee, S., Kim, D., Park, J., Chen, C.C., Campbell, K.P., Shin, H.S. (2007). Attenuated pain responses in mice lacking Ca(V)3.2 T-type channels. *Genes Brain Behav* 6(5):425–431.

125. Kim, D., Park, D., Choi, S., Lee, S., Sun, M., Kim, C., Shin, H.S. (2003). Thalamic control of visceral nociception mediated by T-type Ca2+ channels. *Science* 302(5642):117–119.

126. Llinas, R.R., Ribary, U., Jeanmonod, D., Kronberg, E., Mitra, P.P. (1999). Thalamocortical dysrhythmia: a neurological and neuropsychiatric syndrome characterized by magnetoencephalography. *Proc Natl Acad Sci U S A* 96(26):15222–15227.

127. McGivern, J.G. (2006). Pharmacology and drug discovery for T-type calcium channels. *CNS Neurol Disord Drug Targets* 5(6):587–603.

128. Gomora, J.C., Daud, A.N., Weiergraber, M., Perez-Reyes, E. (2001). Block of cloned human T-type calcium channels by succinimide antiepileptic drugs. *Mol Pharmacol* 60(5):1121–1132.

129. Todorovic, S.M., Lingle, C.J. (1998). Pharmacological properties of T-type Ca2+ current in adult rat sensory neurons: effects of anticonvulsant and anesthetic agents. *J Neurophysiol* 79(1):240–252.

130. Coulter, D.A., Huguenard, J.R., Prince, D.A. (1989). Characterization of ethosuximide reduction of low-threshold calcium current in thalamic neurons. *Ann Neurol* 25(6):582–593.

131. Leresche, N., Parri, H.R., Erdemli, G., Guyon, A., Turner, J.P., Williams, S.R., Asprodini, E., Crunelli, V. (1998). On the action of the anti-absence drug ethosuximide in the rat and cat thalamus. *J Neurosci* 18(13):4842–4853.

132. Matthews, E.A., Dickenson, A.H. (2001). Effects of ethosuximide, a T-type Ca(2+) channel blocker, on dorsal horn neuronal responses in rats. *Eur J Pharmacol* 415(2–3):141–149.

133. Gogas, K.R., Loo, C., Fellows, R., Lewis, R., Secchi, R., Thompson, J., Waligora, D., Jacobson, L., Zhu, Q., Hedley, L.R., Malmberg, A.B., Hunter, J.C., McGivern, J.G. (2002). Effects of the T-type calcium channel blocker, ethosuximide, in rodent models of acute and chronic pain. IASP 10th World Congress on Pain. San Diego, CA, August 17–22.

134. Dogrul, A., Gardell, L.R., Ossipov, M.H., Tulunay, F.C., Lai, J., Porreca, F. (2003). Reversal of experimental neuropathic pain by T-type calcium channel blockers. *Pain* 105(1–2):159–168.

135. Flatters, S.J., Bennett, G.J. (2004). Ethosuximide reverses paclitaxel- and vincristine-induced painful peripheral neuropathy. *Pain* 109(1–2):150–161.

136. Eggers, A.E., Moreno, H. (2002). Suggestion for another anti-epileptic drug to use for migraine prophylaxis. *Headache* 42(7):696–697.

137. Suzuki, S., Kawakami, K., Nishimura, S., Watanabe, Y., Yagi, K., Seino, M., Miyamoto, K. (1992). Zonisamide blocks T-type calcium channel in cultured neurons of rat cerebral cortex. *Epilepsy Res* 12(1):21–27.
138. Kito, M., Maehara, M., Watanabe, K. (1994). Antiepileptic drugs–calcium current interaction in cultured human neuroblastoma cells. *Seizure* 3(2):141–149.
139. Kito, M., Maehara, M., Watanabe, K. (1996). Mechanisms of T-type calcium channel blockade by zonisamide. *Seizure* 5(2):115–119.
140. Tanabe, M., Murakami, T., Ono, H. (2008). Zonisamide suppresses pain symptoms of formalin-induced inflammatory and streptozotocin-induced diabetic neuropathy. *J Pharmacol Sci* 107(2):213–220.
141. Hord, A.H., Denson, D.D., Chalfoun, A.G., Azevedo, M.I. (2003). The effect of systemic zonisamide (Zonegran) on thermal hyperalgesia and mechanical allodynia in rats with an experimental mononeuropathy. *Anesth Analg* 96(6): 1700–1706.
142. Drake, M.E., Jr., Greathouse, N.I., Renner, J.B., Armentbright, A.D. (2004). Open-label zonisamide for refractory migraine. *Clin Neuropharmacol* 27(6):278–280.
143. Takahashi, Y., Hashimoto, K., Tsuji, S. (2004). Successful use of zonisamide for central poststroke pain. *J Pain* 5(3):192–194.
144. Randall, A.D., Tsien, R.W. (1997). Contrasting biophysical and pharmacological properties of T-type and R-type calcium channels. *Neuropharmacology* 36(7):879–893.
145. Arnoult, C., Villaz, M., Florman, H.M. (1998). Pharmacological properties of the T-type Ca2+ current of mouse spermatogenic cells. *Mol Pharmacol* 53(6): 1104–1111.
146. Mishra, S.K., Hermsmeyer, K. (1994). Selective inhibition of T-type Ca2+ channels by Ro 40-5967. *Circ Res* 75(1):144–148.
147. Mehrke, G., Zong, X.G., Flockerzi, V., Hofmann, F. (1994). The Ca(++)-channel blocker Ro 40-5967 blocks differently T-type and L-type Ca++ channels. *J Pharmacol Exp Ther* 271(3):1483–1488.
148. Clozel, J.P., Ertel, E.A., Ertel, S.I. (1997). Discovery and main pharmacological properties of mibefradil (Ro 40-5967), the first selective T-type calcium channel blocker. *J Hypertens Suppl* 15(5):S17–S25.
149. Leuranguer, V., Mangoni, M.E., Nargeot, J., Richard, S. (2001). Inhibition of T-type and L-type calcium channels by mibefradil: physiologic and pharmacologic bases of cardiovascular effects. *J Cardiovasc Pharmacol* 37(6):649–661.
150. Todorovic, S.M., Meyenburg, A., Jevtovic-Todorovic, V. (2002). Mechanical and thermal antinociception in rats following systemic administration of mibefradil, a T-type calcium channel blocker. *Brain Res* 951(2):336–340.
151. Cheng, J.K., Lin, C.S., Chen, C.C., Yang, J.R., Chiou, L.C. (2007). Effects of intrathecal injection of T-type calcium channel blockers in the rat formalin test. *Behav Pharmacol* 18(1):1–8.
152. Todorovic, S.M., Rastogi, A.J., Jevtovic-Todorovic, V. (2003). Potent analgesic effects of anticonvulsants on peripheral thermal nociception in rats. *Br J Pharmacol* 140(2):255–260.

CHAPTER 6

Adenosine Receptors

JANA SAWYNOK

Department of Pharmacology, Dalhousie University

Content

6.1 PERIPHERAL ASPECTS OF SENSORY NERVES

Pain, in a physiological sense, involves a sensory system that conveys important adaptive information about the environment to the organism. This type of signaling is known as nociception. Pain signaling involves several components, including sensory nerve activation, afferent transmission to the spinal cord, spinal integration and modulation, supraspinal signaling, and descending regulation [1,2]. Pain signaling becomes amplified and altered by inflammation and nerve injury, and distinct processes of modulation and modification at peripheral sites have been elaborated [3]. Drugs that modify pain potentially act at several different loci. The focus of this book is on peripheral influences on pain signaling, with a particular intent of considering the potential for targeting this component of action for pain-relieving actions. Inherent in this consideration is appreciating that inhibition of sensory nerve activation at the site of origin of pain can significantly modify pain signaling and that pathologi-

Peripheral Receptor Targets for Analgesia: Novel Approaches to Pain Management, Edited by Brian E. Cairns

cal processes can alter the functioning of the sensory nerve throughout its entire extent. This chapter will consider adenosine receptors as mediators of peripheral pain signaling and the possibility that drugs that target such receptors may be useful analgesics.

Pain afferent fibers include small-diameter, unmyelinated C-fibers and small-diameter, myelinated Aδ-fibers; additional afferent fibers (larger-diameter Aβ-fibers) are recruited following inflammation and nerve injury [1]. Pain is initiated by thermal, mechanical, and chemical stimuli. While the molecular entities (receptors) mediating chemogenic activation of sensory afferent fibers have been appreciated for some time (e.g., receptors for prostaglandin E_2 [PGE_2], bradykinin, histamine, 5-hydroxytryptamine [5-HT]), those transducing thermal and mechanical stimuli began to be characterized with the identification of the transient receptor potential vanilloid 1 (TRPV1) (VR1 receptor for capsaicin) [4,5] and are still being elaborated [6]. Sensory nerves can be modulated by a plethora of excitatory and inhibitory influences as elaborated in other chapters in this book. With the involvement of so many molecules in such signaling, the issue of which targets will provide meaningful analgesia arises. Inhibition of production of prostaglandins, which leads to decreased phosphorylation of Na^+ channels on sensory nerves, is a major mechanism underlying whole classes of analgesic agents (nonsteroidal anti-inflammatory drugs and selective cyclooxygenase-2 inhibitors) [7,8]. The success of this strategy suggests that modulation of Na^+ channels may be a particularly desirable property for novel peripheral analgesics to exert (see Chapter 3). As details of intracellular signaling in sensory afferent fibers unfold [3], these considerations may also be helpful for drug development strategies.

6.2 ADENOSINE RECEPTORS AND SENSORY NEURONS

There are four types of adenosine receptors, A1, A2A, A2B, and A3, with well-characterized signaling via G proteins, cyclic adenosine 5′-monophosphate (AMP), and protein kinase A (PKA) and its response elements (cyclic AMP responsive element binding protein [CREB], dopamine and cyclic AMP-regulated phosphoprotein [DARPP]-32); A1 and A3 receptors inhibit cyclic AMP production, while A2A and A2B receptors stimulate cyclic AMP production [9]. Activation of A1 receptors can also involve increased inositol trisphosphate (IP_3)/diacylglyceride (DAG) via phospholipase C (PLC), increased arachidonate via phospholipase A_2 (PLA_2), increased phosphotidylethanolamine via phospholipase D [9,10] as well as interactions with mitogen-activated protein kinases (MAPKs) [11]. Activation of A2A receptors can involve further G protein-dependent signaling pathways including extracellular signal-regulated kinase (ERK)1/2, and p38, as well as G protein-independent signaling pathways [10,12]. Stimulation of A2B receptors can result in activation of several forms of MAPKs (ERK1/2, p38, c-jun N-terminal kinase [JNK])

[10,13], while A3 receptors interface with ERK1/2, PLC, and several other kinases [10,14]. Many of these signaling pathways have been characterized under conditions of overexpression, and their involvement in more physiological systems has not necessarily been elaborated.

Sensory neurons contain both adenosine A1 and A2A receptors (Figure 6.1). While earlier electrophysiological reports indicated the presence of adenosine A1 receptors on sensory afferent neurons in culture [15,16], it has only been more recently that these receptors have been visualized directly on such afferent fibers by immunohistochemistry in culture [17] or *in situ* [10]. Activation of adenosine A1 receptors on sensory neurons leads to reduced Ca^{2+} entry [15,16,18], decreased cyclic AMP production [17], and decreased release of calcitonin gene-related peptide [17,19,20]. Sensory afferent fibers are characterized as peptidergic and nonpeptidergic [3,21], and the ability of A1 receptors to influence peptide release suggests localization on the peptidergic population of afferent fibers. Adenosine A2A receptors have also been identified directly in dorsal root ganglia using hybridization histochemistry, and these were present in large neuronal cells [22]. There has been little *in vitro* characterization of the cellular actions of A2A receptors in this population of neurons.

Adenosine A2B and A3 receptors have not been identified in sensory neurons. The peripheral distribution of A2B receptors [13] makes it unlikely that this receptor contributes directly to regulation of nociception, but A2B receptor activation could cause release of inflammatory mediators (e.g., from

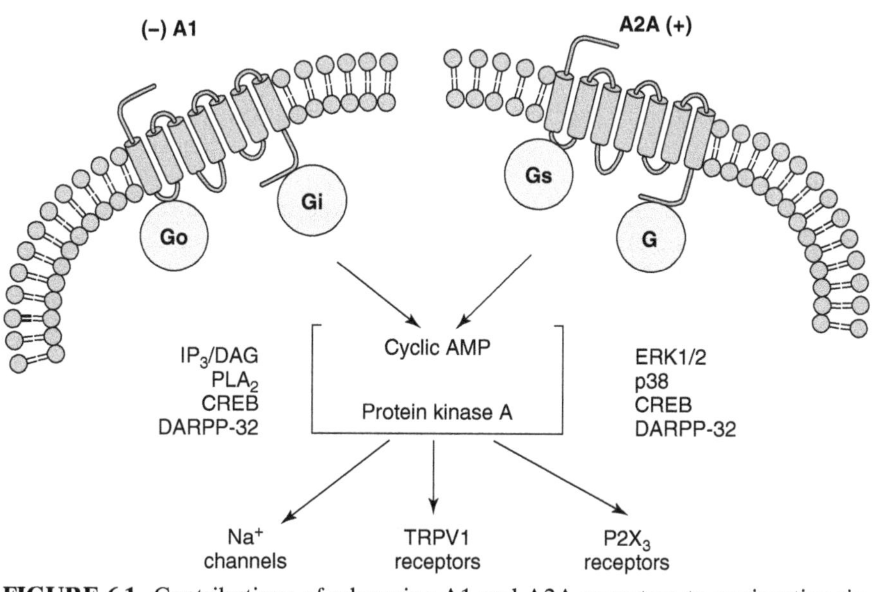

FIGURE 6.1. Contributions of adenosine A1 and A2A receptors to nociceptive signaling on peripheral sensory nerve endings.

mast cells), which then produce indirect influences on nociception. Adenosine A3 receptors are present on several types of immune and inflammatory cells, and exert complex pro- and anti-inflammatory actions [14]. Administered acutely, adenosine A3 receptor agonists promote mast cell degranulation and release of mediators and can also influence nociception indirectly via such mechanisms (see Section 6.4).

6.3 PERIPHERAL PHARMACOLOGY OF ADENOSINE A1 AND A2A RECEPTORS

The peripheral pharmacology of adenosine A1 and A2A receptors has largely been revealed by functional studies (behavioral) in which drugs have been delivered locally to the hind paw (the peripheral sensory field) and pain behaviors and/or thresholds have been determined. In many cases, the localized nature of the effects observed is verified by injections into the contralateral hind paw; actions mimicked by such contralateral administration are mediated by systemic effects that are likely mediated at spinal sites, as spinal regulation of pain transmission by adenosine A1 receptors in particular is prominent [23,24]. However, actions at supraspinal sites can also be important [25].

Local peripheral administration of adenosine A1 receptor agonists leads to antinociception in several models (Table 6.1). This includes the formalin model [26] and the rat PGE_2-induced pressure hyperalgesia model [27–29]. Following nerve injury, adenosine A1 receptor agonists also alleviate thermal hyperalgesia induced by the nerve injury (spinal nerve ligation) but do not affect tactile allodynia (to von Frey hair application); this action is locally mediated and blocked by coadministration of caffeine (adenosine A1 and A2A receptor antagonists) [30]. As thermal hyperalgesia is mediated by C-fibers, while tactile allodynia is mediated by a different population of sensory afferent fibers, likely A-fibers [31], these observations suggest the presence of adenosine A1 receptors on C-fibers.

Adenosine is an endogenous mediator involved in several regulatory processes, and intrinsic effects of antagonists can reveal local regulatory actions on a particular function. In many studies where A1 receptor antagonists are used to characterize agonist actions, A1 receptor antagonists are without intrinsic effects on nociception (e.g., 1,3-dipropyl-8-(2-amino-4-chlorophenyl) xanthine [PACPX] [27]). A1 receptor antagonists, however, can elicit hyperalgesia in rats following repeated administration of A1 receptor agonists (dependence) [27,28], or in the presence of inflammation [32]. Hyperalgesia in response to an A1 receptor antagonist is also seen in the presence of an agent that can augment release of adenosine from sensory afferent fibers (glutamate) and following a sensitizing stimulus (which leads to the activation of microglia in the spinal cord) [33]. In a recent study, local administration of the A1 receptor antagonist 1-butyl-8-(3-noradamatanyl)-3-(3-hydroxypropyl) xanthine (PSB-36) had no effect on pain behaviors produced by 5% formalin

TABLE 6.1. Peripheral Influences of Adenosine Agonists and Antagonists on Nociception.

Agent	Species, Dose	Test	Effect	Reference
A1 agonists				
R-PIA	Mouse, 10 µm	F 1%	Analgesia	[26]
NECA	Mouse, 10 µm	F 1%	Analgesia	[26]
CPA	Rat, 0.1–1 µg	PGE_2 pressure	Analgesia	[27]
CPA	Rat, 1 µg	PGE_2 pressure	Analgesia	[29]
CPA	Rat, 1 µg	PGE_2 pressure	Analgesia	[28]
CPA	Rat, 15–50 nmol	TH-SNL	Analgesia	[30]
L-PIA	Rat, 40 nmol	TH-SNL	Analgesia	[30]
A1 antagonists				
CPT	Rat, 15 nmol	F 2.5%	Hyperalgesia	[32]
CPT	Rat, 150 nmol	F 1.5%/ glutamate	Hyperalgesia	[33]
PSB-36	Mouse	F 5%	No effect	[34]
A2A agonists				
CV1808	Rat, 0.1, 1 µg	Pressure	Hyperalgesia	[21]
NECA	Rat, 0.1, 1 µg	Pressure	Hyperalgesia	[21]
APEC	Mouse, 0.1 µm	F 1%	Hyperalgesia	[26]
CGS21680	Rat, 0.1 µg	Pressure	Hyperalgesia	[29]
CGS21680	Rat, 1 µg	Pressure	Hyperalgesia	[27]
CGS21680	Rat, 1.5 nmol	F 0.5%	Hyperalgesia	[32]
A2A antagonists				
DMPX	Rat, 50 nmol	F 2.5%	Analgesia	[32]
MSX-3	Mouse	F 5%	Analgesia	[34]

R-PIA, R-phenylisopropyl adenosine; L-PIA, L-N^6-phenylisopropyl adenosine; CV1808, 2-phenylaminoadenosine; APEC, 2-(2-aminoethylamino)-carbonylethyl phenylethylamino adenosine; F, formalin; TH-SNL, thermal hyperalgesia–spinal nerve ligation.

[34]; it should, however, be noted that 5% formalin leads to maximal effects and it may be difficult to see facilitatory effects under such conditions.

In contrast to adenosine A1 receptors, local administration of adenosine A2A receptor agonists leads to enhanced nociception (Table 6.1). This has been demonstrated in the formalin model [26] and in the PGE_2 hyperalgesia to pressure model [27–29]. Consistent with this profile of activity, local administration of 3,7-dimethyl-1-propargylxanthine (DMPX), a somewhat selective A2A receptor antagonist, produces antinociception against 2.5% formalin in rats [32], while the more selective antagonist phosphoric acid mono-(3-(8-[2-(3-methoxyphenyl)vinyl]-7-methyl-2,6-dioxo-1-prop-2-ynyl-1,2,6,7-tetrahydropurin-3-yl)propyl) ester (MSX-3) inhibits pain behaviors produced by 5% formalin in mice [34]. Such effects of antagonists reveal a significant contribution of endogenous adenosine to nociception via A2A receptors under inflammatory conditions.

Mouse strains lacking genes for adenosine A1 and A2A receptors have been developed in recent years, and investigation of their phenotypes has been instructive [35]. With respect to nociception, potential alterations in sensory signaling by several different modalities, as well as drug actions have been examined. Mice lacking the adenosine A1 receptor exhibit hyperalgesia to heat but no change in mechanical thresholds (to von Frey hair stimulation) or cold responses [36,37]. Mice lacking A2A receptors exhibit hypoalgesia (i.e., increased thresholds) to heat [38,39] and a reduced response to formalin [40]. While these effects could also reflect central influences on nociception, these observations are generally consistent with the respective peripheral antinociceptive and pronociceptive effects of A1 and A2A receptors noted above.

Some studies have examined potential second messenger systems involved in adenosine A1 and A2A receptor-mediated actions. Hyperalgesia produced by 2-[p(2-carboxyethyl)phenethylamino]-5′-N-ethylcarboxamido adenosine (CGS21680) is blocked by an inhibitor of nitric oxide synthetase, and this implicates nitric oxide in A2A receptor-mediated hyperalgesia [41]. Such hyperalgesia is also attenuated by inhibitors of adenyl cyclase and PKA, implicating increased cyclic AMP production in hyperalgesia [42]. Pretreatment with an A1 receptor agonist (N^6-cyclopentyl-adenosine [CPA]) inhibits CGS21680-induced hyperalgesia, an effect expected from the local antinociceptive actions of adenosine A1 receptor agonists [29]. Curiously, posttreatment with CPA leads to augmentation of hyperalgesia; this paradoxical effect was attributed to an action of $\beta\gamma$-subunits liberated following receptor activation [29].

There are circumstantial data suggesting that adenosine A1 and A2A receptors may be localized on the same sensory neurons. Given that the effects of activating these two receptors are opposite (Figure 6.1), the relationship between these two receptors needs to be considered. There is evidence for functional complexes between A1 and A2A receptors in transfected cells and at certain presynaptic sites [12,43]. At some sites, the activation of A2A receptors leads to decreased affinity of ligands for A1 receptors, and the complex operates as a concentration-dependent switch mechanism [43]. At other sites, the receptor complex may contribute to the actions of caffeine, as caffeine has a similar affinity for A1 receptors alone or with A2A receptors, but a lower affinity for A2A receptors when these are present in dimer form [12]. It is interesting to note that caffeine administered peripherally is largely without intrinsic peripheral actions on sensory function even though selective antagonists for A1 and A2A receptors can reveal intrinsic influences on nociception (cf. References 32 and 34). The issue of potential colocalization, formation of complexes, and functional consequences of A1 and A2A receptors on the same sensory neuron has not been explored directly.

Adenosine A1 receptors may also form heteroreceptor complexes with unrelated receptors, and there is evidence for such complexes on sensory neurons from functional studies. Thus, repeated administration of CPA produced tolerance (loss of response) and dependence (rebound with administration of antagonist); cross-tolerance and cross-dependence between agents interacting with μ-opioid and $\alpha 2$-adrenergic receptors and adenosine A1 receptors was observed [28]. These results led to the suggestion of a tri-receptor functional complex on sensory neurons that could influence sensory nerve activation [28]. Whether peripheral combinations of adenosine agents with opioids or with α2-adrenergic agents would be a useful approach for pain relief remains to be investigated.

6.4 PERIPHERAL PHARMACOLOGY OF ADENOSINE A2B AND A3 RECEPTORS

As noted above (Section 6.2), A2B and A3 receptors may not act directly on sensory afferent fibers but are more likely to influence nociception indirectly via their influences on inflammatory cells (e.g., mast cells) that are in proximity to sensory nerve endings. Mice lacking A3 receptors show no changes in thermal or mechanical thresholds, but they do exhibit a reduced hyperalgesia in response to carrageenan; this is consistent with the involvement of A3 receptors in inflammatory processes mediating pronociceptive actions [44]. Mice lacking A2B receptors were developed more recently; these exhibit enhanced inflammatory responses, suggesting that A2B receptors protect against inflammation [45,46].

Several studies have examined the peripheral pharmacology of these receptors by determining the effects of local administration of selective agonists and antagonists on pain behaviors and edema. The A2B and A3 receptor agonist N^6-benzyl-5′-(N-ethyl)-carboxamido-adenosine (NECA) administered locally to the rat hind paw, alone and in combination with a low concentration of formalin (0.5%), leads to pain behaviors (flinching) as well as producing paw edema; both actions result from histamine and 5-HT release [47]. The selective A3 receptor agonist N^6-(3-iodobenzyl)-N-methyl-5′-carbamyladenosine (IB-MECA) also produces potent paw edema and plasma extravasation via release of mast cell mediators [48,49]. Recently, local administration of a selective antagonist for A2B receptors (1-propyl-8-(4-sulfophenyl) xanthine [PSB-1115]) inhibited both pain behaviors and paw edema produced by local injection of 5% formalin to the mouse hind paw, while a selective A3 receptor antagonist ((R)-8-ethyl-4-methyl-2-[2,3,5-trichlorophenyl)-4,5,7,8-tetrahydro-1H-imidazol[2,1-I]purin-5-one [PSB-10]) inhibited paw edema but had no effect on pain behaviors [34]. These observations for both agonists and antagonists at A2B and A3 receptors are generally consistent with pronociceptive and proinflammatory influences for these receptors, even though there are differences in details (i.e., how inflammation is produced).

6.5 INDIRECTLY ACTING AGENTS INVOLVING ADENOSINE

Local tissue levels of adenosine are regulated by production, transport, and metabolism, and can be altered by inhibition of two key enzymes, adenosine kinase (low capacity, high affinity) and adenosine deaminase (high capacity, low affinity) [50]. Effects of local peripheral administration of inhibitors of adenosine metabolism on sensory function mediated by localized actions are summarized in Table 6.2. Peripheral administration of the adenosine kinase inhibitor 5′-amino-5′-deoxyadenosine (NH_2dAD) results in an intensity-dependent antinociception in the formalin model, whereby antinociception is observed at a low concentration of formalin (0.5%) but not at higher concentrations unless there has been a prior exposure to formalin on the contralateral side [51]. This prior exposure was later shown to amplify peripheral adenosine A1 receptor regulation of sensory signaling, perhaps as a result of activation of spinal microglia [33]. Following nerve injury, NH_2dAD relieved thermal hyperalgesia produced by nerve injury (spinal nerve ligation) but had no effect on mechanical allodynia [51]. Local peripheral administration of 2′-deoxycoformycin (DCF), an inhibitor of adenosine deaminase, had no effect alone in the formalin test but augmented the action of an ineffective dose of NH_2dAD at a low concentration of formalin [51]. However, following spinal nerve ligation, DCF led to a long-lasting relief of thermal hyperalgesia but had no effect on mechanical allodynia [30]. In all instances, antinociception produced by inhibitors of adenosine metabolism could be reduced by coadministration with caffeine, supporting involvement of endogenous adenosine and by implication, adenosine A1 receptors (Section 6.3).

Several other studies have examined potential peripheral effects of inhibitors of adenosine kinase using the carrageenan-induced thermal hyperalgesia model of inflammation. Both NH_2dAD and DCF had little effect at 300 nmol [52]; given that doses lower than this were active in the low-concentration formalin model (Table 6.2), this suggests that such actions occur at milder, but not under strong, inflammatory conditions. Antinociceptive effects *were* seen at a dose of 1 μmol, but these were due to systemic actions as they were also observed with contralateral injections [52]. Several novel adenosine kinase

TABLE 6.2. Peripheral Influences of Inhibitors of Adenosine Kinase and Adenosine Deaminase on Nociception.

Agent	Species, Dose	Test	Effect	Reference
Adenosine kinase inhibitors				
NH_2dAD	Rat, 1–100 nmol	F 0.5%	Antinociception	[51]
		F 1.5% (pretreated)		
NH_2dAD	Rat, 100 nmol	TH-SNL	Antinociception	[30]
		MA-SNL	No effect	
Adenosine deaminase inhibitors				
DCF	Rat, 1–100 nmol	F 0.5%	No effect	[51]
DCF	Rat, 100 nmol	TH-SNL	Antinociception	[30]
		MA-SNL	No effect	

F, formalin; TH-SNL, thermal hyperalgesia–spinal nerve ligation; MA-SNL, mechanical allodynia–spinal nerve ligation.

inhibitors have been developed as part of exploring whether this could be an innovative strategy for analgesia [53]. Effects seen following intraplantar administration of A-134974, one of these novel adenosine kinase inhibitors, were due entirely to systemic actions, as they were also observed following contralateral administration [54]. Effects of intraplantar A-134974 in relieving mechanical allodynia following spinal nerve ligation were similarly due to systemic actions [55].

Microdialysis studies provide further insights into the contributions of endogenous adenosine to peripheral nociceptive regulation. Local peripheral administration of both NH_2dAD and DCF leads to elevated tissue levels of adenosine following formalin, with effects occurring selectively at low (0.5–1.5%, for NH_2dAD) or high (5%, for DCF) concentrations of formalin [56]. At low concentrations, up to 1.5%, the response to formalin is largely neurogenic, while at high concentrations, especially at 5%, there is a prominent tissue inflammation [57]. Furthermore, at a low concentration, adenosine release is largely from sensory afferent fibers, but at a higher concentration, there is additional release from sympathetic nerves [58]. This pattern of influences suggests that a more pronounced degree of tissue inflammation is a condition that allows for involvement of adenosine deaminase in regulating peripheral adenosine levels. Following spinal nerve ligation, there was an enhanced tissue release of adenosine in response to local injections of saline, but NH_2dAD and DCF did not further alter this [59]. This particular nerve injury model is not known to have a prominent inflammatory component, and it would be of interest to explore other nerve injury models, such as the partial sciatic nerve ligation model, in which inflammation is known to contribute to altered sensory signaling. The local effects of these two classes of inhibitors on sensory function and on tissue levels of adenosine clearly depend on the conditions under which they are applied.

These observations collectively highlight the condition-dependent nature of peripheral regulation of nociception by agents that inhibit adenosine metabolism. Two general observations can be made: (1) Regulation occurs at low intensities of formalin (where the response is largely neurogenic) but not at higher concentrations of formalin or following carrageenan, where inflammation is a prominent contributor to hyperalgesia. (2) Peripheral regulation of responses mediated by C-fibers occurs (thermal hyperalgesia), but there is no regulation of responses mediated by fibers less sensitive to capsaicin (i.e., mechanical allodynia).

6.6 ADENOSINE AND OTHER PHARMACOLOGICAL AGENTS

Some pharmacological agents appear to utilize endogenous adenosine systems as part of their antinociceptive actions when administered peripherally. Thus, local peripheral administration of amitriptyline (tricyclic antidepressant used orally as an adjuvant analgesic in chronic pain [60]) produces antinociception in the formalin test [61] and in the spinal nerve ligation model (against thermal hyperalgesia) [62]; in both instances, this local effect is inhibited by coadministration of caffeine (blocks A1 and A2A receptors) or 8-cyclopentyl-1,3-dimethyl xanthine (CPT) (blocks A1 receptors). Microdialysis reveals that amitriptyline increases tissue levels of adenosine, perhaps by blocking cellular uptake [63]. Amitriptyline exerts several pharmacological actions (e.g., block of norepinephrine and 5-HT uptake, block of Na^+ channels, block of N-methyl-D-aspartate [NMDA] glutamate receptors, block of cholinergic, histaminic, and adrenergic receptors), many of which are implicated in antinociception [64], but the ability of methylxanthine adenosine receptor antagonists to inhibit antinociception implicates adenosine-based mechanisms as a component of such actions.

Similar observations have been reported for another drug, carbamazepine, which was introduced as an anticonvulsant agent. Oxcarbazepine, an analog that is better tolerated than the parent compound, exhibits systemic analgesic properties in several preclinical models of nociception [65] and exhibits promise in treatment of neuropathic pain in humans [66]. Oxcarbazepine produces a local peripheral antinociceptive effect in the concanavalin A thermal hyperalgesia model, and both caffeine and 1,3-dipropyl-8-cyclopentylxanthine (DPCPX) (selective A1 receptor antagonist) decrease the antihyperalgesic effect of oxcarbazepine [65]. There are several reports of carbamazepine and its derivatives interacting directly with adenosine A1 receptors [67], and this interaction may reflect agonist actions at such receptors.

6.7 POTENTIAL FOR DEVELOPMENT AS ANALGESICS

The profile of activity of A1 receptor agonists, whereby local administration of agonists produces antinociception in several preclinical tests for nociception, provides a basis for considering whether the localized topical delivery of such agents to peripheral aspects of sensory nerves would be of benefit in inflammatory conditions or in neuropathic pain states. Key observations supporting an antinociceptive potential include the demonstration of antinociception by A1 receptor agonists and an inhibitor of adenosine kinase in preclinical models involving C-fiber activation (low concentrations of formalin; thermal hyperalgesia after nerve injury), and antinociception in a pressure hyperalgesia model (Tables 6.1 and 6.2). Antinociception with such agents, however, is dependent on conditions and end points, and there is no evidence for a localized antinociception under more pronounced conditions of inflammation (higher concentrations of formalin, carrageenan hyperalgesia) or conditions that use other populations of sensory afferent fibers (i.e., with allodynia, which is mediated via A-fibers).

A2A receptors are located on sensory nerves and adjacent inflammatory cells; they play a significant role in inflammation, and selective agonists are considered to be potential novel anti-inflammatory agents. However, local administration of adenosine A2A receptor agonists produces pronociceptive actions (Table 6.1), and knockout mice exhibit a hypoalgesic phenotype [39,40], and this suggests that blockade of A2A receptors would be of benefit to peripheral pain control. The multiplicity of actions of A2A receptors on neuronal versus inflammatory cell targets may confound the potential for agents of this class to be useful peripheral analgesics.

At peripheral sites, adenosine A2B and A3 receptors are not located on sensory neurons but on adjacent inflammatory and immune cells that may release mediators that can indirectly influence sensory nerve function. Effects of local administration of A2B and A3 receptor agonists facilitate nociception and cause edema, while local administration of selective antagonists inhibit edema and, for A2B receptors, nociception as well [34]. Such observations suggest that if there was a role for such receptors in peripheral pain regulation, an antagonist profile would be more beneficial. However, as A3 receptors can have complex effects on inflammatory and immune function [14,34], and recent A2B knockout mice exhibit increased inflammatory responses [45], their multiplicity of actions may confound their usefulness as analgesics.

Some pharmacological agents (amitriptyline, oxcarbazepine), which exhibit several mechanisms of action, also interact with adenosine-based systems as revealed by sensitivity to adenosine receptor antagonists. It is interesting to note that such agents produce peripheral antinociception with higher concentrations of formalin (amitriptyline [61]) and with more pronounced inflammation (concanavalin A-induced thermal hyperalgesia) (oxcarbazepine [65]). Both agents also exhibit other pharmacological actions, in particular, block of Na^+ channels [64,67]. Given that such channels are key in sensory nerve activation (depolarization), modification (by phosphorylation), and modulation (altered ion channel expression), it may be that a duality of action (or even a multiplicity of action, as there are other effects involved as well) is required in order to see the expression of prominent inhibition of sensory nerve activation following the activation of adenosine A1 receptors.

Another final issue to consider is that of receptor complexes involving adenosine. Thus, there is some evidence for adenosine A1 receptors occurring as a receptor complex with μ-opioid and α2-adrenergic receptors on sensory neurons [28]. Given that both of those agents also lead to peripheral pain-relieving effects, the examination of the effects of combinations of agonists for these systems in a range of preclinical models for nociception may be worthwhile.

REFERENCES

1. Millan, M.J. (1999). The induction of pain: an integrative review. *Prog Neurobiol* 57:1–164.
2. Millan, M.J. (2002). Descending control of pain. *Prog Neurobiol* 66:355–474.

3. Woolf, C.J., Ma, Q. (2007). Nociceptors–noxious stimulus detectors. *Neuron* 55:353–364.
4. Caterina, M.J., Julius, D. (2001). The vanilloid receptor: a molecular gateway to the pain receptor. *Annu Rev Neurosci* 24:487–517.
5. Julius, D., Basbaum, A.I. (2001). Molecular mechanisms of nociception. *Nature* 413:203–210.
6. Cortright, D.N., Krause, J.E., Broom, D.C. (2007). TRP channels and pain. *Biochim Biophys Acta* 1772:978–988.
7. England, S., Bevan, S., Docherty, R.J. (1996). PGE2 modulates the tetrodotoxin-resistant sodium current in neonatal rat dorsal root ganglion neurons via the cyclic AMP-protein kinase A cascade. *J Physiol* 495:429–440.
8. Gold, M.S., Reichling, D.B., Schuster, M.J., Levine, J.D. (1996). Hyperalgesic agents increase a tetrodotoxin-resistant Na+ current in nociceptors. *Proc Natl Acad Sci U S A* 93:1108–1112.
9. Fredholm, B.B., Ijzerman, A.P., Jacobson, K.A., Klotz, K.N., Linden, J. (2001). International Union of Pharmacology. XXV. Nomenclature and classification of adenosine receptors. *Pharmacol Rev* 53:527–552.
10. Schulte, G., Fredholm, B.B. (2003). Signalling from adenosine receptors to mitogen-activated protein kinases. *Cell Signal* 15:813–827.
11. Brust, T.B., Cayabyab, F.S., Zhou, N., MacVicar, B.A. (2006). p38 Mitogen-activated protein kinase contributes to adenosine A1 receptor-mediated synaptic depression in area CA1 of the rat hippocampus. *J Neurosci* 26:12427–12438.
12. Fredholm, B.B., Chen, Y., Franco, R., Sitkovsky, M. (2007). Aspects of the general biology of adenosine A2A signaling. *Prog Neurobiol* 83:263–276.
13. Baraldi, P.G., Romagnoli, R., Preti, D., Fruttarolo, F., Carrion, M.D., Tabrizi, M.A. (2006). Ligands for A2B adenosine receptor subtypes. *Curr Med Chem* 13:3467–3482.
14. Gessi, S., Marighi, S., Varani, K., Leung, E., Maclennan, S., Borea, P.A. (2008). The A3 adenosine receptor: an enigmatic player in cell biology. *Pharmacol Ther* 117:123–140.
15. Dolphin, A.C., Forda, S.R., Scott, R.H. (1986). Calcium-dependent currents in cultured rat dorsal root ganglion neurons are inhibited by an adenosine analogue. *J Physiol* 373:47–61.
16. MacDonald, R.I., Skerritt, J.H., Werz, M.A. (1986). Adenosine agonists reduce voltage-dependent calcium conductance of mouse sensory neurons in cell culture. *J Physiol* 370:75–80.
17. Carruthers, A.M., Sellers, L.A., Jenkins, D.W., Jarvie, E.M., Feniuk, W., Humphrey, P.P.A. (2001). Adenosine A1 receptor-mediated inhibition of protein kinase A-induced calcitonin gene-related peptide release from rat trigeminal neurons. *Mol Pharmacol* 59:1533–1541.
18. Haas, H.L., Selbach, O. (2000). Functions of neuronal adenosine receptors. *Naunyn Schmiedebergs Arch Pharmacol* 362:375–381.
19. Mauborgne, A., Polienor, H., Hamon, M., Cesselin, F., Bourgoin, S. (2002). Adenosine receptor-mediated control of in vitro release of pain-related neuropeptides from the rat spinal cord. *Eur J Pharmacol* 441:47–55.

20. Santicioli, P., Del Bianco, E., Maggi, C.A. (1993). Adenosine A1 receptors mediate the presynaptic inhibition of calcitonin gene-related peptide release by adenosine in the rat spinal cord. *Eur J Pharmacol* 231:139–142.
21. Snider, W.D., McMahon, S.B. (1998). Tackling pain at the source: new ideas about nociceptors. *Neuron* 20:629–632.
22. Kaelin-Lang, A., Lauterburg, T., Burgunder, J.M. (1998). Expression of adenosine A2A receptor gene in rat dorsal root and autonomic ganglia. *Neurosci Lett* 246: 21–24.
23. Sawynok, J., Liu, X.J. (2003). Adenosine in the spinal cord and periphery: release and regulation of pain. *Prog Neurobiol* 69:313–340.
24. Sawynok, J. (1998). Adenosine receptor activation and nociception. *Eur J Pharmacol* 347:1–11.
25. Ramos-Zepeda, G., Schröder, W., Rosenow, S., Herrero, J.F. (2004). Spinal vs supraspinal antinociceptive activity of the adenosine A1 receptor agonist cyclopentyladenosine in rats with inflammation. *Eur J Pharmacol* 499:247–256.
26. Karlsten, R., Gordh, T., Post, C. (1992). Local antinociceptive and hyperalgesic effects in the formalin test after peripheral administration of adenosine analogues in mice. *Pharmacol Toxicol* 70:434–438.
27. Aley, K.O., Green, P.G., Levine, J.D. (1995). Opioid and adenosine peripheral antinociception are subject to tolerance and withdrawal. *J Neurosci* 15:8031–8038.
28. Aley, K.O., Levine, J.D. (1997). Multiple receptors involved in peripheral α2, μ and A1 antinociception, tolerance, and withdrawal. *J Neurosci* 17:735–744.
29. Khasar, S.G., Wang, J.F., Taiwo, Y.O., Heller, P.H., Green, P.G., Levine, J.D. (1995). Mu-opioid agonist enhancement of prostaglandin-induced hyperalgesia in the rat: a G-protein beta gamma subunit-mediated effect? *Neuroscience* 67:189–195.
30. Liu, X.J., Sawynok, J. (2000). Peripheral antihyperalgesic effects by adenosine A1 receptor agonists and inhibitors of adenosine metabolism in a rat neuropathic pain model. *Analgesia* 5:19–29.
31. Field, M.J., Bramwell, S., Hughes, J., Singh, L. (1999). Detection of static and dynamic components of mechanical allodynia in rat models of neuropathic pain: are they signaled by distinct primary sensory neurons? *Pain* 83:303–311.
32. Doak, G.J., Sawynok, J. (1995). Complex role of peripheral adenosine in the genesis of the response to subcutaneous formalin in the rat. *Eur J Pharmacol* 281: 311–318.
33. Aumeerally, N., Allen, G., Sawynok, J. (2004). Glutamate-evoked release of adenosine and regulation of peripheral antinociception. *Neuroscience* 127:1–11.
34. Bilkei-Gorzo, A., Abo-Salem, O.M., Hayallah, A.M., Michel, K., Muller, C.E., Zimmer, A. (2008). Adenosine receptor subtype-selective antagonists in inflammation and hyperalgesia. *Naunyn Schmiedebergs Arch Pharmacol* 377:65–76.
35. Fredholm, B.B., Chen, J.F., Masino, S.A., Vaugeois, J.M. (2005). Actions of adenosine at its receptors in the CNS: insights from knockouts and drugs. *Annu Rev Pharmacol Toxicol* 45:385–412.
36. Johansson, B., Halldner, L., Dunwiddie, T.V., Masino, S.A., Poelchen, W., Giménez-Llort, L., Escorihuela, R.M., Fernández-Teruel, A., Weisenfeld-Hallin, Z., Xu, X., Hardemark, A., Betscholtz, C., Herlenius, E., Fredholm, B.B. (2001).

Hyperalgesia, anxiety, and decreased hypoxic neuroprotection in mice lacking the adenosine A1 receptor. *Proc Natl Acad Sci U S A* 98:9407–9412.

37. Wu, W.P., Hao, J.X., Halldner-Henriksson, L., Xu, X.J., Jacobson, M.A., Weisenfeld-Hallin, Z., Fredholm, B.B. (2005). Increased nociceptive response in mice lacking the adenosine A1 receptor. *Pain* 113:395–404.
38. Godfrey, L., Yan, L., Clarke, G.D., Ledent, C., Kitchen, I., Hourani, S.M.O. (2006). Modulation of paracetamol antinociception by caffeine and by selective adenosine A2 receptor antagonists in mice. *Eur J Pharmacol* 531:80–86.
39. Ledent, C., Vaugeois, J.M., Schiffmann, S.N., Pedrazzini, T., El Yacoubi, M., Vanderhaegehen, J.J., Costentin, J., Heath, J.K., Vassart, G., Paremetier, M. (1997). Aggressiveness, hypoalgesia and high blood pressure in mice lacking the adenosine A2A receptor. *Nature* 388:674–678.
40. Hussey, M.J., Clarke, G.D., Ledent, C., Hourani, S.M.O., Kitchen, I. (2007). Reduced response to the formalin test and lowered spinal NMDA glutamate receptor binding in adenosine A2A receptor knockout mice. *Pain* 129:287–294.
41. Aley, K.O., McCarther, G., Levine, J.D. (1998). Nitric oxide signaling in pain and nociceptor sensitization in the rat. *J Neurosci* 18:7008–7014.
42. Aley, K.O., Levine, J.D. (1999). Role of protein kinase A in the maintenance of inflammatory pain. *J Neurosci* 19:2181–2186.
43. Ferré, S., Ciruela, F., Quiroz, C., Luján, R., Popoli, P., Cunha, R.A., Agnati, L.F., Fuxe, K., Woods, A.S., Lluis, C., Franco, R. (2007). Adenosine receptor heteromers and their integrative role in striatal function. *ScientificWorldJournal* 7:74–85.
44. Wu, W.P., Hao, J.X., Halldner-Henricksson, L., Xu, X.-J., Jacobson, M.A., Weisenfeld-Hallin, A., Fredholm, B.B. (2002). Decreased inflammatory pain due to reduced carrageenan-induced inflammation in mice lacking adenosine A3 receptors. *Neuroscience* 114:523–527.
45. Yang, D., Zhang, Y., Nguyen, H.G., Koupenova, M., Chauhan, A.K., Makitalo, M., Jones, M.R., St Hilare, C., Sheldin, D.C., Toselli, P., Lamperti, E., Schreiber, B.M., Gavras, H., Wagner, D.D., Ravid, K. (2006). The A2B adenosine receptor protects against inflammation and excessive vascular adhesion. *J Clin Invest* 116:1913–1923.
46. Hua, X., Kovarova, M., Chasan, K.D., Nguyen, M., Koller, B.H., Tilley, S.L. (2007). Enhanced mast cell activation in mice deficient in the A2B adenosine receptor. *J Exp Med* 204:117–128.
47. Sawynok, J., Zarrindast, M.R., Reid, A., Doak, G. (1997). Adenosine A3 receptor activation produces nociceptive behavior and edema by release of histamine and 5-hydroxytryptamine. *Eur J Pharmacol* 333:1–7.
48. Reeves, J.J., Jones, C.A., Sheehan, M.J., Vardey, C.J., Whelan, C.J. (1997). Adenosine A3 receptors promote degranulation of rat mast cells both in vitro and in vivo. *Inflamm Res* 46:180–184.
49. Esquisatto, L.C.M., Costa, S.K.P., Camargo, E.A., Ribela, M.T.C.P., Brain, S.D., de Nucci, G., Antunes, E. (2001). The plasma protein extravasation induced by adenosine and its analogues in the rat dorsal skin: evidence for the involvement of capsaicin sensitive primary afferent neurones and mast cells. *Brit J Pharmacol* 134:108–115.

50. Fredholm, B.B. (2007). Adenosine, an endogenous distress signal, modulates tissue damage and repair. *Cell Death Differ* 14:1315–1323.
51. Sawynok, J., Reid, A., Poon, A. (1998). Peripheral antinociceptive effect of an adenosine kinase inhibitor, with augmentation by an adenosine deaminase inhibitor, in the rat formalin test. *Pain* 74:75–81.
52. Poon, A., Sawynok, J. (1999). Antinociceptive and anti-inflammatory properties of an adenosine kinase inhibitor and an adenosine deaminase inhibitor. *Eur J Pharmacol* 384:123–138.
53. McGaraughty, S., Cowart, M., Jarvis, M.F., Berman, R.F. (2005). Anticonvulsant and antinociceptive actions of novel adenosine kinase inhibitors. *Curr Top Med Chem* 5:43–58.
54. McGaraughty, S., Chu, K.L., Wismer, C.T., Mikusa, J., Zhu, C.Z., Cowart, M., Kowaluk, E.A., Jarvis, M.F. (2001). Effects of A-134974, a novel adenosine kinase inhibitor, on carrageenan-induced inflammatory hyperalgesia and locomotor activity in rats: evaluation of the sites of action. *J Pharmacol Exp Ther* 296:501–509.
55. Zhu, C.Z., Mikusa, J., Chu, K.L., Cowart, M., Kowaluk, E.A., Jarvis, M.F., McGaraughty, S. (2001). A-134974: a novel adenosine kinase inhibitor, relieves tactile allodynia via spinal sites of action in peripheral nerve injured rats. *Brain Res* 905:104–110.
56. Liu, X.J., White, T.D., Sawynok, J. (2000). Potentiation of formalin-evoked adenosine release by an adenosine kinase inhibitor and an adenosine deaminase inhibitor in the rat hind paw: a microdialysis study. *Eur J Pharmacol* 408:143–152.
57. Sawynok, J., Liu, X.J. (2004). The formalin test: characteristics and usefulness of the model. *Rev Analg* 7:145–163.
58. Liu, X.J., White, T.D., Sawynok, J. (2001). Involvement of primary sensory afferents, postganglionic sympathetic nerves and mast cells in the formalin-evoked peripheral release of adenosine. *Eur J Pharmacol* 429:147–155.
59. Liu, X.J., White, T.D., Sawynok, J. (2002). Enhanced release of adenosine in rat hind paw following spinal nerve ligation: involvement of capsaicin-sensitive sensory afferents. *Neuroscience* 114:379–387.
60. Finnerup, N.B., Otto, M., McQuay, H.J., Jensen, T.S., Sindrup, S.H. (2005). Algorithm for neuropathic pain treatment: an evidence based proposal. *Pain* 118:289–305.
61. Sawynok, J., Reid, A.R., Esser, M.J. (1999). Peripheral antinociceptive action of amitriptyline in the rat formalin test: involvement of adenosine. *Pain* 80:45–55.
62. Esser, M.J., Sawynok, J. (2000). Caffeine block of the thermal antihyperalgesic effect of acute amitriptyline in a rat model of neuropathic pain. *Eur J Pharmacol* 399:131–139.
63. Sawynok, J., Reid, A., Liu, X.J., Parkinson, F.E. (2005). Amitriptyline enhances extracellular levels of adenosine in the rat hindpaw and inhibits adenosine uptake. *Eur J Pharmacol* 518:116–122.
64. Micó, J.A., Ardid, D., Berrocoso, E., Eschalier, A. (2006). Antidepressants and pain. *Trends Pharmacol Sci* 27:348–354.
65. Tomic, M.A., Vucokic, S.M., Stepanovic-Petrovic, R.M., Ugresic, N., Prostran, M.S., Boskovic, B. (2004). The anti-hyperalgesic effects of carbamazepine and oxcarbazepine are attenuated by treatment with adenosine receptor antagonists. *Pain* 111:253–260.

66. Dogra, S., Beydoun, S., Mazzola, J., Hopwood, M., Wan, Y. (2005). Oxcarbazepine in painful diabetic neuropathy: a randomized, placebo-controlled study. *Eur J Pain* 9:543–554.
67. Ambrosio, A.F., Soares-da-Silva, P., Carvalho, C.M., Carvalho, A.P. (2002). Mechanisms of action of carbamazepine and its derivatives, oxcarbazepine, BIA 2-093, and BIA 2-024. *Neurochemical Res* 27:121–130.

CHAPTER 7

Acid-Sensing Ion Channels and Pain

ROXANNE Y. WALDER,[1] CHRISTOPHER J. BENSON,[2] and KATHLEEN A. SLUKA[1]

[1]Graduate Program in Physical Therapy and Rehabilitation Science, Pain Research Program, Neuroscience Graduate Program, University of Iowa
[2]Department of Internal Medicine, University of Iowa

Content

7.1 INTRODUCTION

Pain is a complex experience that is unique to each individual. The International Association for the Study of Pain (www.iasp-pain.org) defines pain as "an unpleasant sensory and emotional experience associated with actual or potential tissue damage, or described in terms of such damage." Pain can arise as a result of damage to any tissue that is innervated by nociceptors. Everyone has

Peripheral Receptor Targets for Analgesia: Novel Approaches to Pain Management, Edited by Brian E. Cairns

or will experience pain at some point in his or her life. Pain can be either acute or chronic. Acute pain occurs as a direct result of tissue damage or potential tissue damage. Acute pain serves to protect oneself from tissue damage and, if tissue damage has occurred, to allow time for healing. Acute pain that requires clinical treatment usually results from observable tissue damage associated with an inflammatory process. Acute pain is usually treated with pharmacological and nonpharmacological remedies aimed at the peripheral tissue damage. For example, nonsteroidal anti-inflammatory drugs (NSAIDs) or ice is commonly used to treat acute inflammation associated with joint or muscle injury.

Unlike acute pain, chronic pain is not protective and does not serve a biologically beneficial purpose. Pain can be considered chronic if (i) it outlasts normal tissue healing time, (ii) the impairment is greater than would be expected from the physical findings or injury, or (iii) pain occurs in the absence of identifiable tissue damage. Most cases of acute pain resolve within 3 months. Acute pain that becomes chronic costs billions of dollars per year in health care and lost wages. When pain becomes chronic, it is no longer a symptom but rather a disease in and of itself.

Pain, either acute or chronic, is the number one reason that people seek medical attention. A Research America survey of 1004 adults from the United States shows that 57% of those surveyed experienced chronic or recurrent pain in the last 12 months [1]. A recent survey of 303 patients with chronic pain shows that they have hardships that far exceed the management of pain itself. This survey quantitatively shows that patients with chronic pain have greater limitations in conducting everyday activities, such as walking, standing, working, participating in sports or physical activities, running errands, doing household chores, taking care of self and others, traveling, and attending a public event, than those with acute pain [2]. The Center for Disease Control and Prevention's National Center for Health Statistics reports that pain is indiscriminately distributed between genders, and across age, ethnic groups, geography, and socioeconomic boundaries. Low back pain is a prevalent form of pain (28%), but a significant percentage of the population suffers from peripheral joint pain (30%), including knee (18%), neck (15%), migraine (15%), and shoulder pain (9%) [3].

Extracellular acidification at the site of tissue injury was recognized many years ago as a major factor in pain associated with conditions that include inflammation, hematomas, exercise, cardiac muscle ischemia, and cancer [4–6]. This led to the hypothesis that nociceptors express receptors that are activated by acidic pH. In the early 1980s, Krishtal and Pidoplichko were the first to study acid-activated ion channels in isolated sensory neurons [7,8]. These channels had the distinct property of being rapidly activated and desensitized by extracellular acidification; they were selectively permeable to Na^+ ions and were blocked by the drug amiloride [9]. It was not until the late 1990s that the molecular identity of these channels became known; several members belonging to the degenerin/epithelial sodium channel (DEG/ENaC) family of channels were cloned [10–14]. When these channels were expressed in heterologous cells, their properties matched those of channels recorded decades earlier by Krishtal in sensory neurons [10–15]. These channels are now called acid-sensing ion channels (ASICs), and this chapter will review our current understanding of the role of the ASICs in the generation and maintenance of pain.

7.2 ASIC ISOTYPES, STRUCTURE, AND LOCALIZATION

Based upon homology, four genes encode ASICs in mammals and these, to date, encode seven isoforms: ASIC1a, ASIC1b, ASIC1b2, ASIC2a, ASIC2b, ASIC3, and ASIC4 (ASIC1 and ASIC2 have splice variants) (see References 9, 16, and 17). Interestingly, ASIC orthologs cloned from fish and the simple chordate *Ciona intestinalis* demonstrate remarkable sequence homology and evolutionary conservation [18–23].

The recent solution of the X-ray crystal structure of the ASIC1a channel confirmed the presumed topology of ASIC proteins [24]. ASICs are relatively small proteins (~500 amino acids) and have two membrane spanning domains that flank a large extracellular loop (making up 70% of the entire protein), with relatively small intracellular N- and C-termini. Perhaps the most novel and unexpected finding revealed by the crystal structure is that ASIC channels are comprised of three subunits (Figure 7.1), as opposed to four or nine subunits based on previous stoichiometric studies of other DEG/ENaC channels [25–27]. The unusually large extracellular domain of ASICs contains multiple cavities and protrusions, including a pocket rich in acidic residues that serves as the proton-binding site. Several asparagine residues within the extracellular domain of ASICs are glycosylated and may be important for the cell-surface expression of the protein [28]. The extracellular domain of ASICs contains several cysteine residues with conserved spacing, which may be important in interactions with the extracellular matrix. This unique structure suggests that ASICs might be particularly poised to sense extracellular signals.

ASICs are found abundantly in the mammalian central (CNS) and peripheral nervous systems (PNS) where they are purported to play a role in synaptic transmission and sensory transduction [16,17]. ASIC1a, ASIC2a, and ASIC2b are widely expressed throughout the brain and PNS [9,13,15,16,29,30]. Although ASICs are expressed in pain regulatory regions such as the cerebral cortex, habenula, basolateral amygdaloid nuclei, and spinal cord, a role for brain ASICs in pain has been largely unexplored. In addition, ASIC1a, ASIC2a, ASIC3, and ASIC4 are expressed in the spinal cord [31–33].

In the PNS, ASICs are primarily localized to sensory neurons and are absent from autonomic and motor neurons. Messenger RNA (mRNA) for most ASIC isoforms is found in the sensory ganglia, and ASIC1 and ASIC3 are predominantly expressed in the periphery. ASIC1 is found in dorsal root ganglion (DRG) neurons that colocalize with substance P (SP) and calcitonin gene-related peptide (CGRP), suggesting a role in nociception [34]. In the

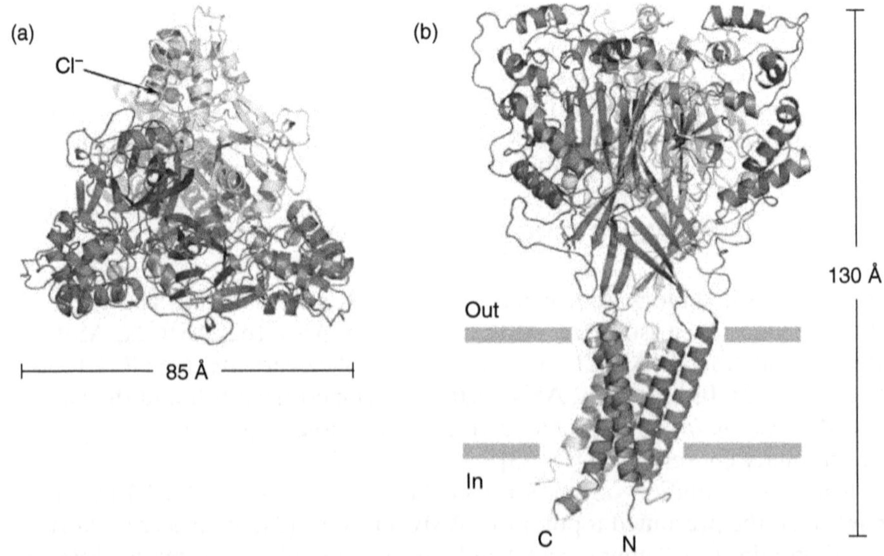

FIGURE 7.1. Trimeric structure of ASIC1. (a) View from the extracellular side. (b) Side view of the three subunits, viewed parallel to the membrane. Reprinted by permission from Jasti, J., Furukawa, H., Gonzales, E.B., Gouaux, E. (2007). Structure of acid-sensing ion channel 1 at 1.9 A resolution and low pH. *Nature* 449:316–323, copyright (2007), with permission from Macmillan Publishers Ltd. See color insert.

skin, ASIC2 and ASIC3 are located in the epidermal nociceptors and in the nerves, innervating specialized sensory structures such as Meissner's corpuscles, lanceolate fibers surrounding hair shafts, and Merkel cells [35,36]. ASIC3 was originally thought to be DRG specific and called DRASIC for "dorsal root ASIC" and is found in primary afferent fibers innervating the skin, muscle, joint, and viscera [36–40]. ASIC3 is located in free nerve endings in the epidermis that colocalize with SP and in free nerve endings innervating the muscle that colocalize with CGRP [36,37]. Interestingly, ASIC3 is found more abundantly in muscle nociceptors (~50%) than in skin nociceptors (~10%) [37]. In the skeletal muscle, ASIC3 is localized to afferent fibers in the adventitia of arterioles and coexpressed with CGRP [37]. In Figure 7.2, we show that ASIC3 is expressed in afferent fibers coursing between individual muscle fascicles. In the knee joint, ASIC3 is located in putative nociceptors innervating the synovium but only after the induction of inflammation [39]. ASICs are also located in non-neuronal cells. For example, ASIC3 is expressed in synoviocytes, intervertebral disk, bone, testis, and in cultured myocytes [39,41–44]. Both ASIC1 and ASIC3 are also expressed in the peripheral chemoreceptive glomus cells of the carotid body [45]. ASIC4 is not expressed in DRG neurons but is found in the testis and in the pituitary gland [46–48]. The role of ASICs in these non-neuronal cells is unclear at present.

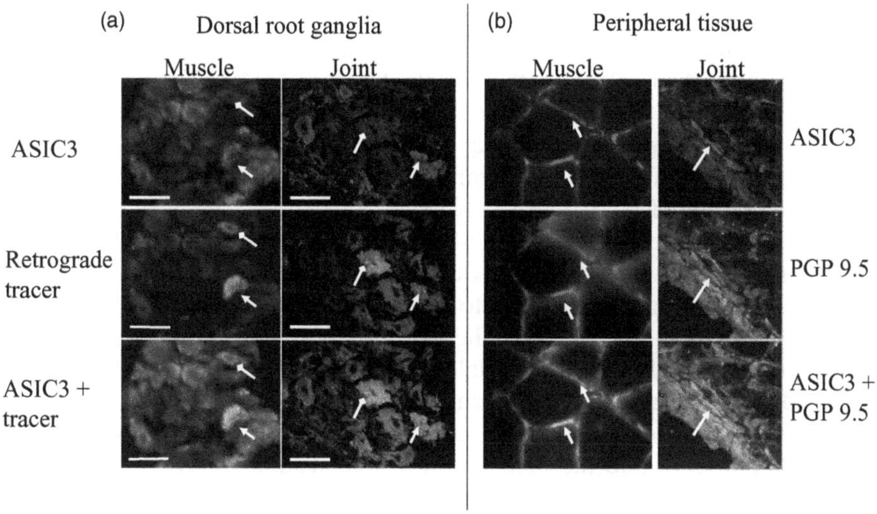

FIGURE 7.2. Immunohistochemical localization of ASIC3 in retrogradely labeled DRG neurons from the muscle and joint, or primary afferent fibers located within the muscle endomysium or joint synovium. (a) Staining for ASIC3 and a retrograde tracer (Fluoro-Gold [muscle]; Fast Blue [joint]) in DRG neurons from the muscle or joint show colocalization of ASIC3 and Fast Blue labeling in DRG neurons from wild-type mice. Muscle DRG neuron pictures are reprinted with permission from the International Association for the Study of Pain; Sluka, K.A., Price, M.P., Breese, N.M., Stucky, C.L., Wemmie, J.A., Welsh, M.J. (2003). Chronic hyperalgesia induced by repeated acid injections in muscle is abolished by the loss of ASIC3, but not ASIC1. *Pain* 106:229–239 [38], copyright 2003. (b) Primary afferent fibers innervating the muscle or joint were labeled with ASIC3 and the neuronal marker PGP 9.5. In the muscle, the endoneurium surrounding individual muscle fibers colabeled with ASIC3 and PGP 9.5. In the synovium of the knee joint 24 hours after inflammation, primary afferent fibers colabeled with ASIC3 and PGP 9.5. Knee joint pictures are reprinted with permission from the International Association for the Study of Pain; Ikeuchi, M., Kolker, S.J., Burnes, L.A., Walder, R.Y., Sluka, K.A. (2008). Role of ASIC3 in the primary and secondary hyperalgesia produced by joint inflammation in mice. *Pain* 137:662–669 [39], copyright 2008. See color insert.

7.3 ASIC FUNCTIONAL PROPERTIES

ASIC1a, ASIC1b, ASIC2a, and ASIC3 form acid-activated homomeric channels when expressed individually in heterologous cells [9,16,17]. ASIC1b2 and ASIC2b cannot be activated when expressed by themselves, but when coexpressed with other isoforms, they modulate their properties [9,16,17,49]. Despite its homology, ASIC4 does not form homomeric functional channels *in vitro* and its function remains unknown [46,47]. When two or more ASIC isoforms are coexpressed, channels are generated with distinct functional properties, indicating that heteromeric channels are formed from different isoforms [50–54]. In fact, studies suggest that the majority of ASICs in both PNS and CNS neurons is comprised of heteromers [50,55,56]. Because ASICs can form channel complexes with multiple different combinations of isoforms, each with their own distinct properties, it suggests that the ASIC subunit composition can be suited to a particular stimulus in a particular tissue.

Unusual for ligand-gated ion channels, ASICs selectively permeate Na^+ but, to a lesser extent, also conduct Li^+, K^+, Ca^{2+}, and H^+ [12]. ASIC1a homomers are most conductive of Ca^{2+}, which might be important for initiating intracellular signaling and neuronal injury during ischemia [57,58]. Most ASICs activate rapidly (within milliseconds) to acidic pH and then rapidly desensitize (within seconds). At first glance, these transient current properties are not congruent with pain, which is usually more persistent. Yagi et al. recently revealed data that address this dilemma; they found that ASIC3 homomers and ASIC2a/3 heteromers generate sustained currents in a more physiological pH range (7.3–6.7), and the mechanism of the sustained current is due to a window of overlap between the activation and desensitization ranges of the transient current [52]. Transient receptor potential vanilloid 1 (TRPV1), the capsaicin receptor, is also activated by protons and might serve as a pain receptor, such as when the pH is <6.0 [59]. However, ASICs are activated by pH changes within the physiological range and are thought to be the major channels involved in acid-induced pain.

There is an increasing body of literature demonstrating the modulatory effects of various compounds and interacting proteins on ASIC function [16,17]. These modulators may have distinct roles in different tissues such as activating and deactivating the channel, ligand binding, second messenger signaling, regulating protein turnover, cell-surface expression, facilitating the trafficking of the subunits to synapses and sensory receptors, and assembly of the subunits into functional channels. Here, we will highlight a few examples as they pertain to the role of ASICs in pain. Lactate and arachidonic acid, both released during tissue ischemia and other painful conditions, potentiate ASIC1a and ASIC3 [60–63]. Regarding lactate, it has been observed in recordings from visceral afferents that protons derived from lactate cause more neural excitation than other acids [64,65]. The molecular mechanism underlying this apparent paradox has now been explained; lactate potentiates ASICs by chelating extracellular Ca^{2+}, which blocks the conduction of Na^+ through the channel [61]. Although the mechanism is less clear, arachidonic acid induces increased acid-evoked currents in CNS and DRG neurons [60,63]. Proinflammatory mediators such as serotonin, nerve growth factor, bradykinin, and interleukin-1 increase ASIC transcript levels *in vivo* [66,67]. Inflammation also induces expression of Phe-Met-Arg-Phe (FMRF) amide-like peptides *in vivo*. FMRF amide potentiates H^+-induced currents from ASIC1 and ASIC3 expressed in heterologous cells and in cultured DRG neurons [56,68,69]. The inflammatory mediator, nitric oxide, also potentiates ASIC activity in DRG neurons and in ASICs expressed in heterologous cells [70]. In contrast, NSAIDs can directly inhibit ASIC1a and ASIC3 activity, which can in part explain their analgesic effects [67]. Finally, phosphorylation and resultant modulation of ASICs by cyclic adenosine monophosphate (cAMP)-dependent protein kinase A (PKA) [71], protein kinase C (PKC) [55], and calcium/calmodulin-dependent protein kinase II (CaMKII) [72] suggest that ASICs might be modulated by multiple signaling pathways, including those that regulate pain signaling.

ASICs share sequence homology with the DEGs in the nematode *Caenorabditis elegans*, such as the mechanosensitive DEG/ENaC channels Mec-4 and Mec-10 [73,74]. However, the role of ASICs as mechanosensors in mammals is controversial. Initial studies using skin nerve preparations of ASIC2 and ASIC3 knockout mice show subtle changes in rapidly adapting mechanosensation and Aδ nociceptors [35,36]. ASIC3 knockout mice, however, show either enhanced or no changes in mechanosensation to von Frey filaments relative to controls [36,75]. Other studies show that ASIC2 knockout mice do not have differences in cutaneous mechanical sensation and visceral mechanonociception relative to wild-type mice [76]. Cultured DRG neurons from ASIC2 knockout and ASIC3 knockout mice show no differences upon mechanical stimulation, compared with DRG neurons from wild-type mice [77]. Transgenic mice expressing a dominant negative mutant form of ASIC3, which inhibits acid-evoked current, show increases in behavioral responses to mechanical stimulation [78]. Recordings from gastrointestinal afferent fibers from ASIC1, ASIC2, and ASIC3 knockout mice show that the lack of any one of the three ASICs causes variable responses, both increased and decreased, to mechanosensitive stimulation, compared with wild-type mice [79]. The role that ASICs play in mechanosensation is complex and unclear. More studies are needed to establish whether they play a direct role in mechanosensation.

ASICs are reversibly blocked by amiloride and related compounds. Their nonselectivity and lack of potency (IC_{50} ~50 μm) has led to the search for better pharmacological agents. The small molecule, A-317567, nonselectively inhibits ASIC currents in DRG neurons, is more potent than amiloride, and does not have amiloride-like diuretic effects [80]. More specific inhibitors of ASICs include the tarantula toxin PcTx1, which blocks the ASIC1a homomeric channel (IC_{50} ~0.9 nM) [81–83]. PcTx1 binds but does not inhibit ASIC1b [84]. At 100 nM, PcTx1 increases the H^+ affinity of ASIC1b and slows the desensitization of the channel and, therefore, actually potentiates ASIC1b [84]. The sea anemone toxin APETx2, blocks homomeric ASIC3 (IC_{50} ~63 nM) as well as ASIC3-containing heteromeric channels (IC_{50} ~0.1–2 μm) [85,86].

7.4 ASICs IN ANIMAL MODELS OF PAIN

Our understanding of the physiological function of ASICs in pain behavior has been facilitated by the use of ASIC blockers and the generation of genetically mutant mice. Knockout mice have been developed for ASIC1a, ASIC2, and ASIC3 [35,36,75,76,87]. Initial studies examining the acid-evoked currents in ASIC knockout and transgenic mice showed significant differences from wild-type controls in cultured neurons [36,50,51,87]. DRG neurons from ASIC1a, ASIC2, or ASIC3 knockout mice still express acid-activated currents, but the pattern of the derived current reveals that the channels are heteromers formed from the remaining ASIC subunits [50]. In addition, DRG neurons from ASIC3 knockout mice show a slower rate of desensitization of acid-activated current, and the current is more sensitive to amiloride, as compared with wild-type controls [51]. Given these alterations in H^+-activated currents in sensory neurons from ASIC knockout mice, subsequent studies examined the genetically modified mice for deficits in nocifensive behaviors in a variety of animal models of pain [35,36,38,39,75,76,78,88].

7.4.1 ASICs in Inflammatory Pain

Peripheral inflammation results in an acute inflammatory process that is associated with decreases in pH, release of inflammatory cytokines, and pain [63,66,89–91]. A number of animal models have been developed to assess mechanisms involving both the PNS and CNS in inflammatory pain and include the injection of inflammatory irritants such as capsaicin, carrageenan, zymosan, formalin, or complete Freund's adjuvant. These irritants are injected into the paw of the animal to produce cutaneous inflammation and hyperalgesia, as well as into the muscle and joints to produce deep tissue injury and associated hyperalgesia. In animals with carrageenan inflammation of the paw, there is an increase in sensitivity to mechanical and heat stimulation of the paw, termed primary hyperalgesia. The injection of carrageenan into the muscle or joint results in increased sensitivity to compression of the muscle or joint, respectively (primary hyperalgesia) as well as increased mechanical and thermal sensitivity of the paw (secondary hyperalgesia) that lasts for weeks [39,88,92–95]. Systemic administration of the nonselective ASIC antagonists amiloride and A-317567 in rats reverses the heat hyperalgesia of the paw (primary hyperalgesia) observed after complete Freund's adjuvant paw inflammation, suggesting a role for ASICs in inflammatory hyperalgesia [80]. In ASIC3 knockout mice, after the induction of paw inflammation, primary hyperalgesia to heat and mechanical stimuli still develops and is similar to wild-type controls [36,75]. Similarly, after joint inflammation, primary hyperalgesia to mechanical compression of the inflamed joint develops to the same extent as wild-type controls [39]. However, secondary hyperalgesia, measured as increased mechanical sensitivity of the paw, induced by carrageenan muscle or joint inflammation, does not develop in ASIC3 knockout mice compared with wild-type controls [39,88]. Figure 7.3 summarizes the changes we have observed in ASIC3 knockout mice and wild-type controls in our models of noninflammatory and inflammatory pain. Based on differences expressed as a percent inhibition, ASIC3 knockout mice still develop primary hyperalgesia but do not develop secondary hyperalgesia, as compared with control mice (Figure 7.3). Similarly, in a dominant negative mutant ASIC3 transgenic mouse,

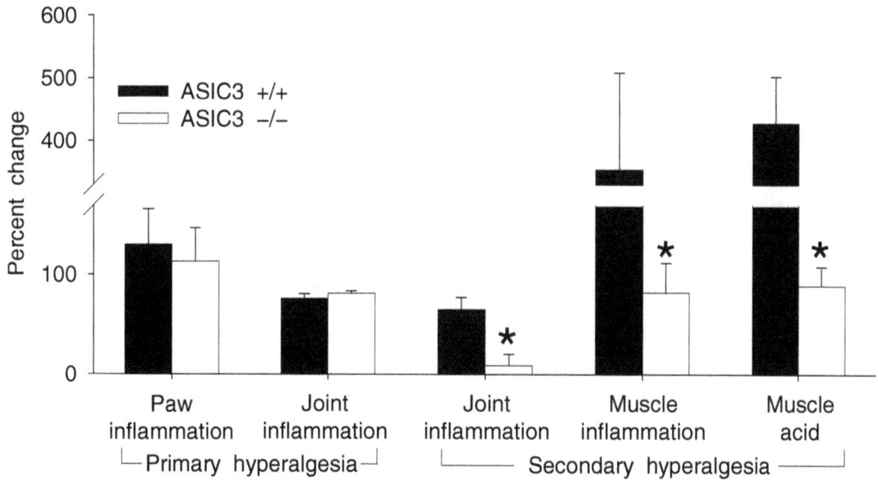

FIGURE 7.3. Behavior of wild-type (black bars; ASIC3 +/+) and ASIC3 knockout (open bars; ASIC3 –/–) mice in models of inflammatory and noninflammatory pain. Data are plotted as a percentage change between the baseline, and the value is measured after the potential development of pain. Primary mechanical hyperalgesia induced by paw or joint inflammation develops similarly in ASIC3 knockout mice. However, secondary mechanical hyperalgesia that develops after joint or muscle inflammation, or repeated intramuscular acid injections, does not develop in ASIC3 knockout mice when compared with wild-type controls. Paw, muscle, or joint inflammation was initiated by injection of carrageenan. Noninflammatory pain developed after two injections of acidic saline (pH 4.0) into the gastrocnemius muscle. Paw sensitivity was measured by mechanical withdrawals to von Frey filaments, and muscle and joint sensitivity was measured by withdrawal threshold. Adapted from data presented in References 36, 38, 39, and 88.

paw inflammation still produces increased sensitivity to mechanical and chemical stimuli [78].

ASIC3 in primary afferent fibers innervating the muscle is important for the generation of secondary hyperalgesia. Reexpression of ASIC3 in primary afferent fibers innervating the gastrocnemius muscle of ASIC3 knockout mice using a recombinant herpes simplex virus-1 (HSV-1) virus expressing ASIC3 restores the secondary mechanical hyperalgesia induced by carrageenan muscle inflammation [88]. In uninjured tissues, there is immunoreactivity for ASIC3 in peripheral terminals of primary afferent fibers innervating skin and muscle, which colocalize with the neuronal markers protein gene product (PGP) 9.5 or CGRP in muscle [37]. In contrast, in uninjured joint tissue, there is no ASIC3 in primary afferent fibers innervating the synovium [39] (Figure 7.2). With the development of joint inflammation, 24 hours after carrageenan injection, there is an upregulation of ASIC3 in the primary afferent fibers innervating the synovium of the knee joint and in retrogradely labeled DRGs from the inflamed knee [39] (Figure 7.2). Further, Mamet et al. and Voilley et al. showed that the application of inflammatory mediators to cultured DRG neurons or induction of inflammation with complete Freund's adjuvant induces an upregulation of ASIC1, ASIC2, and ASIC3 mRNA in the DRG [66,67]. Thus, from these results, we can conclude that peripheral inflammation results in activation and upregulation of ASIC3 in primary afferent fibers, which would increase the excitatory input to the spinal cord, resulting in central sensitization, manifested behaviorally as secondary hyperalgesia of the paw.

7.4.2 ASICs in Noninflammatory Muscle Pain

Our laboratory developed an animal model of noninflammatory pain in rats and mice that mimics chronic noninflammatory pain conditions, such as fibromyalgia. Noninflammatory musculoskeletal pain can be induced by two unilateral intramuscular injections of acidic saline (pH 4.0) spaced 5 days apart [96]. Mechanical sensitivity to noxious stimuli is assessed by examining withdrawal thresholds to mechanical stimuli of the paw and muscle [38,96,97]. The injection of pH 4.0 acidic saline into the left gastrocnemius muscle results in a brief lowering of pH at the injection site to 6.0–6.5 that lasts approximately 6 minutes. Further, injection of acidic saline is not associated with tissue damage or inflammation [96]. After the second injection of acidic saline, there is a long-lasting bilateral mechanical hyperalgesia of the paw and muscle [96,97]. The increased sensitivity of the injected gastrocnemius muscle to mechanical stimuli is considered primary hyperalgesia; the increased sensitivity of the paw to mechanical stimuli after the injection of acidic saline into the gastrocnemius muscle is considered secondary hyperalgesia. Hyperalgesia, both primary and secondary, associated with this two acid injections model is thought to be maintained by changes in the CNS at both spinal and supraspinal sites [97–103].

The nonselective ASIC blocker amiloride, delivered directly into the injected muscle during the second intramuscular acid injection, prevents the onset of secondary mechanical hyperalgesia of the paw 24 hours later, suggesting a role for ASICs in the development of hyperalgesia associated with the repeated acid injection model [38]. In ASIC3 knockout mice, mechanical hyperalgesia of the paw does not develop after the second intramuscular acid injection [38]. Recordings from wide dynamic range dorsal horn neurons do not show the development of central sensitization in ASIC3 knockout mice. Specifically, dorsal horn neurons from ASIC3 knockout mice do not show an expansion of receptive fields or enhanced sensitivity to noxious mechanical stimuli that normally occurs after the second injection saline in dorsal horn neurons recorded from wild-type mice. In ASIC1 knockout mice, however, repeated injections of intramuscular acidic saline still results in the development of mechanical hyperalgesia of the paw [38]. Therefore, ASIC3, and not ASIC1, is involved in the development of secondary mechanical hyperalgesia of the paw and central sensitization.

7.4.3 ASICs in Postoperative Pain

Incision of the hind paw, including the skin, underlying fascia, and muscle, is used to assess mechanisms of postoperative pain [104,105]. In rats after incision, there is a decrease in pH in the incision within 10 minutes to approximately 6.9, compared with pH 7.2 in sham-operated rats, which lasts for 4 days [106]. The decrease in pH in the incised animals coincides with hyperalgesia, measured as decreases in withdrawal threshold to von Frey filaments and a decrease in weight bearing on the incised paw. Both amiloride and A-317567, two nonspecific ASIC inhibitors, improve weight bearing on the incised paw following skin incision [80]. Together, these data suggest that the activation of ASICs may play a role in the development of postoperative pain.

7.4.4 ASICs in Lumbar Disk Herniation Pain

Lumbar disk herniation can result in radicular pain from inflammation and compression of the nerve root as it exits the vertebral foramen. In an animal model of lumbar disk herniation with radiculopathy, nucleus pulposis is collected from the tail of the rat and applied to the L5 nerve root and results in increased mechanical sensitivity of the paw, that is, secondary hyperalgesia, which lasts for 8 days. In these animals, there is an increased expression of ASIC3 in DRG neurons [107]. Lidocaine applied at the same time and at the site of nucleus pulposis application prevents the rats from developing increased mechanical sensitivity and concomitantly prevents the increased expression of ASIC3 in the DRG [107]. Thus, application of nucleus pulposis to the dorsal root upregulates ASIC3 in DRG neurons to produce a long-lasting secondary hyperalgesia, similar to that observed in the inflammatory and noninflammatory pain models.

7.4.5 ASICs in Gastrointestinal Pain

Excess gastric hydrochloric acid (HCl) in the esophagus, stomach, and the upper small intestine can cause tissue injury and pain. Intragastric administration of HCl in rats causes a visceromotor response that resembles visceral pain [108]. To test the role of ASICs on acid-mediated stomach pain, or gastritis, mild inflammatory gastritis was induced in mice by the addition of 0.1% iodoacetamide to the drinking water for 7 days [109]. On day 8, the animals were challenged with an intragastric administration of 0.25 M HCl, which, from previous studies, does not produce tissue damage, but does produce a visceromotor response, and an increase in activation of brainstem neurons, measured by c-fos expression in the nucleus tractus soliarius (NTS) [110]. ASIC3 knockout mice, in comparison to wild-type mice, do not show this increase in c-fos expression in the NTS. In contrast, ASIC2 knockout mice show a 33% enhancement in c-fos expression over that seen in wild-type mice, suggesting a differential role for ASIC3 and ASIC2 in modulation of the central consequences of peripheral HCl application [109]. ASIC3 plays a major role in the sensory hyperresponsiveness to acid in experimental gastritis, while ASIC2 may decrease the acid-induced response that is mediated by changes in the NTS.

In addition to responding to the application of acid, the gastroesophageal afferents may also be involved in mechanical sensitivity and mechanonociception. There are two populations of vagal mechanoreceptor fibers, tension and mucosal afferents, that respond to muscle stretch or mucosal stroking, respectively [111]. Recordings from *in vitro* gastroesophageal nerve preparations from ASIC1 knockout mice show enhanced mechanosensitivity in mucosal afferents to von Frey filaments applied to the mucosal surface and in tension afferents to a mechanical load [79]. In ASIC2 knockout mice, there is an enhanced mechanosensitivity of mucosal afferents suggesting specific roles of ASIC2 in different types of afferents innervating the colon [79]. In ASIC3 knockout mice, however, there is a decreased mechanosensitivity of both the mucosal and tension afferent fibers [79]. Thus, ASICs play a role in mechanosensation from the stomach and esophagus.

Colonic mechanical hypersensitivity is a hallmark of pain associated with conditions such as colitis and irritable bowel syndrome [112]. Distension of the colon in animals serves to model colonic visceral pain conditions and results in activation of colonic afferents and a visceromotor response [112,113]. ASIC3 or TRPV1 knockout mice are less sensitive to distension of the colon than wild-type control mice [40]. The splanchnic afferents innervating the colon are mainly mechanoreceptors with receptive fields in the serosa [111]. Recordings from *in vitro* colonic–splanchnic nerve preparations show that the nonselective antagonist benzamil reduced the mechanosensitivity of serosal colonic afferent fibers [114]. However, recordings from *in vitro* colon nerve preparations from either ASIC1 or ASIC2 knockout mice show an enhanced mechanosensitivity to von Frey filaments applied to the mucosal surface [79,115]. In ASIC3 knockout mice, however, there is a decreased mechanosensitivity in serosal colonic afferents [79]. Similarly, stretch-evoked afferent fiber responses from ASIC3 and TRPV1 knockout mice are significantly less sensitive than fibers from wild-type mice [40]. Thus, these data in colon afferents suggest that ASICs play a role in mechanosensation of the viscera and ASIC3 could be a good pharmacological target for reducing colonic mechanosensitivity and visceral pain.

7.4.6 ASICs in Ischemic Pain

Cardiac pain occurs during myocardial infarction or ischemia and is associated with significant decreases in myocardial pH [64,116]. Recordings from DRG neurons innervating the heart show a large depolarizing current evoked by decreasing pH in a concentration dependent manner [117,118]. These acid-evoked currents in the cardiac afferents possess properties consistent with ASICs. Sutherland et al. demonstrated that ASIC3 can produce the acid sensitivity profile observed in rat cardiac afferents and is thought to be a sensor associated with cardiac pain [118]. A greater understanding of the regulation and inhibition of ASIC3 might be useful in the treatment of cardiac angina and pathological reflexes that are activated in the setting heart disease.

7.4.7 ASICs in Cancer Pain

Severe bone pain often arises in cancer patients with bone metastases. In a rat model of bone pain, MRMT-1 breast cancer cells injected into the tibial bone marrow cavity induces hyperalgesia, as measured by decreases in the mechanical paw withdrawal threshold [119]. Within 7 days of the cancer cell injections, hyperalgesia develops and radiolucent lesions are seen in the proximal tibia. Histological examination of the lesions show that they contain increased numbers of osteoclasts, which secrete acid. ASIC1a and ASIC1b mRNA levels increases in the DRG of tumor-inoculated rats, whereas ASIC3 and TRPV1 mRNA levels were unchanged [119]. In this model of bone pain, colonization of metastatic bone cells in the tibia of rats causes hyperalgesia with associated acidosis and increases in ASIC expression.

7.5 ASICs AND PAIN BEHAVIOR IN HUMANS

In human studies of pain, acidic solutions injected into the skin or muscle evoke pain [120–123]. In skin, infusion of phosphate-buffered saline, pH 5–7.4, into the palmar forearm skin of volunteers produces pain in a pH-dependent manner [121,122]. The pain is detectably more intense as the pH is decreased below pH 7.2, with a pH 5.0 solution producing the greatest pain. Amiloride inhibits the pain induced by acid infusion into the skin, whereas capsazepine, a TRPV1 antagonist, does not [122]. In a less invasive model of acid-induced cutaneous pain, iontophoresis was used to drive protons into the forearm skin of healthy volunteers [124]. Iontophoresis of the pH 2.0 acidic solution produces more pain than pH 7.2 saline. Amiloride and the cyclooxygenase inhibitors ibuprofen or diclofenac inhibit the acid-induced pain, whereas capsaicin application to the skin prior to iontophoresis, in concentrations that would desensitize the TRPV1 receptor, did not change the acid-induced pain [124]. Together, these data suggest that ASICs, and not TRPV1, contribute a greater role in acid-induced pain of human skin.

Similar to injections into the skin, infusion of acid into muscle produces local pain at the site of the injection of acid [120,123]. Intramuscular injections of acid also result in referred pain at the ankle [123]. Similar to our animal model of intramuscular acid injections, the injection of acid into the tibialis anterior muscle in humans causes mechanical hyperalgesia at the site of the injection (primary hyperalgesia) and at the site of the referred pain (secondary hyperalgesia), as measured by decreases in pressure pain thresholds. Intramuscular injections of hypertonic saline or normal pH phosphate buffer similarly produces local and referred pain but does not result in primary or secondary hyperalgesia [123]. While we have not tested a specific role for ASICs as of yet, the results in humans are remarkably similar to our data from mice. Intramuscular acid injections trigger primary and secondary mechanical hyperalgesia and suggest that ASICs might play a role in their development.

7.6 CLINICAL SIGNIFICANCE

The data in this chapter suggest that decreases in pH and activation of ASICs play a significant role in the generation of a wide range of conditions that are associated with pain. Although the majority of studies was done in animal models, there is strong evidence for a role of acid and pain that are mediated by ASICs in human subjects. The greater expression of ASICs in deep tissue afferents and the upregulation of ASICs after inflammatory injury suggest that blockade of these channels after injury to deep tissue such as muscle, joint, or viscera would reduce the associated pain. There is emerging evidence from our laboratory that ASIC3 plays a critical role in deep tissue pain and in the development of secondary hyperalgesia and referred pain. However, we still need a better understanding of the localization and function of all ASIC channels to fully understand their role in nociception and pain. Better animal models of deep tissue pain that are predictive of clinical conditions are essential to further our understanding of the role of ASICs in pain. Our laboratory has begun to assess the role of ASICs in animal models of deep tissue pain from the muscle and joint, and other laboratories are beginning to assess the role of ASICs in models of visceral pain. Interestingly, some NSAIDs produce part of their analgesic effects by blockade of ASICs, and this may, in part, explain their effectiveness for the treatment of pain, especially inflammatory pain. Nonspecific or specific blockade of ASICs may, therefore, be an important pharmacological approach for the treatment of pain particularly that associated with deep tissue injury.

REFERENCES

1. Peter, D. Hart Research Associates. (2003). Americans talk about pain. http://www.researchamerica.org/uploads/poll2003pain.pdf (accessed May 8, 2008).
2. David Michaelson & Company, LLC. (2006). Voices of chronic pain. http://www.painfoundation.org/Voices/VoicesSurveyReport.pdf (accessed May 8, 2008).
3. National Center for Health Statistics. (2007). *Health, United States, 2007 with Chartbooks on Trends in the Health of Americans*. Hyattsville, MD: National Center for Health Statistics.
4. Häbler, C. (1929). Untersuchungen zur Molekularpathologie der Gelenkexsudate und ihre klinischen Ergebnisse. *Arch Klin Chir* 156:20–42.

5. Häbler, C. (1929). Über den K^+- und Ca^{2+}-Gehalt von Eiter und Exsudaten und seine Beziehungen zum Entzündungsschmerz. *Klin Wochenschr* 8:1569–1572.
6. Revici, E., Stoopen, E., Frenk, E., Ravich, R.A. (1949). The painful focus. II. The relation of pain to local physiochemical changes. *Bull Inst Appl Biol* 1:21–38.
7. Krishtal, O.A., Pidoplichko, V.I. (1980). A receptor for protons in the nerve cell membrane. *Neuroscience* 5:2325–2327.
8. Krishtal, O.A., Pidoplichko, V.I. (1981). Receptor for protons in the membrane of sensory neurons. *Brain Res* 214:150–154.
9. Krishtal, O. (2003). The ASICs: signaling molecules? Modulators? *Trends Neurosci* 26:477–483.
10. Price, M.P., Snyder, P.M., Welsh, M.J. (1996). Cloning and expression of a novel human brain Na+ channel. *J Biol Chem* 271:7879–7882.
11. Waldmann, R., Champigny, G., Voilley, N., Lauritzen, I., Lazdunski, M. (1996). The mammalian degenerin MDEG, an amiloride-sensitive cation channel activated by mutations causing neurodegeneration in *Caenorhabditis elegans*. *J Biol Chem* 271:10433–10436.
12. Waldmann, R., Champigny, G., Bassilana, F., Heurteaux, C., Lazdunski, M. (1997). A proton-gated cation channel involved in acid-sensing. *Nature* 386:173–177.
13. Garcia-Anoveros, J., Derfler, B., Neville-Golden, J., Hyman, B.T., Corey, D.P. (1997). BNaC1 and BNaC2 constitute a new family of human neuronal sodium channels related to degenerins and epithelial sodium channels. *Proc Natl Acad Sci U S A* 94:1459–1464.
14. Waldmann, R., Bassilana, F., de Weille, J., Champigny, G., Heurteaux, C., Lazdunski, M. (1997). Molecular cloning of a non-inactivating proton-gated Na+ channel specific for sensory neurons. *J Biol Chem* 272:20975–20978.
15. Lingueglia, E., de Weille, J.R., Bassilana, F., Heurteaux, C., Sakai, H., Waldmann, R., Lazdunski, M. (1997). A modulatory subunit of acid sensing ion channels in brain and dorsal root ganglion cells. *J Biol Chem* 272:29778–29783.
16. Wemmie, J.A., Price, M.P., Welsh, M.J. (2006). Acid-sensing ion channels: advances, questions and therapeutic opportunities. *Trends Neurosci* 29:578–586.
17. Lingueglia, E. (2007). Acid-sensing ion channels in sensory perception. *J Biol Chem* 282:17325–17329.
18. Coric, T., Zhang, P., Todorovic, N., Canessa, C.M. (2003). The extracellular domain determines the kinetics of desensitization in acid-sensitive ion channel 1. *J Biol Chem* 278:45240–45247.
19. Paukert, M., Sidi, S., Russell, C., Siba, M., Wilson, S.W., Nicolson, T., Grunder, S. (2004). A family of acid-sensing ion channels from the zebrafish: widespread expression in the central nervous system suggests a conserved role in neuronal communication. *J Biol Chem* 279:18783–18791.
20. Coric, T., Zheng, D., Gerstein, M., Canessa, C.M. (2005). Proton sensitivity of ASIC1 appeared with the rise of fishes by changes of residues in the region that follows TM1 in the ectodomain of the channel. *J Physiol* 568:725–735.
21. Zhang, P., Sigworth, F.J., Canessa, C.M. (2006). Gating of acid-sensitive ion channel-1: release of Ca2+ block vs. allosteric mechanism. *J Gen Physiol* 127:109–117.
22. Chen, X., Polleichtner, G., Kadurin, I., Grunder, S. (2007). Zebrafish acid-sensing ion channel (ASIC) 4, characterization of homo- and heteromeric channels, and

identification of regions important for activation by H+. *J Biol Chem* 282: 30406–30413.

23. Coric, T., Passamaneck, Y.J., Zhang, P., Di Gregorio, A., Canessa, C.M. (2008). Simple chordates exhibit a proton-independent function of acid-sensing ion channels. *FASEB J* 22:1914–1923.
24. Jasti, J., Furukawa, H., Gonzales, E.B., Gouaux, E. (2007). Structure of acid-sensing ion channel 1 at 1.9 A resolution and low pH. *Nature* 449:316–323.
25. Coscoy, S., Lingueglia, E., Lazdunski, M., Barbry, P. (1998). The Phe-Met-Arg-Phe-amide-activated sodium channel is a tetramer. *J Biol Chem* 273:8317–8322.
26. Firsov, D., Gautschi, I., Merillat, A.M., Rossier, B.C., Schild, L. (1998). The heterotetrameric architecture of the epithelial sodium channel (ENaC). *EMBO J* 17:344–352.
27. Snyder, P.M., Cheng, C., Prince, L.S., Rogers, J.C., Welsh, M.J. (1998). Electrophysiological and biochemical evidence that DEG/ENaC cation channels are composed of nine subunits. *J Biol Chem* 273:681–684.
28. Kadurin, I., Golubovic, A., Leisle, L., Schindelin, H., Grunder, S. (2008). Differential effects of N-glycans on surface expression suggest structural differences between acid-sensing ion channel (ASIC) 1a and ASIC1b. *Biochem J* 412:469–475.
29. Alvarez de la Rosa, D., Krueger, S.R., Kolar, A., Shao, D., Fitzsimonds, R.M., Canessa, C.M. (2003). Distribution, subcellular localization and ontogeny of ASIC1 in the mammalian central nervous system. *J Physiol* 546:77–87.
30. Champigny, G., Voilley, N., Waldmann, R., Lazdunski, M. (1998). Mutations causing neurodegeneration in *Caenorhabditis elegans* drastically alter the pH sensitivity and inactivation of the mammalian H+-gated Na+ channel MDEG1. *J Biol Chem* 273:15418–15422.
31. Wu, L.J., Duan, B., Mei, Y.D., Gao, J., Chen, J.G., Zhuo, M., Xu, L., Wu, M., Xu, T.L. (2004). Characterization of acid-sensing ion channels in dorsal horn neurons of rat spinal cord. *J Biol Chem* 279:43716–43724.
32. Baron, A., Voilley, N., Lazdunski, M., Lingueglia, E. (2008). Acid sensing ion channels in dorsal spinal cord neurons. *J Neurosci* 28:1498–1508.
33. Hruska-Hageman, A.M., Benson, C.J., Leonard, A.S., Price, M.P., Welsh, M.J. (2004). PSD-95 and Lin-7b interact with acid-sensing ion channel-3 and have opposite effects on H+-gated current. *J Biol Chem* 279:46962–46968.
34. Olson, T.H., Riedl, M.S., Vulchanova, L., Ortiz-Gonzalez, X.R., Elde, R. (1998). An acid sensing ion channel (ASIC) localizes to small primary afferent neurons in rats. *Neuroreport* 9:1109–1113.
35. Price, M.P., Lewin, G.R., McIlwrath, S.L., Cheng, C., Xie, J., Heppenstall, P.A., Stucky, C.L., Mannsfeldt, A.G., Brennan, T.J., Drummond, H.A., Qiao, J., Benson, C.J., Tarr, D.E., Hrstka, R.F., Yang, B., Williamson, R.A., Welsh, M.J. (2000). The mammalian sodium channel BNC1 is required for normal touch sensation. *Nature* 407:1007–1011.
36. Price, M.P., McIlwrath, S.L., Xie, J., Cheng, C., Qiao, J., Tarr, D.E., Sluka, K.A., Brennan, T.J., Lewin, G.R., Welsh, M.J. (2001). The DRASIC cation channel contributes to the detection of cutaneous touch and acid stimuli in mice. *Neuron* 32:1071–1083.

37. Molliver, D.C., Immke, D.C., Fierro, L., Pare, M., Rice, F.L., McCleskey, E.W. (2005). ASIC3, an acid-sensing ion channel, is expressed in metaboreceptive sensory neurons. *Mol Pain* 1:35.
38. Sluka, K.A., Price, M.P., Breese, N.M., Stucky, C.L., Wemmie, J.A., Welsh, M.J. (2003). Chronic hyperalgesia induced by repeated acid injections in muscle is abolished by the loss of ASIC3, but not ASIC1. *Pain* 106:229–239.
39. Ikeuchi, M., Kolker, S.J., Burnes, L.A., Walder, R.Y., Sluka, K.A. (2008). Role of ASIC3 in the primary and secondary hyperalgesia produced by joint inflammation in mice. *Pain* 137:662–669.
40. Jones, R.C., 3rd, Xu, L., Gebhart, G.F. (2005). The mechanosensitivity of mouse colon afferent fibers and their sensitization by inflammatory mediators require transient receptor potential vanilloid 1 and acid-sensing ion channel 3. *J Neurosci* 25:10981–10989.
41. Babinski, K., Le, K.T., Seguela, P. (1999). Molecular cloning and regional distribution of a human proton receptor subunit with biphasic functional properties. *J Neurochem* 72:51–57.
42. Jahr, H., van Driel, M., van Osch, G.J., Weinans, H., van Leeuwen, J.P. (2005). Identification of acid-sensing ion channels in bone. *Biochem Biophys Res Commun* 337:349–354.
43. Uchiyama, Y., Cheng, C.C., Danielson, K.G., Mochida, J., Albert, T.J., Shapiro, I.M., Risbud, M.V. (2007). Expression of acid-sensing ion channel 3 (ASIC3) in nucleus pulposus cells of the intervertebral disc is regulated by p75NTR and ERK signaling. *J Bone Miner Res* 22:1996–2006.
44. Gitterman, D.P., Wilson, J., Randall, A.D. (2005). Functional properties and pharmacological inhibition of ASIC channels in the human SJ-RH30 skeletal muscle cell line. *J Physiol* 562:759–769.
45. Tan, Z.Y., Lu, Y., Whiteis, C.A., Benson, C.J., Chapleau, M.W., Abboud, F.M. (2007). Acid-sensing ion channels contribute to transduction of extracellular acidosis in rat carotid body glomus cells. *Circ Res* 101:1009–1019.
46. Akopian, A.N., Chen, C.C., Ding, Y., Cesare, P., Wood, J.N. (2000). A new member of the acid-sensing ion channel family. *Neuroreport* 11:2217–2222.
47. Grunder, S., Geissler, H.S., Bassler, E.L., Ruppersberg, J.P. (2000). A new member of acid-sensing ion channels from pituitary gland. *Neuroreport* 11:1607–1611.
48. Ishibashi, K., Marumo, F. (1998). Molecular cloning of a DEG/ENaC sodium channel cDNA from human testis. *Biochem Biophys Res Commun* 245:589–593.
49. Ugawa, S., Ueda, T., Takahashi, E., Hirabayashi, Y., Yoneda, T., Komai, S., Shimada, S. (2001). Cloning and functional expression of ASIC-beta2, a splice variant of ASIC-beta. *Neuroreport* 12:2865–2869.
50. Benson, C.J., Xie, J., Wemmie, J.A., Price, M.P., Henss, J.M., Welsh, M.J., Snyder, P.M. (2002). Heteromultimers of DEG/ENaC subunits form H+-gated channels in mouse sensory neurons. *Proc Natl Acad Sci U S A* 99:2338–2343.
51. Xie, J., Price, M.P., Berger, A.L., Welsh, M.J. (2002). DRASIC contributes to pH-gated currents in large dorsal root ganglion sensory neurons by forming heteromultimeric channels. *J Neurophysiol* 87:2835–2843.
52. Yagi, J., Wenk, H.N., Naves, L.A., McCleskey, E.W. (2006). Sustained currents through ASIC3 ion channels at the modest pH changes that occur during myocardial ischemia. *Circ Res* 99:501–509.

53. Jiang, N., Rau, K.K., Johnson, R.D., Cooper, B.Y. (2006). Proton sensitivity Ca2+ permeability and molecular basis of acid-sensing ion channels expressed in glabrous and hairy skin afferents. *J Neurophysiol* 95:2466–2478.

54. Hesselager, M., Timmermann, D.B., Ahring, P.K. (2004). pH dependency and desensitization kinetics of heterologously expressed combinations of acid-sensing ion channel subunits. *J Biol Chem* 279:11006–11015.

55. Baron, A., Waldmann, R., Lazdunski, M. (2002). ASIC-like, proton-activated currents in rat hippocampal neurons. *J Physiol* 539:485–494.

56. Askwith, C.C., Wemmie, J.A., Price, M.P., Rokhlina, T., Welsh, M.J. (2004). Acid-sensing ion channel 2 (ASIC2) modulates ASIC1 H+-activated currents in hippocampal neurons. *J Biol Chem* 279:18296–18305.

57. Yermolaieva, O., Leonard, A.S., Schnizler, M.K., Abboud, F.M., Welsh, M.J. (2004). Extracellular acidosis increases neuronal cell calcium by activating acid-sensing ion channel 1a. *Proc Natl Acad Sci U S A* 101:6752–6757.

58. Xiong, Z.G., Zhu, X.M., Chu, X.P., Minami, M., Hey, J., Wei, W.L., MacDonald, J.F., Wemmie, J.A., Price, M.P., Welsh, M.J., Simon, R.P. (2004). Neuroprotection in ischemia: blocking calcium-permeable acid-sensing ion channels. *Cell* 118: 687–698.

59. Caterina, M.J., Schumacher, M.A., Tominaga, M., Rosen, T.A., Levine, J.D., Julius, D. (1997). The capsaicin receptor: a heat-activated ion channel in the pain pathway. *Nature* 389:816–824.

60. Allen, N.J., Attwell, D. (2002). Modulation of ASIC channels in rat cerebellar Purkinje neurons by ischaemia-related signals. *J Physiol* 543:521–529.

61. Immke, D.C., McCleskey, E.W. (2001). Lactate enhances the acid-sensing Na+ channel on ischemia-sensing neurons. *Nat Neurosci* 4:869–870.

62. Immke, D.C., McCleskey, E.W. (2001). ASIC3: a lactic acid sensor for cardiac pain. *ScientificWorldJournal* 1:510–512.

63. Smith, E.S., Cadiou, H., McNaughton, P.A. (2007). Arachidonic acid potentiates acid-sensing ion channels in rat sensory neurons by a direct action. *Neuroscience* 145:686–698.

64. Pan, H.L., Longhurst, J.C., Eisenach, J.C., Chen, S.R. (1999). Role of protons in activation of cardiac sympathetic C-fibre afferents during ischaemia in cats. *J Physiol* 518(Pt 3):857–866.

65. Stahl, G.L., Longhurst, J.C. (1992). Ischemically sensitive visceral afferents: importance of H+ derived from lactic acid and hypercapnia. *Am J Physiol* 262: H748–H753.

66. Mamet, J., Baron, A., Lazdunski, M., Voilley, N. (2002). Proinflammatory mediators, stimulators of sensory neuron excitability via the expression of acid-sensing ion channels. *J Neurosci* 22:10662–10670.

67. Voilley, N., de Weille, J., Mamet, J., Lazdunski, M. (2001). Nonsteroid anti-inflammatory drugs inhibit both the activity and the inflammation-induced expression of acid-sensing ion channels in nociceptors. *J Neurosci* 21:8026–8033.

68. Askwith, C.C., Cheng, C., Ikuma, M., Benson, C., Price, M.P., Welsh, M.J. (2000). Neuropeptide FF and FMRF amide potentiate acid-evoked currents from sensory neurons and proton-gated DEG/ENaC channels. *Neuron* 26:133–141.

69. Catarsi, S., Babinski, K., Seguela, P. (2001). Selective modulation of heteromeric ASIC proton-gated channels by neuropeptide FF. *Neuropharmacology* 41: 592–600.

70. Cadiou, H., Studer, M., Jones, N.G., Smith, E.S., Ballard, A., McMahon, S.B., McNaughton, P.A. (2007). Modulation of acid-sensing ion channel activity by nitric oxide. *J Neurosci* 27:13251–13260.

71. Leonard, A.S., Yermolaieva, O., Hruska-Hageman, A., Askwith, C.C., Price, M.P., Wemmie, J.A., Welsh, M.J. (2003). cAMP-dependent protein kinase phosphorylation of the acid-sensing ion channel-1 regulates its binding to the protein interacting with C-kinase-1. *Proc Natl Acad Sci U S A* 100:2029–2034.

72. Gao, J., Duan, B., Wang, D.G., Deng, X.H., Zhang, G.Y., Xu, L., Xu, T.L. (2005). Coupling between NMDA receptor and acid-sensing ion channel contributes to ischemic neuronal death. *Neuron* 48:635–646.

73. Gu, G., Caldwell, G.A., Chalfie, M. (1996). Genetic interactions affecting touch sensitivity in *Caenorhabditis elegans*. *Proc Natl Acad Sci U S A* 93:6577–6582.

74. O'Hagan, R., Chalfie, M., Goodman, M.B. (2005). The MEC-4 DEG/ENaC channel of *Caenorhabditis elegans* touch receptor neurons transduces mechanical signals. *Nat Neurosci* 8:43–50.

75. Chen, C.C., Zimmer, A., Sun, W.H., Hall, J., Brownstein, M.J., Zimmer, A. (2002). A role for ASIC3 in the modulation of high-intensity pain stimuli. *Proc Natl Acad Sci U S A* 99:8992–8997.

76. Roza, C., Puel, J.L., Kress, M., Baron, A., Diochot, S., Lazdunski, M., Waldmann, R. (2004). Knockout of the ASIC2 channel in mice does not impair cutaneous mechanosensation, visceral mechanonociception and hearing. *J Physiol* 558: 659–669.

77. Drew, L.J., Rohrer, D.K., Price, M.P., Blaver, K.E., Cockayne, D.A., Cesare, P., Wood, J.N. (2004). Acid-sensing ion channels ASIC2 and ASIC3 do not contribute to mechanically activated currents in mammalian sensory neurones. *J Physiol* 556:691–710.

78. Mogil, J.S., Breese, N.M., Witty, M.F., Ritchie, J., Rainville, M.L., Ase, A., Abbadi, N., Stucky, C.L., Seguela, P. (2005). Transgenic expression of a dominant-negative ASIC3 subunit leads to increased sensitivity to mechanical and inflammatory stimuli. *J Neurosci* 25:9893–9901.

79. Page, A.J., Brierley, S.M., Martin, C.M., Price, M.P., Symonds, E., Butler, R., Wemmie, J.A., Blackshaw, L.A. (2005). Different contributions of ASIC channels 1a, 2, and 3 in gastrointestinal mechanosensory function. *Gut* 54:1408–1415.

80. Dube, G.R., Lehto, S.G., Breese, N.M., Baker, S.J., Wang, X., Matulenko, M.A., Honore, P., Stewart, A.O., Moreland, R.B., Brioni, J.D. (2005). Electrophysiological and in vivo characterization of A-317567, a novel blocker of acid sensing ion channels. *Pain* 117:88–96.

81. Chen, X., Kalbacher, H., Grunder, S. (2005). The tarantula toxin psalmotoxin 1 inhibits acid-sensing ion channel (ASIC) 1a by increasing its apparent H+ affinity. *J Gen Physiol* 126:71–79.

82. Escoubas, P., De Weille, J.R., Lecoq, A., Diochot, S., Waldmann, R., Champigny, G., Moinier, D., Menez, A., Lazdunski, M. (2000). Isolation of a tarantula toxin specific for a class of proton-gated Na+ channels. *J Biol Chem* 275:25116–25121.

83. Salinas, M., Rash, L.D., Baron, A., Lambeau, G., Escoubas, P., Lazdunski, M. (2006). The receptor site of the spider toxin PcTx1 on the proton-gated cation channel ASIC1a. *J Physiol* 570:339–354.

84. Chen, X., Kalbacher, H., Grunder, S. (2006). Interaction of acid-sensing ion channel (ASIC) 1 with the tarantula toxin psalmotoxin 1 is state dependent. *J Gen Physiol* 127:267–276.

85. Diochot, S., Baron, A., Rash, L.D., Deval, E., Escoubas, P., Scarzello, S., Salinas, M., Lazdunski, M. (2004). A new sea anemone peptide, APETx2, inhibits ASIC3, a major acid-sensitive channel in sensory neurons. *EMBO J* 23:1516–1525.

86. Diochot, S., Salinas, M., Baron, A., Escoubas, P., Lazdunski, M. (2007). Peptides inhibitors of acid-sensing ion channels. *Toxicon* 49:271–284.

87. Wemmie, J.A., Chen, J., Askwith, C.C., Hruska-Hageman, A.M., Price, M.P., Nolan, B.C., Yoder, P.G., Lamani, E., Hoshi, T., Freeman, J.H., Jr., Welsh, M.J. (2002). The acid-activated ion channel ASIC contributes to synaptic plasticity, learning, and memory. *Neuron* 34:463–477.

88. Sluka, K.A., Radhakrishnan, R., Benson, C.J., Eshcol, J.O., Price, M.P., Babinski, K., Audette, K.M., Yeomans, D.C., Wilson, S.P. (2007). ASIC3 in muscle mediates mechanical, but not heat, hyperalgesia associated with muscle inflammation. *Pain* 129:102–112.

89. Waldmann, R. (2001). Proton-gated cation channels–neuronal acid sensors in the central and peripheral nervous system. *Adv Exp Med Biol* 502:293–304.

90. Ma, C., Greenquist, K.W., Lamotte, R.H. (2006). Inflammatory mediators enhance the excitability of chronically compressed dorsal root ganglion neurons. *J Neurophysiol* 95:2098–2107.

91. Ozaktay, A.C., Kallakuri, S., Takebayashi, T., Cavanaugh, J.M., Asik, I., DeLeo, J.A., Weinstein, J.N. (2006). Effects of interleukin-1 beta, interleukin-6, and tumor necrosis factor on sensitivity of dorsal root ganglion and peripheral receptive fields in rats. *Eur Spine J* 15:1529–1537.

92. Sluka, K.A. (2002). Stimulation of deep somatic tissue with capsaicin produces long-lasting mechanical allodynia and heat hypoalgesia that depends on early activation of the cAMP pathway. *J Neurosci* 22:5687–5693.

93. Radhakrishnan, R., Moore, S.A., Sluka, K.A. (2003). Unilateral carrageenan injection into muscle or joint induces chronic bilateral hyperalgesia in rats. *Pain* 104:567–577.

94. Skyba, D.A., Radhakrishnan, R., Sluka, K.A. (2005). Characterization of a method for measuring primary hyperalgesia of deep somatic tissue. *J Pain* 6:41–47.

95. Vance, C.G., Radhakrishnan, R., Skyba, D.A., Sluka, K.A. (2007). Transcutaneous electrical nerve stimulation at both high and low frequencies reduces primary hyperalgesia in rats with joint inflammation in a time-dependent manner. *Phys Ther* 87:44–51.

96. Sluka, K.A., Kalra, A., Moore, S.A. (2001). Unilateral intramuscular injections of acidic saline produce a bilateral, long-lasting hyperalgesia. *Muscle Nerve* 24:37–46.

97. Tillu, D.V., Gebhart, G.F., Sluka, K.A. (2008). Descending facilitatory pathways from the RVM initiate and maintain bilateral hyperalgesia after muscle insult. *Pain* 136:331–339.

98. Bement, M.K., Sluka, K.A. (2007). Co-localization of p-CREB and p-NR1 in spinothalamic neurons in a chronic muscle pain model. *Neurosci Lett* 418:22–27.
99. Hoeger-Bement, M.K., Sluka, K.A. (2003). Phosphorylation of CREB and mechanical hyperalgesia is reversed by blockade of the cAMP pathway in a time-dependent manner after repeated intramuscular acid injections. *J Neurosci* 23:5437–5445.
100. Yokoyama, T., Maeda, Y., Audette, K.M., Sluka, K.A. (2007). Pregabalin reduces muscle and cutaneous hyperalgesia in two models of chronic muscle pain in rats. *J Pain* 8:422–429.
101. Bement, M.K., Sluka, K.A. (2005). Low-intensity exercise reverses chronic muscle pain in the rat in a naloxone-dependent manner. *Arch Phys Med Rehabil* 86: 1736–1740.
102. Skyba, D.A., King, E.W., Sluka, K.A. (2002). Effects of NMDA and non-NMDA ionotropic glutamate receptor antagonists on the development and maintenance of hyperalgesia induced by repeated intramuscular injection of acidic saline. *Pain* 98:69–78.
103. Nielsen, A.N., Mathiesen, C., Blackburn-Munro, G. (2004). Pharmacological characterisation of acid-induced muscle allodynia in rats. *Eur J Pharmacol* 487:93–103.
104. Brennan, T.J., Zahn, P.K., Pogatzki-Zahn, E.M. (2005). Mechanisms of incisional pain. *Anesthesiol Clin North Am* 23:1–20.
105. Pogatzki-Zahn, E.M., Zahn, P.K., Brennan, T.J. (2007). Postoperative pain–clinical implications of basic research. *Best Pract Res Clin Anaesthesiol* 21:3–13.
106. Woo, Y.C., Park, S.S., Subieta, A.R., Brennan, T.J. (2004). Changes in tissue pH and temperature after incision indicate acidosis may contribute to postoperative pain. *Anesthesiology* 101:468–475.
107. Ohtori, S., Inoue, G., Koshi, T., Ito, T., Doya, H., Saito, T., Moriya, H., Takahashi, K. (2006). Up-regulation of acid-sensing ion channel 3 in dorsal root ganglion neurons following application of nucleus pulposus on nerve root in rats. *Spine* 31: 2048–2052.
108. Lamb, K., Kang, Y.M., Gebhart, G.F., Bielefeldt, K. (2003). Gastric inflammation triggers hypersensitivity to acid in awake rats. *Gastroenterology* 125:1410–1418.
109. Wultsch, T., Painsipp, E., Shahbazian, A., Mitrovic, M., Edelsbrunner, M., Lazdunski, M., Waldmann, R., Holzer, P. (2008). Deletion of the acid-sensing ion channel ASIC3 prevents gastritis-induced acid hyperresponsiveness of the stomach-brainstem axis. *Pain* 134:245–253.
110. Wultsch, T., Painsipp, E., Thoeringer, C.K., Herzog, H., Sperk, G., Holzer, P. (2005). Endogenous neuropeptide Y depresses the afferent signaling of gastric acid challenge to the mouse brainstem via neuropeptide Y type Y2 and Y4 receptors. *Neuroscience* 136:1097–1107.
111. Page, A.J., Martin, C.M., Blackshaw, L.A. (2002). Vagal mechanoreceptors and chemoreceptors in mouse stomach and esophagus. *J Neurophysiol* 87:2095–2103.
112. Ness, T.J., Gebhart, G.F. (1990). Visceral pain: a review of experimental studies. *Pain* 41:167–234.
113. Kamp, E.H., Jones, R.C., 3rd, Tillman, S.R., Gebhart, G.F. (2003). Quantitative assessment and characterization of visceral nociception and hyperalgesia in mice. *Am J Physiol Gastrointest Liver Physiol* 284:G434–G444.

114. Page, A.J., Brierley, S.M., Martin, C.M., Hughes, P.A., Blackshaw, L.A. (2007). Acid sensing ion channels 2 and 3 are required for inhibition of visceral nociceptors by benzamil. *Pain* 133:150–160.

115. Page, A.J., Brierley, S.M., Martin, C.M., Martinez-Salgado, C., Wemmie, J.A., Brennan, T.J., Symonds, E., Omari, T., Lewin, G.R., Welsh, M.J., Blackshaw, L.A. (2004). The ion channel ASIC1 contributes to visceral but not cutaneous mechanoreceptor function. *Gastroenterology* 127:1739–1747.

116. Cobbe, S.M., Poole-Wilson, P.A. (1980). The time of onset and severity of acidosis in myocardial ischaemia. *J Mol Cell Cardiol* 12:745–760.

117. Benson, C.J., Eckert, S.P., McCleskey, E.W. (1999). Acid-evoked currents in cardiac sensory neurons: a possible mediator of myocardial ischemic sensation. *Circ Res* 84:921–928.

118. Sutherland, S.P., Benson, C.J., Adelman, J.P., McCleskey, E.W. (2001). Acid-sensing ion channel 3 matches the acid-gated current in cardiac ischemia-sensing neurons. *Proc Natl Acad Sci U S A* 98:711–716.

119. Nagae, M., Hiraga, T., Yoneda, T. (2007). Acidic microenvironment created by osteoclasts causes bone pain associated with tumor colonization. *J Bone Miner Metab* 25:99–104.

120. Issberner, U., Reeh, P.W., Steen, K.H. (1996). Pain due to tissue acidosis: a mechanism for inflammatory and ischemic myalgia? *Neurosci Lett* 208:191–194.

121. Steen, K.H., Reeh, P.W. (1993). Sustained graded pain and hyperalgesia from harmless experimental tissue acidosis in human skin. *Neurosci Lett* 154:113–116.

122. Ugawa, S., Ueda, T., Ishida, Y., Nishigaki, M., Shibata, Y., Shimada, S. (2002). Amiloride-blockable acid-sensing ion channels are leading acid sensors expressed in human nociceptors. *J Clin Invest* 110:1185–1190.

123. Frey Law, L.A., Sluka, K.A., McMullen, T., Lee, J., Arendt-Nielsen, L., Graven-Nielsen, T. (2008). Acidic buffer induced muscle pain evokes referred pain and mechanical hyperalgesia in humans. *Pain* 140: 254–264.

124. Jones, N.G., Slater, R., Cadiou, H., McNaughton, P., McMahon, S.B. (2004). Acid-induced pain and its modulation in humans. *J Neurosci* 24:10974–10979.

CHAPTER 8

Vanilloid (TRPV1) and Other Transient Receptor Potential Channels

MARCELLO TREVISANI[1] and ARPAD SZALLASI[2,3]

[1]PharmEste
[2]Monmouth Medical Center Long Branch
[3]Drexel University College of Medicine

Content

Peripheral Receptor Targets for Analgesia: Novel Approaches to Pain Management, Edited by Brian E. Cairns

8.1 OVERVIEW

The neuropathic pain market in the United States is expected to nearly double from today's $2.6 billion to $5 billion by 2018 according to a recent report by the market research firm WWMR, Inc. However, despite a substantial increase in the number of clinical trials, the therapy of chronic pain conditions remains an unmet medical need. Preclinical research has uncovered new molecular mechanisms underlying the generation and transduction of pain, many of which represent new targets for pharmacological intervention. A group of proteins expressed on polymodal nociceptive neurons that belong to the transient receptor potential (TRP) family of cation channels is particularly interesting. These proteins are involved in thermosensation (both hot and cold), mediate taste modalities, and, importantly, also act as molecular sensors for a broad variety of unrelated noxious stimuli. These heat-sensitive channels (TRP vanilloid 1 [TRPV1]–TRPV4, TRP ankyrin 1 [TRPA1] and TRP melastatin 8 [TRPM8]), collectively referred to as "thermoTRPs," are believed to represent novel targets for the discovery of the next generation of analgesic agents. Indeed, in contrast to traditional analgesic agents that either suppress inflammation (e.g., nonsteroidal anti-inflammatory drugs [NSAIDs]) or inhibit pain transmission (like opiates), thermoTRP inhibitors aim to prevent pain by blocking a receptor where pain is generated. The capsaicin (vanilloid) receptor TRPV1, the archetypal thermoTRP, was discovered in 1997, and it took less than a decade from channel cloning through antagonist proof of concept to clinical trials. As many proalgesic pathways converge on TRPV1 and this nocisensor is upregulated and sensitized by inflammation and injury, TRPV1 is thought to be a central transducer of hyperalgesia and a prime target for the pharmacological control of pain. This chapter focuses on present evidence that validates TRPV1 and other TRP channels as targets for new-generation analgesic drugs, along with potential adverse effects that may limit their clinical value.

8.2 INTRODUCTION

Acute pain, such as pain resulting from disease, inflammation, or injury to tissues, frequently has a reversible cause and may require only transient measures and correction of the underlying problem. In contrast, chronic pain, defined as pain lasting longer than 3 months, often results from conditions that are difficult to diagnose and treat, and that may take a long time (if at all) to reverse (e.g., cancer, neuropathic and referred pain). Patients suffering from disabling pain conditions often need complex and aggressive treatment plans that combine medical and surgical approaches and yet may provide limited pain relief [1–3]. In recognition of this problem, the U.S. Congress had declared the 10-year period that began on January 1, 2001 as the Decade of Pain Control and Research [4]. Furthermore, the Joint Commission of Accreditation of Healthcare Organizations (JCAHO) has mandated pain as the "fifth vital sign" (the other four being blood pressure, respiration, pulse, and temperature).

Although the Decade of Pain Control and Research has given new impetus to pain research, the differences and overlaps among nociceptive, inflammatory, and neuropathic pain conditions are only beginning to be understood. Furthermore, the translation of preclinical research to clinical practice is slow to occur. This is evident by the limited number of mechanistically novel therapeutic agents that have entered into the clinic for the treatment of pain in recent years. These analgesic drugs include gabapentin, pregabalin, ziconotide, duloxetine, and cyclo-oxygenase-2 (COX-2) inhibitors. Although gabapentin (Neurontin, Pfizer, New York, NY, USA), pregabalin (Lyrica, Pfizer, New York, NY, USA), and duloxetine (Cymbalta, Eli Lilly, Indianapolis, IN, USA) are among the most prescribed pain relief medications for neuropathic conditions, there is still space for improvement in terms of potency, tolerability, and central nervous system (CNS) adverse effects [5]. Ziconotide (Prialt, Elan, Dublin, Ireland), a conopeptide N-type calcium channel blocker, is restricted to intractable (opiate refractory) pain by a combination of side effects and the need for intrathecal delivery [6]. Finally, COX-2 inhibitors provided a promising line of therapy for inflammatory conditions before side effects cast a shadow over the use of this class of drugs.

To date, the mainstay of pain therapy remains agents such as opiates [3] and NSAIDs that have been around for a number of decades, indicating that the current therapeutic approach for pain does not provide adequate relief to patients [7]. Clearly, there is a great need for new therapeutic agents acting via novel mechanisms in this field of medicine.

A recent development in the search for novel analgesics is the advance into clinical testing of small-molecule antagonists of the capsaicin receptor TRPV1 (TRP, vanilloid subfamily member 1) [8,9]. TRPV1 is now recognized as a heat-sensitive nonselective cation channel characterized by a dynamic threshold of activation [10–12]. A multitude of primary activators (e.g., protons and "endovanilloids") and secondary modulators (e.g., nerve growth factor [NGF], bradykinin, eicosanoids, prostaglandins, adenosine triphosphate [ATP], and cytokines) that are present in the "inflammatory soup" act in concert on TRPV1 to reduce its threshold to heat activation; this is in support of the role of TRPV1 as a convergence point of multiple pain-producing stimuli [10–14]. Other temperature-sensitive TRP channels, referred to as thermoTRPs (see Figures 8.1 and 8.2) that are implicated in sensory processing include TRPV2, TRPV3, TRPV4, TRPA1, and TRPM8 [15].

In contrast to traditional analgesic agents that either suppress inflammation (e.g., NSAIDs) or inhibit pain transmission (e.g., opiates), thermoTRP antagonists aim to prevent pain by directly acting on the site where pain is generated (Figures 8.1 and 8.2) [9,16–18]. TRPV1 as a target for novel analgesic drugs has already been validated by genetic deletion [19,20] and pharmacological blockade experiments (reviewed in References 17, 21, and 22), and several small-molecule TRPV1 antagonists are currently undergoing phase I or II clinical trials for indications related to pain [23–28].

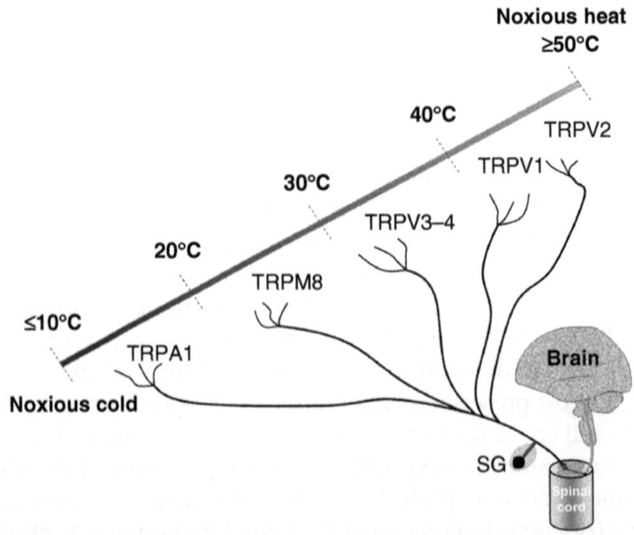

FIGURE 8.1. ThermoTRPs as sensors of the whole spectrum of temperatures, from painful cold (10 °C) to painful heat (53 °C). SG, sensory ganglia. See color insert.

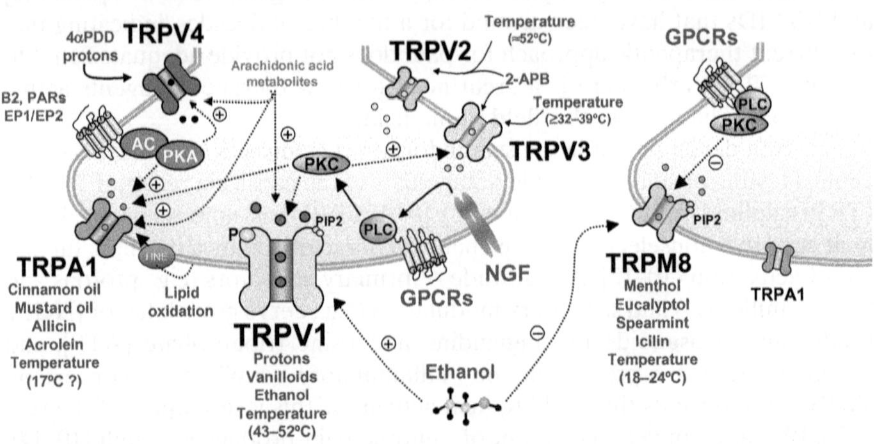

FIGURE 8.2. Schematic diagram of some of the stimuli and intracellular pathways that contribute to the activation/modulation of thermoTRP functions in the sensory nerve terminals.

This chapter focuses on the pivotal role of TRPV1 as a target for the development of next-generation analgesic drugs and highlights the potential adverse effects that may limit its clinical utility. Antagonists targeting non-TRPV1 thermoTRP channels are still in preclinical phase and will be discussed only briefly.

8.3 TEMPERATURE-SENSITIVE TRP (THERMOTRP) CHANNELS ARE MULTIFACETED SENSORS

As discussed above, thermoTRPs represent a group of channels that, combined, cover a broad range of temperatures, from painful cold (10 °C) to painful hot (53 °C) [29–31] (Figure 8.1). Six thermoTRPs have been identified to date, namely TRPV1 to TRPV4, TRPA1, and TRPM8. Generally speaking, these channels are localized on subpopulations of primary sensory neurons referred to as "nociceptors." TRPV1, TRPV2, TRPV3, and TRPV4 sense hot and warm temperatures, while TRPA1 and TRPM8 are activated by cold (Figures 8.1 and 8.2). Of note, some thermoTRPs (e.g., TRPV1 and TRPV3) are also expressed in keratinocytes and urothelial cells where they are believed to play a sensory role.

A nociceptor ("noci" derived from the Latin word for "hurt") is a free nerve ending that sends signals that are perceived as painful in response to potentially damaging stimuli (e.g., painful mechanical stimuli, extreme heat or cold, and chemical damage to tissues) [32]. Nociceptors, discovered by Charles Scott Sherrington more than a century ago, are localized in tissues such as the skin (cutaneous nociceptors), cornea, and mucosa, and also in the muscle, joint, bladder, airways, gut, and along the digestive tract. In other words, nociceptors detect potentially harmful stimuli both from the external milieu and our internal organs.

Primary sensory neurons serve nociceptive functions. These neurons are bipolar cells with bodies located in the sensory ganglia (dorsal root ganglia [DRG], trigeminal ganglia [TG], and nodose ganglia of the vagal nerve) (Figure 8.1) [33]. The central axons of these neurons enter the CNS where they form synapse with second-order neurons of the dorsal horn of the spinal cord (for DRG neurons), the spinal nucleus of the trigeminal tract (for TG neurons), and the area postrema (vagal neurons) (Figure 8.1). The majority of primary sensory neurons possesses unmyelinated axons (so-called C-fibers) and respond to the xenobiotic agent capsaicin, the pungent ingredient in hot chilli peppers [34]. This lack of myelination is the cause of their slow conduction velocity, which is on the order of 2 m/s. C-fiber nociceptor axons branch extensively in human skin to innervate cutaneous areas of approximately one to several square centimeters [35–37]. An orthodromic impulse activated in one branch normally invades every other branch antidromically.

A small subset of neurons with thin myelinated axons (Aδ-fibers) has larger axons in diameter; these neurons have a higher conduction velocity, which is on the order of about 20 m/s. This subset has been brought in the focus of attention by the recent observation that Aδ-fibers that do not normally express TRPV1 do so under inflammatory conditions or following injury neuropathic pain [38,39]. This abnormal, TRPV1-positive Aδ-fiber population was suggested to contribute to pain in patients with diabetic polyneuropathy [40]. Indeed, desensitization to TRPV1 agonists (e.g., capsaicin and its ultrapotent analog resiniferatoxin [RTX], the latter isolated from the latex of the perennial

Euphorbia resinifera) relieves chronic pain in these patients [18] despite the degeneration of C-fibers [41,42].

ThermoTRPs are also operated by a number of natural products [43]. In fact, the TRPV1 channel was previously known as the "capsaicin receptor" (capsaicin is responsible for the spiciness of chili peppers) or the "vanilloid receptor VR1" ("vanilloid" comes from the presence of a vanillyl moiety in both the chemical structures of capsaicin and RTX) [44]. In addition to capsaicin, TRPV1 is also a target for pungent compounds in jellyfish [45] and spider toxins [46]. On the other hand, TRPA1 is activated by both cinnamaldehyde (from cinnamon) [47,48] and allicin (an active ingredient in garlic) [49]. TRPM8 is also referred to as the menthol receptor [50], and TRPV3 represents a target for camphor [51]. TRPV4 is thought to mediate the actions of bisandrographolide, the bioactive ingredient in the Chinese medicinal plant, *Andrographis paniculata* [52].

Some other natural toxins exhibit lower pharmacological selectivity toward thermoTRPs. For instance, citral (a major component and active ingredient in lemongrass oil, lemon peel, citronella, and palmarosa grass) functions as a partial agonist for all TRPs in sensory neurons (TRPV1, TRPV3, TRPA1, and TRPM8) with a lasting blockage of TRPV1, TRPV3, and TRPM8, and a transient inhibition of TRPV4 and TRPA1 [53]. Menthol is an even more interesting compound as it activates TRPM8 (hence its popular cooling effect), but, paradoxically, it also stimulates TRPV3, causing a warm sensation, and blocks TRPA1 [54]. Furthermore, there is a significant "cross-talk" and "cross-desensitization" among the TRP channels that modifies the bioactivity of natural TRP channel agonists. A shared (and controversial) feature of thermoTRP channels, in particular TRPV1 [55] and TRPM8 [56], is their regulation by phosphatidylinositol 4,5-biphosphate (in short, PIP2) [57,58]. Indeed, TRPV1 possesses PIP2-recognition sites [59,60]. Initially, it was postulated that TRPV1 is under the inhibitory control of PIP2 [55], implying a pivotal role for phospholipase C, the enzyme that cleaves PIP2, in TRPV1 activation. The new concept, however, is that PIP2 may be either inhibitory or activating, depending on the context [61]. Of note, recently, it was suggested that ethanol potentiates TRPV1-mediated responses via the PIP2–TRPV1 interaction [62]. This is interesting because ethanol is known to cause a burning pain in patients with reflux esophagitis, a condition in which TRPV1 is upregulated.

There is a strong experimental evidence that thermoTRP channels play a central role (i) in thermal nociception, (ii) in detecting noxious chemicals (Figure 8.1 and 8.2) [63,64], and (iii) in generating and maintaining pain and hypersensitivity that occurs under various pathological conditions.

It is worth mentioning here that many non-neuronal cells (e.g., endothelium and epithelial cells like urothelium and keratinocytes) also express thermoTRP channels, in particular TRPV1 [65–68], TRPV3 [42], and TRPV4 [69,70]; it has been suggested that these cells, too, may function as pain sensors [67,71]. This observation may provide a mechanistic explanation for the efficacy of the selective TRPV3 antagonist GRC-15133 to reverse thermal and mechanical hyperalgesia in the rat despite the absence of TRPV3 in rodent DRG neurons (for further details, please see Section 8.7).

8.4 TRPV1, THE ARCHETYPAL THERMOTRP CHANNEL, IS ACTIVATED BY CAPSAICIN AND ENDOVANILLOIDS

The existence of a receptor for capsaicin and related molecules had long been anticipated based on the specific action of capsaicin on nociceptive afferent neurons: the initial excitation by capsaicin of these neurons is followed by a lasting refractory state, traditionally referred to as "capsaicin desensitization." Owing to their peculiar response to capsaicin, these neurons have become known as "capsaicin-sensitive afferent neurons" [34,44,72,73]. Capsaicin-sensitive (that is, TRPV1 expressing) primary sensory neurons release a variety of proinflammatory neuropeptides (e.g., substance P [SP], calcitonin gene-related peptide [CGRP], and neurokinin A [NKA]) that induce a series of local effects globally defined as neurogenic inflammation [74]. Neurogenic inflammation is thought to play a central role in the pathogenesis of various disease states that range from migraine through asthma to inflammatory bowel disease [74,75].

TRPV1 is a polymodal nocisensor par excellence, sensitive to noxious heat (above 43 °C), acidosis (pH between 5 and 6), endovanilloids (e.g., anandamide, arachidonic acid metabolites such as N-arachidonoyl-dopamine [NADA] 12-hydroperoxyeicosatetraenoic acid, and others), and to a variety of pungent compounds such as capsaicin, RTX, piperine, gingerol, zingerone, camphor, eugenol, ethanol, and venoms from jellyfish and spiders [9,10,46,76–79]. Proinflammatory agents such as prostaglandins, bradykinin, ATP, 5-hydroxytryptamine, and NGF cause allosteric modification of TRPV1 either directly or indirectly (e.g., via phosphorylation by protein kinase C [PKC]) such that the probability of channel opening by heat, protons, and capsaicin is enhanced [9,10,76,80,81]. Thus, TRPV1 functions as a molecular integrator in which each stimulus sensitizes the channel to other stimuli, with the result that TRPV1 acts as a molecular amplifier in the sensory neuron [82]. These findings have implied TRPV1 as a promising target to relieve inflammatory pain (Figure 8.2). Indeed, both genetic deletion [19,20] and pharmacological blockade of TRPV1 ameliorate heat hyperalgesia in rodent models of inflammatory pain [9,16,22].

The property of TRPV1 to become sensitized when exposed to painful stimuli has led to the hypothesis of TRPV1 being a prime factor in hyperalgesia [83]. Sensitization of the ion channel depends on several mechanisms among which phosphorylation of TRPV1 by protein kinase A (PKA), PKC, and other kinases (Figure 8.2) is of pivotal importance [80,84–91]. Bradykinin, NGF, and anandamide increase TRPV1 activity involving phospholipase C-mediated hydrolysis of PIP2 that, as mentioned above, normally inhibits TRPV1 gating by agonists [55]. Dephosphorylation of TRPV1 by protein phosphatases promotes desensitization and represents a major mechanism of inhibitory regulation [92]. Desensitization of TRPV1 to capsaicin involves a number of intracellular components including PKA, ATP, and calmodulin [59,93–96]. It is possible that a dynamic balance between phosphorylation and dephosphorylation of TRPV1 controls the activation/desensitization state of the channel [92,97].

There is a good experimental evidence that TRPV1 is an important mediator of pathological pain (reviewed in References 9, 16, and 98). TRPV1 agonists such as capsaicin and RTX have long been used to probe the function of sensory fibers in a variety of physiological processes, such as the airway and urinary bladder (reviewed in References 16, 74, 98, and 99). It has also been appreciated for some time that capsaicin and RTX treatment can result in persistent, but fully reversible, desensitization of the sensory fibers (reviewed in References 16, 34, 44, and 98). The mechanism of desensitization likely involves both channel desensitization as well as a change in the expression profile of neuropeptides and receptors involved in pain perception and processing, the latter referred to as "vanilloid-induced messenger plasticity" (reviewed in Reference 44). This results in analgesia *in vivo*, a therapeutic effect that justifies the continued efforts to develop site-specific capsaicin formulations as analgesics (e.g., Adlea by Anesiva (San Francisco, CA, USA) and NGX-4010 by NeurogesX (San Mateo, CA, USA), reviewed in References 18 and 100). The treatment of overactive bladder/urinary incontinence represents another clinical indication for topical capsaicin therapy (reviewed in References 99 and 101). Other approaches include formulations of RTX and synthetic capsaicin congeners like olvanil (reviewed in References 44 and 98). For instance, rats desensitized to RTX are devoid of the thermal hyperalgesia and guarding behavior that develops following mechanical damage of the sciatic nerve (Bennett model) (A. Szallasi, M. Tal, and G. Bennett, unpublished observations). In mice and dogs, topical RTX ameliorates bone cancer pain [102,103]. Additional indications for topical treatment with TRPV1 agonists include migraine, cluster headache, osteoarthritis, lateral epicondylitis (e.g., "tennis elbow"), Morton's neuroma, and postsurgical pain (e.g., bunionectomy and hernia repair) [16,18,98].

8.4.1 Evidence Derived from TRPV1-Deficient Animals

TRPV1 knockout mice generated in recent years have been studied extensively to determine the role of the receptor in normal physiological signaling and pathological processes. Two independent gene-targeting studies deleting TRPV1 alleles conclusively showed that TRPV1 is a critical channel that mediates thermal hyperalgesia under inflammatory pain conditions in mice [19,20,104]. In addition, one study showed that TRPV1 null mice are significantly less sensitive to acute noxious heat stimulation; TRPV1 (–/–) mice exhibit significantly larger withdrawal latencies in response to noxious heat in the hot-plate assay than their wild-type littermates [19]. The phenotype of the

TRPV1 knockout mice generated tremendous interest in developing small-molecule antagonists with an antihyperalgesic profile. In wild-type mice, the endogenous fatty acid oleoylethanolamide (OEA), which is synthesized and released from the intestine upon feeding, evokes visceral pain-related behavior. This effect was prevented by TRPV1 antagonism and was absent in TRPV1 (–/–) mice [105]. Interestingly, TRPV1 (–/–) mice also show less weight gain than their wild-type littermates when kept on high-fat diet. This beneficial effect might also be related to lack of response of these mice to OEA, a substance that was also implicated in feeding behavior.

Other loss-of-function studies such as transgenic mice expressing TRPV1 short hairpin RNA (shRNA) have shown that silencing the gene encoding for TRPV1 by RNA interference significantly attenuates capsaicin-induced nocifensive behavior and sensitivity toward noxious heat, a similar phenotype that was observed in the TRPV1 "knockout" mice [106]. Interestingly, and unlike the TRPV1 (–/–) mice, the TRPV1 shRNA mice did not develop mechanical hypersensitivity in the spinal nerve injury model of neuropathic pain. This is in accord with the reversal by capsazepine of mechanical hyperalgesia following sciatic nerve injury (chronic constriction injury [CCI] model) in the rat. In addition, antisense oligonucleotides and short interfering RNAs (siRNAs) have been reported and used to characterize the role of TRPV1 in pain [107–109]. Surprisingly, the injection of short interference RNA targeting TRPV1 significantly reduced the sensitivity of the rats to noxious heat but had no effect on the development of thermal hyperalgesia, which is highly impaired in the knockout mice. This finding may be interpreted to suggest marked species-related differences in the contribution of TRPV1 to pain states that may hinder the extrapolation of animal studies to man. An antibody directed at the extracellular loop that precedes the pore domain is an antagonist *in vitro*, but no *in vivo* characterization was reported [110].

Another study has reported that TRPV1 mice lacking a functional *TRPV1* gene did not display nocifensive behavior following intraplantar injection of phorbol 12-myristate 13-acetate (PMA), a PKC activator, suggesting that PMA-induced nocifensive behavior was exclusively dependent on TRPV1 [104].

Taken together, the above-mentioned evidence strongly implicates TRPV1 as an important polymodal receptor whose function is to combine multiple noxious physical and chemical stimuli in a nociceptive response predominantly during inflammatory conditions and tissue damage.

8.4.2 Brain TRPV1 Receptors and Pain

The presence and function of TRPV1 in the brain remains controversial. In Northern blot experiments, no TRPV1-encoding mRNA was detected in brain preparations. This negative result most likely reflects the low level of TRPV1 signal in brain nuclei compared with DRG. Now the presence of TRPV1 mRNA and protein is well-established throughout the whole neuroaxis of the rat, from the olfactory bulb through cortex, limbic system, and basal ganglia down to the brain stem and cerebellum [111–113]. TRPV1 receptors have been identified in various central regions known for their role in pain transmission or modulation [111,113,114]. These regions include (but are not restricted to) the amygdala, solitary tract nucleus, somatosensory cortex, anterior cingulated cortex, and insula [115]. Importantly, the presence of TRPV1 was also demonstrated in the human cortex and basal ganglia [113]. The TRPV1 receptor is localized in the cell bodies and dendrites of sensory neurons, in astrocytes, and in perivascular structures within the brain [113,114,116,117]. The latter finding is intriguing in the light of the recent concept that glial cells and astrocytes contribute to the maintenance of neuropathic pain. Intracerebroventricular (ICV) capsaicin injection was shown to decrease nociceptive threshold and to reduce morphine- and stress-induced analgesia [118,119]. Moreover, the ICV administration of TRPV1 receptor antagonists attenuated nocifensive behavior induced by an intradermal injection of capsaicin or formalin in mice [120].

A recent study showed that systemic administration of TRPV1 antagonists can reduce the spontaneous firing of spinal wide dynamic range (WDR) neurons in inflamed, but not control, rats. Spontaneous firing is elevated after injury and may reflect ongoing pain in the animal [121].

The locus coeruleus (LC) is activated by painful stimuli, and its stimulation produces antinociception. Systemic capsaicin increased LC firing activity even after sensory nerve fiber destruction, confirming a central effect of capsaicin [122,123]. In accord, TRPV1 receptor activation with capsaicin increased glutamatergic miniature excitatory postsynaptic currents in LC [124]. TRPV1 receptor stimulation by capsaicin application into the ventral tegmental area was shown to enhance dopaminergic output to the nucleus accumbens following peripheral noxious stimulation, suggesting a novel role for TRPV1 channels in the mesencephalon [125].

Of note, TRPV1 antagonists that enter the CNS are superior as analgesic drugs to their peripherally restricted analogs. TRPV1 is present at high densities in the dorsal horn of the spinal cord, and a spinal action is long believed to contribute to desensitization to vanilloids. However, it is feasible that pharmacological blockade of TRPV1 expressed in brain nuclei (that are believed to be involved in pain processing) also contributes to the analgesic activity of brain-penetrant TRPV1 antagonists.

8.5 TRPV1 ANTAGONISTS: A PRECLINICAL OVERVIEW

The rational for using potent and selective small-molecule TRPV1 antagonists to relieve inflammatory pain is the recognition that TRPV1 is activated by agents present in the inflammatory soup, the so-called endovanilloids (reviewed in References 9 and 13). In other words, TRPV1 antagonists prevent activation by endovanilloids of TRPV1. It is well established that capsaicin "silences" TRPV1-expressing neurons via ill-defined molecular processes (reviewed in References 16, 34, 44, and 98). Indeed, neurons desensitized to capsaicin are also unresponsive to mustard oil [126] though this chemical agent acts on

TRPA1 and not TRPV1 [127]. As TRPV1 agonists like capsaicin and RTX block neuropathic pain both in preclinical models [16,34,44,98] and patients [18,100], and as TRPV1 antagonists are effective therapeutics in models of inflammatory pain [17,21,22], it has been tempting to postulate that TRPV1 antagonists will be new therapeutics in neuropathic pain.

A number of pharmaceutical companies have initiated drug discovery programs to identify new TRPV1 modulators for the treatment of different pain states by mass-screening of compound libraries. This has resulted in the identification of a variety of potent and efficacious small-molecule TRPV1 antagonists (see Table 8.1). However, the first TRPV1 antagonist of significant potency, capsazepine, was obtained by systematic chemical modification of capsaicin [128]. It is important to note that capsazepine is not selective for TRPV1. In fact, capsazepine inhibits nicotinic acetylcholine and voltage-gated calcium channels (reviewed in References 9 and 44), as well as TRPM8 [129,130]. This is a problem as many studies had employed capsazepine as a "selective capsaicin antagonist."

Recently, many small-molecule TRPV1 antagonists with great potency and selectivity have been described (reviewed in References 17, 21, 22, and 131). As discussed above, TRPV1 is activated by multiple stimuli that interact with different domains of the channel protein. Therefore, it is hardly surprising that some TRPV1 blockers appear to be stimulus specific [132,133]. For instance, AMG-0610 [(2E)-3-(6-tert-butyl-2-methylpyridin-3-yl)-N-(1H-indol-6-yl)acrylamide, by Amgen, Thousand Oaks, CA, USA] and SB-366791 [N-(3-methoxyphenyl)-4-chlorocinnamide, by GlaxoSmithKline, Harlow, Essex, UK] inhibit the activation of rat TRPV1 by capsaicin, but not by acid, whereas I-RTX, N-(4-tertiarybutylphenyl)-4(3-cholorphyridin-2-yl)-tetrahydropyrazine-1(2H)-carboxamide (BCTC), (2E)-3-[2-piperidin-1-yl-6-(trifluoromethyl) pyridin-3-yl]-N-quinolin-7-ylacrylamide (AMG-6880, by Amgen), 5-chloro-6-{(3R)-3-methyl-4-[6-(trifluoromethyl)-4-(3,4,5-trifluorophenyl)-1Hbenzimidazol-2-yl]piperazin-1-yl}pyridin-3-yl)methanol (AMG-7472, by Amgen), (E)-3-(4-t-butylphenyl)-N-(2,3-dihydrobenzo[b][1,4]dioxin-6-yl)acrylamide (AMG-9810), and 1-isoquinolin-5-yl-3-(4-trifluoromethyl-benzyl)-urea (A-425619) are TRPV1 antagonists that do not differentiate between capsaicin and protons [132,134–136]. These compounds were referred to as profile A (blocks TRPV1 activation by both capsaicin and protons) and B (selective for capsaicin) antagonists, respectively.

The situation is, however, even more complex. For example, (R,E)-N-(2-hydroxy-2,3-dihydro-1H-inden-4-yl)-3-(2-(piperidin-1-yl)-4-(trifluoromethyl) phenyl)acrylamide (AMG-8562) blocks capsaicin-induced activation of TRPV1 but paradoxically potentiates activation by protons of rat TRPV1 [133]. This behavior was designated as profile C antagonist. In the rat, profile A and B antagonists are associated with a hyperthermic (febrile) response, whereas profile C compounds are devoid of this adverse effect. However, there are marked species-related differences in pharmacological profile of TRPV1 blockers. Most importantly, AMG-8562 functions as a profile B antagonist (and causes hyperthermia) in nonrodents. Other examples include capsazepine and

TABLE 8.1. Profiles of Selected Competitive TRPV1 Antagonists.

	rIC_{50} (Capsaicin)	hIC_{50} (Capsaicin)	**Effective Dose** (Acute Inflammatory Pain)	Effective Dose (Neuropathic Pain)	Development Status	Hyperthermia (in Rats)	References
A-425619 (Abbott)	9 nM	5 nM	4–10 mg/kg (p.o.)	>100 mg/kg (p.o.)	Preclinic	√	[142,231,232,233]
A-784168 (Abbott)	10 nM	23 nM	6–76 µmol/kg (p.o.)	86 µmol (i.t.)	Preclinic	N/A	[144,145]
ABT-102 (Abbott)	1 nM	7 nM	30–300 nmol (i.pl.)	N/A	Clinical candidate	√	[148,149]
AMG-517 (Amgen)	1 nM	0.76–1 nM	0.3–30 mg/kg (p.o.)	N/A	Phase II (abandoned)	√	[155,234]
AMG-8562 (Amgen)	1.75 nM		1–100 mg/kg (p.o.)	N/A	Preclinic	No effect	[133]
AMG-9810 (Amgen)	86 nM	25 nM	30–100 mg/kg (i.p.)	N/A	Preclinic	√	[9,152,235]
BCTC (Neurogen)	35 nM	0.3 nM	3–30 mg/kg (p.o.)	10–30 mg/kg (p.o.)	Preclinic	√	[140,152,236]
Capsazepine (Sandoz-NVS, now Novartis)	420 nM	149 nM	30–100 mg/kg (s.c.)	30 mg/kg (s.c.)	Preclinic	√	[131,139]

GRC-6211 (Glenmark/Lilly)	9.9 nM	3.6 nM	1–10 mg/kg (p.o.)	0.3–3 mg/kg (p.o.)	Phase II	No effect	[26,146]
JNJ-17203212 (J&J-PRD)	35 nM	65 nM	N/A	30 mg/kg (s.c.) (cancer pain)	Preclinic	√	[9,143]
JYL-1421 (Schwarz Pharma)	8 nM	N/A	>2 mg/kg (p.o.)	N/A	Preclinic	No effect	[131,237]
SB-705498 (GlaxoSmithKline)	32 nM	3 nM	2–10 mg/kg (p.o.)	Active	Phase II	√	[238,239,131]
V377 (PharmEste)	6 nM	N/A	2–30 mg/kg (p.o.)	3–30 mg/kg (p.o.)	Preclinic	No effect	[147]

√indicates that hyperthermia has been observed in rats.

A-425619, 1-isoquinolin-5-yl-3-(4-trifluoromethyl-benzyl)-urea; A-784168, 1-(3-(trifluoromethyl)pyridin-2-yl)-N-(4-(trifluoromethylsulfonyl)phenyl)-1,2,3,6-tetrahydropyridine-4-carboxamide; ABT-102, (R)-1-(5-tert-butyl-2,3-dihydro-1H-inden-1-yl)-3-(1H-indazol-4-yl)urea; AMG-517, N-(4-[6-(4-trifluoromethyl-phenyl)-pyrimidin-4-yloxy]-benzothiazol-2-yl)-acetamide; AMG-8562, (R,E)-N-(2-hydroxy-2,3-dihydro-1H-inden-4-yl)-3-(2-(piperidin-1-yl)-4-(trifluoromethyl)phenyl)acrylamide; AMG-9810, (E)-3-(4-t-butylphenyl)-N-(2,3-dihydrobenzo[b][1,4]dioxin-6-yl)acrylamide; BCTC, N-(4-tertiarybutylphenyl)-4(3-cholorphyridin-2-yl)-tetrahydropyrazine-1(2H)-carboxamide; GRC-6211, chemical structure undisclosed; JNJ-17203212, 4-(3-trifluoromethyl-pyridin-2-yl)-piperazine-1-carboxylic acid (5-trifluoromethyl-pyridin-2-yl)-amide; JYL-1421, *N*-(4-*tert*-butylbenzyl)-*N'*-[3-fluoro-4-(methylsulfonylamino) benzyl]thiourea; SB-705498, N-(2-bromophenyl)-N'-[((R)-1-(5-trifluoromethyl-2-pyridyl)pyrrolidin-3-yl)] urea; V377, chemical structure undisclosed; rIC_{50} and hIC_{50}, concentration of antagonists that prevent 50% of capsaicin-induced response on rat or human TRPV1 receptor, respectively; N/A, not available; p.o., *per os*; i.pl., intraplantar; i.p., intraperitoneal; s.c., subcutaneous, i.t., intrathecal.

SB-366791 that are more effective in blocking proton-induced gating of human TRPV1 than of rat TRPV1 [132,137]. Among these inhibitors, I-RTX, the urea analog BCTC, and the cinnamide analog SB-366791 are the best characterized. Within this group, I-RTX and SB-366791 are selective for TRPV1 compared with other receptors and channels, whereas BCTC is an inhibitor of TRPM8 [138]. These results warrant caution when extrapolating the results of animal experiments (and in particular rodent experiments) with TRPV1 antagonists to humans.

Several structurally different TRPV1 antagonists such as capsazepine, BCTC, A-425619, 1-(3-(trifluoromethyl)pyridin-2-yl)-N-(4-(trifluoromethylsulfonyl)phenyl)-1,2,3,6-tetrahydropyridine-4-carboxamide (A-784168), GRC-6211 (clinical candidate by Glenmark (Chakala, Mumbai, India)/Lilly (Indianapolis, IN, USA)), V377 (lead molecule by PharmEste, Ferrara, Italy), and the quinazolinone "compound 26" are reported to decrease hypersensitivity in rat neuropathic pain models [139–147] (Table 8.1). A recent study showed that a new TRPV1 receptor antagonist, (R)-1-(5-tert-butyl-2,3-dihydro-1H-inden-1-yl)-3-(1H-indazol-4-yl)urea (ABT-102) (Table 8.1), which has just entered in clinical trials, exhibits analgesic properties in several rodent pain models, including chronic inflammatory, bone cancer, and post-operative pain [148,149].

It should be mentioned that preclinical models of pain may underestimate the clinical value of TRPV1 antagonist in that they do not adequately address the extent of spontaneous or ongoing pain in rodents [6]. It is also worth noting that while pain due to cancer may only partly arise from neuropathy, TRPV1 antagonists have exhibited utility in models of cancer pain [102,103].

8.5.1 TRPV1 and Body Temperature Regulation

On-target (type I) side effects due to TRPV1 antagonism were believed to be relatively benign, and no idiosyncratic (type II) adverse effects have been reported to date. Agonists of TRPV1, such as capsaicin and RTX, have long been known to decrease body temperature in multiple species including humans [44,150]; this effect was attributed to skin vasodilation and reduction in metabolism (a decreased VO2 reflects decreased heat production).

A new (and debated) concept suggests that a predominant function of TRPV1 is body temperature regulation [151]. This concept is based on the profound hyperthermic action of some (but not all) TRPV1 antagonists, implying an endogenous tone for TRPV1 involved in thermoregulation [151,152]. The initial observation was that the urea analog TRPV1 antagonist ("compound 41") increased core body temperature when administered to rats [143]. Subsequently, another study reported that the low CNS-penetrant TRPV1 antagonist AMG-0347 [(E)-N-(7-hydroxy-5,6,7,8-tetrahydronaphthalen-1-yl)-3-(2-(piperidin-1-yl)-6-(trifluoromethyl)pyridin-3-yl)acrylamide, by Amgen] was no more effective in causing hyperthermia when administered into the brain (intracerebroventricularly) or spinal cord (intrathecally) than when given systemically (intravenously) [153]. This evidence suggested that TRPV1 expressed on a peripheral site (i.e., outside the blood-brain barrier) mediated the effect of TRPV1 antagonist on core body temperature [153]. Subchronic administration of TRPV1 antagonists results in desensitization of the hyperthermic effect, consistent with the observation that core body temperature in TRPV1 knockout mice is identical to wild-type mice. Although it was initially believed that the transient hyperthermic activity of TRPV1 antagonists could be reversed by acetaminophen and other common antipyretics, later it turned out not to be the case for all compounds.

Additional investigations comparing limited CNS exposure compounds [e.g., A-795614, (N-1H-indazol-4-yl-N′-[(1R)-5-piperidin-1-yl-2,3-dihydro-1H-inden-1-yl]urea), by Abbott] to their brain-penetrant analogs [e.g., A-784168, (1-[3-(trifluoromethyl)pyridin-2-yl]-N-[4-(trifluoromethylsulfonyl) phenyl]-1,2,3,6-tetrahydropyridine-4-carboxamide), by Abbott] suggest that CNS exposure improves the analgesic efficacy of TRPV1 antagonists [145]. However, rats treated with compounds with very low CNS exposure exhibited core body temperature increases that were comparable to brain-penetrant compounds [154]. These data support the hypothesis that TRPV1 expressed in the CNS (perhaps in terminals of sensory neuron projections to the spinal cord dorsal horn) is important for mediating nociception, but that TRPV1 in CNS sites such as the hypothalamus may not be involved in regulating core body temperature [151]. The site of action for antagonist-induced hyperthermia to be present outside the blood-brain barrier was further confirmed by TRPV1 desensitization experiments (with RTX) that demonstrated that visceral TRPV1 channels were responsible for antagonist-induced hyperthermia [153].

Compound N-(4-[6-(4-trifluoromethyl-phenyl)-pyrimidin-4-yloxy]-benzothiazol-2-yl)-acetamide (AMG-517) (Amgen, see Table 8.1) is a highly selective TRPV1 antagonist whose clinical trials were terminated due to the undesirable magnitude of hyperthermia [155]. Other potent TRPV1 antagonists (e.g., AMG-8562, GRC-6211, and V377), however, have no effect on body temperature (S. Narayanan and M. Trevisani, pers. comm.) or, conversely, cause hypothermia following a very mild and circadian-dependent hyperthermic response [133].

An experimental approach aimed to eliminate TRPV1 antagonist-induced hyperthermia was to evaluate compounds that display *in vitro* differential pharmacologies (i.e., compounds that differentially modulate distinct modes of *in vitro* TRPV1 activation such as capsaicin, pH 5, and heat) [133]. Letho and coworkers reported results concerning four potent and selective TRPV1 modulators with unique *in vitro* pharmacology profiles and their respective effects on body temperature. They concluded that it is feasible to eliminate hyperthermia while preserving antihyperalgesia by differential modulation of distinct modes of TRPV1 activation. From this investigation, potentiation of pH (5) activation alone seems to negate the classic TRPV1 blockade-mediated hyperthermia [133]. Obviously, more research is needed to resolve these conflicting findings and to appreciate the impact of TRPV1 antagonism on body temperature.

8.5.2 TRPV1 Antagonist Undergoing Clinical Trials for Indications Related to Pain

Several small-molecule TRPV1 antagonists are currently undergoing phase I and II clinical trials for indications related to pain. Phase I data obtained with N-(2-bromophenyl)-N′-[((R)-1-(5-trifluoromethyl-2-pyridyl)pyrrolidin-3-yl)] urea (SB-705498) (GlaxoSmithKline) have been reported [23]. In the first part of the study, single doses of SB-705498 ranging from 2 to 200 mg did not display efficacy in the capsaicin-evoked flare test. However, in the second part of the study, a single oral dose of 400 mg SB-705498 substantially reduced pain from cutaneous capsaicin challenge (0.075% capsaicin cream applied to the forearm) compared with placebo. In December 2005, an active-controlled, placebo-controlled, randomized, single-blind, phase II trial (NCT00281684, VRA105345) was initiated in subjects with dental pain following third molar tooth extraction. The subjects were to receive a single oral dose of SB-705498, placebo or co-codamol. The study was completed in February 2008, and no results have been revealed yet [25].

AstraZeneca (Wilmington, DE, USA) is developing AZD-1386, a TRPV1 antagonist, for the potential oral treatment of chronic nociceptive pain and gastroesophageal reflux disease (GERD). In April 2008, an active-controlled, placebo-controlled, randomized, double-blind phase II trial (NCT00672646, D5090C00010) was initiated in subjects with pain. The study was expected to be complete in June 2008 [28].

A phase II trial with the TRPV1 antagonist, GRC-6211 (Glenmark/Lilly) is still ongoing for incontinence [26], but the osteoarthritis trial was terminated owing to undisclosed reasons.

Merck (Whitehouse, NJ, USA) is developing MK-2295 (NGD-8243, MRK-2295), the lead from a series of orally active small-molecule TRPV1 antagonists, for the potential treatment of pain and cough [27,156].

Japan Tobacco (Tokyo, Japan) is developing an oral TRPV1 antagonist, namely JTS-653, for the potential treatment of pain and overactive bladder. In February 2008, a Japanese phase I study was ongoing [157].

8.6 TRPV2, A STRUCTURAL HOMOLOG OF TRPV1

TRPV2, originally named “vanilloid receptor-like protein 1” (VR-L1), was discovered as a structural homolog of TRPV1 with 50% amino acid identity [158]. It is insensitive to capsaicin and protons but is activated by high temperature (52 °C and higher) [158], 2-aminoethoxydiphenyl borate (2-APB) [159], probenicid [160], swelling, and high concentrations of delta9-tetrahydrocannabinol (Figures 8.1 and 8.2) [161]. TRPV2 exhibits a much broader tissue distribution than TRPV1, and its expression in sensory neuron subpopulations is largely distinct from other TRP channels [162,163]. TRPV2 is also expressed in certain hypothalamic brain nuclei and in some non-neuronal tissues including the heart, gastrointestinal (GI) tract, macrophages, lymphocytes, and smooth muscle [164–166]. Because of its very high heat threshold as well as its differential distribution compared with TRPV1, there have been fewer studies related to pain that focus on TRPV2.

TRPV2 is found in myelinated sensory fibers that are mechanically sensitive, and its expression is increased in DRG neurons in response to nerve injury and peripheral inflammation [167]. In certain cellular contexts, the intracellular localization of TRPV2 is affected by growth factors [168]; however, these observations have not been extended to sensory neurons. A study with TRPV2 antisense oligonucleotide provided evidence that TRPV2 mediated membrane stretch-activated currents in Chinese hamster ovary (CHO) cells overexpressing TRPV2 and aortic myocytes [165]. Additionally, a TRPV2 siRNA has been reported to block fMLF (N-formyl-Met-Leu-Phe)-activated calcium entry in a macrophage cell line [169]. The generation of mice lacking functional *TRPV2* gene would be very useful to further investigate its role in inflammatory and neuropathic pain.

8.7 TRPV3, A WARM-SENSITIVE RELATIVE OF TRPV1

TRPV3 shares 40% identity with TRPV1 and is activated by warm temperature (32–39 °C), with increased responses to higher noxious thermal stimuli and enhanced current following repetitive heat stimulation [170,171]. TRPV3 is also activated and sensitized (to heat) by 2-APB and monoterpenes, including camphor, carvacrol, and thymol, as well as the vanilloid compounds eugenol, vanillin, and ethyl-vanillin [159,172,173] (Figure 8.2). TRPV3 exhibits both homologous and heterologous sensitization [174,175]; this characteristic supports the potential role of TRPV3 as a molecular thermal nociceptor. Moreover, TRPV3 activation by 2-APB is potentiated by unsaturated fatty acids including arachidonic acid as well as by protein kinase activation [173].

Adding to the complexity of the potential role of TRPV3 in pain, its tissue expression varies depending on the species considered. While it is specific to the skin (e.g., keratinocytes) in mice [176], in humans, it is expressed in the TG, spinal cord, brain, keratinocytes, tongue, and DRG neurons [171]. It is worth mentioning that TRPV3 is downregulated in the skin of patients with diabetic polyneuropathy [42] while its expression is enhanced in skin biopsies obtained from the breast of women with mastalgia (e.g., breast tenderness due to macromastia) [177].

The proof of concept for the role of TRPV3 in thermal nociception and hyperalgesia was furnished by knockout experiments [51]. Indeed, GRC-15133, a selective TRPV3 antagonist developed at Glenmark, was shown to relieve both inflammatory and neuropathic pain in animal models [178]. Surprisingly, GRC-15133 also caused mechanical hyperalgesia in rats following nerve injury. These results are difficult to reconcile with the apparent lack of TRPV3 expression in rodent sensory ganglia. It is possible that rodent DRG neurons start expressing TRPV3 under pathological conditions, similar to the abnormal expression by Aδ-fibers of TRPV1 in murine models of diabetic neuropathy. It is also possible that TRPV3 expressed on keratinocytes is somehow involved in the development of hyperalgesia.

Of note, TRPV3 knockout mice have a fairly unremarkable phenotype with only mild alterations in hair texture (G. Story, pers. comm.). This is in sharp contrast to animals with gain of function TRPV3 mutations that suffer from severe alopecia and an atopic dermatitis-like skin condition [179,180]. Most recently, incensole acetate (an ingredient in incense) was shown to possess anxiolytic- and antidepressant-like activity in wild-type, but not in TRPV3 knockout, mice, implying a role for TRPV3 in mood disorders [181]. Finally, it should be mentioned that TRPV3 antagonists exert a hypothermic effect in the brain that may be exploited for neuroprotection [182,183].

8.8 TRPV4, A POLYMODAL CHANNEL WITH A WIDESPREAD DIVERSITY OF ACTIVATION MECHANISMS

TRPV4 is activated by a variety of physical (moderate heat, cell swelling, mechanical stimuli) and chemical stimuli. Indeed, initially characterized as an osmolarity-sensitive channel, TRPV4 is now known to be activated by increases in temperatures (with a threshold between 25 and 34 °C), by 4α-phorbol 12,13-didecanoate (4αPDD), and by epoxyeicosatrienoic acids (cytochrome P450 metabolites of anandamide and arachidonic acid) [184–186] (Figure 8.2). Activation of TRPV4 by cell swelling is caused by phospholipase A2 (PLA2) activation [185,187]. PLA2-mediated release of arachidonic acid from membrane lipids and its subsequent metabolization by cytochrome P450 epoxygenase activity lead to the formation of epoxyeicosatrienoic acids, which activate TRPV4 directly.

While TRPV4 is widely expressed in the brain, heart, placenta, bladder, kidney, lung, and skeletal muscle [188,189], its distribution in the cochlear hair cells, Merkel cells, and sensory ganglia [66,145,190,191] as well as in the free nerve endings and cutaneous A- and C-fiber terminals [192] suggest a role for TRPV4 in mechanotransduction beyond osmosensation.

Unlike TRPV3, TRPV4 channels get desensitized in response to prolonged suprathreshold heat stimuli [193]. Experiments with TRPV4 (–/–) mice suggest that (i) TRPV4 plays a role in normal warm sensation [194] and (ii) it acts as a mechanosensor [192]. In fact, TRPV4 knockout mice show reduced mechanical hyperalgesia [195]. Surprisingly, TRPV4 mutant and wild-type mice behaved similarly in the hot-plate assay (latency to escape; 35–50 °C) or when their paws were exposed to radiant heat, suggesting this channel is not involved in acute noxious thermal sensation [196]. In contrast, TRPV4 mutant mice exhibit higher withdrawal latency in response to heat in a tail immersion assay performed at 45–46 °C [194]. While the same group showed that TRPV4 mutant mice behaved normally in the temperature gradient assay after intraplantar complete Freund's adjuvant (CFA) injection, others concluded that TRPV4 plays an essential role in models of carrageenan-induced thermal hyperalgesia and inflammatory mediator-induced mechanical hyperalgesia [196,197]. Furthermore, spinal administration of antisense oligodeoxynucleotides to TRPV4 abolished taxol-induced mechanical hyperalgeisa in a model of chemotherapy-induced neuropathic pain [198].

Although current knowledge on TRPV4 function suggests that it may play a role complementary to that of TRPV1 in producing peripheral sensitization, more investigation is needed to better elucidate its pathophysiological functions. Moreover, the severe phenotype of TRPV4 knockout mice (deaf [199], incontinent [70], and deficient in osmoregulation [200]) questions the clinical utility of TRPV4 antagonists.

8.9 TRPA1, THE COLD RECEPTOR HIGHLY COEXPRESSED WITH THE HOT TRPV1

TRPA1 was first identified as a protein overexpressed in a liposarcoma cell line (Ankyrin-like Protein with Transmembrane Domains 1, ANKTM1 [201]). Eventually, TRPA1 was recognized as the as yet sole member of a new TRP subfamily, the ankyrin family. TRPA1 was originally characterized as a noxious, cold-activated ion channel with a threshold of activation of about 17 °C [202], although this finding remains controversial. TRPA1 is highly coexpressed with TRPV1 in small-diameter peptidergic nociceptors, while it is rarely expressed with TRPM8 [202–204] (Figure 8.2). This evidence led to the proposal that noxious cold might consist of two components: cold sensation that may be processed by TRPM8-expressing neurons and a painful component that might be brought by activation of TRPA1-expressing polymodal nociceptors [205].

Several reports showed that TRPA1 can also be activated by pungent compounds and irritants such as cinnamaldehyde (cinnamon oil), isothiocyanates (such as those found in mustard oil), allicin (from garlic), acrolein (a metabolized by-product of chemotherapeutic agents and also present in tear gas and vehicle exhaust), and formalin that can induce acute pain, hyperalgesia, or neurogenic inflammation in animals and humans [47–49,204,206–209] (Figure 8.2). For example, mustard oil has been historically used as a chemical algogen resulting in neurogenic inflammation and was shown to evoke a sharp pain and hyperalgesia in human subjects [210–213]. Cinnamaldehyde was shown to induce acute nociception and hyperalgesia in mice and human subjects [47,48]. More recently, the α,β-unsaturated aldehyde, 4-hydroxy-2-nonenal (HNE), and the electrophilic carbon-containing prostaglandin J2 (PGJ2) metabolite 15-deoxy-delta-12,14-PGJ2 (15dPGJ2) released in response to tissue injury, inflammation, and oxidative stress, were reported to be the first endogenous activators of TRPA1 [214–217]. TRPA1 can also be activated by bradykinin and has been recently proposed as a candidate mechanically activated channel involved in hearing [29,218]. Finally, TRPA1 appears to be sensitized by NGF and proteinase-activated receptor-2 (PAR-2) [219,220], both of which are known to play a role in inflammatory pain.

TRPA1 is expressed in the dorsal root, trigeminal, and nodose ganglia in a specific subpopulation of neurons that coexpress TRPV1 [202,220] (Figure 8.2). TRPA1 was also shown to be expressed in the hair cells of the inner ear; however, a role for TRPA1 in hearing has not been established to date [218].

TRPA1 mRNA expression was reported to increase in tyrosine kinase receptor A (trkA)-expressing (i.e., NGF responsive) small- to medium-diameter neurons in L5 DRG following spinal nerve ligation (SNL), contributing to the exaggerated response to cold observed in the neuropathic pain model [221]. In models of inflammatory and neuropathic pain, knockdown of TRPA1 by intrathecal administration of specific antisense oligodeoxynucleotides suppresses SNL- and CFA-induced cold hyperalgesia [221]. Antisense and knockout studies have identified a role for TRPA1 in pain mechanism. TRPA1 expression is induced following both inflammatory and nerve injuries, and TRPM8 antisense knockdown resulted in decreased cold hyperalgesia with little effect on thermal (heat) hyperalgesia or mechanical allodynia [222]. Moreover, in contrast to TRPV1 mutant mice, which exhibit strong deficits in thermal hyperalgesia irrespective of the methods used to induce inflammation, TRPA1 null mice developed a robust and normal thermal and mechanical hyperalgesia upon CFA injection [207,223,224].

Given its expression on polymodal nociceptor neurons and its activation by proalgesic compounds and, possibly, noxious cold temperatures, TRPA1 is proposed to have a pivotal role in integrating nociceptive stimuli. The first pharmacological evidence implicating the TRPA1 in mediating pain under inflammatory conditions came recently when it was shown that AP18 [(Z)-4-(4-chlorophynyl)-3-methylbut-3-en-2-oxime], a TRPA1 small-molecule antagonist, can significantly attenuate CFA-induced inflammatory pain [224]. AP18 is a selective TRPA1 antagonist that inhibits both the mouse and the human receptors. Acute pharmacological inhibition of TRPA1 using intraplantar (local) injection of AP18 significantly reduced the CFA-induced mechanical hypersensitivity and cold allodynia. AP18 has no effect in TRPA1 (–/–) mice, strongly suggesting that AP18-induced analgesia results from on-target activities [224]. Moreover, local preadministration of AP18 in the hind paw reversed cinnamaldehyde-induced nocifensor behavior, again indicating that AP18 acts on the TRPA1 receptors.

Another selective TRPA1 antagonist, HC-030031 [2-(1,3-dimethyl-2,6-dioxo-1,2,3,6-tetrahydro-7H-purin-7-yl)-N-(4-isopropylphenyl)acetamide], [208] was shown to significantly and dose-dependently (100 and 300 mg/kg) reduce flinching in both phases of the formalin response *in vivo* and to abolish allyl isothiocyanate (AITC)-induced mechanical hypersensitivity in a dose-dependent manner. Other TRPA1 antagonists have been reported [e.g. 4-nitro-N-(2,2,2-trichloro-1-((4-chlorophenyl)sulfanyl)ethyl)benzamide, AMG-2504, by Amgen] but have not yet been characterized *in vivo* [225]. Moreover, oral HC-030031 (100 mg/kg) significantly reversed mechanical hypersensitivity [226] in the models CFA-induced inflammatory pain and the SNL model of neuropathic pain. If many questions remain on the exact modalities of TRPA1 activation, its contribution to nociception is reasonably well established.

8.10 TRPM8, THE COOL MENTHOL RECEPTOR

The cold menthol receptor TRPM8 belongs to the "melastatin" TRP family. First identified in the prostate gland as an androgen-responsive channel, TRPM8 is now described as a cold- and menthol-activated channel [50,225,227]. The cloning and characterization of TRPM8 marked a milestone in our understanding the molecular mechanisms underlying cold temperature transduction. TRPM8 is expressed in ~15% of small-diameter DRG and trigeminal neurons [50,225]. It is a nonselective cation channel that permeates Ca2+, Cs+, K+, and Na+ and can be activated by cold temperatures (threshold of 18–24 °C), menthol, and icilin, a monoterpene synthetic supercooling compound (Figures 8.1 and 8.2). Activation of TRPM8 is followed by desensitization of the channel that depends on extracellular Ca2+. TRPM8 is also activated by numerous other cooling compounds such as eucalyptol, spearmint, and WS-3 (N-Ethyl-5-methyl-2-(1-methylethyl)cyclohexanecarboxamide).

In analogy to the synergistic effect of capsaicin and heat on the activation of TRPV1, menthol and other agonists were shown to activate and sensitize the TRPM8 channel, rendering the channel active at higher temperatures [50,225]. Interestingly, when compared with TRPV1, TRPM8 exhibits opposite mechanisms of activation: PIP2 acts as an enhancer of the channel activation by cold and menthol preventing its desensitization, while PKC leads to its dephosphorylation [56,228].

While *in vitro* data provided strong evidence of a possible role for TRPM8 in cold sensation, the validation of TRPM8 role in cold transduction *in vivo* came after three independent studies on TRPM8-deficient mice [205,227,229]. All three working groups used the two temperature preference assay and challenged the mice to choose between a preferred warm temperature (30–34 °C) and a cool temperature usually avoided by mice. Strikingly, and unlike the wild-type mice, mice lacking TRPM8 function lost their preference to warm temperatures (or avoidance of cool temperatures). It is noteworthy that while two studies showed that TRPM8 knockout mice regained aversion to cold temperatures at or below 10 °C [205,227], one study showed that the deficit in cold temperatures detection persists down to 0 °C [229]. Nevertheless, all three studies indicate that TRPM8 plays a central and essential role in cold temperature transduction and perception.

Sensitivity to cold is heightened in certain inflammatory and neuropathic pain conditions. This results in the development of cold allodynia, a painful hypersensitivity to innocuous cold temperature stimulation. The role of TRPM8 in mediating cold, mechanical, and thermal hypersensitivity under pathophysiological conditions remains elusive. TRPM8 expression is increased in the ipsilateral DRG neurons after the development of neuropathic pain

[130,167,230]. But different studies indicate that both agonism and antagonism of TRPM8 may be involved in mediating its analgesic effect.

Two recent studies investigated a potential role of TRPM8 in pain hypersensitivity. Katsura and colleagues [221] reported that cold hyperalgesia induced by L5 SNL is not affected by TRPM8 antisense. Proudfoot and colleagues [230] reported that TRPM8 activation by icilin in sensory neurons elicited analgesia in three different models of inflammatory and neuropathic pain. TRPM8 agonism was also effective in reversing both thermal and mechanical hypersensitivity in the CFA model of inflammatory pain and in the cinnamaldehyde-induced hypersensitivity [230]. A more recent study, using a subtle modification of the formalin test, elegantly showed that while wild-type mice exhibit reduced formalin-induced nocifensor behavior when placed on plates set at 17 °C, mice lacking TRPM8 develop similar nociceptive responses at 17 °C and room temperature [205].

While these studies clearly implicate TRPM8 agonism in reversing the hypersensitivity observed across a wide spectrum of pain models, recent data suggest that TRPM8 blockade may lead to an analgesic effect as well. TRPM8 deficient homozygous mice were reported to develop virtually no cold allodynia in both CCI and CFA models, while tactile allodynia is not affected in both genotypes [229].

Although current knowledge on TRPM8 distribution and function implies a role for TRPM8 in nociception, further studies are needed to confirm whether agonism or antagonism of this target should be pursued to treat clinical pain indications.

8.11 CONCLUSIONS

Since their discovery, temperature-sensitive TRP channels (so-called thermoTRP) have been implicated in a number of physiological functions such as heat sensation and taste perception. At present, six temperature-sensitive TRP channels (TRPV1-4, TRPA1, and TRPM8) are known to be expressed in the sensory neurons. Many thermoTRP channels also serve as receptors for sensory-active substances such as capsaicin, menthol, mustard oil, and venoms. The high level of expression of these channels (especially TRPV1, TRPA1, and TRPM8) in the sensory neurons has led many investigators to embrace the hypothesis that modulators of TRP channels expressed on the sensory neurons might yield effective therapeutics for pain. Targeting thermoTRP channels on nociceptive neurons is an attractive new and logical strategy in drug development: thermoTRP channel antagonists aim to prevent pain by blocking a receptor where pain is generated. Genetic deletion and pharmacological blockade of TRPV1 furnished the first proof of concept that TRP inhibitors may relieve hyperalgesia and pain. Most importantly, potent and selective small-molecule TRPV1 antagonists were the first to move into clinical trials as potential analgesic drugs. Other thermoTRPs such as TRPA1 and TRPV3 are now recognized to play an important role in the mechanisms responsible for hypersensitivity observed in inflammatory and neuropathic pain conditions. Selective TRPV3 and TRPA1 antagonists are currently being tried in preclinical models of pain.

In conclusion, results from pharmacological antagonism and knockdown strategies and their ability to sense thermal and mechanical stimuli in physiopathological conditions suggest that thermoTRP channels play a crucial role in postinflammatory hyperalgesia and spontaneous (ongoing) pain.

REFERENCES

1. Campbell, J., Basbaum, A., Dray, A., Dubner, R., Dworkin, R., Sang, C. (2006). *Emerging Strategies for the Treatment of Neuropathic Pain.* Seattle, WA: IASP Press.
2. Gidal, B.E. (2006). New and emerging treatment options for neuropathic pain. *Am J Manag Care* 12:S269–S278.
3. Katz, W.A., Barkin, R.L. (2008). Dilemmas in chronic/persistent pain management. *Am J Ther* 15:256–264.
4. http://www.ampainsoc.org/decadeofthepain (accessed October 30, 2008).
5. Owen, R.T. (2007). Pregabalin: its efficacy, safety and tolerability profile in generalized anxiety. *Drugs Today (Barc)* 43:601–610.
6. Wallace, M.S. (2006). Ziconotide: a new nonopioid intrathecal analgesic for the treatment of chronic pain. *Expert Rev Neurother* 6:1423–1428.
7. Basbaum, A.I., Julius, D. (2006). Toward better pain control. *Sci Am* 294:60–67.
8. Caterina, M.J., Schumacher, M.A., Tominaga, M., Rosen, T.A., Levine, J.D., Julius, D. (1997). The capsaicin receptor: a heat-activated ion channel in the pain pathway. *Nature* 389:816–824.
9. Szallasi, A., Cortright, D.N., Blum, C.A., Eid, S.R. (2007). The vanilloid receptor TRPV1: 10 years from channel cloning to antagonist proof-of-concept. *Nat Rev Drug Discov* 6:357–372.
10. Caterina, M.J., Julius, D. (2001). The vanilloid receptor: a molecular gateway to the pain pathway. *Annu Rev Neurosci* 24:487–517.
11. Ferrer-Montiel, A., Garcia-Martinez, C., Morenilla-Palao, C., Garcia-Sanz, N., Fernandez-Carvajal, A., Fernandez-Ballester, G., Planells-Cases, R. (2004). Molecular architecture of the vanilloid receptor. Insights for drug design. *Eur J Biochem* 271:1820–1826.
12. Immke, D.C., Gavva, N.R. (2006). The TRPV1 receptor and nociception. *Semin Cell Dev Biol* 17:582–591.
13. Di Marzo, V., Blumberg, P.M., Szallasi, A. (2002). Endovanilloid signaling in pain. *Curr Opin Neurobiol* 12:372–379.
14. Suh, Y.G., Oh, U. (2005). Activation and activators of TRPV1 and their pharmaceutical implication. *Curr Pharm Des* 11:2687–2698.

15. Wang, H., Woolf, C.J. (2005). Pain TRPs. *Neuron* 46:9–12.
16. Malmberg, A., Bley, K. (2005). *Turning Up the Heat on Pain: TRPV1 Receptors in Pain and Inflammation*. Basel, Switzerland: Birkhäuser.
17. Roberts, L.A., Connor, M. (2006). TRPV1 antagonists as a potential treatment for hyperalgesia. *Recent Patents CNS Drug Discov* 1:65–76.
18. Knotkova, H., Pappagallo, M., Szallasi, A. (2008). Capsaicin (TRPV1 agonist) therapy for pain relief: farewell or revival? *Clin J Pain* 24:142–154.
19. Caterina, M.J., Leffler, A., Malmberg, A.B., Martin, W.J., Trafton, J., Petersen-Zeitz, K.R., Koltzenburg, M., Basbaum, A.I., Julius, D. (2000). Impaired nociception and pain sensation in mice lacking the capsaicin receptor. *Science* 288:306–313.
20. Davis, J.B., Gray, J., Gunthorpe, M.J., Hatcher, J.P., Davey, P.T., Overend, P., Harries, M.H., Latcham, J., Clapham, C., Atkinson, K., Hughes, S.A., Rance, K., Grau, E., Harper, A.J., Pugh, P.L., Rogers, D.C., Bingham, S., Randall, A., Sheardown, S.A. (2000). Vanilloid receptor-1 is essential for inflammatory thermal hyperalgesia. *Nature* 405:183–187.
21. Gharat, L., Szallasi, A. (2008). Advances in the design and therapeutic use of capsaicin receptor TRPV1 agonists and antagonists. *Expert Opin Ther Pat* 18:159–209.
22. Gunthorpe, M.J., Szallasi, A. (2008). Peripheral TRPV1 receptors as targets for drug development: new molecules and mechanisms. *Curr Pharm Des* 14:32–41.
23. Chizh, B.A., O'Donnell, M.B., Napolitano, A., Wang, J., Brooke, A.C., Aylott, M.C., Bullman, J.N., Gray, E.J., Lai, R.Y., Williams, P.M., Appleby, J.M. (2007). The effects of the TRPV1 antagonist SB-705498 on TRPV1 receptor-mediated activity and inflammatory hyperalgesia in humans. *Pain* 132:132–141.
24. Feltynek, C., Gomtsyan, A. (2009). *Vanilloid Receptor TRPV1 in Drug Discovery: Targeting Pain and Other Pathological Disorders*. John Wiley & Sons (in press).
25. http://clinicaltrials.gov/ct2/show/NCT00281684?cond (accessed October 30, 2008).
26. http://www.glenmarkpharma.com/research/clinical.html (accessed October 30, 2008).
27. http://www.merck.com/finance/pipeline.swf (accessed October 30, 2008).
28. http://clinicaltrials.gov/ct2/results?term=NCT00672646 (accessed October 30, 2008).
29. Dhaka, A., Viswanath, V., Patapoutian, A. (2006). Trp ion channels and temperature sensation. *Annu Rev Neurosci* 29:135–161.
30. Bandell, M., Macpherson, L.J., Patapoutian, A. (2007). From chills to chilis: mechanisms for thermosensation and chemesthesis via thermoTRPs. *Curr Opin Neurobiol* 17:490–497.
31. Talavera, K., Nilius, B., Voets, T. (2008). Neuronal TRP channels: thermometers, pathfinders and life-savers. *Trends Neurosci* 31:287–295.
32. Belmonte, C., Cervero, F. (1996). *Neurobiology of Nociceptors*. New York: Oxford University Press.
33. Kandel, E.R., Schwartz, J., Jessell, T. (1991). *Principles of Neural Science*. Norwalk, CT: Appleton and Lange.

34. Holzer, P. (1991). Capsaicin: cellular targets, mechanisms of action, and selectivity for thin sensory neurons. *Pharmacol Rev* 43:143–201.
35. Messlinger, K. (1996). Functional morphology of nociceptive and other fine sensory endings (free nerve endings) in different tissues. *Prog Brain Res* 113:273–298.
36. Schmidt, R., Schmelz, M., Ringkamp, M., Handwerker, H.O., Torebjork, H.E. (1997). Innervation territories of mechanically activated C nociceptor units in human skin. *J Neurophysiol* 78:2641–2648.
37. Schmidt, R., Schmelz, M., Weidner, C., Handwerker, H.O., Torebjork, H.E. (2002). Innervation territories of mechano-insensitive C nociceptors in human skin. *J Neurophysiol* 88:1859–1866.
38. Ma, Q.P. (2002). Expression of capsaicin receptor (VR1) by myelinated primary afferent neurons in rats. *Neurosci Lett* 319:87–90.
39. Rashid, M.H., Inoue, M., Kondo, S., Kawashima, T., Bakoshi, S., Ueda, H. (2003). Novel expression of vanilloid receptor 1 on capsaicin-insensitive fibers accounts for the analgesic effect of capsaicin cream in neuropathic pain. *J Pharmacol Exp Ther* 304:940–948.
40. Rashid, M.H., Inoue, M., Bakoshi, S., Ueda, H. (2003). Increased expression of vanilloid receptor 1 on myelinated primary afferent neurons contributes to the antihyperalgesic effect of capsaicin cream in diabetic neuropathic pain in mice. *J Pharmacol Exp Ther* 306:709–717.
41. Lauria, G., Morbin, M., Lombardi, R., Capobianco, R., Camozzi, F., Pareyson, D., Manconi, M., Geppetti, P. (2006). Expression of capsaicin receptor immunoreactivity in human peripheral nervous system and in painful neuropathies. *J Peripher Nerv Syst* 11:262–271.
42. Facer, P., Casula, M.A., Smith, G.D., Benham, C.D., Chessell, I.P., Bountra, C., Sinisi, M., Birch, R., Anand, P. (2007). Differential expression of the capsaicin receptor TRPV1 and related novel receptors TRPV3, TRPV4 and TRPM8 in normal human tissues and changes in traumatic and diabetic neuropathy. *BMC Neurol* 7:11.
43. Appendino, G., Minassi, A., Pagani, A., Ech-Chahad, A. (2008). The role of natural products in the ligand deorphanization of TRP channels. *Curr Pharm Des* 14:2–17.
44. Szallasi, A., Blumberg, P.M. (1999). Vanilloid (capsaicin) receptors and mechanisms. *Pharmacol Rev* 51:159–212.
45. Cuypers, E., Yanagihara, A., Karlsson, E., Tytgat, J. (2006). Jellyfish and other cnidarian envenomations cause pain by affecting TRPV1 channels. *FEBS Lett* 580:5728–5732.
46. Siemens, J., Zhou, S., Piskorowski, R., Nikai, T., Lumpkin, E.A., Basbaum, A.I., King, D., Julius, D. (2006). Spider toxins activate the capsaicin receptor to produce inflammatory pain. *Nature* 444:208–212.
47. Bandell, M., Story, G.M., Hwang, S.W., Viswanath, V., Eid, S.R., Petrus, M.J., Earley, T.J., Patapoutian, A. (2004). Noxious cold ion channel TRPA1 is activated by pungent compounds and bradykinin. *Neuron* 41:849–857.
48. Namer, B., Seifert, F., Handwerker, H.O., Maihofner, C. (2005). TRPA1 and TRPM8 activation in humans: effects of cinnamaldehyde and menthol. *Neuroreport* 16:955–959.

49. Macpherson, L.J., Geierstanger, B.H., Viswanath, V., Bandell, M., Eid, S.R., Hwang, S., Patapoutian, A. (2005). The pungency of garlic: activation of TRPA1 and TRPV1 in response to allicin. *Curr Biol* 15:929–934.

50. Peier, A.M., Moqrich, A., Hergarden, A.C., Reeve, A.J., Andersson, D.A., Story, G.M., Earley, T.J., Dragoni, I., McIntyre, P., Bevan, S., Patapoutian, A. (2002). A TRP channel that senses cold stimuli and menthol. *Cell* 108:705–715.

51. Moqrich, A., Hwang, S.W., Earley, T.J., Petrus, M.J., Murray, A.N., Spencer, K.S., Andahazy, M., Story, G.M., Patapoutian, A. (2005). Impaired thermosensation in mice lacking TRPV3, a heat and camphor sensor in the skin. *Science* 307:1468–1472.

52. Smith, P.L., Maloney, K.N., Pothen, R.G., Clardy, J., Clapham, D.E. (2006). Bisandrographolide from *Andrographis paniculata* activates TRPV4 channels. *J Biol Chem* 281:29897–29904.

53. Stotz, S.C., Vriens, J., Martyn, D., Clardy, J., Clapham, D.E. (2008). Citral sensing by TRANSient receptor potential channels in dorsal root ganglion neurons. *PLoS ONE* 3:e2082.

54. Macpherson, L.J., Hwang, S.W., Miyamoto, T., Dubin, A.E., Patapoutian, A., Story, G.M. (2006). More than cool: promiscuous relationships of menthol and other sensory compounds. *Mol Cell Neurosci* 32:335–343.

55. Prescott, E.D., Julius, D. (2003). A modular PIP2 binding site as a determinant of capsaicin receptor sensitivity. *Science* 300:1284–1288.

56. Liu, B., Qin, F. (2005). Functional control of cold- and menthol-sensitive TRPM8 ion channels by phosphatidylinositol 4,5-bisphosphate. *J Neurosci* 25:1674–1681.

57. Brauchi, S., Orta, G., Mascayano, C., Salazar, M., Raddatz, N., Urbina, H., Rosenmann, E., Gonzalez-Nilo, F., Latorre, R. (2007). Dissection of the components for PIP2 activation and thermosensation in TRP channels. *Proc Natl Acad Sci U S A* 104:10246–10251.

58. Qin, F. (2007). Regulation of TRP ion channels by phosphatidylinositol-4,5-bisphosphate. *Handb Exp Pharmacol* 179:509–525.

59. Lishko, P.V., Procko, E., Jin, X., Phelps, C.B., Gaudet, R. (2007). The ankyrin repeats of TRPV1 bind multiple ligands and modulate channel sensitivity. *Neuron* 54:905–918.

60. Kim, A.Y., Tang, Z., Liu, Q., Patel, K.N., Maag, D., Geng, Y., Dong, X. (2008). Pirt, a phosphoinositide-binding protein, functions as a regulatory subunit of TRPV1. *Cell* 133:475–485.

61. Lukacs, V., Thyagarajan, B., Varnai, P., Balla, A., Balla, T., Rohacs, T. (2007). Dual regulation of TRPV1 by phosphoinositides. *J Neurosci* 27:7070–7080.

62. Vetter, I., Wyse, B.D., Roberts-Thomson, S.J., Monteith, G.R., Cabot, P.J. (2008). Mechanisms involved in potentiation of transient receptor potential vanilloid 1 responses by ethanol. *Eur J Pain* 12:441–454.

63. Liedtke, W., Heller, S. (2007). *TRP Ion Channel Function in Sensory Transduction and Cellular Signaling Cascades*. Boca Raton, FL: Taylor & Francis.

64. Nilius, B. (2007). TRP channels in disease. *Biochim Biophys Acta* 1772:805–812.

65. Denda, M., Fuziwara, S., Inoue, K., Denda, S., Akamatsu, H., Tomitaka, A., Matsunaga, K. (2001). Immunoreactivity of VR1 on epidermal keratinocyte of human skin. *Biochem Biophys Res Commun* 285:1250–1252.

66. Birder, L.A., Nakamura, Y., Kiss, S., Nealen, M.L., Barrick, S., Kanai, A.J., Wang, E., Ruiz, G., De Groat, W.C., Apodaca, G., Watkins, S., Caterina, M.J. (2002). Altered urinary bladder function in mice lacking the vanilloid receptor TRPV1. *Nat Neurosci* 5:856–860.

67. Southall, M.D., Li, T., Gharibova, L.S., Pei, Y., Nicol, G.D., Travers, J.B. (2003). Activation of epidermal vanilloid receptor-1 induces release of proinflammatory mediators in human keratinocytes. *J Pharmacol Exp Ther* 304:217–222.

68. Wilder-Smith, E.P., Ong, W.Y., Guo, Y., Chow, A.W. (2007). Epidermal transient receptor potential vanilloid 1 in idiopathic small nerve fibre disease, diabetic neuropathy and healthy human subjects. *Histopathology* 51:674–680.

69. Chung, M.K., Lee, H., Caterina, M.J. (2003). Warm temperatures activate TRPV4 in mouse 308 keratinocytes. *J Biol Chem* 278:32037–32046.

70. Gevaert, T., Vriens, J., Segal, A., Everaerts, W., Roskams, T., Talavera, K., Owsianik, G., Liedtke, W., Daelemans, D., Dewachter, I., Van Leuven, F., Voets, T., De Ridder, D., Nilius, B. (2007). Deletion of the transient receptor potential cation channel TRPV4 impairs murine bladder voiding. *J Clin Invest* 117:3453–3462.

71. Birder, L.A. (2005). More than just a barrier: urothelium as a drug target for urinary bladder pain. *Am J Physiol Renal Physiol* 289:F489–F495.

72. Szolcsanyi, J., Bartho, L. (1982). Capsaicin-sensitive non-cholinergic excitatory innervation of the guinea-pig tracheobronchial smooth muscle. *Neurosci Lett* 34:247–251.

73. Maggi, C.A., Meli, A. (1988). The sensory-efferent function of capsaicin-sensitive sensory neurons. *Gen Pharmacol* 19:1–43.

74. Geppetti, P., Holzer, P. (1996). *Neurogenic Inflammation*. Boca Raton, FL: CRC Press.

75. Butler, C.A., Heaney, L.G. (2007). Neurogenic inflammation and asthma. *Inflamm Allergy Drug Targets* 6:127–132.

76. Trevisani, M., Smart, D., Gunthorpe, M.J., Tognetto, M., Barbieri, M., Campi, B., Amadesi, S., Gray, J., Jerman, J.C., Brough, S.J., Owen, D., Smith, G.D., Randall, A.D., Harrison, S., Bianchi, A., Davis, J.B., Geppetti, P. (2002). Ethanol elicits and potentiates nociceptor responses via the vanilloid receptor-1. *Nat Neurosci* 5:546–551.

77. Patapoutian, A., Peier, A.M., Story, G.M., Viswanath, V. (2003). ThermoTRP channels and beyond: mechanisms of temperature sensation. *Nat Rev Neurosci* 4:529–539.

78. Cromer, B.A., McIntyre, P. (2008). Painful toxins acting at TRPV1. *Toxicon* 51:163–173.

79. Pingle, S.C., Matta, J.A., Ahern, G.P. (2007). Capsaicin receptor: TRPV1 a promiscuous TRP channel. *Handb Exp Pharmacol* 179:155–171.

80. Vellani, V., Mapplebeck, S., Moriondo, A., Davis, J.B., McNaughton, P.A. (2001). Protein kinase C activation potentiates gating of the vanilloid receptor VR1 by capsaicin, protons, heat and anandamide. *J Physiol* 534:813–825.

81. Gunthorpe, M.J., Benham, C.D., Randall, A., Davis, J.B. (2002). The diversity in the vanilloid (TRPV) receptor family of ion channels. *Trends Pharmacol Sci* 23:183–191.

82. Crandall, M., Kwash, J., Yu, W., White, G. (2002). Activation of protein kinase C sensitizes human VR1 to capsaicin and to moderate decreases in pH at physiological temperatures in *Xenopus* oocytes. *Pain* 98:109–117.
83. Reeh, P.W., Petho, G. (2000). Nociceptor excitation by thermal sensitization—a hypothesis. *Prog Brain Res* 129:39–50.
84. Premkumar, L.S., Ahern, G.P. (2000). Induction of vanilloid receptor channel activity by protein kinase C. *Nature* 408:985–990.
85. Tominaga, M., Wada, M., Masu, M. (2001). Potentiation of capsaicin receptor activity by metabotropic ATP receptors as a possible mechanism for ATP-evoked pain and hyperalgesia. *Proc Natl Acad Sci U S A* 98:6951–6956.
86. Kagaya, M., Lamb, J., Robbins, J., Page, C.P., Spina, D. (2002). Characterization of the anandamide induced depolarization of guinea-pig isolated vagus nerve. *Br J Pharmacol* 137:39–48.
87. Olah, Z., Karai, L., Iadarola, M.J. (2002). Protein kinase C(alpha) is required for vanilloid receptor 1 activation. Evidence for multiple signaling pathways. *J Biol Chem* 277:35752–35759.
88. Bhave, G., Hu, H.J., Glauner, K.S., Zhu, W., Wang, H., Brasier, D.J., Oxford, G.S., Gereau, R.W.T. (2003). Protein kinase C phosphorylation sensitizes but does not activate the capsaicin receptor transient receptor potential vanilloid 1 (TRPV1). *Proc Natl Acad Sci U S A* 100:12480–12485.
89. Varga, A., Bolcskei, K., Szoke, E., Almasi, R., Czeh, G., Szolcsanyi, J., Petho, G. (2006). Relative roles of protein kinase A and protein kinase C in modulation of transient receptor potential vanilloid type 1 receptor responsiveness in rat sensory neurons in vitro and peripheral nociceptors in vivo. *Neuroscience* 140:645–657.
90. Vetter, I., Wyse, B.D., Monteith, G.R., Roberts-Thomson, S.J., Cabot, P.J. (2006). The mu opioid agonist morphine modulates potentiation of capsaicin-evoked TRPV1 responses through a cyclic AMP-dependent protein kinase A pathway. *Mol Pain* 2:22.
91. Zhang, X., McNaughton, P.A. (2006). Why pain gets worse: the mechanism of heat hyperalgesia. *J Gen Physiol* 128:491–493.
92. Mohapatra, D.P., Nau, C. (2005). Regulation of Ca2+-dependent desensitization in the vanilloid receptor TRPV1 by calcineurin and cAMP-dependent protein kinase. *J Biol Chem* 280:13424–13432.
93. Bhave, G., Zhu, W., Wang, H., Brasier, D.J., Oxford, G.S., Gereau, R.W.T. (2002). cAMP-dependent protein kinase regulates desensitization of the capsaicin receptor (VR1) by direct phosphorylation. *Neuron* 35:721–731.
94. Mohapatra, D.P., Nau, C. (2003). Desensitization of capsaicin-activated currents in the vanilloid receptor TRPV1 is decreased by the cyclic AMP-dependent protein kinase pathway. *J Biol Chem* 278:50080–50090.
95. Numazaki, M., Tominaga, T., Takeuchi, K., Murayama, N., Toyooka, H., Tominaga, M. (2003). Structural determinant of TRPV1 desensitization interacts with calmodulin. *Proc Natl Acad Sci U S A* 100:8002–8006.
96. Rosenbaum, T., Gordon-Shaag, A., Munari, M., Gordon, S.E. (2004). Ca2+/calmodulin modulates TRPV1 activation by capsaicin. *J Gen Physiol* 123:53–62.
97. Jung, J., Shin, J.S., Lee, S.Y., Hwang, S.W., Koo, J., Cho, H., Oh, U. (2004). Phosphorylation of vanilloid receptor 1 by Ca2+/calmodulin-dependent kinase II regulates its vanilloid binding. *J Biol Chem* 279:7048–7054.

98. Wood, J. (1993). *Capsaicin in the Study of Pain*. New York: Academic Press.
99. Szallasi, A., Cruz, F., Geppetti, P. (2006). TRPV1: a therapeutic target for novel analgesic drugs? *Trends Mol Med* 12:545–554.
100. Remadevi, R., Szallisi, A. (2008). Adlea (ALGRX-4975), an injectable capsaicin (TRPV1 receptor agonist) formulation for longlasting pain relief. *IDrugs* 11:120–132.
101. Avelino, A., Cruz, F. (2006). TRPV1 (vanilloid receptor) in the urinary tract: expression, function and clinical applications. *Naunyn Schmiedebergs Arch Pharmacol* 373:287–299.
102. Brown, D.C., Iadarola, M.J., Perkowski, S.Z., Erin, H., Shofer, F., Laszlo, K.J., Olah, Z., Mannes, A.J. (2005). Physiologic and antinociceptive effects of intrathecal resiniferatoxin in a canine bone cancer model. *Anesthesiology* 103: 1052–1059.
103. Menendez, L., Juarez, L., Garcia, E., Garcia-Suarez, O., Hidalgo, A., Baamonde, A. (2006). Analgesic effects of capsazepine and resiniferatoxin on bone cancer pain in mice. *Neurosci Lett* 393:70–73.
104. Bolcskei, K., Helyes, Z., Szabo, A., Sandor, K., Elekes, K., Nemeth, J., Almasi, R., Pinter, E., Petho, G., Szolcsanyi, J. (2005). Investigation of the role of TRPV1 receptors in acute and chronic nociceptive processes using gene-deficient mice. *Pain* 117:368–376.
105. Wang, X., Miyares, R.L., Ahern, G.P. (2005). Oleoylethanolamide excites vagal sensory neurones, induces visceral pain and reduces short-term food intake in mice via capsaicin receptor TRPV1. *J Physiol* 564:541–547.
106. Christoph, T., Bahrenberg, G., De Vry, J., Englberger, W., Erdmann, V.A., Frech, M., Kogel, B., Rohl, T., Schiene, K., Schroder, W., Seibler, J., Kurreck, J. (2008). Investigation of TRPV1 loss-of-function phenotypes in transgenic shRNA expressing and knockout mice. *Mol Cell Neurosci* 37:579–589.
107. Christoph, T., Gillen, C., Mika, J., Grunweller, A., Schafer, M.K., Schiene, K., Frank, R., Jostock, R., Bahrenberg, G., Weihe, E., Erdmann, V.A., Kurreck, J. (2007). Antinociceptive effect of antisense oligonucleotides against the vanilloid receptor VR1/TRPV1. *Neurochem Int* 50:281–290.
108. Christoph, T., Grunweller, A., Mika, J., Schafer, M.K., Wade, E.J., Weihe, E., Erdmann, V.A., Frank, R., Gillen, C., Kurreck, J. (2006). Silencing of vanilloid receptor TRPV1 by RNAi reduces neuropathic and visceral pain in vivo. *Biochem Biophys Res Commun* 350:238–243.
109. Kasama, S., Kawakubo, M., Suzuki, T., Nishizawa, T., Ishida, A., Nakayama, J. (2007). RNA interference-mediated knock-down of transient receptor potential vanilloid 1 prevents forepaw inflammatory hyperalgesia in rat. *Eur J Neurosci* 25:2956–2963.
110. Klionsky, L., Tamir, R., Holzinger, B., Bi, X., Talvenheimo, J., Kim, H., Martin, F., Louis, J.C., Treanor, J.J., Gavva, N.R. (2006). A polyclonal antibody to the prepore loop of transient receptor potential vanilloid type 1 blocks channel activation. *J Pharmacol Exp Ther* 319:192–198.
111. Szabo, T., Biro, T., Gonzalez, A.F., Palkovits, M., Blumberg, P.M. (2002). Pharmacological characterization of vanilloid receptor located in the brain. *Brain Res Mol Brain Res* 98:51–57.

112. Acs, G., Palkovits, M., Blumberg, P.M. (1996). Specific binding of [3H]resiniferatoxin by human and rat preoptic area, locus ceruleus, medial hypothalamus, reticular formation and ventral thalamus membrane preparations. *Life Sci* 59:1899–1908.

113. Mezey, E., Toth, Z.E., Cortright, D.N., Arzubi, M.K., Krause, J.E., Elde, R., Guo, A., Blumberg, P.M., Szallasi, A. (2000). Distribution of mRNA for vanilloid receptor subtype 1 (VR1), and VR1-like immunoreactivity, in the central nervous system of the rat and human. *Proc Natl Acad Sci U S A* 97:3655–3660.

114. Roberts, J.C., Davis, J.B., Benham, C.D. (2004). [3H]resiniferatoxin autoradiography in the CNS of wild-type and TRPV1 null mice defines TRPV1 (VR-1) protein distribution. *Brain Res* 995:176–183.

115. Millan, M.J. (1999). The induction of pain: an integrative review. *Prog Neurobiol* 57:1–164.

116. Liapi, A., Wood, J.N. (2005). Extensive co-localization and heteromultimer formation of the vanilloid receptor-like protein TRPV2 and the capsaicin receptor TRPV1 in the adult rat cerebral cortex. *Eur J Neurosci* 22:825–834.

117. Sasamura, T., Sasaki, M., Tohda, C., Kuraishi, Y. (1998). Existence of capsaicin-sensitive glutamatergic terminals in rat hypothalamus. *Neuroreport* 9:2045–2048.

118. Bodnar, R.J., Kirchgessner, A., Nilaver, G., Mulhern, J., Zimmerman, E.A. (1982). Intraventricular capsaicin: alterations in analgesic responsivity without depletion of substance P. *Neuroscience* 7:631–638.

119. Bodnar, R.J., Simone, D.A., Kordower, J.H., Kirchgessner, A.L., Nilaver, G. (1983). Capsaicin treatment and stress-induced analgesia. *Pharmacol Biochem Behav* 18:65–71.

120. Santos, A.R., Calixto, J.B. (1997). Ruthenium red and capsazepine antinociceptive effect in formalin and capsaicin models of pain in mice. *Neurosci Lett* 235:73–76.

121. McGaraughty, S., Chu, K.L., Brown, B.S., Zhu, C.Z., Zhong, C., Joshi, S.K., Honre, P., Faltynek, C.R., Jarvis, M.F. (2008). Contributions of central and peripheral TRPV1 receptors to mechanically evoked and spontaneous firing of spinal neurons in inflamed rats. *J Neurophysiol* 1:1.

122. Hajos, M., Engberg, G., Elam, M. (1986). Reduced responsiveness of locus coeruleus neurons to cutaneous thermal stimuli in capsaicin-treated rats. *Neurosci Lett* 70:382–387.

123. Hajos, M., Jancso, G., Engberg, G. (1987). Capsaicin-induced excitation of locus coeruleus neurons. *Acta Physiol Scand* 129:415–420.

124. Marinelli, S., Vaughan, C.W., Christie, M.J., Connor, M. (2002). Capsaicin activation of glutamatergic synaptic transmission in the rat locus coeruleus in vitro. *J Physiol* 543:531–540.

125. Marinelli, S., Pascucci, T., Bernardi, G., Puglisi-Allegra, S., Mercuri, N.B. (2005). Activation of TRPV1 in the VTA excites dopaminergic neurons and increases chemical- and noxious-induced dopamine release in the nucleus accumbens. *Neuropsychopharmacology* 30:864–870.

126. Jancso, G., Obal, F., Jr., Toth-Kasa, I., Katona, M., Husz, S. (1985). The modulation of cutaneous inflammatory reactions by peptide-containing sensory nerves. *Int J Tissue React* 7:449–457.

127. Jordt, S.E., Bautista, D.M., Chuang, H.H., McKemy, D.D., Zygmunt, P.M., Hogestatt, E.D., Meng, I.D., Julius, D. (2004). Mustard oils and cannabinoids excite sensory nerve fibres through the TRP channel ANKTM1. *Nature* 427:260–265.

128. Bevan, S., Hothi, S., Hughes, G., James, I.F., Rang, H.P., Shah, K., Walpole, C.S., Yeats, J.C. (1992). Capsazepine: a competitive antagonist of the sensory neurone excitant capsaicin. *Br J Pharmacol* 107:544–552.

129. Weil, A., Moore, S.E., Waite, N.J., Randall, A., Gunthorpe, M.J. (2005). Conservation of functional and pharmacological properties in the distantly related temperature sensors TRVP1 and TRPM8. *Mol Pharmacol* 68:518–527.

130. Xing, H., Chen, M., Ling, J., Tan, W., Gu, J.G. (2007). TRPM8 mechanism of cold allodynia after chronic nerve injury. *J Neurosci* 27:13680–13690.

131. Holzer, P. (2008). The pharmacological challenge to tame the transient receptor potential vanilloid-1 (TRPV1) nocisensor. *Br J Pharmacol* 22:22.

132. Gavva, N.R., Tamir, R., Klionsky, L., Norman, M.H., Louis, J.C., Wild, K.D., Treanor, J.J. (2005). Proton activation does not alter antagonist interaction with the capsaicin-binding pocket of TRPV1. *Mol Pharmacol* 68:1524–1533.

133. Lehto, S.G., Tamir, R., Deng, H., Klionsky, L., Kuang, R., Le, A., Lee, D., Louis, J.C., Magal, E., Manning, B.H., Rubino, J., Surapaneni, S., Tamayo, N., Wang, T., Wang, J., Wang, W., Youngblood, B., Zhang, M., Zhu, D., Norman, M.H., Gavva, N.R. (2008). Antihyperalgesic effects of (R,E)-N-(2-hydroxy-2,3-dihydro-1H-inden-4-yl)-3-(2-(piperidin-1-yl)-4-(trifluorom ethyl)phenyl)-acrylamide (AMG8562), a novel transient receptor potential vanilloid type 1 modulator that does not cause hyperthermia in rats. *J Pharmacol Exp Ther* 326:218–229.

134. Seabrook, G.R., Sutton, K.G., Jarolimek, W., Hollingworth, G.J., Teague, S., Webb, J., Clark, N., Boyce, S., Kerby, J., Ali, Z., Chou, M., Middleton, R., Kaczorowski, G., Jones, A.B. (2002). Functional properties of the high-affinity TRPV1 (VR1) vanilloid receptor antagonist (4-hydroxy-5-iodo-3-methoxyphenylacetate ester) iodo-resiniferatoxin. *J Pharmacol Exp Ther* 303:1052–1060.

135. Gavva, N.R., Klionsky, L., Qu, Y., Shi, L., Tamir, R., Edenson, S., Zhang, T.J., Viswanadhan, V.N., Toth, A., Pearce, L.V., Vanderah, T.W., Porreca, F., Blumberg, P.M., Lile, J., Sun, Y., Wild, K., Louis, J.C., Treanor, J.J. (2004). Molecular determinants of vanilloid sensitivity in TRPV1. *J Biol Chem* 279:20283–20295.

136. Neelands, T.R., Jarvis, M.F., Han, P., Faltynek, C.R., Surowy, C.S. (2005). Acidification of rat TRPV1 alters the kinetics of capsaicin responses. *Mol Pain* 1:28.

137. Gunthorpe, M.J., Rami, H.K., Jerman, J.C., Smart, D., Gill, C.H., Soffin, E.M., Luis Hannan, S., Lappin, S.C., Egerton, J., Smith, G.D., Worby, A., Howett, L., Owen, D., Nasir, S., Davies, C.H., Thompson, M., Wyman, P.A., Randall, A.D., Davis, J.B. (2004). Identification and characterisation of SB-366791, a potent and selective vanilloid receptor (VR1/TRPV1) antagonist. *Neuropharmacology* 46:133–149.

138. Behrendt, H.J., Germann, T., Gillen, C., Hatt, H., Jostock, R. (2004). Characterization of the mouse cold-menthol receptor TRPM8 and vanilloid receptor type-1 VR1 using a fluorometric imaging plate reader (FLIPR) assay. *Br J Pharmacol* 141:737–745.

139. Walker, K.M., Urban, L., Medhurst, S.J., Patel, S., Panesar, M., Fox, A.J., McIntyre, P. (2003). The VR1 antagonist capsazepine reverses mechanical hyperalgesia in models of inflammatory and neuropathic pain. *J Pharmacol Exp Ther* 304:56–62.

140. Pomonis, J.D., Harrison, J.E., Mark, L., Bristol, D.R., Valenzano, K.J., Walker, K. (2003). N-(4-tertiarybutylphenyl)-4-(3-cholorphyridin-2-yl)tetrahydropyrazine -1(2H)-carbox-amide (BCTC), a novel, orally effective vanilloid receptor 1 antagonist with analgesic properties: II. In vivo characterization in rat models of inflammatory and neuropathic pain. *J Pharmacol Exp Ther* 306:387–393.

141. Yamamoto, W., Sugiura, A., Nakazato-Imasato, E., Kita, Y. (2008). Characterization of primary sensory neurons mediating static and dynamic allodynia in rat chronic constriction injury model. *J Pharm Pharmacol* 60:717–722.

142. Honore, P., Wismer, C.T., Mikusa, J., Zhu, C.Z., Zhong, C., Gauvin, D.M., Gomtsyan, A., El Kouhen, R., Lee, C.H., Marsh, K., Sullivan, J.P., Faltynek, C.R., Jarvis, M.F. (2005). A-425619 [1-isoquinolin-5-yl-3-(4-trifluoromethyl-benzyl)-urea], a novel transient receptor potential type V1 receptor antagonist, relieves pathophysiological pain associated with inflammation and tissue injury in rats. *J Pharmacol Exp Ther* 314:410–421.

143. Swanson, D.M., Dubin, A.E., Shah, C., Nasser, N., Chang, L., Dax, S.L., Jetter, M., Breitenbucher, J.G., Liu, C., Mazur, C., Lord, B., Gonzales, L., Hoey, K., Rizzolio, M., Bogenstaetter, M., Codd, E.E., Lee, D.H., Zhang, S.P., Chaplan, S.R., Carruthers, N.I. (2005). Identification and biological evaluation of 4-(3-trifluoromethylpyridin-2-yl)piperazine-1-carboxylic acid (5-trifluoromethylpyridin-2-yl)amide, a high affinity TRPV1 (VR1) vanilloid receptor antagonist. *J Med Chem* 48:1857–1872.

144. Zhong, C., Gauvin, D., Mikusa, J., Chandran, P., Hernandez, G., Lee, L., Brown, B., McDonald, H., Moreland, R., Decker, M.W., Honore, M., Cui, M., Faltynek, C.R. (2005). The novel and potent TRPV1 antagonist, A-784168, is a broad-spectrum analgesic in preclinical pain models. Society for Neuroscience Annual Meeting. Washington, DC, November 12–16.

145. Cui, M., Honore, P., Zhong, C., Gauvin, D., Mikusa, J., Hernandez, G., Chandran, P., Gomtsyan, A., Brown, B., Bayburt, E.K., Marsh, K., Bianchi, B., McDonald, H., Niforatos, W., Neelands, T.R., Moreland, R.B., Decker, M.W., Lee, C.H., Sullivan, J.P., Faltynek, C.R. (2006). TRPV1 receptors in the CNS play a key role in broad-spectrum analgesia of TRPV1 antagonists. *J Neurosci* 26:9385–9393.

146. http://www.glenmarkpharma.com/research/pdf/GRC6127_n_GRC6211_Ion_Channeltargetsposter2006.pdf (accessed October 30, 2008).

147. Trevisani, M., Fruttarolo, F., Pavani, M., Campi, B., Gatti, R., De Siena, G., Prosdocimi, M., Napoletano, M., Varani, K., Borea, P., Baraldi, P.G., Semeraro, C., Geppetti, P. (2008). V377, a potent TRPV1 antagonist for pain management. European Opioid Conference (EOC)–European Neuropeptide Club (ENC) Joint Meeting. Ferrara, Italy, April 8–11.

148. Surowy, C.S., Neelands, T.R., Bianchi, B.R., McGaraughty, S., El Kouhen, R., Han, P., Chu, K.L., McDonald, H.A., Vos, M., Niforatos, W., Bayburt, E.K., Gomtsyan, A., Lee, C.H., Honore, P., Sullivan, J.P., Jarvis, M.F., Faltynek, C.R. (2008). (R)-(5-tert-butyl-2,3-dihydro-1H-inden-1-yl)-3-(1H-indazol-4-yl)-urea (ABT-102) blocks polymodal activation of transient receptor potential vanilloid

1 receptors in vitro and heat-evoked firing of spinal dorsal horn neurons in vivo. *J Pharmacol Exp Ther* 326:879–888.

149. Gomtsyan, A., Bayburt, E.K., Schmidt, R.G., Surowy, C.S., Honore, P., Marsh, K.C., Hannick, S.M., McDonald, H.A., Wetter, J.M., Sullivan, J.P., Jarvis, M.F., Faltynek, C.R., Lee, C.H. (2008). Identification of (R)-1-(5-tert-butyl-2,3-dihydro-1H-inden-1-yl)-3-(1H-indazol-4-yl)urea (ABT-102) as a potent TRPV1 antagonist for pain management. *J Med Chem* 51:392–395.
150. Hori, T. (1984). Capsaicin and central control of thermoregulation. *Pharmacol Ther* 26:389–416.
151. Gavva, N.R. (2008). Body-temperature maintenance as the predominant function of the vanilloid receptor TRPV1. *Trends Pharmacol Sci* 19:19.
152. Gavva, N.R., Bannon, A.W., Surapaneni, S., Hovland, D.N., Jr., Lehto, S.G., Gore, A., Juan, T., Deng, H., Han, B., Klionsky, L., Kuang, R., Le, A., Tamir, R., Wang, J., Youngblood, B., Zhu, D., Norman, M.H., Magal, E., Treanor, J.J., Louis, J.C. (2007). The vanilloid receptor TRPV1 is tonically activated in vivo and involved in body temperature regulation. *J Neurosci* 27:3366–3374.
153. Steiner, A.A., Turek, V.F., Almeida, M.C., Burmeister, J.J., Oliveira, D.L., Roberts, J.L., Bannon, A.W., Norman, M.H., Louis, J.C., Treanor, J.J., Gavva, N.R., Romanovsky, A.A. (2007). Nonthermal activation of transient receptor potential vanilloid-1 channels in abdominal viscera tonically inhibits autonomic cold-defense effectors. *J Neurosci* 27:7459–7468.
154. Tamayo, N., Liao, H., Stec, M.M., Wang, X., Chakrabarti, P., Retz, D., Doherty, E.M., Surapaneni, S., Tamir, R., Bannon, A.W., Gavva, N.R., Norman, M.H. (2008). Design and synthesis of peripherally restricted transient receptor potential vanilloid 1 (TRPV1) antagonists. *J Med Chem* 51:2744–2757.
155. Gavva, N.R., Treanor, J.J., Garami, A., Fang, L., Surapaneni, S., Akrami, A., Alvarez, F., Bak, A., Darling, M., Gore, A., Jang, G.R., Kesslak, J.P., Ni, L., Norman, M.H., Palluconi, G., Rose, M.J., Salfi, M., Tan, E., Romanovsky, A.A., Banfield, C., Davar, G. (2008). Pharmacological blockade of the vanilloid receptor TRPV1 elicits marked hyperthermia in humans. *Pain* 136:202–210.
156. http://www.clinicaltrials.gov/ct2/show/NCT00387140? (accessed October 30, 2008).
157. http://www.jti.co.jp/JTI_E/IR/08/P.L.20080207_E.pdf (accessed October 30, 2008).
158. Caterina, M.J., Rosen, T.A., Tominaga, M., Brake, A.J., Julius, D. (1999). A capsaicin-receptor homologue with a high threshold for noxious heat. *Nature* 398:436–441.
159. Hu, H.Z., Gu, Q., Wang, C., Colton, C.K., Tang, J., Kinoshita-Kawada, M., Lee, L.Y., Wood, J.D., Zhu, M.X. (2004). 2-Aminoethoxydiphenyl borate is a common activator of TRPV1, TRPV2, and TRPV3. *J Biol Chem* 279:35741–35748.
160. Bang, S., Kim, K.Y., Yoo, S., Lee, S.H., Hwang, S.W. (2007). Transient receptor potential V2 expressed in sensory neurons is activated by probenecid. *Neurosci Lett* 425:120–125.
161. Neeper, M.P., Liu, Y., Hutchinson, T.L., Wang, Y., Flores, C.M., Qin, N. (2007). Activation properties of heterologously expressed mammalian TRPV2: evidence for species dependence. *J Biol Chem* 282:15894–15902.

162. Lewinter, R.D., Skinner, K., Julius, D., Basbaum, A.I. (2004). Immunoreactive TRPV-2 (VRL-1), a capsaicin receptor homolog, in the spinal cord of the rat. *J Comp Neurol* 470:400–408.

163. Lewinter, R.D., Scherrer, G., Basbaum, A.I. (2008). Dense transient receptor potential cation channel, vanilloid family, type 2 (TRPV2) immunoreactivity defines a subset of motoneurons in the dorsal lateral nucleus of the spinal cord, the nucleus ambiguus and the trigeminal motor nucleus in rat. *Neuroscience* 151:164–173.

164. Montell, C., Birnbaumer, L., Flockerzi, V., Bindels, R.J., Bruford, E.A., Caterina, M.J., Clapham, D.E., Harteneck, C., Heller, S., Julius, D., Kojima, I., Mori, Y., Penner, R., Prawitt, D., Scharenberg, A.M., Schultz, G., Shimizu, N., Zhu, M.X. (2002). A unified nomenclature for the superfamily of TRP cation channels. *Mol Cell* 9:229–231.

165. Muraki, K., Iwata, Y., Katanosaka, Y., Ito, T., Ohya, S., Shigekawa, M., Imaizumi, Y. (2003). TRPV2 is a component of osmotically sensitive cation channels in murine aortic myocytes. *Circ Res* 93:829–838.

166. Beech, D.J., Muraki, K., Flemming, R. (2004). Non-selective cationic channels of smooth muscle and the mammalian homologues of *Drosophila* TRP. *J Physiol* 559:685–706.

167. Frederick, J., Buck, M.E., Matson, D.J., Cortright, D.N. (2007). Increased TRPA1, TRPM8, and TRPV2 expression in dorsal root ganglia by nerve injury. *Biochem Biophys Res Commun* 358:1058–1064.

168. Kanzaki, M., Zhang, Y.Q., Mashima, H., Li, L., Shibata, H., Kojima, I. (1999). Translocation of a calcium-permeable cation channel induced by insulin-like growth factor-I. *Nat Cell Biol* 1:165–170.

169. Nagasawa, M., Nakagawa, Y., Tanaka, S., Kojima, I. (2007). Chemotactic peptide fMetLeuPhe induces translocation of the TRPV2 channel in macrophages. *J Cell Physiol* 210:692–702.

170. Smith, G.D., Gunthorpe, M.J., Kelsell, R.E., Hayes, P.D., Reilly, P., Facer, P., Wright, J.E., Jerman, J.C., Walhin, J.P., Ooi, L., Egerton, J., Charles, K.J., Smart, D., Randall, A.D., Anand, P., Davis, J.B. (2002). TRPV3 is a temperature-sensitive vanilloid receptor-like protein. *Nature* 418:186–190.

171. Xu, H., Ramsey, I.S., Kotecha, S.A., Moran, M.M., Chong, J.A., Lawson, D., Ge, P., Lilly, J., Silos-Santiago, I., Xie, Y., DiStefano, P.S., Curtis, R., Clapham, D.E. (2002). TRPV3 is a calcium-permeable temperature-sensitive cation channel. *Nature* 418:181–186.

172. Vogt-Eisele, A.K., Weber, K., Sherkheli, M.A., Vielhaber, G., Panten, J., Gisselmann, G., Hatt, H. (2007). Monoterpenoid agonists of TRPV3. *Br J Pharmacol* 151:530–540.

173. Xu, H., Delling, M., Jun, J.C., Clapham, D.E. (2006). Oregano, thyme and clove-derived flavors and skin sensitizers activate specific TRP channels. *Nat Neurosci* 9:628–635

174. Chung, M.K., Lee, H., Mizuno, A., Suzuki, M., Caterina, M.J. (2004). TRPV3 and TRPV4 mediate warmth-evoked currents in primary mouse keratinocytes. *J Biol Chem* 279:21569–21575.

175. Xiao, R., Tang, J., Wang, C., Colton, C.K., Tian, J., Zhu, M.X. (2008). Calcium plays a central role in the sensitization of TRPV3 channel to repetitive stimulations. *J Biol Chem* 283:6162–6174.

176. Peier, A.M., Reeve, A.J., Andersson, D.A., Moqrich, A., Earley, T.J., Hergarden, A.C., Story, G.M., Colley, S., Hogenesch, J.B., McIntyre, P., Bevan, S., Patapoutian, A. (2002). A heat-sensitive TRP channel expressed in keratinocytes. *Science* 296:2046–2049.

177. Gopinath, P., Wan, E., Holdcroft, A., Facer, P., Davis, J.B., Smith, G.D., Bountra, C., Anand, P. (2005). Increased capsaicin receptor TRPV1 in skin nerve fibres and related vanilloid receptors TRPV3 and TRPV4 in keratinocytes in human breast pain. *BMC Womens Health* 5:2.

178. Gullapalli, S., Thomas, A., Kattige, V., Gudi, G., Khairatkar-Joshi, N. (2008). GRC-15133: a novel, selective TRPV3 antagonist with antihyperalgesic effects in inflammatory and neuropathic pain. World Pharmaceutical Congress. Philadelphia, PA, May 12–14.

179. Asakawa, M., Yoshioka, T., Matsutani, T., Hikita, I., Suzuki, M., Oshima, I., Tsukahara, K., Arimura, A., Horikawa, T., Hirasawa, T., Sakata, T. (2006). Association of a mutation in TRPV3 with defective hair growth in rodents. *J Invest Dermatol* 126:2664–2672.

180. Imura, K., Yoshioka, T., Hikita, I., Tsukahara, K., Hirasawa, T., Higashino, K., Gahara, Y., Arimura, A., Sakata, T. (2007). Influence of TRPV3 mutation on hair growth cycle in mice. *Biochem Biophys Res Commun* 363:479–483.

181. Moussaieff, A., Rimmerman, N., Bregman, T., Straiker, A., Felder, C.C., Shoham, S., Kashman, Y., Huang, S.M., Lee, H., Shohami, E., Mackie, K., Caterina, M.J., Walker, J.M., Fride, E., Mechoulam, R. (2008). Incensole acetate, an incense component, elicits psychoactivity by activating TRPV3 channels in the brain. *FASEB J* 22:3024–3034.

182. Guatteo, E., Chung, K.K., Bowala, T.K., Bernardi, G., Mercuri, N.B., Lipski, J. (2005). Temperature sensitivity of dopaminergic neurons of the substantia nigra pars compacta: involvement of transient receptor potential channels. *J Neurophysiol* 94:3069–3080.

183. Lipski, J., Park, T.I., Li, D., Lee, S.C., Trevarton, A.J., Chung, K.K., Freestone, P.S., Bai, J.Z. (2006). Involvement of TRP-like channels in the acute ischemic response of hippocampal CA1 neurons in brain slices. *Brain Res* 1077:187–199.

184. Nilius, B., Vriens, J., Prenen, J., Droogmans, G., Voets, T. (2004). TRPV4 calcium entry channel: a paradigm for gating diversity. *Am J Physiol Cell Physiol* 286:C195–C205.

185. Watanabe, H., Vriens, J., Prenen, J., Droogmans, G., Voets, T., Nilius, B. (2003). Anandamide and arachidonic acid use epoxyeicosatrienoic acids to activate TRPV4 channels. *Nature* 424:434–438.

186. Watanabe, H., Vriens, J., Suh, S.H., Benham, C.D., Droogmans, G., Nilius, B. (2002). Heat-evoked activation of TRPV4 channels in a HEK293 cell expression system and in native mouse aorta endothelial cells. *J Biol Chem* 277:47044–47051.

187. Vriens, J., Owsianik, G., Fisslthaler, B., Suzuki, M., Janssens, A., Voets, T., Morisseau, C., Hammock, B.D., Fleming, I., Busse, R., Nilius, B. (2005). Modulation of the Ca2 permeable cation channel TRPV4 by cytochrome P450 epoxygenases in vascular endothelium. *Circ Res* 97:908–915.

188. Delany, N.S., Hurle, M., Facer, P., Alnadaf, T., Plumpton, C., Kinghorn, I., See, C.G., Costigan, M., Anand, P., Woolf, C.J., Crowther, D., Sanseau, P., Tate, S.N.

(2001). Identification and characterization of a novel human vanilloid receptor-like protein, VRL-2. *Physiol Genomics* 4:165–174.

189. Liedtke, W., Choe, Y., Marti-Renom, M.A., Bell, A.M., Denis, C.S., Sali, A., Hudspeth, A.J., Friedman, J.M., Heller, S. (2000). Vanilloid receptor-related osmotically activated channel (VR-OAC), a candidate vertebrate osmoreceptor. *Cell* 103:525–535.
190. Goadsby, P.J. (2005). Calcitonin gene-related peptide antagonists as treatments of migraine and other primary headaches. *Drugs* 65:2557–2567.
191. Sugiuar, T., Bielefeldt, K., Gebhart, G.F. (2004). TRPV1 function in mouse colon sensory neurons is enhanced by metabotropic 5-hydroxytryptamine receptor activation. *J Neurosci* 24:9521–9530.
192. Suzuki, M., Watanabe, Y., Oyama, Y., Mizuno, A., Kusano, E., Hirao, A., Ookawara, S. (2003). Localization of mechanosensitive channel TRPV4 in mouse skin. *Neurosci Lett* 353:189–192.
193. Guler, A.D., Lee, H., Iida, T., Shimizu, I., Tominaga, M., Caterina, M. (2002). Heat-evoked activation of the ion channel, TRPV4. *J Neurosci* 22:6408–6414.
194. Lee, H., Iida, T., Mizuno, A., Suzuki, M., Caterina, M.J. (2005). Altered thermal selection behavior in mice lacking transient receptor potential vanilloid 4. *J Neurosci* 25:1304–1310.
195. Chen, X., Alessandri-Haber, N., Levine, J.D. (2007). Marked attenuation of inflammatory mediator-induced C-fiber sensitization for mechanical and hypotonic stimuli in TRPV4-/- mice. *Mol Pain* 3:31.
196. Todaka, H., Taniguchi, J., Satoh, J., Mizuno, A., Suzuki, M. (2004). Warm temperature-sensitive transient receptor potential vanilloid 4 (TRPV4) plays an essential role in thermal hyperalgesia. *J Biol Chem* 279:35133–35138.
197. Alessandri-Haber, N., Dina, O.A., Joseph, E.K., Reichling, D., Levine, J.D. (2006). A transient receptor potential vanilloid 4-dependent mechanism of hyperalgesia is engaged by concerted action of inflammatory mediators. *J Neurosci* 26:3864–3874.
198. Alessandri-Haber, N., Dina, O.A., Yeh, J.J., Parada, C.A., Reichling, D.B., Levine, J.D. (2004). Transient receptor potential vanilloid 4 is essential in chemotherapy-induced neuropathic pain in the rat. *J Neurosci* 24:4444–4452.
199. Tabuchi, K., Suzuki, M., Mizuno, A., Hara, A. (2005). Hearing impairment in TRPV4 knockout mice. *Neurosci Lett* 382:304–308.
200. Liedtke, W. (2007). TRPV channels' role in osmotransduction and mechanotransduction. *Handb Exp Pharmacol* 179:473–487.
201. Jaquemar, D., Schenker, T., Trueb, B. (1999). An ankyrin-like protein with transmembrane domains is specifically lost after oncogenic transformation of human fibroblasts. *J Biol Chem* 274:7325–7333.
202. Story, G.M., Peier, A.M., Reeve, A.J., Eid, S.R., Mosbacher, J., Hricik, T.R., Earley, T.J., Hergarden, A.C., Andersson, D.A., Hwang, S.W., McIntyre, P., Jegla, T., Bevan, S., Patapoutian, A. (2003). ANKTM1, a TRP-like channel expressed in nociceptive neurons, is activated by cold temperatures. *Cell* 112:819–829.
203. Kobayashi, K., Fukuoka, T., Obata, K., Yamanaka, H., Dai, Y., Tokunaga, A., Noguchi, K. (2005). Distinct expression of TRPM8, TRPA1, and TRPV1 mRNAs

in rat primary afferent neurons with adelta/c-fibers and colocalization with trk receptors. *J Comp Neurol* 493:596–606.

204. Bautista, D.M., Movahed, P., Hinman, A., Axelsson, H.E., Sterner, O., Hogestatt, E.D., Julius, D., Jordt, S.E., Zygmunt, P.M. (2005). Pungent products from garlic activate the sensory ion channel TRPA1. *Proc Natl Acad Sci U S A* 102:12248–12252.
205. Dhaka, A., Murray, A.N., Mathur, J., Earley, T.J., Petrus, M.J., Patapoutian, A. (2007). TRPM8 is required for cold sensation in mice. *Neuron* 54:371–378.
206. Macpherson, L.J., Dubin, A.E., Evans, M.J., Marr, F., Schultz, P.G., Cravatt, B.F., Patapoutian, A. (2007). Noxious compounds activate TRPA1 ion channels through covalent modification of cysteines. *Nature* 445:541–545.
207. Bautista, D.M., Jordt, S.E., Nikai, T., Tsuruda, P.R., Read, A.J., Poblete, J., Yamoah, E.N., Basbaum, A.I., Julius, D. (2006). TRPA1 mediates the inflammatory actions of environmental irritants and proalgesic agents. *Cell* 124:1269–1282.
208. McNamara, C.R., Mandel-Brehm, J., Bautista, D.M., Siemens, J., Deranian, K.L., Zhao, M., Hayward, N.J., Chong, J.A., Julius, D., Moran, M.M., Fanger, C.M. (2007). TRPA1 mediates formalin-induced pain. *Proc Natl Acad Sci U S A* 104:13525–13530.
209. Ward, L., Wright, E., McMahon, S.B. (1996). A comparison of the effects of noxious and innocuous counterstimuli on experimentally induced itch and pain. *Pain* 64:129–138.
210. Handwerker, H.O., Forster, C., Kirchhoff, C. (1991). Discharge patterns of human C-fibers induced by itching and burning stimuli. *J Neurophysiol* 66:307–315.
211. Koltzenburg, M., Lundberg, L.E., Torebjork, H.E. (1992). Dynamic and static components of mechanical hyperalgesia in human hairy skin. *Pain* 51:207–219.
212. McMahon, S.B., Wood, J.N. (2006). Increasingly irritable and close to tears: TRPA1 in inflammatory pain. *Cell* 124:1123–1125.
213. Reeh, P.W., Kocher, L., Jung, S. (1986). Does neurogenic inflammation alter the sensitivity of unmyelinated nociceptors in the rat? *Brain Res* 384:42–50.
214. Macpherson, L.J., Xiao, B., Kwan, K.Y., Petrus, M.J., Dubin, A.E., Hwang, S., Cravatt, B., Corey, D.P., Patapoutian, A. (2007). An ion channel essential for sensing chemical damage. *J Neurosci* 27:11412–11415.
215. Taylor-Clark, T.E., Undem, B.J., Macglashan, D.W., Jr., Ghatta, S., Carr, M.J., McAlexander, M.A. (2008). Prostaglandin-induced activation of nociceptive neurons via direct interaction with transient receptor potential A1 (TRPA1). *Mol Pharmacol* 73:274–281.
216. Trevisani, M., Siemens, J., Materazzi, S., Bautista, D.M., Nassini, R., Campi, B., Imamachi, N., Andre, E., Patacchini, R., Cottrell, G.S., Gatti, R., Basbaum, A.I., Bunnett, N.W., Julius, D., Geppetti, P. (2007). 4-Hydroxynonenal, an endogenous aldehyde, causes pain and neurogenic inflammation through activation of the irritant receptor TRPA1. *Proc Natl Acad Sci U S A* 104:13519–13524.
217. Materazzi, S., Nassini, R., Andre, E., Campi, B., Amadesi, S., Trevisani, M., Bunnett, N.W., Patacchini, R., Geppetti, P. (2008). Cox-dependent fatty acid metabolites cause pain through activation of the irritant receptor TRPA1. *Proc Natl Acad Sci U S A* 105:12045–12050.

218. Corey, D.P., Garcia-Anoveros, J., Holt, J.R., Kwan, K.Y., Lin, S.Y., Vollrath, M.A., Amalfitano, A., Cheung, E.L., Derfler, B.H., Duggan, A., Geleoc, G.S., Gray, P.A., Hoffman, M.P., Rehm, H.L., Tamasauskas, D., Zhang, D.S. (2004). TRPA1 is a candidate for the mechanosensitive transduction channel of vertebrate hair cells. *Nature* 432:723–730.

219. Dai, Y., Wang, S., Tominaga, M., Yamamoto, S., Fukuoka, T., Higashi, T., Kobayashi, K., Obata, K., Yamanaka, H., Noguchi, K. (2007). Sensitization of TRPA1 by PAR2 contributes to the sensation of inflammatory pain. *J Clin Invest* 117:1979–1987.

220. Diogenes, A., Akopian, A.N., Hargreaves, K.M. (2007). NGF up-regulates TRPA1: implications for orofacial pain. *J Dent Res* 86:550–555.

221. Katsura, H., Obata, K., Mizushima, T., Yamanaka, H., Kobayashi, K., Dai, Y., Fukuoka, T., Tokunaga, A., Sakagami, M., Noguchi, K. (2006). Antisense knock down of TRPA1, but not TRPM8, alleviates cold hyperalgesia after spinal nerve ligation in rats. *Exp Neurol* 200:112–123.

222. Obata, K., Katsura, H., Mizushima, T., Yamanaka, H., Kobayashi, K., Dai, Y., Fukuoka, T., Tokunaga, A., Tominaga, M., Noguchi, K. (2005). TRPA1 induced in sensory neurons contributes to cold hyperalgesia after inflammation and nerve injury. *J Clin Invest* 115:2393–2401.

223. Kwan, K.Y., Allchorne, A.J., Vollrath, M.A., Christensen, A.P., Zhang, D.S., Woolf, C.J., Corey, D.P. (2006). TRPA1 contributes to cold, mechanical, and chemical nociception but is not essential for hair-cell transduction. *Neuron* 50:277–289.

224. Klionsky, L., Tamir, R., Gao, B., Wang, W., Immke, D.C., Nishimura, N., Gavva, N.R. (2007). Species-specific pharmacology of trichloro(sulfanyl)ethyl benzamides as transient receptor potential ankyrin 1 (TRPA1) antagonists. *Mol Pain* 3:39.

225. McKemy, D.D., Neuhausser, W.M., Julius, D. (2002). Identification of a cold receptor reveals a general role for TRP channels in thermosensation. *Nature* 416: 52–58.

226. Eid, S.R., Crown, E.D., Moore, E.L., Liang, H.A., Choong, K.C., Dima, S., Henze, D.A., Kane, S.A., Urban, M.O. (2008). HC-030031, a TRPA1 selective antagonist, attenuates inflammatory- and neuropathy-induced mechanical hypersensitivity. *Mol Pain* 4:48.

227. Bautista, D.M., Siemens, J., Glazer, J.M., Tsuruda, P.R., Basbaum, A.I., Stucky, C.L., Jordt, S.E., Julius, D. (2007). The menthol receptor TRPM8 is the principal detector of environmental cold. *Nature* 448:204–208.

228. Rohacs, T., Lopes, C.M., Michailidis, I., Logothetis, D.E. (2005). PI(4,5)P2 regulates the activation and desensitization of TRPM8 channels through the TRP domain. *Nat Neurosci* 8:626–634.

229. Colburn, R.W., Lubin, M.L., Stone, D.J., Jr., Wang, Y., Lawrence, D., D'Andrea, M.R., Brandt, M.R., Liu, Y., Flores, C.M., Qin, N. (2007). Attenuated cold sensitivity in TRPM8 null mice. *Neuron* 54:379–386.

230. Proudfoot, C.J., Garry, E.M., Cottrell, D.F., Rosie, R., Anderson, H., Robertson, D.C., Fleetwood-Walker, S.M., Mitchell, R. (2006). Analgesia mediated by the TRPM8 cold receptor in chronic neuropathic pain. *Curr Biol* 16:1591–1605.

231. El Kouhen, R., Surowy, C.S., Bianchi, B.R., Neelands, T.R., McDonald, H.A., Niforatos, W., Gomtsyan, A., Lee, C.H., Honore, P., Sullivan, J.P., Jarvis, M.F., Faltynek, C.R. (2005). A-425619 [1-isoquinolin-5-yl-3-(4-trifluoromethyl-benzyl)-urea], a novel and selective transient receptor potential type V1 receptor antagonist, blocks channel activation by vanilloids, heat, and acid. *J Pharmacol Exp Ther* 314:400–409.

232. Mills, C., McMackin, M., Jaffe, R., Yu, J., Zininberg, E., Slee, D., Gogas, K., Bradbury, M. (2008). Effects of the transient receptor potential vanilloid 1 antagonist A-425619 on body temperature and thermoregulation in the rat. *Neuroscience* 156:165–174.

233. Joshi, S.K., Hernandez, G., Mikusa, J.P., Zhu, C.Z., Zhong, C., Salyers, A., Wismer, C.T., Chandran, P., Decker, M.W., Honore, P. (2006). Comparison of antinociceptive actions of standard analgesics in attenuating capsaicin and nerve-injury-induced mechanical hypersensitivity. *Neuroscience* 143:587–596.

234. Doherty, E.M., Retz, D., Gavva, N.R., Tamir, R., Treanor, J.J., Norman, M.H. (2008). 4-Aminopyrimidine tetrahydronaphthols: a series of novel vanilloid receptor-1 antagonists with improved solubility properties. *Bioorg Med Chem Lett* 18: 1830–1834.

235. Gavva, N.R., Tamir, R., Qu, Y., Klionsky, L., Zhang, T.J., Immke, D., Wang, J., Zhu, D., Vanderah, T.W., Porreca, F., Doherty, E.M., Norman, M.H., Wild, K.D., Bannon, A.W., Louis, J.C., Treanor, J.J. (2005). AMG 9810 [(E)-3-(4-t-butylphenyl)-N-(2,3-dihydrobenzo[b][1,4] dioxin-6-yl)acrylamide], a novel vanilloid receptor 1 (TRPV1) antagonist with antihyperalgesic properties. *J Pharmacol Exp Ther* 313:474–484.

236. Valenzano, K.J., Grant, E.R., Wu, G., Hachicha, M., Schmid, L., Tafesse, L., Sun, Q., Rotshteyn, Y., Francis, J., Limberis, J., Malik, S., Whittemore, E.R., Hodges, D. (2003). N-(4-tertiarybutylphenyl)-4-(3-chloropyridin-2-yl)tetrahydropyrazine -1(2H)-carbox-amide (BCTC), a novel, orally effective vanilloid receptor 1 antagonist with analgesic properties: I. In vitro characterization and pharmacokinetic properties. *J Pharmacol Exp Ther* 306:377–386.

237. Jakab, B., Helyes, Z., Varga, A., Bolcskei, K., Szabo, A., Sandor, K., Elekes, K., Borzsei, R., Keszthelyi, D., Pinter, E., Petho, G., Nemeth, J., Szolcsanyi, J. (2005). Pharmacological characterization of the TRPV1 receptor antagonist JYL1421 (SC0030) in vitro and in vivo in the rat. *Eur J Pharmacol* 517:35–44.

238. Rami, H.K., Thompson, M., Stemp, G., Fell, S., Jerman, J.C., Stevens, A.J., Smart, D., Sargent, B., Sanderson, D., Randall, A.D., Gunthorpe, M.J., Davis, J.B. (2006). Discovery of SB-705498: a potent, selective and orally bioavailable TRPV1 antagonist suitable for clinical development. *Bioorg Med Chem Lett* 16:3287–3291.

239. Gunthorpe, M.J., Hannan, S.L., Smart, D., Jerman, J.C., Arpino, S., Smith, G.D., Brough, S., Wright, J., Egerton, J., Lappin, S.C., Holland, V.A., Winborn, K., Thompson, M., Rami, H.K., Randall, A., Davis, J.B. (2007). Characterization of SB-705498, a potent and selective vanilloid receptor-1 (VR1/TRPV1) antagonist that inhibits the capsaicin-, acid-, and heat-mediated activation of the receptor. *J Pharmacol Exp Ther* 321:1183–1192.

CHAPTER 9

Glutamate Receptors

BRIAN E. CAIRNS

Faculty of Pharmaceutical Sciences, The University of British Columbia

Content

9.1 INTRODUCTION

The excitatory amino acid receptors are composed of two distinct types of receptors: mixed cation channels known as inotropic receptors and a group of G protein-coupled receptors, which are known collectively as metabotropic

Peripheral Receptor Targets for Analgesia: Novel Approaches to Pain Management, Edited by Brian E. Cairns

receptors (mGluRs). There are multiple subtypes of both the inotropic receptors and mGluRs, each with their own unique molecular composition, pharmacology, and distribution. Nevertheless, the common denominator for all of these receptors is that they can be activated by the excitatory amino acid glutamate, which is one of the major excitatory neurotransmitters in the central nervous system. Recent evidence indicates that glutamate concentrations become elevated in tissues such as skin, skeletal muscle, and viscera in association with potential or actual tissue injury and thus may play an important role in the modulation of nociceptor excitability in these tissues. Indeed, artificial elevation of glutamate concentrations in various tissues results in nocifensive behavior in animals and pain in humans that can be attenuated by ionotropic receptor and mGluR antagonists, which further strengthens the link between peripheral glutamate receptor (GluR) activation and pain transduction mechanisms. The following sections provide an overview of GluR pharmacology, followed by a discussion of the potential role of peripheral GluRs in various painful conditions and the potential utility of peripheral GluR agonists and antagonists in the treatment of these conditions.

9.2 GluR PHARMACOLOGY

The GluRs can be divided into ionotropic receptor and mGluR subtypes [1–6]. The former are mixed cation channels, which allow the passage of Na+, K+, and, in some cases, Ca++ across cell membranes, while the latter are G protein linked. There are three ionotropic GluR subtypes, which have been named for the agonist first describe to be selective for them: the N-methyl-D-aspartate (NMDA) receptor and two non-NMDA GluRs, the kainate receptor and the α-amino-3-hydroxy-5-methyl-5-isoxazolepropionate (AMPA) receptor [1–6]. There are eight subtypes of mGluR, which have been grouped into three families on the basis of the G proteins and downstream signaling mechanisms they activate. Group I mGluRs mediate their effects through Gq/G11 G proteins and stimulate the activity of phospholipase C. Group II and Group III mGluRs are coupled to Gi/Go G proteins and inhibit the activation of adenylate cyclase. The following sections provide a brief overview of the pharmacology of GluRs.

9.2.1 NMDA Receptors (NRs)

The NR is a mixed cation channel that is permeable to Na^+, K^+, and Ca^+ [2,7]. The NR ion channel is heteromeric and is a made up of combinations of NR_1, NR_2 (A, B, C, D), and NR_3 (A, B) subunits [2,7–11]. The structure is likely a tetramer, and functional receptors are composed of dimers of NR_1/NR_2 subunits although an NR_3 subunit can replace one of the NR_2 subunits, which results in some decrease in receptor conductance and permeability to calcium compared with the NR_1/NR_2 receptor [2,7,9,10]. The agonist binding site for glutamate is located on the NR_2 subunit, and NR receptor activation requires the binding of two glutamate molecules [2,7,9–11]. In addition to glutamate, the NR requires glycine as a coagonist, with a binding site on the NR_1 subunit [2,7,9–11]. The opening of the NR ion channel is voltage dependent because a magnesium ion blocks the pore at resting membrane potentials [2,7,9–11]. The NR is also subject to modulation by protons, which act at a site located on the NR_1 subunit and tend to keep the receptor in a low-conductance state [12,13]. Certain compounds, such as spermine and spermidine, can occlude access of protons to their binding site on the NR_1 subunit and thus attenuate inhibition of NR current flow by protons [2]. On the other hand, phosphorylation of the NR_2 subunit increases current flow through the NR [11,14]. NRs have been found on dorsal root and trigeminal ganglion neurons [15–17] as well as on the peripheral ends of small-diameter primary afferents fibers [18,19]. In humans, NR_{2B} and NR_{2D} subunits have been found in the skin [20,21], and NR_1 subunits in tendons [22,23]. It has been suggested that NRs comprised of NR_1/NR_{2B} subunits may be the dominant functional form of the NR on primary afferent fibers [15–17].

9.2.1.1 Selective Agonists. Glutamate is an endogenous agonist for NRs; however, aspartate, which shows greater affinity for NRs than GluRs, may also be released by some synapses (Table 9.1) [2]. NMDA is selective for NRs; however, it does not exhibit receptor subtype (e.g., NR_{2A} over NR_{2B}) selectivity. Although NMDA is somewhat less potent than glutamate, it is not a substrate for glutamate transporters and thus is often much more effective than

TABLE 9.1. Summary of the Glutamate Receptor Selective Agonists and Antagonists Discussed in This Chapter.

Compound	Action	Receptor Specificity
Glutamate	Agonist	Nonselective (endogenous)
Aspartate	Agonist	Slightly greater affinity for NRs
NMDA	Agonist	NR selective
Kainate	Agonist	$GluR_{1-7}$, KA_{1-2}
AMPA	Agonist	$GluR_{1-7}$, KA_{1-2}
(S)-2-Me-Tet-AMPA	Agonist	$GluR_{1-4}$
Domoic acid	Agonist	$GluR_{1-7}$, KA_{1-2}
(S ATPA)	Agonist	$GluR_5$
1S,3R-ACPD	Agonist	$mGluR_{1-8}$
DHPG	Agonist	$mGluR_{1,5}$
LY354740	Agonist	$mGluR_{2,3}$
NAAG	Agonist	$mGluR_{2,3}$
L-AP4	Agonist	$mGluR_{4,6,8}$
Cyclothiazide	Positive allosteric modulator	$GluR_{1-4}$
CX516	Positive allosteric modulator	$GluR_{1-4}$

TABLE 9.1. ***Continued***

Compound	Action	Receptor Specificity
Concanavalin A, soybean agglutinin, and wheat germ agglutinin	Positive allosteric modulator	$GluR_{5-7}$, KA_{1-2}
2-Phenyl-1-benzenesulfonyl-pyrrolidine derivatives	Positive allosteric modulator	$mGluR_1$
CPPHA	Positive allosteric modulator	$mGluR_5$
Kynurenic acid	Competitive antagonist Noncompetitive antagonist	$GluR_{1-7}$, KA_{1-2} NR (glycine site)
AP-5	Competitive antagonist	NR selective
CNQX	Competitive antagonist Noncompetitive antagonist	$GluR_{1-7}$, KA_{1-2} NR (glycine site)
DNQX	Competitive antagonist Noncompetitive antagonist	$GluR_{1-7}$, KA_{1-2} NR (glycine site)
NBQX	Competitive antagonist	$GluR_{1-4}$
LY382884	Competitive antagonist	$GluR_5$
MPEP	Competitive antagonist	$mGluR_5$ (and NR)
MTEP	Competitive antagonist	$mGluR_5$
LY341495	Competitive antagonist	$mGluR_{2,3}$
CPPG	Competitive antagonist	$mGluR_{4,6,8}$
MSOP	Competitive antagonist	$mGluR_{4,6,8}$
7-Chlorokynurenic acid	Noncompetitive antagonist	NR selective (glycine site)
Ifenprodil	Noncompetitive partial antagonist	NR_{2B} subtype selective (polyamine site)
Haloperidol	Noncompetitive partial antagonist	NR_{2B} subtype selective (polyamine site)
Zn^{+2}	Noncompetitive partial antagonist	NR_{2A} subtype selective
Memantine	Noncompetitive antagonist	NR selective (*phencyclidine site*)
Ketamine	Noncompetitive antagonist	NR selective (*phencyclidine site*)
Amantidine	Noncompetitive antagonist	NR selective (*phencyclidine site*)
Dextromethorphan	Noncompetitive antagonist	NR selective (*phencyclidine site*)
GYKI 53655	Negative allosteric modulator	$GluR_{1-4}$
CPCCOEt	Negative allosteric modulator	$mGluR_1$

glutamate when administered to intact preparations [2]. Activation of NRs also requires that glycine be bound to the coagonist site on the NR_1 subunit, and D-serine has approximately the same affinity and intrinsic activity as glycine itself in this capacity.

9.2.1.2 Selective Antagonists. The first selective competitive antagonists for the NR were conformationally constrained amino acid derivatives containing an ω-phosphonic group. One of the most commonly used of these antagonists is 2-amino-5-phosphonopentanoic acid (AP-5) [2]. Some competitive antagonists exhibit modest subunit selectivity; however, much better selectivity is achieved with antagonists at the polyamine site (see below).

9.2.1.3 Noncompetitive Antagonists. Kynurenic acid is a noncompetitive antagonist of NRs, which acts at the glycine site. It is also a competitive antagonist at GluRs, and thus, its actions are not selective for NRs over other GluRs [24]. A derivate of kynurenic acid, 7-chlorokynurenic acid, is the prototypical NR-selective noncompetitive glycine site antagonist [24,25]. There appears to be no subunit selectivity for glycine site antagonists, possibly because the binding site for glycine resides on the NR_1 subunit, which is required for functional activity [25].

Other antagonists, which include drugs such as ifenprodil and the neuroleptic agent haloperidol, act at the polyamine site and display significant (~100-fold) selectivity for NR_{2B}-containing NRs over NRs with $NR_{2A,\ B,\ or\ D}$ subunits [10,12,13,24]. These agents bind the N-terminal region of the NR_{2B} subunit, are noncompetitive, and show no voltage dependence. Interestingly, ifenprodil exerts only partial antagonist effects, with a maximum of 90% inhibition of NR_{2B} currents [12,13]. Ifenprodil, in addition to its inhibitory effect, also produces an increase in the receptor affinity for glutamate, thus is only effective at high glutamate concentration [8].

As mentioned, Mg^{+2} ions block the NR pore, and elevated levels of Mg^{+2} can act to inhibit the NR. In addition, Zn^{+2} is a highly selective antagonist of NR_{2A}-containing NRs; however, as with the polyamine site antagonists, it acts primarily as a partial antagonist, with about 70% maximal inhibition of NR_{2A} currents [2,8,9].

Most clinically employed NR antagonists, which include memantine, amantidine, ketamine, and dextromethorphan, fall into the category of NR channel blockers and act at the so-called *phencyclidine site* [2,8,9,24]. These agents exhibit use dependency because their block of the channel requires it to be in the open state. All are positively charged and have voltage-dependent blocking ability but differ in their ability to sustain channel blockade.

9.2.2 AMPA Receptors

Glutamate is an endogenous agonist for AMPA receptors, which are composed of $GluR_{1-4}$ subunits in a tetrameric structure (Table 9.1) [26,27]. Naturally occurring AMPA receptors are mixed cation channels permeable to Na^+, K^+, and Ca^+; however, AMPA receptors with the $GluR_2$ subunit have low permeability to Ca^+ [9,28]. In addition to AMPA, these receptors are readily activated by kainate. The AMPA receptor exhibits desensitization to sustained agonist activation by either AMPA or glutamate but does not desensitize when activated by kainate [2,27]. Subunits can exist in two alternatively spliced isoforms, designated flip and flop, which exhibit differences in their desensitization properties [9,28,29]. Dorsal root and trigeminal ganglion neurons express $GluR_{1-4}$ subunits [30–33], and $GluR_1$ subunits have been identified on afferent fibers in various nerves and in human skin [19,21].

9.2.2.1 Selective Agonists. Although AMPA is a selective agonist for this receptor, it can also activate kainate receptors at higher concentrations [34]. Additional modification of AMPA has led to more selective agonists, such as (S)-2-Me-Tet-AMPA, which activates AMPA receptors at concentrations two orders of magnitude lower than those at which it activates kainate receptors [27,28,34].

9.2.2.2 Allosteric Modulators. Certain compounds have been identified that can modify the rapid desensitization and/or deactivation of AMPA receptors through binding at an allosteric site. These benzamide compounds are not agonists (do not open the receptor) but instead act to facilitate AMPA-mediated currents and have been termed "AMPA-kines" [26,34]. Cyclothiazide and many related benzamides appear to act primarily by inhibiting receptor desensitization, whereas other benzamides, such as 1-(quinoxalin-6-ylcarbonyl)-piperidine (CX516), appear to inhibit both desensitization and deactivation [26,34].

9.2.2.3 Selective Competitive Antagonists. Early competitive antagonists, such as 6-cyano-7-nitroquinoxaline-2,3-dione (CNQX) and 6,7-dinitroquinoxalin-2,3-dione (DNQX), were not selective for AMPA receptors over kainate receptors and had the added disadvantage of acting as noncompetitive antagonists at the glycine site of the NR at higher concentrations [28,34]. This appears to be due to significant structural similarities between the AMPA receptor and the glycine site of the NR. However, 2,3-dihydroxy-6-nitro-7-sulfamoyl-benzo(F)quinoxaline (NBQX) has more than 100-fold selectivity for AMPA versus kainate receptors and does not act at the glycine site of the NR [28,34].

9.2.2.4 Noncompetitive Antagonists. AMPA receptor negative allosteric modulators, for example, 2,3-disubstituted benzodiazepines, such as GYKI 53655 (1-[4-aminophenyl]-4-methyl-7,8-methylenedioxy-5H-2,3,-benzodiazepine), which act as AMPA-receptor-selective, noncompetitive antagonists (over kainic acid [KA] and NR) [26,28,34]. These compounds exhibit little selectivity among different subunit-containing AMPA receptors [28,34].

9.2.3 Kainate Receptors

Although glutamate is also the endogenous agonist for kainate receptors, natural agonists for this receptor include kainic and domoic acids, although all these compounds also interact with AMPA receptors (Table 9.1) [6,35,36]. Naturally occurring kainate receptors are composed of homomeric and heteromeric tetramers of the $GluR_{5-7}$ and KA_1 and KA_2 subunits [2,6,9,36,37]. While $GluR_{5-7}$ are able to form functional homomeric and heteromeric channels, functional receptors with the KA_1 and KA_2 subunits are heteromeric [2,6,9,36,37]. Kainate receptors are also mixed cation channels; however, they exhibit rapid and strong desensitization upon activation, and desensitization can occur at agonist concentrations lower than those required for channel opening. Prolonged exposure to agonists may actually cause antagonism through desensitization [2,6,36]. Dorsal root and trigeminal ganglion neurons express $GluR_{5-7}$ as well as KA_1 and KA_2 subunits [32,33,36]. Antibodies directed against $GluR_{5-7}$ suggest that these receptors are also expressed in human skin [21].

9.2.3.1 Selective Agonists. The similarities between kainate and AMPA receptors have limited the number of agonists available that have selective actions at the kainate receptor. Some selective agonists, such as (S)-2-amino-3(3-hydroxy-5-tert.-butylisox-azol-4-yl) propanoic acid (S ATPA), are part of a group of $GluR_5$ subunit selective kainic acid receptor agonists that have been developed [2,6,36,37]. These $GluR_5$-preferring agonists have activity at homomeric $GluR_5$ kainate receptors and naturally occurring receptors in dorsal root ganglion neurons.

9.2.3.2 Allosteric Modulators. Certain naturally occurring compounds from plants, for example, concanavalin A, soybean agglutinin, and wheat germ agglutinin, appear to decrease the rapid desensitization of kainate receptors [2,6,35,37]. These compounds bind to the carbohydrate side chain of the kainate receptor through N-glycosylation to modulate channel activity [6,35,37]. Protons also appear to inhibit native kainate receptors in a voltage-dependent manner [6,35,37]. This inhibition can be relieved by compounds such as spermine, which have a similar effect on the polyamine site of NRs [2,6,35,37].

9.2.3.3 Selective Antagonists. Although the decahydroxyisoquinoline carboxylate group-containing competitive antagonists, such as DNQX, block kainate receptor activation, they are also effective AMPA receptor antagonists. A derivative of this group of antagonists, LY382884 ([3S,4aR,6S, 8aR]-6-[4-carboxyphenyl]methyl-1,2,3,4,4a,5,6,7,8,8a-decahydroisoquinoline-3-carboxylic acid), is a selective $GluR_5$ subunit containing kainate receptor antagonist [2,6,35,37]. The $GluR_5$ subunit is the most common subunit expressed by peripheral nerve fibers [2].

9.2.4 mGluRs

There are currently eight G protein-coupled mGluRs, designated $mGluR_{1–8}$, at which glutamate acts as an agonist (Table 9.1) [2,38,39]. These receptors have been divided into three families based on the G proteins they couple to, their molecular structure, and their sensitivity to different agonists. Functional mGluRs are thought to be homodimers [2,38,39]. Group I mGluRs ($mGluR_{1\ and\ 5}$) are coupled to couple to Gq/G11 G proteins to stimulate phospholipase C and are often located postsynaptically in the central nervous systems [2,38]. Group II ($mGluR_{2\ and\ 3}$) and Group III mGluRs ($mGluR_{4,6,7,\ and\ 8}$) are coupled to Gi/Go G proteins and inhibit adenylyl cyclase [2,38,39] and, in the central nervous system, appear to modulate G protein-coupled, inwardly rectifying potassium channels and/or voltage-gated calcium channels. Group II and III mGluRs are more often associated with presynaptic terminals in the central nervous system [38,40]. All mGluRs appear to be found peripherally except for $mGluR_6$, which is not expressed to any great extent outside of the retina [41–44]. Recent evidence suggests a very high expression of the $mGluR_8$ subunit [45].

9.2.4.1 Selective Agonists. As with the inotropic receptors, the endogenous agonist for mGluRs is glutamate [2,9]. The compound (1S,3R)-1-aminocyclopentane-1,3-dicarboxylic acid (1S,3R-ACPD) was one of the first agonists to exhibit selectivity for mGluRs over NRs and GluRs; however, it has no selectivity for the various mGluR subtypes and has low potency at mGluRs [2,9,39]. There are, however, an increasing number of agonists that appear relatively selective for specific groups of mGluRs. For example, 3,5-dihydroxyphenylglycine (DHPG) is somewhat more selective for group I mGluRs, (1S,2S,5R,6S)-(1)-2-aminobicyclo[3.1.0]hexane-2,6-dicarboxylic acid (LY354740) and N-acetylaspartylglutamate (NAAG) are fairly selective for group II receptors, and L-(1)-2-amino-4-phosphonobutyric acid (L-AP4) is selective for $mGluR_{4,6,\ and\ 8}$ but is a poor agonist for the $mGluR_7$ receptor [39,40].

9.2.4.2 mGluR Positive Allosteric Modulators. As with the inotropic receptors, group I mGluR function is modifiable through an allosteric binding site, which can markedly facilitate agonist-induced activity. Examples of such compounds include 2-phenyl-1-benzenesulfonyl-pyrrolidine derivatives ($mGluR_1$ selective) and N-{4-chloro-2-[(1,3-dioxo-1,3-dihydro-2H-isoindol-2-yl) methyl]phenyl}-2-hydroxybenzamide (CPPHA; $mGluR_5$ selective) [2]. These allosteric modulators are thought to act by stabilizing activated receptors states [2].

9.2.4.3 Antagonists. For group I, the compound (S)-2-methyl-4-carboxyphenylglycine (LY367385) exhibits selective antagonism for $mGlu_1$ over $mGluR_5$ [2]. Selective $mGluR_5$ antagonists include 2-methyl-6-

(phenylethynyl)pyridine (MPEP), which is unfortunately also an effective antagonist at NR_{2A}- and NR_{2B}-containing NRs, and $GluR_6$-containing KAs [46], as well as 3-[(2-methyl-1,3-thiazol-4-yl)ethynyl]pyridine (MTEP), which appears to be much more selective for $mGluR_5$ over inotropic GluRs [2,46]. The most potent group II mGluR antagonist identified to date is 2S-2-amino-2-(1S,2S-2-carboxycycloprop-1-yl)-3-(xanth-9-yl) propanoic acid (LY341495), which exhibits nanomolar affinity at both $mGluR_{2\ \text{and}\ 3}$ but is only approximately 10-fold selective at $mGluR_8$ [2,39]. Selective competitive group III mGluR antagonists have been identified including (R,S)-α-cyclopropyl-4-phosphonophenyl-glycine (CPPG) and (R,S)-α-methylserine-O-phosphate (MSOP) [2,39].

9.2.4.4 Noncompetitive Antagonists. Recent research has revealed that at least some of the mGluRs ($mGluR_5$, $mGluR_1$) can also be noncompetitively inhibited by allosteric modulators, which appear to act by reducing the efficacy of glutamate-stimulated phosphoinositide (PI) hydrolysis. One of the first of these compounds is 7-hydroxyiminocyclopropan[b]chromen-1a-carboxylic acid ethyl ester (CPCCOEt), an $mGlu_1$-selective antagonist that has no activity at $mGluR_5$, group II and III mGluRs, or inotropic GluRs [2,39].

9.3 PERIPHERAL GluRs AND PAIN PROCESSING

9.3.1 Cutaneous Pain

It has been about 15 years since it was initially suggested that peripheral GluRs might contribute to cutaneous pain processing based on findings that glutamate and kainate application to the tail skin could evoke a putative nociceptive reflex in the neonatal rat isolated spinal cord–tail preparation [47]. It was reported that cutaneously administered glutamate could evoke ventral root reflexes by activating peripheral kainate receptors [47]. Subsequent behavioral investigations in adult rats have found that subcutaneously administered glutamate likely activates all three subtypes of inotropic receptors as well as mGluRs (Figure 9.1). Subcutaneous or intradermal injection of glutamate (~1 mM) or selective agonists (NMDA, AMPA, or kainate) as well as group I mGluRs (DHPG) into the rat paw results in sensitization of the skin to noxious mechanical and/or thermal stimulation [18,41,43,48–51], while injection of a high concentration of glutamate (100–3000 mM) also results in nocifensive (pain-related) behaviors, such as paw licking [52,53]. These findings indicate that there are functional inotropic receptors and mGluRs in the cutaneous tissue and that their activation in animals results in nocifensive behavior.

Glutamate, through activation of peripheral GluRs, also contributes to inflammatory pain mechanisms in cutaneous tissues. Inflammation of the skin with agents such as formalin or capsaicin increased baseline glutamate con-

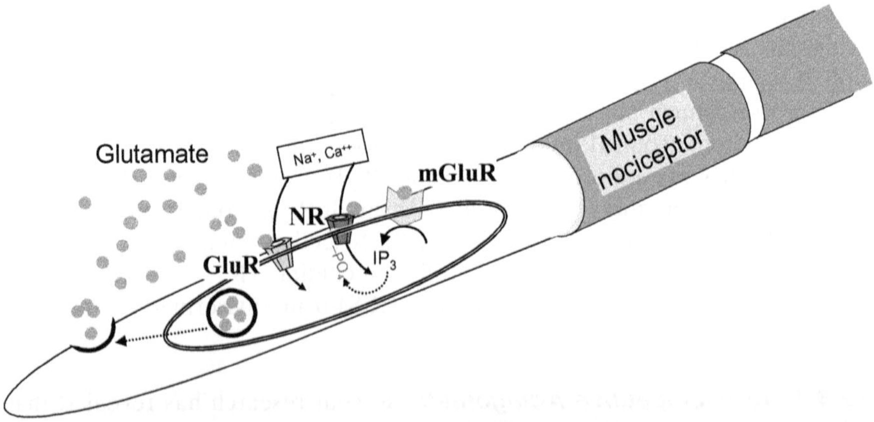

FIGURE 9.1. A model of how elevation of interstitial glutamate concentration could interact with peripheral excitatory amino acid (EAA) receptors to excite and sensitize masticatory muscle nociceptors. Glutamate could be released by nociceptor endings and act on either NRs or GluRs to depolarize the terminal ending or mGluRs to increase intracellular phosphoinositol (IP_3) and affect downstream targets through phosphorylation ($-PO_4$).

centrations, reported to be about 14 μM in rat skin, by 30–300% [54,55]. There is good evidence that NR antagonists attenuate nocifensive behaviors as well as thermal and mechanical sensitization, which results from irritant chemical application to the skin [56–59]. In addition, behavioral evidence also indicates that the group I mGluR antagonists (MPEP, (RS)-1-aminoindan-1,5-dicarboxylic acid) can attenuate nocifensive behavior induced by irritant chemicals or surgical incision, which suggests that in addition to inotropic GluRs, the activation of group I mGluRs also contributes to inflammatory pain mechanisms in the skin [44,60]. It is important to note, however, that MPEP is also an NR antagonist and that NMDA and glutamate are more potent sensitizers of rat skin than DHPG [43,46], which suggests that NRs may be more important than mGluRs in mediating nocifensive behavioral responses to elevated cutaneous glutamate levels.

In the skin, glutamate appears to be effective in activating slowly conducting, putative nociceptive afferent fibers as well as faster conducting fibers believed to convey innocuous sensory input. In the rat, subcutaneous injection of glutamate (300 μM, 10 μL) under the skin of the back activates roughly 80% of mechanoreceptive C-, Aδ-, and Aβ-fibers [61,62]. Glutamate also excites slowly conducting corneal afferent fibers *in vivo*, and this excitation can be blocked by ketamine [63]. In contrast, *in vitro*, using a rat paw skin nerve preparation, glutamate (300 μM) was reported not to excite Aβ-fibers but did increase the spontaneous discharge of about 40% of Aδ- and 70% of C-fibers, and also induced thermal but not mechanical sensitization [64]. Similar findings have been reported for NMDA and kainate in this *in vitro* model [65,66], which is in agreement with earlier reports of expression of GluRs and NRs in cutaneous tissues [18,19]. However, the response of slowly adapting type 1 mechanoreceptive afferents of rat whiskers to sustained mechanical stimulation is attenuated by kyurenic acid and the NR antagonists memantine, MK-801, and ifenprodil, which suggests that glutamate excites both fast and slowly conducting cutaneous fibers [67,68]. *In vivo*, there is also evidence that the activation of group I mGluRs contributes to inflammation-induced sensitization of slowly conducting skin afferent fibers [69]. The differential effect of glutamate on Aβ discharge may reflect differences between the *in vitro* and *in vivo* models and/or differences in the sensitivity of nerve fibers that innervate the paw compared with those that innervate the back and whiskers. Nevertheless, it appears that in the skin, glutamate is not a selective activator of nociceptors. Taken together, these findings suggest that elevated interstitial glutamate acts to increase the excitability of a broad range of cutaneous afferent fibers through activation of both inotropic receptors and metabotropic GluRs.

In healthy humans, subcutaneous injection of a fairly high concentration of glutamate (0.1 mL; 100 mM) is necessary to induce pain, mechanical sensitization, and vasomotor responses, while lower concentrations of glutamate (1 and 10 mM) are not significantly different from isotonic saline injections [70]. However, despite the finding that glutamate can evoke pain, induce mechanical sensitization, and increase blood flow when injected subcutaneously [70], human experimental and clinical studies that have employed topical or subdermal ketamine have not consistently identified a role for peripheral GluRs in human cutaneous pain mechanisms. After experimental burns to the legs of healthy subjects, it was reported in one study that ketamine (3 mM) inhibited the development of secondary mechanical hyperalgesia and thermal sensitization to a similar extent as subcutaneously administered lidocaine (0.5%) [71,72]. However, another study on experimental burn pain reported little effect of ketamine on these parameters at a slightly higher concentration (5 mM) [73]. Other experimental pain studies, in parallel to the animal studies, have used capsaicin to inflame the skin [74–77]. Intradermal injection of capsaicin evokes acute pain and also induces mechanical sensitization at the site of injection. Local ketamine infiltration had no effect on capsaicin-evoked pain or secondary hyperalgesia in these studies [74–76], and where a gel (5%) did appear to decrease capsaicin-induced mechanical sensitization, this was shown due to the systemic rather than the local effect of the drug [77]. In addition to its ability to block NRs, ketamine can exert local anesthetic-like actions [78], which makes it difficult to interpret the limited analgesic effects of ketamine noted in these studies as due only to NR antagonism.

9.3.2 Musculoskeletal Pain

Animal behavioral models, though employed less often than for the skin, have demonstrated the contribution of peripheral GluRs to joint and muscle nociceptive processing. Functional inotropic GluRs have been found in the temporomandibular (jaw) joint, where intra-articular injection of glutamate evoked a reflex jaw muscle response that could be mimicked by injection of

NMDA, AMPA, or kainate and be attenuated by coinjection of AP-5 and CNQX [79]. Behavioral evidence for the involvement of mGluRs in muscle pain is derived from experiments where the injection of glutamate or the group I mGluR agonist DHPG into the masseter muscle evoked nocifensive behavior and induced mechanical sensitization [42,80]. These findings indicate that there are functional peripheral inotropic receptors and mGluRs within both joints and muscles.

Research also indicates that elevated glutamate concentrations, through activation of peripheral GluRs, contribute to inflammatory pain mechanisms in joints and muscles as they do in the skin. Experimental induction of arthritis in the rat knee joint produced mechanical sensitization and increased synovial glutamate concentrations by approximately 300% [81–83]. Intra-articular injection of AP-7 (2-amino-7-phosphonoheptanoate), ketamine, CNQX, or AIDA (1-aminoindan-1,5 dicarboxylic acid)/MPEP attenuates mechanical sensitization associated with experimental arthritis, which suggests that the activation of peripheral inotropic and group I metabotropic glutamate mediates the effects of elevated synovial glutamate concentration [81,83]. Jaw muscle reflexes evoked by injection of inflammatory irritants, such as mustard oil or capsaicin, into the rat temporomandibular joint were also attenuated by NR antagonists (MK-801 and APV [2-amino-5-phosphonopentanoate]), which provides further evidence for a role of peripheral NR receptors in nociceptive mechanisms related to acutely induced experimental arthritis [84,85]. Nocifensive behavior related to the experimental induction of myositis, which can be produced in the masseter muscle injection of mustard oil or CFA, was attenuated by MK-801 and APV as well as MPEP [81,86,87]. As MPEP is also an NR antagonist [46], these results suggest that the activation of peripheral NRs, GluRs, and, perhaps to a lesser extent, peripheral mGluRs contributes to nociceptive mechanisms that underlie experimentally induced arthritis and myositis.

Similar to the skin, the injection of glutamate into the joint and muscle excites slowly conducting (Aδ and C) afferent fibers as well as Aβ-fibers (Figure 9.2) [88–90]. However, the injection of glutamate into the masseter muscle also significantly decreases the mechanical threshold of afferent fibers that innervate this muscle [89], an effect that has not been directly demonstrated for cutaneous afferent fibers, although behavioral evidence suggests that this does occur. The basal interstitial concentration of glutamate in the masseter muscle (~25 μM) *in vivo* is higher than that reported in the skin, which may, in part, explain why higher concentrations of exogenously applied glutamate appear to be required to excite and sensitize afferent fibers in the muscle as compared with the skin [91]. Current evidence suggests that the excitatory effect of elevated interstitial glutamate concentrations on muscle and joint afferent fibers is mediated primarily through the activation of peripheral NRs, as glutamate-evoked discharge and mechanical sensitization of muscle afferent fibers can be completely attenuated by local or systemic administration of NR antagonists such as APV and ketamine, and muscle

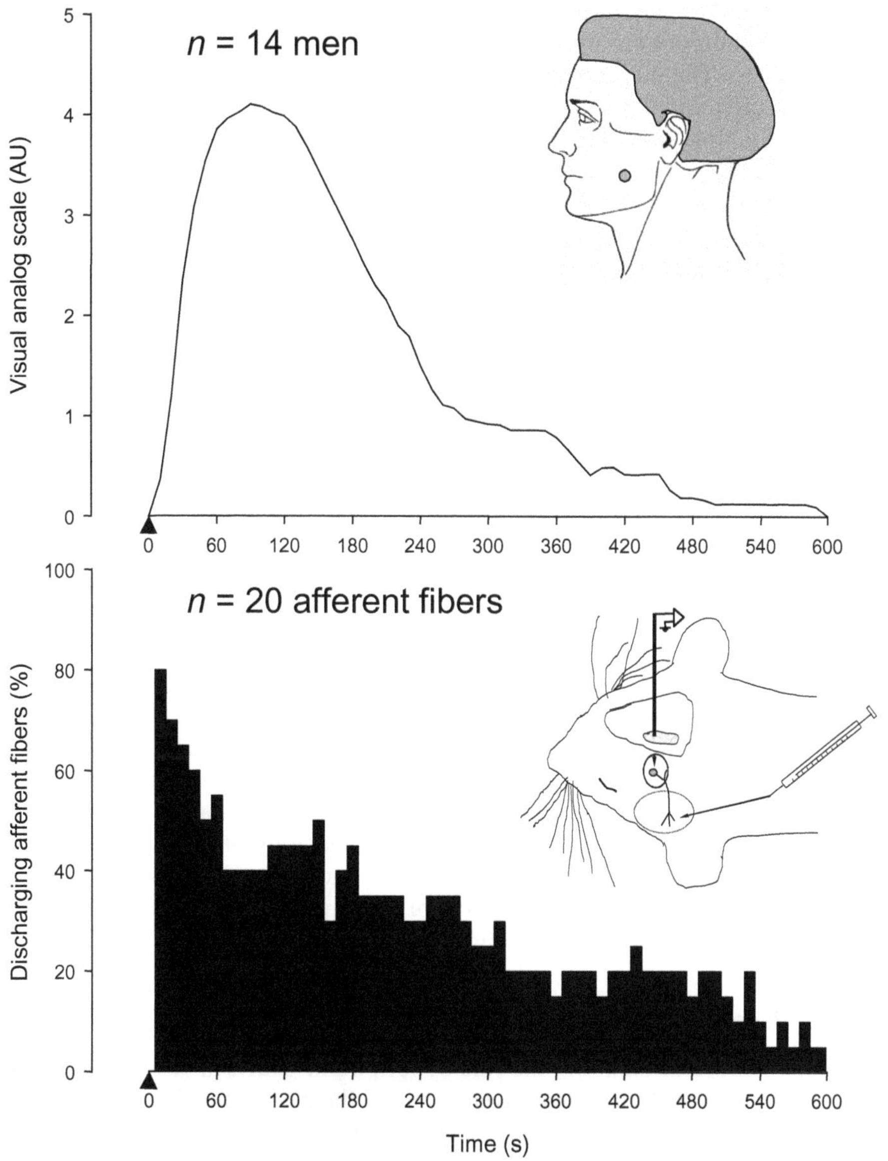

FIGURE 9.2. The top trace illustrates the mean pain rating of 14 men given an injection of glutamate (1 M) in the masseter muscle. The poststimulus histogram below shows the response of a group of 20 rat masseter nociceptors to injection of the same concentration of glutamate into the masseter muscle. There is a similar time course of pain in humans and nociceptor discharge in rats, which suggests that rat nociceptor discharges can be used to model glutamate-induced muscle pain.

afferent fibers are activated by NMDA [17,91–93]. It also appears that only certain NR subtypes are important for the peripheral actions of glutamate on afferent fibers. The majority of the peripheral NRs expressed by muscle afferent fibers contains the NR_{2B} subunit with far fewer that express the NR_{2A} subunit, and NMDA-evoked muscle afferent discharge is significantly attenuated by the NR_{2B}-selective antagonist ifenprodil [17,89,91–94].

The endogenous release of glutamate from muscle afferent fiber terminals could be one source for the elevated glutamate concentrations observed in the skeletal muscle and joints. Recent evidence suggests that vesicular release of glutamate from large-diameter skeletal muscle afferent fibers may occur, although it is not known whether smaller-diameter, putative nociceptive afferent fibers can also release glutamate [95,96]. In rats, a dose of 50 mg/kg monosodium glutamate (MSG) given intravenously raised interstitial concentrations of glutamate in the masseter muscle from 25 to 65 μM, and this degree of elevation of interstitial glutamate in the muscle was associated with significant mechanical sensitization of nociceptors [91].

In humans, the injection of a pharmacological dose of glutamate (1 M, 0.2 mL) into the masseter, splenius, or trapezius muscles produces short-lasting muscle pain and is also associated with mechanical sensitization localized to the site of injection [88,92,97–102]. Glutamate-evoked pain and glutamate-induced mechanical sensitization are attenuated by coinjection of the NR antagonist ketamine (10 mM) in men [92,102]. This concentration of ketamine is without effect on hypertonic saline-evoked muscle pain, which suggests that the effect is not due to a local analgesic effect of ketamine but rather to antagonism of peripheral NRs, as has been demonstrated in animal models [92,102]. Unfortunately, the paucity of GluR antagonists approved for use in humans has limited investigation of the pharmacology of peripheral GluRs. Thus, while animal work suggests that other inotropic receptors as well as metabotropic contribute to the effects of elevated glutamate in muscle and joint tissues, this has yet to be confirmed in human subjects.

9.3.3 Visceral Pain

Almost all information about the role of peripheral GluRs in visceral pain has been derived from studies that have examined the gastrointestinal tract. It has been suggested that nocifensive behavior in response to colonic distension is attenuated by peripheral and, in some cases, central NRs [103,104]. Behavioral studies in mice also suggest a role for peripheral $mGluR_5$ receptor activation in the behavioral response to colonic distention [105].

Vagal afferent fibers, which innervate the duodenum and stomach, have their cell bodies in the nodose ganglion, while colorectal afferent fibers of the splanchnic and pelvic nerves have their cell bodies in the dorsal root ganglion. A number of studies have demonstrated that nodose ganglion and dorsal root neurons express most, if not all, NRs, GluRs, and mGlurs [16,103,106–109]. The ongoing discharge and mechanically evoked responses of vagal afferent fibers are enhanced by NMDA and AMPA and decreased by antagonists for

NRs (MK-801, memantine, AP-5) and GluRs (CNQX) [110,111], which suggests that inotopic GluR activation modulates vagal afferent sensitivity. Anatomical evidence suggests that NR_{2B}-containing NRs are the most likely candidate receptor that mediate the effect of NR activation on the properties of vagal afferent fibers [16,106,107]. Mechanical responsiveness of colorectal afferent fibers of the pelvic nerve can also be reduced by NR antagonists, and this effect is mediated principally through activation of the NR_{2B} subtype [15,16,104,109]. Interestingly, the group I mGluR agonist S 3,5-DHPG reportedly did not affect vagal mechanical sensitivity [112], although a different group I agonist (1S,3R-ACPD) has been shown to inhibit nodose ganglion potassium currents [113], an action that would be predicted to lead to increased vagal afferent excitability. Indeed, the $mGluR_5$-selective antagonists MPEP and MTEP decreased the response of vagal and colorectal afferents to mechanical stimuli [105,111,114], which does suggest that $mGluR_5$ receptor activation sensitizes these mechanoreceptors. Activation of either group II or group III mGluRs results in decreased afferent mechanical sensitivity [112]. Taken together, these findings indicate that as with cutaneous and musculoskeletal afferent fibers, visceral afferent fiber excitability can be modulated by peripheral GluR activation.

9.4 PERIPHERAL GluR ANTAGONISTS FOR ANALGESIA

9.4.1 Neuropathic Pain

Open-label clinical studies have reported that topical ketamine-containing gels (~1.5% ketamine) may be effective in the treatment of neuropathic pain including that suffered by complex regional pain syndrome (CRPS) I patients [115–117]. However, in some of these studies, the most effective topical product contained a combination of amitriptyline (a tricyclic antidepressant agent) and ketamine, which makes it difficult to assess what component of this analgesic effect is due to peripheral NR block [115,116]. It has been difficult, however, to demonstrate the effectiveness of topical ketamine for the treatment of neuropathic pain in double-blind, placebo-controlled trials [115,118]. Unfortunately, ketamine is the only NR antagonist that appears to have been tried as a topical analgesic in human clinical studies to date. Although immunohistochemical studies have found evidence for the expression of all three inotropic receptors in the skin [20,21], almost nothing is known about the role of other GluRs in cutaneous pain processing. A single study has reported that the competitive mixed AMPA–kainate receptor antagonist LY293558 ([3S,4aR,6R,8aR]-6-[2-(1(2)H-tetrazole-5-yl)ethyl]decahydroisoquinoline-3-carboxylic acid) could attenuate capsaicin-induced pain and mechanical sensitization; however, the administration of this drug was associated with significant central side effects, and thus, the extent to which antagonism of peripheral GluRs contributed to the effects of LY293558 on experimental cutaneous pain is not known [119].

9.4.2 Arthritis/Arthralgia

Synovial glutamate concentrations in osteoarthritis exceed 200 μM, and in gouty arthritis and rheumatoid arthritis exceed 300 μM and are significantly greater than reported for synovial fluid from individuals who do not have arthritis [120]. The association between elevated glutamate concentration and pain in these various musculoskeletal pain conditions suggests that the local administration of GluR antagonists could offer a potential therapeutic option. However, intra-articular injection of ketamine (5–10 mM) was without effect on postoperative pain after arthroscopic knee surgery or ongoing pain and sensitivity in patients with temporomandibular joint arthralgia [121–123]. To date, ketamine is the only NR antagonist that has been administered by intra-articular injection.

9.4.3 Muscle Pain

In healthy humans without symptoms of chronic muscle pain, the concentration of the glutamate in tendons and muscles has been estimated to be between 20 and 70 μM [22,124–130]. Interstitial glutamate concentrations have been reported to increase dramatically in several noninflammatory pain conditions involving the skeletal muscle and/or tendons [124,127,128]. In tendons, such as the extensor carpi radialis brevis tendon of patients with tennis elbow and the patellar tendon of patients with "jumper's knee," glutamate concentrations of greater than 200 μM have been found [22,124,127,128]. In the skeletal muscle, it has been reported that baseline pain pressure thresholds showed a significant negative correlation with muscle glutamate concentration in women with chronic work-related trapezius myalgia [124]. During a low-force exercise that resulted in muscle pain, glutamate concentrations were positively correlated to the magnitude of muscle pain reported by both healthy subjects and those with chronic trapezius myalgia [124]. In other studies, no differences in interstitial glutamate concentrations in the trapezius muscle between healthy controls and pain patients have been identified [129,130].

Myofascial temporomandibular disorder (TMD) is a noninflammatory chronic muscle pain condition characterized by pain in the masticatory muscles with palpation and during function (e.g., chewing, mouth opening, speech). Preliminary data suggest that interstitial glutamate concentration in the masseter muscle of patients suffering from a myofascial TMD is two to three times higher than those measured in healthy controls. Taken together, these various findings suggest that elevated interstitial concentrations of glutamate may be associated with certain types of noninflammatory muscle pain.

Despite the association between elevated glutamate concentrations and muscle pain, few investigations have been made to assess the potential benefit of local NR antagonist administration. A single study has examined the effect of injection of ketamine (10 mM) into the most painful part of the masseter muscle of myofascial TMD patients [131]. However, this concentration of ketamine did not decrease ongoing muscle pain or alter mechanical sensitivity in these patients, who were mostly women. It now appears that one of the reasons for a lack of effect of ketamine in this study may have been that women are less sensitive than men to the local effects of this concentration of ketamine [100].

9.4.4 Visceral Pain

At present, only a few experimental pain studies and no clinical studies have been undertaken to examine the effect of NR antagonists on visceral pain. The administration of oral ketamine (25 or 50 mg) or dextromethorphan (10 or 30 mg) did not alter pain sensitivity of healthy volunteers to controlled gastric distension with a barostat [132,133]. In another study, intravenous infusion of ketamine was undertaken to achieve steady-state serum levels of 0, 60, or 120 ng/mL ketamine in healthy volunteers exposed to graded esophageal distension and thermal cutaneous stimuli in a randomized, blinded study [134]. In this study, ketamine did significantly attenuate esophageal distension pain but was less effective against cutaneous pain. While this result suggests that ketamine might be more effective against visceral than cutaneous pain, taken together, these studies seem to indicate that any effect of ketamine is probably due to a central nervous system action as opposed to a peripheral effect. Thus, the current experimental studies do not seem to support a large role for peripheral NR activation in human visceral pain [135].

9.5 PERIPHERAL GluRs; TARGETS FOR ANALGESIC DEVELOPMENT?

As discussed, a large body of basic research supports the concept that peripheral GluRs play a role in the mechanisms that underlie cutaneous and deep tissue pain. Despite this, the results of clinical trials with GluR antagonists have been relatively disappointing. Does this mean that peripheral GluRs are an unlikely target for the development of useful peripherally acting analgesic agents? It is important to consider that only a few, rather small clinical trials have been completed and that all of these trials have employed ketamine as an NR antagonist. This, of course, reflects an important limitation to studies of peripheral GluR function in humans, namely that there are very few GluR antagonists approved for use in human subjects, despite interest in the potential of these compounds for analgesia. Of the drugs that are currently available for use in humans, all have been designed for actions in the central nervous system. Indeed, one of the problems with using ketamine to investigate the role of peripheral NRs, is that the drug is rapidly cleared from the site of administration (this is particularly true for the skeletal muscle and the gastrointestinal tract) into the systemic circulation, and thus, it is difficult *in vivo* to maintain, for any length of time, the elevated tissue concentrations that appear to be necessary to block peripheral NRs. Indeed, some positive results have been reported for local ketamine analgesia when it is delivered topically in an ointment, a situation where sustained elevated concentrations of ketamine in the skin may be maintained. Clearly, though, additional research that examines other NR receptor antagonists, particularly those with NR subunit selectivity, is required before the potential utility of peripherally acting GluR antagonists for pain treatment will be well understood.

The role of kainate and AMPA receptors in human peripheral pain mechanisms is unknown. Again, basic research suggests that these receptors contribute to the modulation of nociceptors in the skin and also joints; however, the lack of available antagonist compounds coupled with the undesirable effects of systemically administered agents has stymied research into the role of these receptors in human pain.

Another underexplored area is the possibility of using agonists to activate group II or III mGluRs to cause peripheral analgesia. There is a reasonable body of basic scientific findings that support the hypothesis that the activation of these mGluRs could decrease afferent excitability under certain conditions. At present, this concept has not been tested in human experimental pain models or in clinical pain conditions. A related and potentially promising approach might be to instead use locally acting inhibitors to artificially elevate the level of inhibitory substances, for example, kynurenic acid (nonselective inotropic receptor antagonist) or NAAG, a naturally occurring $mGluR_2$ agonist. A recent animal study found that inhibition of NAAG peptidase results in analgesia in animal models of inflammatory and neuropathic pain [136]. These approaches may prove to be more easily translated into human experimental research than the administration of receptor antagonists.

There remains much to discover about the functional role that peripheral GluRs may play in pain processing. As research better defines the roles of various inotropic receptors and mGluRs in a number of different tissue pain mechanisms, it will become possible to better test whether any of these receptors are viable targets for the development of a peripherally acting analgesic for human use.

REFERENCES

1. Collingridge, G.L., Lester, R.A. (1989). Excitatory amino acid receptors in the vertebrate central nervous system. *Pharmacol Rev* 41:143–210.
2. Kew, J.N., Kemp, J.A. (2005). Ionotropic and metabotropic glutamate receptor structure and pharmacology. *Psychopharmacology (Berl)* 179:4–29.
3. Dingledine, R., Conn, P.J. (2000). Peripheral glutamate receptors: molecular biology and role in taste sensation. *J Nutr* 130(Suppl. 4S):1039S–1042S.
4. Monaghan, D.T., Bridges, R.J., Cotman, C.W. (1989). The excitatory amino acid receptors: their classes, pharmacology, and distinct properties in the function of the central nervous system. *Annu Rev Pharmacol Toxicol* 29:365–402.

5. Neugebauer, V. (2002). Metabotropic glutamate receptors—important modulators of nociception and pain behavior. *Pain* 98:1–8.
6. Pinheiro, P., Mulle, C. (2006). Kainate receptors. *Cell Tissue Res* 326:457–482.
7. Paoletti, P., Neyton, J. (2007). NMDA receptor subunits: function and pharmacology. *Curr Opin Pharmacol* 7:39–47.
8. Neyton, J., Paoletti, P. (2006). Relating NMDA receptor function to receptor subunit composition: limitations of the pharmacological approach. *J Neurosci* 26:1331–1333.
9. Bleakman, D., Alt, A., Nisenbaum, E.S. (2006). Glutamate receptors and pain. *Semin Cell Dev Biol* 17:592–604.
10. Gogas, K.R. (2006). Glutamate-based therapeutic approaches: NR2B receptor antagonists. *Curr Opin Pharmacol* 6:68–74.
11. Chen, B.S., Roche, K.W. (2007). Regulation of NMDA receptors by phosphorylation. *Neuropharmacology* 53:362–368.
12. Mott, D.D., Doherty, J.J., Zhang, S., Washburn, M.S., Fendley, M.J., Lyuboslavsky, P., Traynelis, S.F., Dingledine, R. (1998). Phenylethanolamines inhibit NMDA receptors by enhancing proton inhibition. *Nat Neurosci* 1:659–667.
13. Williams, K. (2001). Ifenprodil, a novel NMDA receptor antagonist: site and mechanism of action. *Curr Drug Targets* 2:285–298.
14. Salter, M.W., Kalia, L.V. (2004). Src kinases: a hub for NMDA receptor regulation. *Nat Rev Neurosci* 5:317–328.
15. Li, J., McRoberts, J.A., Nie, J., Ennes, H.S., Mayer, E.A. (2004). Electrophysiological characterization of N-methyl-D-aspartate receptors in rat dorsal root ganglia neurons. *Pain* 109:443–452.
16. Marvizon, J.C., McRoberts, J.A., Ennes, H.S., Song, B., Wang, X., Jinton, L., Corneliussen, B., Mayer, E.A. (2002). Two N-methyl-D-aspartate receptors in rat dorsal root ganglia with different subunit composition and localization. *J Comp Neurol* 446:325–441.
17. Dong, X.D., Mann, M.K., Kumar, U., Svensson, P., Arendt-Nielsen, L., Hu, J.W., Sessle, B.J., Cairns, B.E. (2007). Sex-related differences in NMDA-evoked rat masseter muscle afferent discharge result from estrogen-mediated modulation of peripheral NMDA receptor activity. *Neuroscience* 146:822–832.
18. Carlton, S.M., Hargett, G.L., Coggeshall, R.E. (1995). Localization and activation of glutamate receptors in unmyelinated axons of rat glabrous skin. *Neurosci Lett* 197:25–28.
19. Coggeshall, R.E., Carlton, S.M. (1998). Ultrastructural analysis of NMDA, AMPA, and kainate receptors on unmyelinated and myelinated axons in the periphery. *J Comp Neurol* 391:78–86.
20. Kim, S.H., Jang, T.J., Moon, I.S. (2006). Increased expression of N-methyl-D-aspartate receptor subunit 2D in the skin of patients with fibromyalgia. *J Rheumatol* 33:785–788.
21. Kinkelin, I., Bröcker, E.B., Koltzenburg, M., Carlton, S.M. (2000). Localization of ionotropic glutamate receptors in peripheral axons of human skin. *Neurosci Lett* 283:149–152.
22. Alfredson, H., Forsgren, S., Thorsen, K., Lorentzon, R. (2001). In vivo microdialysis and immunohistochemical analyses of tendon tissue demonstrated high amounts

of free glutamate and glutamate NMDAR1 receptors, but no signs of inflammation, in jumper's knee. *J Orthop Res* 19:881–886.

23. Alfredson, H., Forsgren, S., Thorsen, K., Fahlström, M., Johansson, H., Lorentzon, R. (2001). Glutamate NMDAR1 receptors localised to nerves in human Achilles tendons. Implications for treatment? *Knee Surg Sports Traumatol Arthrosc* 9:123–126.
24. Parsons, C.G. (2001). NMDA receptors as targets for drug action in neuropathic pain. *Eur J Pharmacol* 429:71–78.
25. Jansen, M., Dannhardt, G. (2003). Antagonists and agonists at the glycine site of the NMDA receptor for therapeutic interventions. *Eur J Med Chem* 38:661–670.
26. Lynch, G. (2006). Glutamate-based therapeutic approaches: ampakines. *Curr Opin Pharmacol* 6:82–88.
27. Johansen, T.N., Greenwood, J.R., Frydenvang, K., Madsen, U., Krogsgaard-Larsen, P. (2003). Stereostructure-activity studies on agonists at the AMPA and kainate subtypes of ionotropic glutamate receptors. *Chirality* 15:167–179.
28. Catarzi, D., Colotta, V., Varano, F. (2007). Competitive AMPA receptor antagonists. *Med Res Rev* 27:239–278.
29. Palmer, C.L., Cotton, L., Henley, J.M. (2005). The molecular pharmacology and cell biology of alpha-amino-3-hydroxy-5-methyl-4-isoxazolepropionic acid receptors. *Pharmacol Rev* 57:253–277.
30. Lee, C.J., Bardoni, R., Tong, C.K., Engelman, H.S., Joseph, D.J., Magherini, P.C., MacDermott, A.B. (2002). Functional expression of AMPA receptors on central terminals of rat dorsal root ganglion neurons and presynaptic inhibition of glutamate release. *Neuron* 35:135–146.
31. Lu, C.R., Hwang, S.J., Phend, K.D., Rustioni, A., Valtschanoff, J.G. (2002). Primary afferent terminals in spinal cord express presynaptic AMPA receptors. *J Neurosci* 22:9522–9529.
32. Sato, K., Kiyama, H., Park, H.T., Tohyama, M. (1993). AMPA, KA and NMDA receptors are expressed in the rat DRG neurones. *Neuroreport* 4:1263–1265.
33. Sahara, Y., Noro, N., Iida, Y., Soma, K., Nakamura, Y. (1997). Glutamate receptor subunits GluR5 and KA-2 are co-expressed in rat trigeminal ganglion neurons. *J Neurosci* 17:6611–6625.
34. Kemp, J.A., McKernan, R.M. (2002). NMDA receptors as drug targets. *Nature Neurosci* 5:1039–1042.
35. Conti, P., De Amici, M., De Micheli, C. (2002). Selective agonists and antagonists for kainate receptors. *Mini Rev Med Chem* 2:177–184.
36. Ruscheweyh, R., Sandkühler, J. (2002). Role of kainate receptors in nociception. *Brain Res Brain Res Rev* 40:215–222.
37. Bleakman, D., Gates, M.R., Ogden, A.M., Mackowiak, M. (2002). Kainate receptor agonists, antagonists and allosteric modulators. *Curr Pharm Des* 8:873–885.
38. Palucha, A., Pilc, A. (2007). Metabotropic glutamate receptor ligands as possible anxiolytic and antidepressant drugs. *Pharmacol Ther* 115:116–147.
39. Cartmell, J., Schoepp, D.D. (2000). Regulation of neurotransmitter release by metabotropic glutamate receptors. *J Neurochem* 75:889–907.
40. Gasparini, F., Kuhn, R., Pin, J.P. (2002). Allosteric modulators of group I metabotropic glutamate receptors: novel subtype-selective ligands and therapeutic perspectives. *Curr Opin Pharmacol* 2:43–49.

41. Bhave, G., Karim, F., Carlton, S.M., Gereau, R.W.T. (2001). Peripheral group I metabotropic glutamate receptors modulate nociception in mice. *Nat Neurosci* 4:417–423.
42. Lee, J.S., Ro, J.Y. (2007). Peripheral metabotropic glutamate receptor 5 mediates mechanical hypersensitivity in craniofacial muscle via protein kinase C dependent mechanisms. *Neuroscience* 146:375–383.
43. Walker, K., Reeve, A., Bowes, M., Winter, J., Wotherspoon, G., Davis, A., Schmid, P., Gasparini, F., Kuhn, R., Urban, L. (2001). mGlu5 receptors and nociceptive function II. mGlu5 receptors functionally expressed on peripheral sensory neurones mediate inflammatory hyperalgesia. *Neuropharmacology* 40:10–19.
44. Zhou, S., Komak, S., Du, J., Carlton, S.M. (2001). Metabotropic glutamate 1alpha receptors on peripheral primary afferent fibers: their role in nociception. *Brain Res* 913:18–26.
45. Carlton, S.M., Hargett, G.L. (2007). Colocalization of metabotropic glutamate receptors in rat dorsal root ganglion cells. *J Comp Neurol* 501:780–789.
46. Lea, P.M.T., Faden, A.I. (2006). Metabotropic glutamate receptor subtype 5 antagonists MPEP and MTEP. *CNS Drug Rev* 12:149–166.
47. Ault, B., Hildebrand, L.M. (1993). L-glutamate activates peripheral nociceptors. *Agents Actions* 39:C142–C144.
48. Carlton, S.M., Zhou, S., Coggeshall, R.E. (1998). Evidence for the interaction of glutamate and NK1 receptors in the periphery. *Brain Res* 790:160–169.
49. Davidson, E.M., Coggeshall, R.E., Carlton, S.M. (1997). Peripheral NMDA and non-NMDA glutamate receptors contribute to nociceptive behaviors in the rat formalin test. *Neuroreport* 8:941–946.
50. Zhou, S., Bonasera, L., Carlton, S.M. (1996). Peripheral administration of NMDA, AMPA or KA results in pain behaviors in rats. *Neuroreport* 7:895–900.
51. Aumeerally, N., Allen, G., Sawynok, J. (2004). Glutamate-evoked release of adenosine and regulation of peripheral nociception. *Neuroscience* 127:1–11.
52. Beirith, A., Santos, A.R.S., Calixto, J.B. (2002). Mechanisms underlying the nociception and paw oedema caused by injection of glutamate into the mouse paw. *Brain Res* 924:219–228.
53. Beirith, A., Santos, A.R.S., Calixto, J.B. (2003). The role of neuropeptides and capsaicin-sensitive fibres in glutamate-induced nociception and paw oedema in mice. *Brain Res* 969:110–116.
54. Omote, K., Kawamata, T., Kawamata, M., Namiki, A. (1998). Formalin-induced release of excitatory amino acids in the skin of the rat hindpaw. *Brain Res* 787:161–164.
55. deGroot, J., Zhou, S., Carlton, S.M. (2000). Peripheral glutamate release in the hindpaw following low and high intensity sciatic stimulation. *Neuroreport* 11:497–502.
56. Sawynok, J., Reid, A. (2002). Modulation of formalin-induced behaviors and edema by local and systemic administration of dextromethorphan, memantine and ketamine. *Eur J Pharmacol* 450:153–162.
57. Christoph, T., Reissmüller, E., Schiene, K., Englberger, W., Chizh, B.A. (2005). Antiallodynic effects of NMDA glycine(B) antagonists in neuropathic pain: possible peripheral mechanisms. *Brain Res* 1048:218–227.

58. Davidson, E.M., Carlton, S.M. (1998). Intraplantar injection of dextrorphan, ketamine or memantine attenuates formalin-induced behaviors. *Brain Res* 785:136–142.

59. Jackson, D.L., Graff, C.B., Richardson, J.D., Hargreaves, K.M. (1995). Glutamate participates in the peripheral modulation of thermal hyperalgesia in rats. *Eur J Pharmacol* 284:321–325.

60. Walker, K., Bowes, M., Panesar, M., Davis, A., Gentry, C., Kesingland, A., Gasparini, F., Spooren, W., Stoehr, N., Pagano, A., Flor, P.J., Vranesic, I., Lingenhoehl, K., Johnson, E.C., Varney, M., Urban, L., Kuhn, R. (2001). Metabotropic glutamate receptor subtype 5 (mGlu5) and nociceptive function. I. Selective blockade of mGlu5 receptors in models of acute, persistent and chronic pain. *Neuropharmacology* 40:1–9.

61. Tian, Y.L., Guo, Y., Cao, D.Y., Zhang, Q., Wang, H.S., Zhao, Y. (2005). Local application of morphine suppresses glutamate-evoked activities of C and Aδ afferent fibers in rat hairy skin. *Brain Res* 1059:28–34.

62. Zhang, Q., Zhao, Y., Guo, Y., Cao, D.Y., Tian, Y.L., Yao, F.R., Wang, H.S. (2006). Electrophysiological evidence for the interaction of substance P and glutamate on Aδ and C afferent fibre activity in rat hairy skin. *Clin Exp Pharmacol Physiol* 33:1128–1133.

63. MacIver, M.B., Tanelian, D.L. (1993). Structural and functional specialization of A delta and C fiber free nerve endings innervating rabbit corneal epithelium. *J Neurosci* 13:4511–4524.

64. Du, J., Koltzenburg, M., Carlton, S.M. (2001). Glutamate-induced excitation and sensitization of nociceptors in rat glabrous skin. *Pain* 89:187–198.

65. Du, J., Zhou, S., Coggeshall, R.E., Carlton, S.M. (2003). N-methyl-D-aspartate-induced excitation and sensitization of normal and inflamed nociceptors. *Neuroscience* 118:547–562.

66. Du, J., Zhou, S., Carlton, S.M. (2006). Kainate-induced excitation and sensitization of nociceptors in normal and inflamed rat glabrous skin. *Neuroscience* 137: 999–1013.

67. Cahusac, P.M., Senok, S.S., Hitchcock, I.S., Genever, P.G., Baumann, K.I. (2005). Are unconventional NMDA receptors involved in slowly adapting type I mechanoreceptor responses? *Neuroscience* 133:763–773.

68. Fagan, B.M., Cahusac, P.M. (2001). Evidence for glutamate receptor mediated transmission at mechanoreceptors in the skin. *Neuroreport* 12:341–347.

69. Su, X., Urban, M.O. (2005). Effect of metabotropic glutamate receptor subtype 5 antagonist, 2-methyl-6-(phenylethynyl)-pyridine on mechanosensory afferents innervating rat hind paw following inflammation. *Neurosci Lett* 390:123–128.

70. Gazerani, P., Wang, K., Cairns, B.E., Svensson, P., Arendt-Nielsen, L. (2006). Effects of subcutaneous administration of glutamate on pain, sensitization and vasomotor responses in healthy men and women. *Pain* 124:338–348.

71. Warncke, T., Stubhaug, A., Jørum, E. (1997). Ketamine, an NMDA receptor antagonist, suppresses spatial and temporal properties of burn-induced secondary hyperalgesia in man: a double-blind, cross-over comparison with morphine and placebo. *Pain* 72:99–106.

72. Warncke, T., Jorum, E., Stubhaug, A. (1997). Local treatment with the N-methyl-D-aspartate receptor antagonist ketamine, inhibit development of secondary hyperalgesia in man by a peripheral action. *Neurosci Lett* 227:1–4.
73. Pedersen, J.L., Galle, T.S., Kehlet, H. (1998). Peripheral analgesic effects of ketamine in acute inflammatory pain. *Anesthesiology* 89:58–66.
74. Gottrup, H., Bach, F.W., Arendt-Nielsen, L., Jensen, T.S. (2000). Peripheral lidocaine but not ketamine inhibits capsaicin-induced hyperalgesia in humans. *Br J Anaesth* 85:520–528.
75. Gottrup, H., Bach, F.W., Juhl, G., Jensen, T.S. (2006). Differential effect of ketamine and lidocaine on spontaneous and mechanical evoked pain in patients with nerve injury pain. *Anesthesiology* 104:527–536.
76. Koppert, W., Zeck, S., Blunk, J.A., Schmelz, M., Likar, R., Sittl, R. (1999). The effects of intradermal fentanyl and ketamine on capsaicin-induced secondary hyperalgesia and flare reaction. *Anesth Analg* 89:1521–1527.
77. Pöyhiä, R., Vainio, A. (2006). Topically administered ketamine reduces capsaicin-evoked mechanical hyperalgesia. *Clin J Pain* 22:32–36.
78. Frenkel, C., Urban, B.W. (1992). Molecular actions of racemic ketamine on human CNS sodium channels. *Br J Anaesth* 69:292–297.
79. Cairns, B.E., Sessle, B.J., Hu, J.W. (1998). Evidence that excitatory amino acid receptors within the temporomandibular joint region are involved in the reflex activation of the jaw muscles. *J Neurosci* 18:8056–8064.
80. Ro, J.Y., Capra, N.F. (2006). Assessing mechanical sensitivity of masseter muscle in lightly anesthetized rats: a model for craniofacial muscle hyperalgesia. *Neurosci Res* 56:119–123.
81. Lee, H.J., Choi, H.S., Ju, J.S., Bae, Y.C., Kim, S.K., Yoon, Y.W., Ahn, D.K. (2006). Peripheral mGluR5 antagonist attenuated craniofacial muscle pain and inflammation but not mGluR1 antagonist in lightly anesthetized rats. *Brain Res Bull* 70:378–385.
82. Lawand, N.B., McNearney, T., Westlund, K.N. (2000). Amino acid release into the knee joint: key role in nociception and inflammation. *Pain* 86:69–74.
83. Lawand, N.B., Willis, W.D., Westlund, K.N. (1997). Excitatory amino acid receptor involvement in peripheral nociceptive transmission in rats. *Eur J Pharmacol* 324:169–177.
84. Yu, X.M., Sessle, B.J., Haas, D.A., Izzo, A., Vernon, H., Hu, J.W. (1996). Involvement of NMDA receptor mechanisms in jaw electromyographic activity and plasma extravasation induced by inflammatory irritant application to temporomandibular joint region of rats. *Pain* 68:169–178.
85. Lam, D.K., Sessle, B.J., Cairns, B.E., Hu, J.W. (2005). Peripheral NMDA receptor modulation of jaw muscle electromyographic activity induced by capsaicin injection into the temporomandibular joint of rats. *Brain Res* 1046:68–76.
86. Ro, J.Y., Nies, M., Zhang, Y. (2005). The role of peripheral N-methyl-D-aspartate receptors in muscle hyperalgesia. *Neuroreport* 16:485–489.
87. Ro, J.Y. (2003). Contribution of peripheral NMDA receptors in craniofacial muscle nociception and edema formation. *Brain Res* 979:78–84.
88. Cairns, B.E., Hu, J.W., Arendt-Nielsen, L., Sessle, B.J., Svensson, P. (2001). Sex-related differences in human pain perception and rat afferent discharge evoked by injection of glutamate into the masseter muscle. *J Neurophysiol* 86:782–791.

89. Cairns, B.E., Gambarota, G., Svensson, P., Arendt-Nielsen, L., Berde, C.B. (2002). Glutamate-induced sensitization of rat masseter muscle fibers. *Neuroscience* 109:389–399.

90. Cairns, B.E., Sessle, B.J., Hu, J.W. (2001). Characteristics of glutamate-evoked temporomandibular joint afferent activity in the rat. *J Neurophysiol* 85: 2446–2454.

91. Cairns, B.E., Dong, X.D., Mann, M.K., Svensson, P., Sessle, B.J., Arendt-Nielsen, L., McErlane, K.M. (2007). Systemic administration of monosodium glutamate elevates intramuscular glutamate levels and sensitizes rat masseter muscle afferent fibers. *Pain* 132:33–41.

92. Cairns, B.E., Svensson, P., Wang, K., Hupfeld, S., Graven-Nielsen, T., Sessle, B.J., Berde, C.B., Arendt-Nielsen, L. (2003). Activation of peripheral NMDA receptors contributes to human pain and rat afferent discharges evoked by injection of glutamate into the masseter muscle. *J Neurophysiol* 90:2098–2105.

93. Dong, X.D., Mann, M.K., Sessle, B.J., Arendt-Nielsen, L., Svensson, P., Cairns, B.E. (2006). Sensitivity of rat temporalis muscle afferent fibers to peripheral N-methyl-D-aspartate receptor activation. *Neuroscience* 141:939–945.

94. Dong, X.D., Mann, M.K., Kumar, U., Svensson, P., Arendt-Nielsen, L., Hu, J.W., Sessle, B.J., Cairns, B.E. (2007). Sex-related differences in glutamate evoked rat muscle nociceptor discharge result from estrogen-mediated modulation of peripheral NMDA receptors. *Neuroscience* 146:822–832.

95. Banks, R.W., Bewick, G.S., Reid, B., Richardson, C. (2002). Evidence for activity-dependent modulation of sensory-terminal excitability in spindles by glutamate release from synaptic-like vesicles. *Adv Exp Med Biol* 508:13–18.

96. Bewick, G.S., Reid, B., Richardson, C., Banks, R.W. (2005). Autogenic modulation of mechanoreceptor excitability by glutamate release from synaptic-like vesicles: evidence from the rat muscle spindle primary sensory ending. *J Physiol* 562(Pt 2):381–394.

97. Wang, K., Sessle, B.J., Svensson, P., Arendt-Nielsen, L. (2004). Glutamate evoked neck and jaw muscle pain facilitate the human jaw stretch reflex. *Clin Neurophysiol* 115:1288–1295.

98. Svensson, P., Wang, K., Arendt-Nielsen, L., Cairns, B.E., Sessle, B.J. (2005). Pain effects of glutamate injections into human jaw or neck muscles. *J Orofac Pain* 19:109–118.

99. Svensson, P., Cairns, B.E., Wang, K., Hu, J.W., Graven-Nielsen, T., Arendt-Nielsen, L., Sessle, B.J. (2003). Glutamate-evoked pain and mechanical allodynia in the human masseter muscle. *Pain* 101:221–227.

100. Castrillon, E., Cairns, B.E., Ernberg, M., Wang, K., Sessle, B.J., Arendt-Nielsen, L., Svensson, P. (2007). Effect of peripheral NMDA receptor blockade on glutamate-evoked masseter muscle pain and mechanical sensitization in women. *J Orofac Pain* 21:216–224.

101. Cairns, B.E., Wang, K., Hu, J.W., Sessle, B.J., Arendt-Nielsen, L., Svensson, P. (2003). The effect of glutamate-evoked masseter muscle pain on the human jaw-stretch reflex differs in men and women. *J Orofac Pain* 17:317–325.

102. Cairns, B.E., Svensson, P., Wang, K., Castrillon, E., Hupfeld, S., Sessle, B.J., Arendt-Nielsen, L. (2006). Ketamine attenuates glutamate-induced mechanical sensitization of the masseter muscle in human males. *Exp Brain Res* 169:467–472.

103. Gaudreau, G.A., Plourde, V. (2004). Involvement of N-methyl-d-aspartate (NMDA) receptors in a rat model of visceral hypersensitivity. *Behav Brain Res* 150:185–189.

104. McRoberts, J.A., Coutinho, S.V., Marvizon, J.C., Grady, E.F., Tognetto, M., Sengupta, J.N., Ennes, H.S., Chaban, V.V., Amadesi, S., Creminon, C., Lanthorn, T., Geppetti, P., Bunnett, N.W., Mayer, E.A. (2001). Role of peripheral N-methyl-D-aspartate (NMDA) receptors in visceral nociception in rats. *Gastroenterology* 120: 1737–1748.

105. Lindström, E., Brusberg, M., Hughes, P.A., Martin, C.M., Brierley, S.M., Phillis, B.D., Martinsson, R., Abrahamsson, C., Larsson, H., Martinez, V., Ashley Blackshaw, L. (2007). Involvement of metabotropic glutamate 5 receptor in visceral pain. *Pain* 137(2):295–305.

106. Czaja, K., Ritter, R.C., Burns, G.A. (2006). Vagal afferent neurons projecting to the stomach and small intestine exhibit multiple N-methyl-D-aspartate receptor subunit phenotypes. *Brain Res* 1119:86–93.

107. Czaja, K., Ritter, R.C., Burns, G.A. (2006). N-methyl-D-aspartate receptor subunit phenotypes of vagal afferent neurons in nodose ganglia of the rat. *J Comp Neurol* 496:877–885.

108. Hoang, C.J., Hay, M. (2001). Expression of metabotropic glutamate receptors in nodose ganglia and the nucleus of the solitary tract. *Am J Physiol Heart Circ Physiol* 281:H457–H462.

109. Li, J., McRoberts, J.A., Ennes, H.S., Trevisani, M., Nicoletti, P., Mittal, Y., Mayer, E.A. (2006). Experimental colitis modulates the functional properties of NMDA receptors in dorsal root ganglia neurons. *Am J Physiol Gastrointest Liver Physiol* 291:G219–G228.

110. Sengupta, J.N., Petersen, J., Peles, S., Shaker, R. (2004). Response properties of antral mechanosensitive afferent fibers and effects of ionotropic glutamate receptor antagonists. *Neuroscience* 125:711–723.

111. Slattery, J.A., Page, A.J., Dorian, C.L., Brierley, S.M., Blackshaw, L.A. (2006). Potentiation of mouse vagal afferent mechanosensitivity by ionotropic and metabotropic glutamate receptors. *J Physiol* 577:295–306.

112. Page, A.J., Young, R.L., Martin, C.M., Umaerus, M., O'Donnell, T.A., Cooper, N.J., Coldwell, J.R., Hulander, M., Mattsson, J.P., Lehmann, A., Blackshaw, L.A. (2005). Metabotropic glutamate receptors inhibit mechanosensitivity in vagal sensory neurons. *Gastroenterology* 128:402–410.

113. Hay, M., Lindsley, K.A. (1995). Metabotropic glutamate receptor inhibition of visceral afferent potassium currents. *Brain Res* 698:169–174.

114. Young, R.L., Page, A.J., O'Donnell, T.A., Cooper, N.J., Blackshaw, L.A. (2007). Peripheral versus central modulation of gastric vagal pathways by metabotropic glutamate receptor 5. *Am J Physiol Gastrointest Liver Physiol* 292:G501–G511.

115. Lynch, M.E., Clark, A.J., Sawynok, J. (2003). A pilot study examining topical amitriptyline, ketamine, and a combination of both in the treatment of neuropathic pain. *Clin J Pain* 19:323–328.

116. Lynch, M.E., Clark, A.J., Sawynok, J., Sullivan, M.J. (2005). Topical amitriptyline and ketamine in neuropathic pain syndromes: an open-label study. *J Pain* 6:644–649.

117. Ushida, T., Tani, T., Kanbara, T., Zinchuk, V.S., Kawasaki, M., Yamamoto, H. (2002). Analgesic effects of ketamine ointment in patients with complex regional pain syndrome type 1. *Reg Anesth Pain Med* 27:524–528.

118. Lynch, M.E., Clark, A.J., Sawynok, J., Sullivan, M.J. (2005). Topical 2% amitriptyline and 1% ketamine in neuropathic pain syndromes: a randomized, double-blind, placebo-controlled trial. *Anesthesiology* 103:140–146.

119. Sang, C.N., Hostetter, M.P., Gracely, R.H., Chappell, A.S., Schoepp, D.D., Lee, G., Whitcup, S., Caruso, R., Max, M.B. (1998). AMPA/kainate antagonist LY293558 reduces capsaicin-evoked hyperalgesia but not pain in normal skin in humans. *Anesthesiology* 89:1060–1067.

120. McNearney, T., Baethge, B.A., Cao, S., Alam, R., Lisse, J.R., Westlund, K.N. (2004). Excitatory amino acids, TNF-alpha, and chemokine levels in synovial fluids of patients with active arthropathies. *Clin Exp Immunol* 137:621–627.

121. Ayesh, E.E., Jensen, T.S., Svensson, P. (2007). Effects of intra-articular ketamine on pain and somatosensory function in temporomandibular joint arthralgia patients. *Pain* 137:286–294.

122. Huang, G.S., Yeh, C.C., Kong, S.S., Lin, T.C., Ho, S.T., Wong, C.S. (2000). Intra-articular ketamine for pain control following arthroscopic knee surgery. *Acta Anaesthesiol Sin* 38:131–136.

123. Rosseland, L.A., Stubhaug, A., Sandberg, L., Breivik, H. (2003). Intra-articular (IA) catheter administration of postoperative analgesics. A new trial design allows evaluation of baseline pain, demonstrates large variation in need of analgesics, and finds no analgesic effect of IA ketamine compared with IA saline. *Pain* 104:25–34.

124. Rosendal, L., Larsson, B., Kristiansen, J., Peolsson, M., Søgaard, K., Kjær, M., Sørensen, J., Gerdle, B. (2004). Increase in muscle nociceptive substances and anaerobic metabolism in patients with trapezius myalgia: microdialysis in rest and during exercise. *Pain* 112:324–334.

125. Tegeder, L., Zimmermann, J., Meller, S.T., Geisslinger, G. (2002). Release of algesic substances in human experimental muscle pain. *Inflamm Res* 51:393–402.

126. Ashina, M., Stallknecht, B., Bendtsen, L., Pedersen, J.F., Schifter, S., Galbo, H., Olesen, J. (2003). Tender points are not sites of ongoing inflammation: in vivo evidence in patients with chronic tension-type headache. *Cephalalgia* 23: 109–116.

127. Alfredson, H., Lorentzon, R.J. (2002). Chronic tendon pain: no signs of chemical inflammation but high concentrations of the neurotransmitter glutamate. Implications for treatment? *Curr Drug Targets* 3:43–54.

128. Alfredson, H., Ljung, B.O., Thorsen, K., Lorentzon, R.J. (2000). In vivo investigation of ECRB tendons with microdialysis technique—no signs of inflammation but high amounts of glutamate in tennis elbow. *Acta Orthop Scand* 71:475–479.

129. Flodgren, G.M., Crenshaw, A.G., Alfredson, H., Fahlstrom, M., Hellstrom, F.B., Bronemo, L., Djupsjobacka, M. (2005). Glutamate and prostaglandin E2 in the trapezius muscle of female subjects with chronic muscle pain and controls determined by microdialysis. *Eur J Pain* 9:511–515.

130. Ashina, M., Jorgensen, M., Stallknecht, B., Mork, H., Bendtsen, L., Pedersen, J.F., Olesen, J., Jensen, R. (2005). No release of interstitial glutamate in experimental human model of muscle pain. *Eur J Pain* 9:337–343.

131. Castrillon, E.E., Cairns, B.E., Ernberg, M., Wang, K., Sessle, B.J., Arendt-Nielsen, L., Svensson, P. (2008). Effect of peripheral NMDA receptor blockade with ketamine on chronic myofascial TMD pain. *J Orofac Pain* 21:216–224.

132. Kuiken, S.D., Lei, A., Tytgat, G.N., Holman, R., Boeckxstaens, G.E. (2002). Effect of the low-affinity, noncompetitive N-methyl-d-aspartate receptor antagonist dextromethorphan on visceral perception in healthy volunteers. *Aliment Pharmacol Ther* 16:1955–1962.

133. Kuiken, S.D., van den Berg, S.J., Tytgat, G.N., Boeckxstaens, G.E. (2004). Oral S(+)-ketamine does not change visceral perception in health. *Dig Dis Sci* 49:1745–1751.

134. Strigo, I.A., Duncan, G.H., Bushnell, M.C., Boivin, M., Wainer, I., Rodriguez Rosas, M.E., Persson, J. (2005). The effects of racemic ketamine on painful stimulation of skin and viscera in human subjects. *Pain* 113:255–264.

135. Willert, R.P., Woolf, C.J., Hobson, A.R., Delaney, C., Thompson, D.G., Aziz, Q. (2004). The development and maintenance of human visceral pain hypersensitivity is dependent on the N-methyl-D-aspartate receptor. *Gastroenterology* 126:683–692.

136. Yamamoto, T., Saito, O., Aoe, T., Bartolozzi, A., Sarva, J., Zhou, J., Kozikowski, A., Wroblewska, B., Bzdega, T., Neale, J.H. (2007). Local administration of N-acetylaspartylglutamate (NAAG) peptidase inhibitors is analgesic in peripheral pain in rats. *Eur J Neurosci* 25:147–158.

CHAPTER 10

Serotonin Receptors

MALIN ERNBERG

Division of Clinical Oral Physiology, Department of Dental Medicine, Karolinska Institutet

Content

Peripheral Receptor Targets for Analgesia: Novel Approaches to Pain Management, Edited by Brian E. Cairns

10.1 INTRODUCTION

5-Hydroxytryptamine (5-HT), also known as serotonin, is an important mediator of pain and inflammation that may excite and sensitize peripheral and central sensory nerves, and also modulates pain processes, especially at spinal levels. It is widely distributed throughout the body and is found in the central nervous system (CNS) and peripheral nervous system (PNS), in the intestines, and in the platelets and mast cells as well as certain immune cells. The interest in 5-HT evolved by the end of the nineteenth century when it was noted that a substance with vasoactive properties was released from the platelets during blood clotting. This substance was identified in 1948 and named serotonin due to its presence in the blood serum [1]. Today, 5-HT is known to have profound biological effects in the human body by modulating physiological processes in the vascular and the nervous systems.

5-HT is synthesized from the essential amino acid tryptophan, derived from the diet, but only 1% of dietary tryptophan is converted to 5-HT [2]. The major synthesis of 5-HT occurs peripherally in the enterochromaffin cells of the small intestines, where 90% of the 5-HT is located, but it is also synthesized in certain regions of the CNS. The first step in this reaction is the synthesis of 5-hydroxytryptophan (5-HTP) by the enzyme tryptophan hydroxylase. 5-HTP is further converted to 5-HT by the enzyme L-amino acid decarboxylase. Degradation of 5-HT occurs mainly in the CNS and liver by different pathways including various enzymes, for example, monoamine oxidase (MAO), and results in several metabolites. The main metabolite is 5-hydroxyindoleacetic acid (5-HIAA) that is excreted in the urine, but 5-HT may also be metabolized to melatonin [3]. An alternative route in the synthesis of tryptophan is the conversion to kynurenine that is further metabolized to the N-methyl-D-aspartate (NMDA) agonist quinolinic acid [4].

When 5-HT is released, it exerts its biological effects by acting on several receptors that are distributed throughout the human body. Inactivation of 5-HT occurs not only by metabolism but also by reuptake by the binding of 5-HT to a specific serotonin transporter (SERT). SERT has been identified on platelets and presynaptic nerve terminals as well as on endothelial cells [5]. Before, it was believed that 5-HT does not pass the blood-brain barrier (BBB), but this has recently been refuted as SERT has been found also on BBB endothelial cells. This suggests a role in the inactivation of brain 5-HT into endothelial cells and also an uptake of 5-HT from the circulating blood [6], which indicates that 5-HT indeed may pass the BBB.

The aim of this chapter is to review the current knowledge of 5-HT and its receptors with respect to pain mechanisms. Although the focus is on the peripheral effects of 5-HT receptor activation in pain transduction, central actions by 5-HT receptors with respect to pain mediation and modulation are also reviewed, and drugs that target these receptors peripherally and centrally as potential analgesics are discussed.

10.2 THE SEROTONIN RECEPTORS

5-HT receptors were first classified in the 1950s, when the so-called D- and M-receptors were identified. Later, when radioligand binding studies using rat brain membranes identified 5-HT_1 and 5-HT_2 receptors, the classification was revised, since it then became apparent that these receptors were not identical to the D- and M-receptors [2].

Fifteen 5-HT receptors belonging to seven receptor classes (5-HT_1 to 5-HT_7) have so far been identified in the mammalian brain. The 5-HT_{1-2} and 5-HT_{4-7} receptors are metabotropic, that is, linked to a G protein to alter neuronal activity through a second messenger, and can be categorized according to their second messenger into four groups [7]. The 5-HT_1 receptors are coupled to $G\alpha_{i/o}$ proteins and contain five subclasses (5-$HT_{1A-B,D-F}$). The 5-HT_{1C} receptor has been reclassified into 5-HT_{2C} due to its sequence and functional similarity with the 5-HT_2 receptors [8]. The 5-HT_2 receptors (the former D-receptors) are coupled to $G\alpha_q$ proteins (5-HT_{2A-C}). The 5-HT_4, 5-HT_6, and 5-HT_7 receptors are all coupled to Gs proteins. For the 5-HT_{5A-B} receptors, the coupling has not been determined. The metabotropic receptors have a high affinity for 5-HT but a slow activation constant.

The 5-HT_3 receptor (the former M-receptor) is a ligand-gated cation channel belonging to the nicotine/γ-aminobutyrate (GABA) family [9]. The activation of the receptor causes a rapid depolarization dependent on the opening of cation-selective channels that permit the passage of N^+, K^+, and Ca^{2+} from the extracellular space [10]. The 5-HT_3 receptor has two subunits that are well characterized, 5-$HT_{3A\text{ and }B}$. The 5-HT_{3A} subunit forms functional homomeric 5-HT_{3A} receptors, while the 5-HT_{3B} subunit alone cannot assemble into complete receptors. Instead, it forms functional heteromeric receptors with the 5-HT_{3A} receptor (5-$HT_{3A/B}$ complex). A few years ago, genes for three new subunits were cloned (5-HT_{3C-E}), and these have been shown very recently to be able to form heteromeric 5-HT_3 receptor complexes with the 5-HT_{3A} subunit, which exhibit quantitatively different functional properties compared with homomeric 5-HT_{3A} receptors [11]. The 5-HT_3 receptors have low affinity for 5-HT but have a rapid activation constant [7].

10.2.1 5-HT_1 Receptors

5-HT_1 receptors are mainly found on presynaptic nerve terminals within the CNS and in the endothelium of the blood vessels. They are widely distributed throughout the CNS and are found in the hippocampus, amygdala, raphe nucleus, basal ganglia (globus pallidus and in substantia nigra), and spinal cord [2]. 5-HT_{1B}, 5-HT_{1D}, and 5-HT_{1F} receptors are also found on peripheral afferents [12–14]. The activation of the 5-HT_1 receptors appears to inhibit neuronal firing and 5-HT release. In the CNS, they are involved in cerebral circulation (5-HT_{1B} and 5-HT_{1D}) as well as anxiety, depression, and sleep (5-HT_{1A}) [10,15]. The activation of 5-HT_{1B} and 5-HT_{1D} receptors can attenuate migraine headache through a mechanism that involves the reduction of cerebral vasodilation and neurogenic inflammation induced by the release of certain neuropeptides, for example, calcitonin gene-related peptide (CGRP) [2,16]. In the periphery, they are involved in the modulation of the microcirculation, acting as vasodilators [17]. They also cause local edema by increasing blood vessel permeability [18]. Many of the 5-HT_1 receptors also seem to be involved in pain processing at peripheral and spinal levels.

10.2.2 5-HT_2 Receptors

5-HT_2 receptors are found at several CNS sites, for example, cortex, hippocampus, striatum, cerebellum, and spinal cord. Similar to 5-HT_1 receptors, they are involved in the etiology of anxiety and depression [2]. They are further suggested to be involved in cerebrospinal fluid production, locomotion, obsessive–compulsive disorders, and anorexia nervosa [10]. In the peripheral tissue, 5-HT_2 receptors are mainly found in the smooth muscles in the gastrointestinal tract, in the bronchi, in the blood vessels, and in the uterus, but they are also found in the endothelial cells and platelets and on the peripheral nerve terminals [14,19,20]. They exert excitatory effects on neural activity and mediate potent vasoconstrictive effects on larger arterial vessels (5-HT_{2A}) and may also relax blood vessels (5-HT_{2B}) by the production of nitric oxide [15,17,21]. Although selective ligands for the 5-HT_{2A} receptor have been developed, few studies have tested these in pain-related experiments. However, ketanserin has a high affinity for 5-HT_{2A} receptors and hence, may be pharmacologically distinguished from 5-HT_{2B} and 5-HT_{2C} receptors. Several lines of evidence suggest a role for this receptor in pain processing.

10.2.3 5-HT_3 Receptors

5-HT_3 receptors have been exclusively identified in the neural tissue of the CNS and PNS. In the CNS, they are distributed in the area postrema, lower brain stem, hippocampus, amygdala, and basal ganglia. Peripherally, they are found on the primary sensory neurons and enteric neurons as well as on pre- and postganglionic sympathetic neurons [10,14,20,22]. The 5-HT_3 receptors have a great influence on many events in the body. In the CNS, they are involved in the etiology of psychosis, anxiety, cognition, and eating disorders. They also have a well-known role in emetic pathways [23]. In the periphery, they have major effects on the heart and blood vessels, causing vasodilation [24]. They are also important receptors in the gastrointestinal tract, where they contribute to intestinal tone [10]. The 5-HT_3 receptors are probably the most important 5-HT receptor for pain transduction in the periphery.

10.2.4 5-HT_4 Receptors

5-HT_4 receptors have been identified in many species and tissues. Centrally, they are found in the neurons in the hippocampus, cortex, and limbic areas. This implies that they may have a role in affective disorders and psychoses, but they may also be involved in memory and learning. In the periphery, they are found in the heart, where they appear to evoke tachycardia, and in the urinary bladder, where they enhance smooth muscle contraction in humans, as well as in the smooth muscle cells of the intestines, where they seem to mediate gastric motility [8,10]. They are also found in the dorsal root ganglion cells, suggesting that they may be transported to their peripheral and central nerve terminals [14,20]. They seem to have a role for pain processing, especially in visceral hypersensitivity [25] by modulating the pain signal [23].

10.2.5 5-HT_{5-7} Receptors

The 5-HT_{5A} receptors seem to be widely distributed throughout the CNS and have been found in the cortex, hippocampus, cerebellum, and spinal cord. The 5-HT_{5B} receptors on the other hand, are much less limited in their distribution and have been found only in the habenula and certain regions of the hippocampus [10] but have not been identified in human tissue. Because of lack of specific antagonists and agonists for the 5-HT_5 receptors, their function is largely unknown, but the 5-HT_{5A} receptor has been suggested to be involved in mental disorders. It has been indicated that they may be involved in pain processing as they show high analogy to 5-HT_{1A} receptors, and if located on the inhibitory spinal interneuron, they may mimic 5-HT_{1A} effects [20]. However, this has to be confirmed. In addition, there are no reports that they are present in the peripheral tissue, and they will not be further discussed in this chapter.

Likewise, the 5-HT_6 receptors are present in the central neurons in the hypothalamus, hippocampus, nucleus accumbens, and striatum. They have been implicated in mental disorders and memory and cognitive dysfunctions [26]. Peripherally, they have so far only been identified in the cervical ganglion cells [19] but not in humans, and it is unclear if they have a role in pain processing.

Peripherally, 5-HT_7 receptors are found on the smooth muscle cells in the gastrointestinal tract, spleen, and sympathetic ganglion [8], where they seem to mediate the relaxation of the smooth muscle cells [27,28]. They are also found in the myelinated and unmyelinated axons of the peripheral nerves and in the dorsal spinal cord [20,29], and there is a growing evidence for their role in pain processes. It has been suggested that the 5-HT_7 receptors are similar to a group of previously unidentified 5-HT_1-like "orphan" receptors [10].

10.3 PERIPHERAL EFFECTS BY SEROTONIN ON PAIN TRANSMISSION

The involvement of 5-HT in pain processing is well known. As mentioned above, the 5-$HT_{1–4}$ and 5-HT_7 receptors seem to be involved in pain transmission by 5-HT as they have been identified on the sensory afferent nerves and in the dorsal root ganglia in both rats [14,19,30] and humans [31–33]. The presence of 5-$HT_{1B/D/F}$ and 5-HT_3 receptors is also reported in the sensory trigeminal ganglion cells in rats and humans [32–35] (Figure 10.1).

The main sources of 5-HT in the periphery are the platelets and mast cells, but lymphocytes, monocytes, and macrophages have also been shown to contain 5-HT [36]. 5-HT is released from its stores as a result of tissue trauma, ischemia, or inflammation. This is a direct release of 5-HT due to disruption of blood vessels and neurons, but there may also be an indirect release of 5-HT due to production of proinflammatory vasodilative substances, for example, arachidonic acid, prostaglandins, and cytokines that cause platelet degranulation [22,37].

Activated platelets are reported to excite and sensitize nociceptors by the release of 5-HT [38], which supports the idea that the pronociceptive (excitatory) effect by 5-HT may be attributed to direct activation of peripheral afferents [22,39]. But the algesic effect of 5-HT may also be caused indirectly, as a result of the release of other mediators, such as substance P (SP) and glutamate [40]. 5-HT also sensitizes peripheral mechanoreceptive afferent fibers to other chemicals by enhancing the efficiency of tetrodotoxin (TTX)-resistant sodium channels and lowering the threshold of the transient receptor potential vanilloid 1 (TRPV1) receptor, causing primary hyperalgesia [37].

Studies using *in vitro* nerve preparations have shown that exogenous 5-HT excites and sensitizes afferent nerve fibers [38,41,42]. This is also supported by numerous animal studies in which local administration of 5-HT has been shown to induce nociceptive responses (see below). In humans, intradermal application of 5-HT (1 mM) induced burning pain and itching [43,44]. 5-HT (10 μm) injected into the temporalis muscle did not affect pain or pressure pain thresholds (PPTs), but a combination of 5-HT and bradykinin induced pain and reduced PPTs [45]. Babenko et al. reported that the injection of 5-HT (2–20 nmol) into the tibialis anterior muscle induced mild pain but did not affect PPTs [46]. However, a combination of 5-HT and bradykinin induced even more pain and also reduced the PPTs. In a third study, it was reported that 5-HT at 1 mM, but not a lower concentration, when injected into the masseter muscle, induced pain and that a concentration of at least 10 μm was needed to

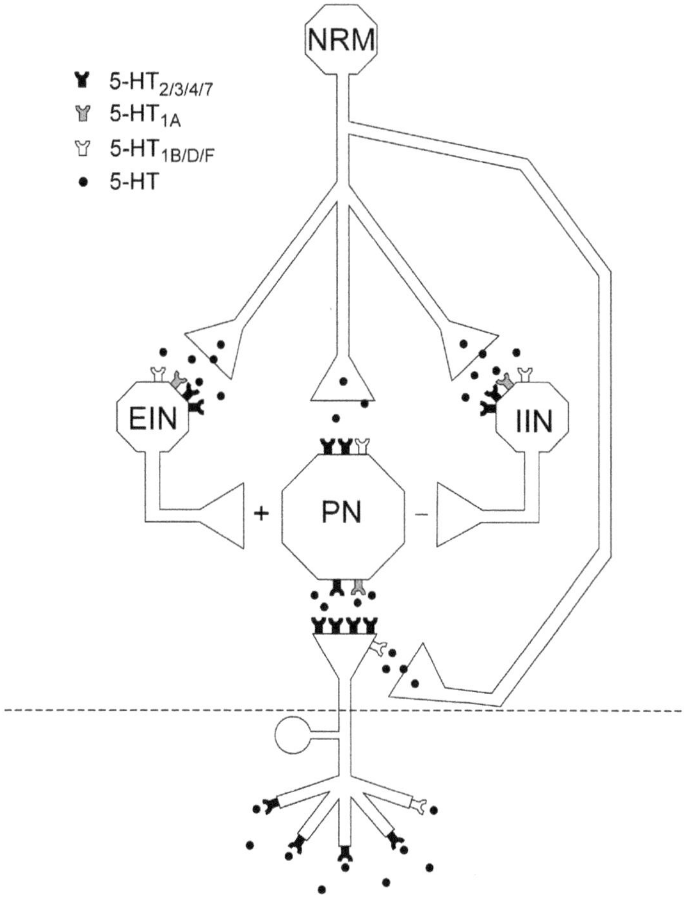

FIGURE 10.1. Distribution of 5-HT receptors on the peripheral afferent nociceptive neurons, projecting (secondary) neuron (PN) in the spinal cord/trigeminal sensory nucleus, and at the excitatory interneurons (EINs) and inhibitory interneurons (IINs) according to present knowledge. EINs contain, for example, substance P and calcitonin gene-related peptide, and IINs contain γ-aminobutyrate (GABA) and opioids (enkephalin and dynorphin). The nucleus raphe magnum (NRM) in the brain stem modulates pain transmission via descending serotonergic neurons. 5-HT receptors facilitating pain transmission (5-HT_2, 5-HT_3, 5-HT_4, and 5-HT_7) are depicted in black color, while 5-HT receptors inhibiting pain transmission (5-$HT_{1B/D/F}$) are depicted in white color. 5-HT_{1A} receptors are depicted in gray color to distinguish them from 5-$HT_{1B/D/F}$ receptors, as they differ somehow in their distribution. At the peripheral level, 5-HT pain transmission may be mediated by 5-HT_2, 5-HT_3, 5-HT_4, and 5-HT_7 receptors, while 5-$HT_{1B/D/F}$ evidently modulate pain transmission. Projecting neurons express 5-HT_{1A}, 5-$HT_{1B/D/F}$, and 5-HT_2 and possibly 5-HT_3 and 5-HT_4 receptors, while interneurons express 5-HT_{1A}, 5-$HT_{1B/D/F}$, and 5-HT_2 as well as 5-HT_3 receptors.

reduce PPTs [47]. The difference between studies is probably attributed to the different concentrations of 5-HT used in the studies, but this may also be due to the anatomical or physiological differences between the muscles. Gender differences offer a third explanation, as this is reported for intramuscular injection of glutamate into the masseter muscle. In two former studies, all subjects were men [45,46], while in the latter study only women participated [47].

10.3.1 5-HT Effects on 5-HT_1 Receptors

In rats, the nociceptive response to intraplantar (i.pl.) injections of 5-HT (assessed as lifts of and licks to the affected paw) increased with increased concentration of 5-HT and was blocked by 5-HT_1, 5-HT_2, and 5-HT_3 receptor antagonists (methysergide, ketanserin, and ondansetron, respectively) [48]. Intradermally injected 5-HT and the 5-$HT_{1A/7}$ agonists 8-OH-DPAT (8-Hydroxy-2-(di-n-propylamino) tetralin) and DP-5-CT (N,N-dipropyl-5-carboxamidotryptamine) in rats produced mechanical hyperalgesia assessed as paw withdrawal threshold, which was blocked by the 5-HT_{1A} receptor antagonists spiroxatrine and spiperone but not 5-HT_{1B}, 5-HT_2, or 5-HT_3 antagonists [49], an effect that was reported to be due to an increase of cyclic adenosine monophosphate (cAMP) [50]. 5-HT_{1A} knockout mice are reported to differ from wild types by higher thermal sensitivity (hot-plate test only) [51]. However, subcutaneous injection of the partial 5-HT_{1A} receptor agonists buspirone, ipsapirone, and gepirone had no effect on heat pain thresholds in the tail-flick test but attenuated morphine-induced analgesia [52]. In another study, intraplantar injection of the 5-HT_{1A} receptor antagonist N-[2-[4-(2-methoxyphenyl)-1-piperazinyl]ethyl]-N-2-pyridinylcyclohexanecarboxamide at maximally effective doses (30 and 100 micro grams; i.pl.) did not alter carrageenan-induced hyperalgesia to noxious heat in rats [53]. Only one study has investigated the effect of 5-HT_{1A} receptors in humans and reported no effect of intramuscular injection of the nonselective 5-HT_{1A} antagonist propranolol on 5-HT-induced pain or allodynia in the masseter muscle [54]. Later, it was reported that 5-HT_{1A} receptors are not expressed in the dorsal root ganglia but rather 5-HT_7 receptors, which have a pharmacological profile that resembles 5-HT_{1A} receptors [19,33]. Hence, many of the 5-HT_{1A} agonists and antagonists also have affinity for the 5-HT_7 receptor. This may indicate that the pronociceptive effect by peripheral 5-HT_{1A} receptors is in fact mediated by 5-HT_7 receptors [55]. This is further supported by findings that the coupling to the second messenger $G\alpha_{i/o}$ supports an inhibitory role for the 5-HT_{1A} receptor in pain signaling [56]. Indeed, an inhibitory link between cloned 5-HT_{1A} receptors and cAMP production is also reported [57].

Similar to 5-HT_{1A} knockout mice, 5-HT_{1B} knockout mice differ from wild types by higher thermal sensitivity, but they also differ with respect to formalin sensitivity [51]. But in contrast to 5-HT_{1A} receptors, the activation of peripheral 5-$HT_{1B/D}$ receptors may alleviate pain by reducing neurogenic inflammation, as the 5-$HT_{1B/D}$ receptor agonist sumatriptan was shown to inhibit capsaicin-induced plasma extravasation [58]. This effect seems to be caused by blocking of presynaptic $5\text{-HT}_{1B/D}$ receptors on the peripheral trigeminovascular neurons, which prevents synaptic transmission to central second-order neurons [59]. In addition, the hypersensitivity to noxious thermal stimuli induced by intraplantar injection of carrageenan in mice was attenuated by the subcutaneous injection of sumatriptan, but the drug had no effect on thermal hyperalgesia induced by sciatic nerve ligation in rats [60]. In contrast, subcutaneous injection of sumatripan induced allodynia to mechanical and thermal stimuli in healthy subjects, which may indicate a sensitization of peripheral $5\text{-HT}_{1B/D}$ receptors [61].

There is now ample support for a role of 5-HT_{1F} receptors in migraine pathophysiology. For example, the activation of 5-HT_{1F} receptors is reported to block migraine pain transmission in the trigeminal ganglion and nucleus caudalis by inhibiting glutamate release [62]. In an animal model of migraine, the activation of 5-HT_{1F} receptors was found to inhibit neurogenic inflammation [63]. Further, intravenous administration of the selective 5-HT_{1F} agonist LY334370 (4-fluoro-N-(3-(1-methyl-4-piperidinyl)-1H-indol-5-yl)benzamide) dose-dependently inhibited neuronal firing in the trigeminal nucleus caudalis, following electrical stimulation of the dura mater without altering dural blood vessel diameter [64]. Oral and intravenous administration of LY344864 (N-[(3R)-3-(Dimethylamino)-2,3,4,9-tetrahydro-1H-carbazo 1-6-yl]-4-fluorobenzamide) potently inhibited dural protein extravasation caused by electrical stimulation of the trigeminal ganglion in rats [65]. It seems that the effect of 5-HT_{1F} receptors is mainly peripheral as they were devoid of any significant vasocontractile activity in cerebral arteries, or did not affect the sumatriptan-induced vasoconstriction [66].

10.3.2 5-HT Effects on 5-HT_2 Receptors

The 5-HT_{2A} receptor seems to be involved in peripheral thermal and chemical hyperalgesia. Intraplantar injection of 5-HT and the 5-HT_2 agonist α-methyl-5-HT in rats induced behavioral effects (lifting of and licking of the affected paw), which was attenuated by the 5-HT_{2A} antagonists ketanserin, ritanserin, and spiperone [67]. Similarly, intradermal injection of 5-HT and α-methyl-5-HT into the rat hind paw increased thermal hyperalgesia, which was attenuated by ketanserin [68], and primary thermal hyperalgesia as well as secondary mechanical allodynia was attenuated by the 5-HT_{2A} antagonist sarpogrelate [69]. Another study in rats showed that 5-HT_{2A} receptor mRNA is colocalized with CGRP in dorsal root ganglion cells, that these receptors are upregulated in inflammatory conditions and that sarpogrelate produced analgesic effects on thermal hyperalgesia caused by peripheral inflammation, but failed to attenuate thermal hyperalgesia in the chronic constriction injury model [70]. In rats, thermal hyperalgesia induced by carrageenan injection was reduced by ketanserin, and in 5-HT_{2A} mutant mice, a dramatic increase of the late formalin-induced nociceptive response compared with wild-type mice was reported [51]. Also, topical application of ketanserin produced significant antihyperalgesia, as well as a remarkable anti-inflammatory effect in a rat model of knee joint arthritis [71].

There are no reports that 5-HT_{2B} receptors are expressed in the primary afferent neurons, but they are selectively expressed in the brain vessels and endothelial cells [72]. Therefore, they may not be directly involved in pain transmission. On the other hand, pharmacological testing has suggested that activation of peripheral and central 5-HT_{2B} receptors causes vasodilation and initiates plasma protein extravasation, which promotes the synthesis of nitric oxide [73–75]. This points to a role for these receptors in migraine pain, and selective 5-HT_{2B} antagonists might therefore be effective prophylactic therapies for migraine.

Most data point to a role for 5-HT_{2C} receptors in nociception at spinal levels but not peripherally. However, it was reported that the selective 5-HT_{2C} receptor agonist RO 60-0175 ((aS)-6-Chloro-5-fluoro-a-methyl-1H-indole-1-ethanamine fumarate) potentiated 5-HT_{1A}-receptor-mediated spontaneous tail-flick responses in rats and that the 5-HT_{1C} antagonist SB 206,553 (3,5-Dihydro-5-methyl-N-3-pyridinylbenzo[1,2-b:4,5-b′]di pyrrole-1(2H)-carboxamide hydrochloride) abolished the effect. This indicates that peripheral activation of 5-HT_{2C} receptors may facilitate pain responses and supports the existence of functional interactions between these receptors [76].

10.3.3 5-HT Effects on 5-HT_3 Receptors

Several lines of evidence from animal research have shown that peripheral 5-HT_3 receptors mediate inflammatory pain. An early study reported that the 5-HT_3 antagonist ondansetron reduced behavioral effects (lifting of and licking of the affected paw) in acute inflammation induced by complete Freund's adjuvant (CFA), but it was even more effective in reducing behavioral effects to chronic inflammation induced by formalin [77]. This is partly due to reduced neurogenic inflammation as blocking of 5-HT_3 receptors in the dorsal root ganglion and on peripheral afferent nerves by ondansetron diminished 5-HT-induced release of SP [22]. Another study found that the nociceptive responses to intraplantar injection of 5-HT were reduced by ondansetron [48]. In 5-HT_3 knockout mice, no difference was found compared with wild-type mice in either acute thermal, inflammatory, or mechanical nociception, or mechanical allodynia to CFA or partial nerve ligation. However, there was a difference in the response to chronic inflammation (late phase formalin test), which was attenuated by ondansetron [78]. Similarly, 5-HT_{3A} knockout mice differed from wild types by a dramatic decrease in the formalin-induced nociceptive responses in the late inflammatory phase [51]. In a recent study, the presence of 5-HT_3 receptors in trigeminal ganglion cells from masticatory afferent fibers and their role in muscle nociception and hyperalgesia was investigated [35]. It was found that 52% of the afferent cell bodies expressed 5-HT_3 receptors. 5-HT (0–10 mM) injected into the rat masseter muscle dose-dependently increased the neuronal firing but did not affect the mechanical pain threshold. Further, afferent discharge induced by intramuscular injection of 5-HT and the 5-HT_3 agonist 2-methyl-5-HT into the masseter muscle was attenuated by tropisetron [35].

Animal studies have shown that 5-HT_3 receptors are also involved in visceral hypersensitivity by activating afferent neurons (for a review, see De Ponti and Malagelada [79]). However, it is not known if this is due to the activation of peripheral and central neurons, as 5-HT_3 antagonists administered both intravenously and intracerebroventricularly reduced visceral hypersensitivity to rectal distension in cats [80]. In humans, intravenous administration of granisetron was reported to reduce rectal sensitivity in patients with irritable bowel syndrome (IBS), which is a functional disorder characterized by abdominal pain associated with diarrhea and/or constipation in the absence of any organic abnormality [81]. In contrast, another study showed no effect by oral ondansetron on colonic distension in healthy subjects but less abdominal pain in patients with IBS [82].

In humans, 5-HT applied to a blister-induced pain that was attenuated by a 5-HT_3 antagonist [83] and topical administration of ondansetron reduced inflammatory pain induced by intradermal capsaicin [84].

We have found that the plasma level of 5-HT was negatively correlated to the PPT in healthy subjects, which might indicate that unbound 5-HT in the blood may sensitize nociceptors to mechanical stimulation [85]. In healthy subjects, oral granisetron increased the PPT over the trapezius and anterior tibialis muscles but not over the masseter and anterior tibialis muscles, indicating a difference between orofacial and locomotor muscles [86]. However, in another study, intramuscular injection of granisetron into the masseter muscle increased the PPT in healthy subjects [87]. The difference between these two studies with respect to the masseter muscle may be attributed to a higher local dose in the latter study. Pretreatment with intramuscular injection of granisetron also significantly reduced visual analog scale (VAS) pain as well as peak pain, pain area, and pain duration induced by hypertonic saline (Figure 10.2).

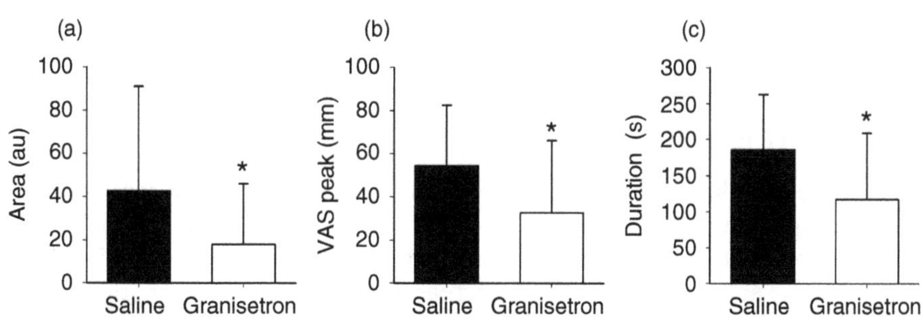

FIGURE 10.2. Bar graph showing the mean (SD) pain area (a), peak pain intensity (b), and pain duration (c) in 30 healthy individuals who received pretreatment with intramuscular injection of granisetron on one side and isotonic saline on the other side 2 minutes before hypertonic saline injections into the masseter muscles. The pain area was measured in arbitrary units (AU), the peak pain intensity on a 0- to 100-mm visual analog scale (VAS), and the pain duration in seconds (s). There was a significant difference between sides for all three variables ($*p < 0.002$). Adapted from reference [88].

It also increased the PPT but only in males [88]. In patients with myofascial temporomandibular disorders, intramuscular injection of granisetron in an experimental setting increased the PPT [87]. However, in patients with fibromyalgia, granisetron was ineffective in reducing pain [89].

10.3.4 5-HT Effects on 5-HT_4 Receptors

As mentioned previously, 5-HT_4 receptors appear to modulate visceral pain in the gastrointestinal system due to activation of afferent neurons [23]. One study reported that 5-HT_4 receptor activation has an inhibitory effect on intramural mechanoreceptors in the cat's rectum [90], and in a recent study, electroacupuncture was reported to attenuate behavioral hyperalgesia and stress-induced colonic motor dysfunction via 5-HT_4 receptors serotonergic pathway [91]. In contrast, the 5-HT_4 receptor antagonist SDZ 205-557 (2-methoxy-4-amino-5-chloro-benzoic acid 2-(diethylamino) ethyl ester) was shown to mediate antinociception in enteric viscera (writhing) and, to a lesser extent, in cutaneous terminals (hot-plate test), but a combination of SDZ 205-557 and the 5-HT_3 antagonist MDL 72222 (tropanyl 3,5-dichlorobenzoate) reduced visceral analgesia [92]. The 5-HT_4 partial agonist tegaserod was reported to reduce the sensitivity to rectal distension in healthy subjects as assessed by the nociceptive flexion reflex (RIII) [93] and improved the esophageal pain threshold to mechanical distension and distressing upper gastrointestinal symptoms, in patients with functional heartburn. It has also been shown to relieve abdominal pain in patients with IBS [94]. However, it is not known if the effects by 5-HT_4 agonists on visceral sensitivity are due to activation of 5-HT_4 receptors as partial agonists may also act as functional antagonists if there is excess of 5-HT [23]. Hence, the effect may also be due to blocking of 5-HT_4 receptors. One study also implied a role for 5-HT_4 receptors in nociceptive behavior in formalin-induced paw inflammation in the rat, as the selective 5-HT_4 agonist methoxytryptamine augmented the nociceptive behavior, while the selective antagonist GR113808A ([1-[2-[(-methylsulphonyl) amino] ethyl]4-piperinidyl]methyl1-methyl-1H-indole-3-carboxylate succinate) blocked the response [95].

10.3.5 5-HT Effects on 5-HT_7 Receptors

5-HT_7 receptors have been found to be expressed in primary afferent neurons terminating in superficial laminae I–II in the dorsal spinal cord, that is, in regions where nociceptive afferents usually terminate. Injection of 5-HT or the 5-$HT_{1A/7}$ agonist 8-OH-DPAT increased c-fos expression in the spinal dorsal horn, which was attenuated by the 5-HT_7 antagonist methiothepin [55]. Local administration by subcutaneous injection of 5-HT and the 5-$HT_{1A/7}$ receptor agonist 5-carboxamidotryptamine (5-CT) dose-dependently augmented formalin-induced nociceptive behavior in rats, while the 5-HT_7 receptor antagonist SB-269970 ((2R)-1-[(3-hydroxyphenyl)sulfonyl]-2-[2-(4-methyl-1-piperidinyl)ethyl]pyrrolidine), but not the 5-HT_{1A} receptor antagonist WAY-100635 (*N*-[2-[4-(2-methoxyphenyl)-1-piperazinyl]ethyl]-*N*-(2-pyridyl)cyclohexanecarboxamide), significantly reduced formalin-induced flinching [29]. While intra-articular injection of low concentrations of sumatriptan reduces capsaicin-induced plasma extravasation in rats, high concentrations (>200 nM) seem to enhance neurogenic inflammation, possibly by activation of 5-HT_7 receptors, for which sumatriptan displays moderate binding affinity [58]. 5-HT_7 receptors are also believed to be involved in migraine headache by causing vasodilation that in turn activates trigeminovascular afferents and thus initiate neurogenic inflammation [74]. Further, 5-HT_7 receptors are upregulated in a rat model of IBS with constipation, which indicate that they might play a role in the pathogenesis of IBS [96].

10.3.6 5-HT Effects on SERT

Recently, there has been a great interest in the role of SERT in pain processes. SERT-deficient mice show reduced 5-HT content in the peripheral nerves and did not develop thermal hyperalgesia due to chronic constriction injury of the sciatic nerve, or chemical inflammation (Freund's complete adjuvant) [97]. This shows that 5-HT in the peripheral nerves is essential for the development of thermal hyperalgesia. One study showed that visceral sensitivity to colorectal distension was suppressed in mice treated with the SERT antagonist paroxetine [98]. In patients with IBS, SERT immunoreactivity was reduced in rectal biopsy specimens [99], and in rats with chronic visceral hypersensitivity, the expression of SERT in the colon mucosa increased after electroacupuncture [91]. This indicates that defects in 5-HT signaling may underlie the altered motility, secretion, and sensitivity.

10.3.7 Section Summary

In summary, peripheral effects by 5-HT in general are pronociceptive by activating and sensitizing afferent neurons. However, although some evidence indicates that 5-HT effects on 5-HT_{1A} and 5-$HT_{1B/D}$ receptors are pronociceptive, peripheral activation of 5-HT_1 receptors in general seems to mediate antinociceptive effects. In addition, as pointed out previously, the pronociceptive effect reported by peripheral 5-HT_{1A} receptors may very well be mediated by 5-HT_7 receptors. By activation of 5-HT_{2A} receptors on peripheral afferents, 5-HT evidently mediates pronociceptive effects, while activation of 5-HT_{2B} and 5-HT_{2C} receptors may not be directly pronociceptive but indirectly pronociceptive as a result of the release of other mediators. On the contrary, 5-HT effects on 5-HT_3, 5-HT_4, and 5-HT_7 receptors are routinely pronociceptive.

10.4 SPINAL AND SUPRASPINAL EFFECTS BY 5-HT RECEPTORS

For a long time, it has been acknowledged that the central effect of 5-HT, as part of the descending endogenous pain inhibitory system, is analgesia. Large quantities of 5-HT are found in the nucleus raphe magnum (NRM) and periaqueductal gray (PAG), and the stimulation of these areas release 5-HT that activates inhibitory interneurons and thus inhibits pain transmission [40]. However, recent research suggests that 5-HT can produce both anti- and pronociceptive effects via the endogenous pain inhibitory system depending on which receptor subclass is activated [20,100]. Thus, it is now believed that tonic activation of central 5-HT neurons that mediate facilitatory responses may contribute to central sensitization in chronic pain conditions [101]. As the scope of this book is peripheral targets for analgesia, this section provides only a summary of 5-HT effects at spinal and supraspinal levels. For more detailed information, the reader is referred to a recent comprehensive review [20].

10.4.1 Effects by 5-HT$_1$ Receptors

As mentioned previously, 5-HT at spinal and supraspinal levels may be both anti- and pronociceptive. 5-HT$_{1A}$ receptors are highly expressed by neurons in the dorsal horn, especially in the superficial laminae. As they do not appear to be present at the peripheral nerves, their location in the spinal dorsal horn indicates that their effects are mediated by the intrinsic spinal neurons and projecting neurons [20]. The stimulation of 5-HT$_{1A}$ receptors in the spinal cord seems to inhibit nociceptive transmission [30,102]. For example, subcutaneous administration of the 8-OH-DPAT reduced both the paw licking and paw elevation induced by formalin injection into the plantar surface of the rat hind paw [103]. In another study, 8-OH-DPAT increased the threshold for flinching, jumping, and vocalizing in rats, an effect that was blocked by propranolol and WAY-100135 ((S)-N-tert-butyl-3-(4-(2-methoxyphenyl)-piperazin-1-yl)-2-phenylpropanamide dihydrochloride) [104]. As previously noted, 5-HT$_{1A}$ receptors have not been found on peripheral afferent fibers, so these effects most probably involve postsynaptic receptors on projection neurons or actions on excitatory interneurons. However, spinal administration of 5-HT$_{1A}$ agonists has been shown to induce spontaneous nociceptive behavior and to facilitate nociceptive responses in rats after carrageenan inflammation [76,105]. This has been explained to be due to the blocking of inhibitory interneurons [20], as intrathecal administration of GABA agonists blocked mechanical allodynia induced by subcutaneous injection of 8-OH-DPAT [106]. It is also possible that inhibition of opioid-containing interneurons by 5-HT$_{1A}$ receptors may occur, as intrathecal administration of the 5-HT$_{1A}$ agonist spioxatrine attenuated allodynia induced by intra-PAG injection of morphine in rats [107]. Supraspinal 5-HT$_{1A}$ receptors seem to facilitate noradrenergic actions and to suppress 5-HT$_{2C}$ receptors at GABAergic interneurons via inhibitory autoreceptors. Indeed, inhibitory 5-HT$_{1A}$ autoreceptors in the NRM attenuate central and spinal 5-HT release [20,108]. However, as the action of 5-HT$_{1A}$ receptors depends on which type of neuron they exert their effect on, supraspinal 5-HT$_{1A}$ receptors may also be pronociceptive.

5-HT$_{1B}$ and 5-HT$_{1D}$ receptors are distributed throughout the dorsal horn on intrinsic neurons especially in the trigeminal nucleus, where they are colocalized with SP- and CGRP-containing neurons [109], but they are also present in the spinal cord [20]. They seem to be located mainly postsynaptic to serotonergic fibers. 5-HT_{1D} receptors differ from 5-HT_{1B} receptors in that they are not present in the endothelium of cerebral blood vessels. However, their density on intrinsic neurons is sparse, which indicates that they exert their inhibitory effect mainly on the central terminals of peripheral afferents, although evidence for a functional role of 5-$HT_{1B/1D}$ receptors on projecting neurons also exists [110]. In contrast, there is no evidence that 5-HT_{1F} receptors are also located in the intrinsic neurons in the spinal cord, although they are present on the intrinsic neurons in the trigeminal nucleus [12]. 5-HT_{1B} receptors also function as autoreceptors on serotonergic terminals, and they are the subclass of 5-HT receptors that show the most robust antinociceptive effects [20]. There seems to be no evidence for a role of any of these receptors in supraspinal antinociception, with the exception of 5-HT_{1F} receptors that have been found in the PAG [12]. However, the significance of this finding is unexplored. As studies with selective ligands that can distinguish 5-HT_{1B}, 5-HT_{1D}, and 5-HT_{1F} receptors have not been carried out, it is to date not possible to determine their exact role.

10.4.2 Activation of 5-HT_2 Receptors

The expression of 5-HT_{2A} and 5-HT_{2B} receptors in the dorsal horn have been found to be low and probably mainly include central terminals of peripheral afferents [20]. However, the expression of these receptors in the dorsal root ganglion was reported to increase during capsaicin-induced peripheral inflammation [111]. In contrast, 5-HT_{2C} receptors are expressed in the superficial and deep laminae of the dorsal horn by intrinsic neurons, but also by dorsal ganglion cells, at least in animals [19,112]. Little is known about the function of spinal 5-HT_{2B} receptors, but the presence of 5-HT_{2A} and 5-HT_{2C} receptors on peripheral afferents and their excitatory effects indicate that they increase nociception, an effect that may be related to the release of SP from presynaptic terminals [30,113]. 5-HT_{2C} receptors have also been shown to reinforce the pronociceptive effects of 5-HT_{1A} receptors in the dorsal horn [114]. However, as there is also evidence for their distribution on intrinsic neurons (especially 5-HT_{2C} receptors), they may also activate inhibitory interneurons and hence reduce nociception. This is supported by reports that spinal 5-HT_{2A} receptors suppressed formalin-induced nociception [115]. 5-$HT_{2A/C}$ receptors are reported to be a binding site for SSRIs and by this mechanism may exert antinociceptive effects [113]. 5-$HT_{2A/C}$ receptors also mediate excitatory influence of autonomic and motor neurons in the ventral spinal horn [76]. At the supraspinal level, 5-$HT2_{A/C}$ receptors seem to modulate nociception via serotonergic and noradrenergic descending pathways. For the 5-HT_{2C} receptor, this is via activation of GABAergic interneurons [20].

10.4.3 Activation of 5-HT_3 Receptors

Spinal 5-HT_3 receptors are located in the superficial laminae of the dorsal horn, but mRNA for 5-HT_3 receptors is also expressed by intrinsic neurons in the dorsal horn [112,116]. A large part of the receptors, however, seem to be located on the central terminals of peripheral afferent fibers. As indicated above, the activation of 5-HT_3 receptors excites neurons and hence increases nociception. As they also stimulate the release of SP from the central terminals of primary afferent fibers, it has been debated if the pronociceptive effect is direct or indirect. However, by recruitment of inhibitory GABAergic and opioidic interneurons, 5-HT_3 receptor-mediated effects are also antinociceptive [117]. For example, intrathecal perfusion of the selective 5-HT_3 receptor agonist 1-phenylbiguanide dose-dependently increased GABA concentration in the spinal cord, and naloxone-induced antinociception is reported to be attenuated by 5-HT_3 agonists [118,119]. The activation of 5-HT_3 receptors has also been shown to reduce hyperexcitability after spinal cord hemisection [102]. On the contrary, there is now a growing evidence that a facilitatory action of spinal 5-HT_3 receptors may enhance nociception, as intrathecal administration of ondansetron reduced second phase nociceptive behavior in the formalin test in rats and mice [78,120] and nociceptive behavior to mechanical stimuli in spinally ligated rats [100]. This facilitatory action may not only be due to direct effects on projecting spinal neurons but may also involve excitatory interneurons [20]. 5-HT_3 receptors have also been identified in the ventral horn, which may explain the report of activation of motor neurons, following intrathecal administration of the 5-HT_3 agonist 2-methyl-5-HT [121]. Although 5-HT_3 receptors are distributed in many brain areas, they do not seem to influence serotonergic descending pathways [20,112].

10.4.4 Activation of 5-HT_4 Receptors

5-HT_4 receptors have been shown to be expressed in the superficial laminae of the dorsal horn, but their anatomical distribution has not been fully established. They are probably located on intrinsic neurons, but they are also likely expressed in the dorsal root ganglion and therefore may be present at the central terminals of peripheral afferent fibers [92]. Similar to 5-HT_3 receptors, they mediate excitatory effects, and they have been shown to augment 5-HT_3 effects [122]. Thus, they may also have a facilitatory effect. Indeed, intrathecal administration of the combined 5-HT_3/5-HT_4 antagonist metoclopramide attenuated paw edema in rats, while ondansetron was not effective, which may support this concept [123]. At supraspinal levels, 5-HT_4 receptors are highly expressed by neurons in the PAG, but their distribution in the NRM is sparse. This indicates that they do not interact with serotonergic descending pathways, although there is some evidence for a role in descending cholinergic transmission [20].

10.4.5 Activation of 5-HT_7 Receptors

There is evidence that 5-HT_7 receptors in the spinal cord are mainly expressed on the central terminals of peripheral afferent fibers, as mRNA for 5-HT_7

receptors have so far not been identified in the spinal cord. However, as mentioned earlier, the pronociceptive role of 5-HT_{1A} receptors may very well be mediated by 5-HT_7 receptors, and if 5-HT_7 receptors were expressed on intrinsic neurons, it is tempting to believe that they would mediate excitatory effects. Indeed, 5-HT_7 receptor activation was reported to mediate 5-HT-evoked facilitation of deep dorsal horn neurons, which may lend support to this hypothesis [124]. There is to date no evidence for a role of 5-HT_7 receptors in supraspinal modulation of serotonergic pathways.

10.4.6 Section Summary

Spinal and supraspinal effects of 5-HT are complex and depend on which receptor subtypes are activated and the interplay between them. 5-HT_{1A}, 5-HT_2, and 5-HT_3 receptors exert excitatory effects and may induce pronociceptive or antinociceptive actions depending on whether excitatory or inhibitory interneurons in the spinal cord are activated. $5\text{-HT}_{1B/D/F}$ receptors, which are mainly expressed on peripheral afferents, mediate antinociceptive effects. 5-HT_{1B} receptors also function as autoreceptors and show their strongest inhibitory effect on 5-HT release in the spinal cord. Likewise, 5-HT_4 and 5-HT_7 receptors are mainly expressed on peripheral nerve terminals, but as they have excitatory actions, they mainly mediate pronociceptive effects.

10.5 CLINICAL IMPLICATION

10.5.1 Serotonin Levels in Pain Disorders

In migraine patients with aura and at the beginning of attacks in both migraineurs with and without aura, the serum 5-HT and 5-HIAA concentration was significantly increased, which was suggested to be due to a downregulation of 5-HT_2 receptors [125]. In patients with spondyloarthropathies, the serum levels of 5-HT did not correspond to disease activity measured by C-reactive protein, interleukin-6, or activity in the joints in skeletal scintigraphy, and it was concluded that "the measurement of serum 5-HT provides no relevant information about disease activity in synovial inflammation" [126].

Patients with fibromyalgia are reported to show decreased cerebrospinal fluid (CSF) levels of 5-HIAA [127,128]. Also, the serum level of 5-HT, which is suggested to mirror the CNS content [129] is reduced in patients with fibromyalgia [130,131] and was found to be negatively correlated to hyperalgesia in fibromyalgia and craniofacial myalgia [132]. Further, a negative correlation between plasma tryptophan and the level of pain [133], as well as a reduced level of plasma tryptophan and a decreased transport ratio of tryptophan across the BBB [134], has been reported in fibromyalgia. Together, these results suggest that descending pain inhibition may be disturbed due to reduced central 5-HT content in chronic muscle pain states, which may be a consequence of an interaction between 5-HT and SP [134]. This is supported by findings of elevated levels of SP in the CSF of patients with fibromyalgia [135,136]. It has been proposed that this may partly be due to an enhanced reuptake of 5-HT, as platelet tritiated imipramine binding was reported to be increased in fibromyalgia patients [130], although this could not be confirmed in another study [128]. Taken together this might indicate that measurements of serum or plasma 5-HT could be a useful tool for the diagnosis of fibromyalgia. However, large interindividual variation of serotonin levels in fibromyalgia patients limits the usefulness of 5-HT levels for the diagnosis of this disorder [137].

A few studies have used microdialysis, which offers a unique possibility to study the release of various mediators *in vivo*, to study intramuscular levels of 5-HT in patients with chronic pain. Via a thin catheter inserted into the tissue that is very slowly perfused with a buffer, substances are recovered due to passive diffusion and can be collected for later analyses (Figure 10.3). Patients with fibromyalgia were shown to release more 5-HT upon puncture trauma than healthy subjects, and a higher muscle level of 5-HT was associated with higher pain levels and hyperalgesia [138]. Increased levels of 5-HT were further reported in myofascial trigger points in patients with neck pain [139]. Recently, the same group reported that the muscle level of 5-HT (and other mediators) was increased also in the gastrocnemius muscle in patients with myofascial trapezius myalgia [140]. In patients with chronic work-related trapezius myalgia, intramuscular levels of 5-HT were increased and positively

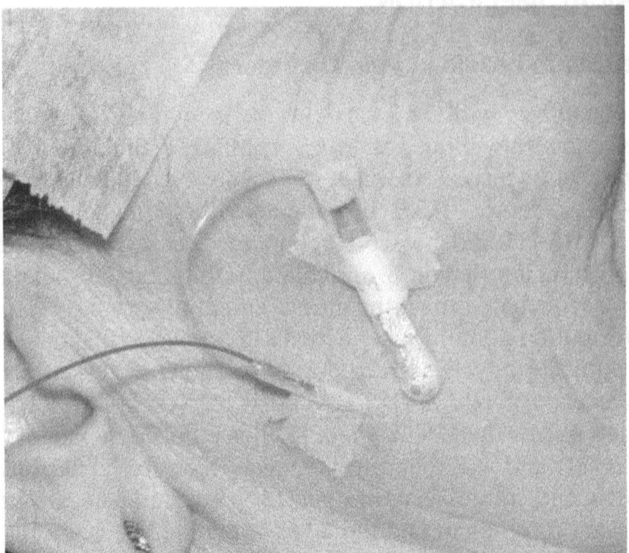

FIGURE 10.3. Intramuscular microdialysis performed to sample 5-HT from the masseter muscle. The probe was perfused with a saline buffer and had a membrane length of 10mm and a diameter of 0.5mm.

correlated with resting pain [141]. Similar findings were recently reported by the same group in patients with whiplash-associated disorders [142].

10.5.2 Serotonin Receptor Agonists and Antagonists for Clinical Use

Several drugs with more or less specific affinity for the various 5-HT receptors have been developed and are in clinical use. The triptans, which show agonist activity at 5-$HT_{1A/B/D/F}$ receptors, have been used the last 20 years due to their effectiveness as antimigraine drugs. However, their vasoconstrictive effect mediated by 5-HT_{1B} receptors leads to side effects such as chest pain. Recently, 5-HT_{1F} receptor agonists have been developed and tested as antimigraine drugs. Several studies have confirmed that the 5-HT_{1F} receptor agonists LY334370 was indeed effective in acute migraine without associated cardiovascular vasoconstrictor effects [62].

Many drugs with anxiolytic and antidepressive effects have affinity to 5-HT receptors, for example, buspirone, which is a partial 5-HT_{1A} agonist. Perhaps, more well-known antidepressant drugs that interfere with 5-HT are the selective serotonin reuptake inhibitors (SSRIs), such as fluoxetine and citalopram. These drugs are reported to exert their effects by blocking SERT. However, recent studies suggest that they also directly activate 5-HT_2 receptors and perhaps also 5-HT_7 receptors [143] and that this effect may be more potent than the effect on SERT [144]. SSRIs are also used to reduce pain in many chronic pain disorders. Although they are less efficacious than tricyclic antidepressants that inhibit both norepinephrine and serotonin reuptake, citalopram was shown to have moderate analgesic effects in patients with chronic pain, which was not dependent on changes in depressive scores [145].

The antidepressive drugs ketanserin and mianserin, which are 5-HT_2 antagonists, have also been shown to exhibit anxiolytic effects in humans [2]. Moreover, ketanserin is also used clinically for the treatment of hypertension [146]. In a double-blind, cross-over study in patients with chronic regional pain syndrome, intravenous administration of ketanserin (10 mg) was effective in reducing pain during exercise, and in an open longitudinal study with oral ketanserin (80–120 mg daily), a positive effect on pain at rest and upon movement was reported after 3 and 6 months of treatment [147].

Several beta-blockers, such as propranolol, have been found to also be nonselective 5-HT_1 receptor antagonists with affinity for the 5-HT_{1A} and 5-HT_{1B} receptors [148]. However, their role in pain disorders have not been evaluated.

Because of their role in the gastrointestinal system, several selective 5-HT_3 and 5-HT_4 receptor ligands have been developed for the treatment of IBS. The 5-HT_4 partial agonist tegaserod is now used for the treatment of the constipation-type IBS, while the 5-HT_3 antagonist alosetron is used clinically for treatment of the diarrhea-type IBS [23,149]. For the newly developed 5-HT_3 antagonist cilansetron and the mixed 5-HT_3 antagonist/5-HT_4 agonist renzapride, further evaluation is needed before their utility can be appraised [149].

Several drugs have been recently developed for the treatment of chemotherapy- and radiotherapy-induced emesis, for example, ondansetron, tropisetron, granisetron, and alosetron [2]. Although they all block the 5-HT_3 receptor, they have somewhat different pharmacological profiles and affinity for the receptor. Granisetron is reported to have an effect that is equivalent to, or better than that of, ondansetron and tropisetron [150]. In addition, ondansetron and tropisetron also show affinity for the 5-HT_4 receptor. These antagonists freely penetrate the BBB and, by blocking the central 5-HT_3 receptors in the area postrema, hippocampus, and limbic regions, reduce emesis and anxiety. Due to their efficiency in reducing emesis, these drugs are now also used for nausea and vomiting induced by general anesthesia. However, they have also garnered interest as potential treatments for various chronic pain states. Their effects have been evaluated in several trials, of which some were randomized controlled trials (RCTs), although none of them yet have been approved for the management of chronic pain. This will be reviewed below.

10.5.3 5-HT_3 Antagonists in Clinical Studies

Most of the treatment trials of 5-HT_3 antagonists for chronic pain have involved fibromyalgia patients, and both local and systemic administrations of 5-HT_3 antagonists have been found effective in relieving pain in these patients. In two open treatment trials with tropisetron, patients showed a clinical improvement in pain score; tender point count, fatigue, and sleep disturbances were reported [151,152]. In a double-blind, cross-over pilot study, oral ondansetron significantly reduced VAS pain, pain score, tender point score, and PPT in patients with fibromyalgia [153]. Finally, in a large-scale, multicenter treatment trial, oral tropisetron (5 mg daily) for 10 days improved VAS, pain score, tender point count, ancillary symptoms, and global pain assessment. However, blood levels of dopamine, norepinephrine, adrenaline, or serotonin did not change [154]. Gastrointestinal adverse events (mostly constipation) were frequent but were mostly mild to moderate. Although pain intensity increased within 1 month after treatment, patients showed a less pronounced increase and pain was still reduced compared with before treatment after 12 months [155].

In a randomized, double-blind, and placebo-controlled study, 2 mg tropisetron administered intravenously for 5 days decreased VAS pain and pain scores in 18 patients with fibromyalgia [156]. In another study, in 20 fibromyalgia patients, tropisetron (5 mg) given intravenously during 5 successive days significantly reduced the serum level of SP in 50% of the patients [157].

There are some studies that have used local administration of 5-HT_3 antagonists for managing pain conditions. In an open study, including 12 patients with low back tendinosis or myofascial pain, intramuscular trigger point injections of tropisetron (5 mg) decreased VAS pain by 36%. No side effects were reported with the exception of short-term burning pain at the injection site

[158]. In an RCT study, tropisetron (2 mg) or prilocaine (10 mg) injected around the tendon in 40 patients with tendinopathies immediately improved pain in both groups. However, after 3 days, only the tropisetron group reported a significant improvement [159]. In another RCT study, tropisetron (5 mg tropisetron) or a combination of dexamethasone (10 mg) and lidocaine (60 mg) administered around the tendon in 40 patients with tendinopathies improved pain without difference between groups after 7 days [160]. In 20 patients with whiplash-associated pain in the head–neck region, repeated trigger point injections decreased pain >50%, an effect that lasted for more than 2 months in 10% [161]. In a randomized and double-blind study, trigger point injection with tropisetron (5 mg) was compared with prilocaine (50 mg) in 33 patients with myofascial pain in the neck–shoulder region [162]. VAS pain decreased significantly in the tropisetron group (n = 17), while it decreased nonsignificantly in the prilocaine group.

Positive effects of 5-HT_3 antagonists are also reported for the treatment of inflammatory conditions. In an open study with 13 patients with low back pain due to arthritis or "nonspecific nature," intravenous tropisetron (5 mg) daily for 5 days decreased the pain score by almost 50% after 2 weeks [158]. In an RCT study including 16 patients with temporomandibular joint inflammatory arthritis, granisetron (1 mg) was reported to have an immediate, short-lasting, and specific pain-reducing effect [163]. In another double-blind study, intra-articular injection with either tropisetron (5 mg) or methylprednisolone (40 mg) in 18 patients with rheumatoid arthritis and 16 patients with osteoarthritis significantly reduced VAS pain was still reported 2 weeks after injection in both groups without difference between groups [164]. Furthermore, in a case report, two patients with systemic sclerosis were reported to be improved regarding skin score, mobility of joints, and pain after 6 weeks of treatment with tropisetron (10 mg) daily [165]. Finally, in a double-blind, placebo-controlled, cross-over study, a single dose of ondansetron (8 mg) administered intravenously was reported to reduce pain 2 hours after injection in 26 patients with chronic neuropathic pain [166].

10.6 SUMMARY

Increasing evidence shows that 5-HT has an important impact in pain transmission and modulation. Several 5-HT receptors are involved peripherally and at the spinal and higher center levels in these processes, and drugs that target central 5-HT receptors are thus of interest. Indeed, during the last 20 years, several such drugs have been developed and are now in clinical use, for example, triptans (5-$HT_{1A/D/F}$ agonists) and 5-HT_4 antagonists. However, the receptor ligands that seem to possess the greatest interest for pain treatment are the 5-HT_3 antagonists. They are especially interesting as they may not only block pain at peripheral sites but may also be effective potentiators of GABAergic and opioid-induced analgesia at spinal and higher levels. Indeed, several pilot studies and a few treatment RCTs have shown that 5-HT_3 antagonists effectively reduce pain and pain-related symptoms in patients with various pain and inflammatory disorders, such as rheumatoid arthritis, tendinopathies, and myofascial pain. However, large-scale RCTs are needed before any firm conclusions can be drawn regarding their efficacy.

REFERENCES

1. Rapport, M.M. (1997). The discovery of serotonin. *Perspect Biol Med* 40:260–273.
2. Hindle, A.T. (1994). Recent developments in the physiology and pharmacology of 5-hydroxytryptamine. *Br J Anaesth* 73:395–407.
3. Gyermek, L. (1996). Pharmacology of serotonin as related to anesthesia. *J Clin Anesth* 8:402–425.
4. Russell, I.J. (1993). A metabolic basis for fibromyalgia syndrome. In: Vaeroy, H., Merskey, H. (eds.). *Progress in Fibromyalgia and Myofascial Pain*. Amsterdam: Elsevier Publisher B.V., pp. 283–309.
5. Brenner, B., Harney, J.T., Ahmed, B.A., Jeffus, B.C., Unal, R., Mehta, J.L., Kilic, F. (2007). Plasma serotonin levels and the platelet serotonin transporter. *J Neurochem* 102:206–215.
6. Wakayama, K., Ohtsuki, S., Takanaga, H., Hosoya, K., Terasaki, T. (2002). Localization of norepinephrine and serotonin transporter in mouse brain capillary endothelial cells. *Neurosci Res* 44:173–180.
7. Bockaert, J., Claeysen, S., Becamel, C., Dumuis, A., Marin, P. (2006). Neuronal 5-HT metabotropic receptors: fine-tuning of their structure, signaling, and roles in synaptic modulation. *Cell Tissue Res* 326:553–572.
8. Boess, F.G., Martin, I.L. (1994). Molecular biology of 5-HT receptors. *Neuropharmacology* 33:275–317.
9. Faerber, L., Drechsler, S., Ladenburger, S., Gschaidmeier, H., Fischer, W. (2007). The neuronal 5-HT3 receptor network after 20 years of research–evolving concepts in management of pain and inflammation. *Eur J Pharmacol* 560:1–8.
10. Hoyer, D., Clarke, D.E., Fozard, J.R., Hartig, P.R., Martin, G.R., Mylecharane, E.J., Saxena, P.R., Humphrey, P.P. (1994). International Union of Pharmacology classification of receptors for 5-hydroxytryptamine (serotonin). *Pharmacol Rev* 46:157–203.
11. Niesler, B., Walstab, J., Combrink, S., Möller, D., Kapeller, J., Rietdorf, J., Bönisch, H., Göthert, M., Rappold, G., Brüss, M. (2007). Characterization of the novel human serotonin receptor subunits 5-HT3C, 5-HT3D, and 5-HT3E. *Mol Pharmacol* 72:8–17.
12. Adham, N., Bard, J.A., Zgombick, J.M., Durkin, M.M., Kucharewicz, S., Weinshank, R.L., Branchek, T.A. (1997). Cloning and characterization of the guinea pig 5-HT1F receptor subtype: a comparison of the pharmacological profile to the human species homolog. *Neuropharmacology* 36:569–576.
13. Potrebic, S., Ahn, A.H., Skinner, K., Fields, H.L., Basbaum, A.I. (2003). Peptidergic nociceptors of both trigeminal and dorsal root ganglia express serotonin 1D

receptors: implications for the selective antimigraine action of triptans. *J Neurosci* 23:10988–10997.

14. Nicholson, R., Small, J., Dixon, A.K., Spanswick, D., Lee, K. (2003). Serotonin receptor mRNA expression in rat dorsal root ganglion neurons. *Neurosci Lett* 337:119–122.
15. Leonard, B.E. (1992). Sub-types of serotonin receptors: biochemical changes and pharmacological consequences. *Int Clin Psychopharmacol* 7:13–21.
16. Buzzi, M.G., Moskowitz, M.A., Peroutka, S.J., Byun, B. (1991). Further characterization of the putative 5-HT receptor which mediates blockade of neurogenic plasma extravasation in rat dura mater. *Br J Pharmacol* 103:1421–1428.
17. Alsip, N.L., Harris, P.D. (1991). Receptor mediation of microvascular responses to serotonin in striated muscle. *Am J Physiol* 261:H1525–H1533.
18. Caillet, R. (1992). *Myofascial pain syndromes*. In: Anonymous (ed.). *Head and Face Pain Syndromes*. Philadelphia: FA Davis, pp. 100–124.
19. Pierce, P.A., Xie, G.X., Levine, J.D., Peroutka, S.J. (1996). 5-Hydroxytryptamine receptor subtype messenger RNAs in rat peripheral sensory and sympathetic ganglia: a polymerase chain reaction study. *Neuroscience* 70:553–559.
20. Millan, M.J. (2002). Descending control of pain. *Prog Neurobiol* 66:355–474.
21. Kurita, H., Ernberg, M., Tominaga, K., Alstergren, P., Kopp, S. (1999). Effect of 5-hydroxytryptamine infusion on microcirculation in the rabbit masseter muscle measured by laser-Doppler flowmetry. *Arch Oral Biol* 44:377–382.
22. Giordano, J., Schultea, T. (2004). Serotonin 5-HT3 receptor mediation of pain and anti-nociception: implications for clinical therapeutics. *Pain Physician* 7:141–147.
23. De Ponti, F. (2004). Pharmacology of serotonin: what a clinician should know. *Gut* 53:1520–1535.
24. Blauw, G.J., van Brummelen, P., Chang, P.C., Vermeij, P., van Zwieten, P.A. (1988). 5HT3 receptor-mediated vasodilation in the human forearm. *J Hypertens Suppl* 6:S33–S35.
25. Bueno, L., De Ponti, F., Fried, M., Kullak-Ublick, G.A., Kwiatek, M.A., Pohl, D., Quigley, E.M., Tack, J., Talley, N.J. (2007). Serotonergic and non-serotonergic targets in the pharmacotherapy of visceral hypersensitivity. *Neurogastroenterol Motil* 19:89–119.
26. Glennon, R.A. (2003). Higher-end serotonin receptors: 5-HT(5), 5-HT(6), and 5-HT(7). *J Med Chem* 46:2795–2812.
27. Prins, N.H., Briejer, M.R., Van Bergen, P.J., Akkermans, L.M., Schuurkes, J.A. (1999). Evidence for 5-HT7 receptors mediating relaxation of human colonic circular smooth muscle. *Br J Pharmacol* 128:849–852.
28. Hedlund, P.B., Sutcliffe, J.G. (2004). Functional, molecular and pharmacological advances in 5-HT7 receptor research. *Trends Pharmacol Sci* 25:481–486.
29. Rocha-Gonzalez, H.I., Meneses, A., Carlton, S.M., Granados-Soto, V. (2005). Pronociceptive role of peripheral and spinal 5-HT7 receptors in the formalin test. *Pain* 117:182–192.
30. Eide, P.K., Hole, K. (1993). The role of 5-hydroxytryptamine (5-HT) receptor subtypes and plasticity in the 5-HT systems in the regulation of nociceptive sensitivity. *Cephalalgia* 13:75–85.

31. Rebeck, G.W., Maynard, K.I., Hyman, B.T., Moskowitz, M.A. (1994). Selective 5-HT1D alpha serotonin receptor gene expression in trigeminal ganglia: implications for antimigraine drug development. *Proc Natl Acad Sci U S A* 91: 3666–3669.

32. Bouchelet, I., Cohen, Z., Case, B., Seguela, P., Hamel, E. (1996). Differential expression of sumatriptan-sensitive 5-hydroxytryptamine receptors in human trigeminal ganglia and cerebral blood vessels. *Mol Pharmacol* 50:219–223.

33. Pierce, P.A., Xie, G.X., Meuser, T., Peroutka, S.J. (1997). 5-Hydroxytryptamine receptor subtype messenger RNAs in human dorsal root ganglia: a polymerase chain reaction study. *Neuroscience* 81:813–819.

34. Doucet, E., Latremoliere, A., Darmon, M., Hamon, M., Emerit, M.B. (2007). Immunolabelling of the 5-HT 3B receptor subunit in the central and peripheral nervous systems in rodents. *Eur J Neurosci* 26:355–366.

35. Sung, D., Dong, X., Ernberg, M., Kumar, U., Cairns, B.E. (2008). Serotonin (5-HT) excites rat masticatory muscle afferent fibers through activation of peripheral 5-HT3 receptors. *Pain* 134:41–50.

36. Mössner, R., Lesch, K.P. (1998). Role of serotonin in the immune system and in neuroimmune interactions. *Brain Behav Immun* 12:249–271.

37. Coutaux, A., Adam, F., Willer, J.C., Le Bars, D. (2005). Hyperalgesia and allodynia: peripheral mechanisms. *Joint Bone Spine* 72:359–371.

38. Ringkamp, M., Schmelz, M., Kress, M., Allwang, M., Ogilvie, A., Reeh, P.W. (1994). Activated human platelets in plasma excite nociceptors in rat skin, in vitro. *Neurosci Lett* 170:103–106.

39. Sommer, C. (2006). Is serotonin hyperalgesic or analgesic? *Curr Pain Headache Rep* 10:101–106.

40. Saria, A., Javorsky, F., Humpel, C., Gamse, R. (1990). 5-HT3 receptor antagonists inhibit sensory neuropeptide release from the rat spinal cord. *Neuroreport* 1:104–106.

41. Kessler, W., Kirchhoff, C., Reeh, P.W., Handwerker, H.O. (1992). Excitation of cutaneous afferent nerve endings in vitro by a combination of inflammatory mediators and conditioning effect of substance P. *Exp Brain Res* 91:467–476.

42. Michaelis, M., Vogel, C., Blenk, K.H., Jänig, W. (1997). Algesics excite axotomised afferent nerve fibres within the first hours following nerve transection in rats. *Pain* 72:347–354.

43. Lischetzki, G., Rukwied, R., Handwerker, H.O., Schmelz, M. (2001). Nociceptor activation and protein extravasation induced by inflammatory mediators in human skin. *Eur J Pain* 5:49–57.

44. Schmelz, M., Schmidt, R., Weidner, C., Hilliges, M., Torebjörk, H.E., Handwerker, H.O. (2003). Chemical response pattern of different classes of C-nociceptors to pruritogens and algogens. *J Neurophysiol* 89:2441–2448.

45. Jensen, K., Tuxen, C., Pedersen-Bjergaard, U., Jansen, I., Edvinsson, L., Olesen, J. (1990). Pain and tenderness in human temporal muscle induced by bradykinin and 5-hydroxytryptamine. *Peptides* 11:1127–1132.

46. Babenko, V., Graven-Nielsen, T., Svensson, P., Drewes, A.M., Jensen, T.S., Arendt-Nielsen, L. (1999). Experimental human muscle pain induced by intramuscular injections of bradykinin, serotonin, and substance P. *Eur J Pain* 3:93–102.

47. Ernberg, M., Lundeberg, T., Kopp, S. (2000). Pain and allodynia/hyperalgesia induced by intramuscular injection of serotonin in patients with fibromyalgia and healthy individuals. *Pain* 85:31–39.
48. Sufka, K.J., Schomburg, F.M., Giordano, J. (1992). Receptor mediation of 5-HT-induced inflammation and nociception in rats. *Pharmacol Biochem Behav* 41:53–56.
49. Taiwo, Y.O., Levine, J.D. (1992). Serotonin is a directly-acting hyperalgesic agent in the rat. *Neuroscience* 48:485–490.
50. Taiwo, Y.O., Heller, P.H., Levine, J.D. (1992). Mediation of serotonin hyperalgesia by the cAMP second messenger system. *Neuroscience* 48:479–483.
51. Kayser, V., Elfassi, I.E., Aubel, B., Melfort, M., Julius, D., Gingrich, J.A., Hamon, M., Bourgoin, S. (2007). Mechanical, thermal and formalin-induced nociception is differentially altered in 5-HT(1A)-/-, 5-HT(1B)-/-, 5-HT(2A)-/-, 5-HT(3A)-/- and 5-HTT-/- knock-out male mice. *Pain* 130:235–248.
52. Millan, M.J., Colpaert, F.C. (1990). Attenuation of opioid induced antinociception by 5-HT1A partial agonists in the rat. *Neuropharmacology* 29:315–318.
53. Wei, H., Chen, Y., Hong, Y. (2005). The contribution of peripheral 5-hydroxytryptamine2A receptor to carrageenan-evoked hyperalgesia, inflammation and spinal Fos protein expression in the rat. *Neuroscience* 132:1073–1082.
54. Ernberg, M., Lundeberg, T., Kopp, S. (2000). Effect of propranolol and granisetron on experimentally induced pain and allodynia/hyperalgesia by intramuscular injection of serotonin into the human masseter muscle. *Pain* 84:339–346.
55. Meuser, T., Pietruck, C., Gabriel, A., Xie, G.X., Lim, K.J., Pierce Palmer, P. (2002). 5-HT7 receptors are involved in mediating 5-HT-induced activation of rat primary afferent neurons. *Life Sci* 71:2279–2289.
56. Fink, K.B., Göthert, M. (2007). 5-HT receptor regulation of neurotransmitter release. *Pharmacol Rev* 59:360–417.
57. Albert, P.R., Zhou, Q.Y., Van Tol, H.H., Bunzow, J.R., Civelli, O. (1990). Cloning, functional expression, and mRNA tissue distribution of the rat 5-hydroxytryptamine1A receptor gene. *J Biol Chem* 265:5825–5832.
58. Pierce, P.A., Xie, G.X., Peroutka, S.J., Levine, J.D. (1996). Dual effect of the serotonin agonist, sumatriptan, on peripheral neurogenic inflammation. *Reg Anesth* 21:219–225.
59. Levy, D., Jakubowski, M., Burstein, R. (2004). Disruption of communication between peripheral and central trigeminovascular neurons mediates the antimigraine action of 5HT 1B/1D receptor agonists. *Proc Natl Acad Sci U S A* 101:4274–4279.
60. Bingham, S., Davey, P.T., Sammons, M., Raval, P., Overend, P., Parsons, A.A. (2001). Inhibition of inflammation-induced thermal hypersensitivity by sumatriptan through activation of 5-HT(1B/1D) receptors. *Exp Neurol* 167:65–73.
61. Linde, M., Elam, M., Lundblad, L., Olausson, H., Dahlof, C.G. (2004). Sumatriptan (5-HT1B/1D-agonist) causes a transient allodynia. *Cephalalgia* 24:1057–1066.
62. Ramadan, N.M., Skljarevski, V., Phebus, L.A., Johnson, K.W. (2003). 5-HT1F receptor agonists in acute migraine treatment: a hypothesis. *Cephalalgia* 23:776–785.
63. Johnson, K.W., Schaus, J.M., Durkin, M.M., Audia, J.E., Kaldor, S.W., Flaugh, M.E., Adham, N., Zgombick, J.M., Cohen, M.L., Branchek, T.A., Phebus, L.A. (1997).

5-HT1F receptor agonists inhibit neurogenic dural inflammation in guinea pigs. *Neuroreport* 8:2237–2240.

64. Mitsikostas, D.D., Sanchez del Rio, M., Moskowitz, M.A., Waeber, C. (1999). Both 5-HT1B and 5-HT1F receptors modulate c-fos expression within rat trigeminal nucleus caudalis. *Eur J Pharmacol* 369:271–277.
65. Phebus, L.A., Johnson, K.W., Zgombick, J.M., Gilbert, P.J., Van Belle, K., Mancuso, V., Nelson, D.L., Calligaro, D.O., Kiefer, A.D., Jr., Branchek, T.A., Flaugh, M.E. (1997). Characterization of LY344864 as a pharmacological tool to study 5-HT1F receptors: binding affinities, brain penetration and activity in the neurogenic dural inflammation model of migraine. *Life Sci* 61:2117–2126.
66. Bouchelet, I., Case, B., Olivier, A., Hamel, E. (2000). No contractile effect for 5-HT1D and 5-HT1F receptor agonists in human and bovine cerebral arteries: similarity with human coronary artery. *Br J Pharmacol* 129:501–508.
67. Abbott, F.V., Hong, Y., Blier, P. (1996). Activation of 5-HT2A receptors potentiates pain produced by inflammatory mediators. *Neuropharmacology* 35:99–110.
68. Tokunaga, A., Saika, M., Senba, E. (1998). 5-HT2A receptor subtype is involved in the thermal hyperalgesic mechanism of serotonin in the periphery. *Pain* 76: 349–355.
69. Sasaki, M., Obata, H., Kawahara, K., Saito, S., Goto, F. (2006). Peripheral 5-HT2A receptor antagonism attenuates primary thermal hyperalgesia and secondary mechanical allodynia after thermal injury in rats. *Pain* 122:130–136.
70. Okamoto, K., Imbe, H., Morikawa, Y., Itoh, M., Sekimoto, M., Nemoto, K., Senba, E. (2002). 5-HT2A receptor subtype in the peripheral branch of sensory fibers is involved in the potentiation of inflammatory pain in rats. *Pain* 99:133–143.
71. Hong, Y., Ji, H., Wei, H. (2006). Topical ketanserin attenuates hyperalgesia and inflammation in arthritis in rats. *Pain* 124:27–33.
72. Cohen, Z., Bouchelet, I., Olivier, A., Villemure, J.G., Ball, R., Stanimirovic, D.B., Hamel, E. (1999). Multiple microvascular and astroglial 5-hydroxytryptamine receptor subtypes in human brain: molecular and pharmacologic characterization. *J Cereb Blood Flow Metab* 19:908–917.
73. Schmuck, K., Ullmer, C., Kalkman, H.O., Probst, A., Lübbert, H. (1996). Activation of meningeal 5-HT2B receptors: an early step in the generation of migraine headache? *Eur J Neurosci* 8:959–967.
74. Hamel, E. (1999). The biology of serotonin receptors: focus on migraine pathophysiology and treatment. *Can J Neurol Sci* 26(Suppl. 3):S2–S6.
75. Johnson, K.W., Nelson, D.L., Dieckman, D.K., Wainscott, D.B., Lucaites, V.L., Audia, J.E., Owton, W.M., Phebus, L.A. (2003). Neurogenic dural protein extravasation induced by meta-chlorophenylpiperazine (mCPP) involves nitric oxide and 5-HT2B receptor activation. *Cephalalgia* 23:117–123.
76. Millan, M.J., Girardon, S., Bervoets, K. (1997). 8-OH-DPAT-induced spontaneous tail-flicks in the rat are facilitated by the selective serotonin (5-HT)2C agonist, RO 60-0175: blockade of its actions by the novel 5-HT2C receptor antagonist SB 206,553. *Neuropharmacology* 36:743–745.
77. Giordano, J., Rogers, L.V. (1989). Peripherally administered serotonin 5-HT3 receptor antagonists reduce inflammatory pain in rats. *Eur J Pharmacol* 170: 83–86.

78. Zeitz, K.P., Guy, N., Malmberg, A.B., Dirajlal, S., Martin, W.J., Sun, L., Bonhaus, D.W., Stucky, C.L., Julius, D., Basbaum, A.I. (2002). The 5-HT3 subtype of serotonin receptor contributes to nociceptive processing via a novel subset of myelinated and unmyelinated nociceptors. *J Neurosci* 22:1010–1019.
79. De Ponti, F., Malagelada, J.R. (1998). Functional gut disorders: from motility to sensitivity disorders. A review of current and investigational drugs for their management. *Pharmacol Ther* 80:49–88.
80. Miura, M., Lawson, D.C., Clary, E.M., Mangel, A.W., Pappas, T.N. (1999). Central modulation of rectal distension-induced blood pressure changes by alosetron, a 5-HT3 receptor antagonist. *Dig Dis Sci* 44:20–24.
81. Prior, A., Read, N.W. (1993). Reduction of rectal sensitivity and post-prandial motility by granisetron, a 5 HT3-receptor antagonist, in patients with irritable bowel syndrome. *Aliment Pharmacol Ther* 7:175–180.
82. Goldberg, P.A., Kamm, M.A., Setti-Carraro, P., van der Sijp, J.R., Roth, C. (1996). Modification of visceral sensitivity and pain in irritable bowel syndrome by 5-HT3 antagonism (ondansetron). *Digestion* 57:478–483.
83. Richardson, B.P., Engel, G., Donatsch, P., Stadler, P.A. (1985). Identification of serotonin M-receptor subtypes and their specific blockade by a new class of drugs. *Nature* 316:126–131.
84. Giordano, J., Daleo, C., Sacks, S.M. (1998). Topical ondansetron attenuates nociceptive and inflammatory effects of intradermal capsaicin in humans. *Eur J Pharmacol* 354:R13–R14.
85. Ernberg, M., Voog, U., Alstergren, P., Lundeberg, T., Kopp, S. (2000). Plasma and serum serotonin levels and their relationship to orofacial pain and anxiety in fibromyalgia. *J Orofac Pain* 14:37–46.
86. Christidis, N., Kopp, S., Ernberg, M. (2005). The effect on mechanical pain threshold over human muscles by oral administration of granisetron and diclofenac-sodium. *Pain* 113:265–270.
87. Christidis, N., Nilsson, A., Kopp, S., Ernberg, M. (2007). Intramuscular injection of granisetron into the masseter muscle increases the pressure pain threshold in healthy participants and patients with localized myalgia. *Clin J Pain* 23: 467–472.
88. Christidis, N., Ioannidou, K., Milosevic, M., Segerdahl, M., Ernberg, M. (2008). Changes of hypertonic saline-induced masseter muscle pain characteristics, by an infusion of the serotonin receptor type 3 antagonist granisetron. *J Pain* 9:892–901.
89. Ernberg, M., Lundeberg, T., Kopp, S. (2003). Effects on muscle pain by intramuscular injection of granisetron in patients with fibromyalgia. *Pain* 101:275–282.
90. Schikowski, A., Thewissen, M., Mathis, C., Ross, H.G., Enck, P. (2002). Serotonin type-4 receptors modulate the sensitivity of intramural mechanoreceptive afferents of the cat rectum. *Neurogastroenterol Motil* 14:221–227.
91. Tian, X.Y., Bian, Z.X., Hu, X.G., Zhang, X.J., Liu, L., Zhang, H. (2006). Electroacupuncture attenuates stress-induced defecation in rats with chronic visceral hypersensitivity via serotonergic pathway. *Brain Res* 1088:101–108.
92. Espejo, E.F., Gil, E. (1998). Antagonism of peripheral 5-HT4 receptors reduces visceral and cutaneous pain in mice, and induces visceral analgesia after simultaneous inactivation of 5-HT3 receptors. *Brain Res* 788:20–24.

93. Coffin, B., Farmachidi, J.P., Rueegg, P., Bastie, A., Bouhassira, D. (2003). Tegaserod, a 5-HT4 receptor partial agonist, decreases sensitivity to rectal distension in healthy subjects. *Aliment Pharmacol Ther* 17:577–585.

94. Müller-Lissner, S.A., Fumagalli, I., Bardhan, K.D., Pace, F., Pecher, E., Nault, B., Rüegg, P. (2001). Tegaserod, a 5-HT(4) receptor partial agonist, relieves symptoms in irritable bowel syndrome patients with abdominal pain, bloating and constipation. *Aliment Pharmacol Ther* 15:1655–1666.

95. Doak, G.J., Sawynok, J. (1997). Formalin-induced nociceptive behavior and edema: involvement of multiple peripheral 5-hydroxytryptamine receptor subtypes. *Neuroscience* 80:939–949.

96. Zou, B.C., Dong, L., Wang, Y., Wang, S.H., Cao, M.B. (2007). Expression and role of 5-HT7 receptor in brain and intestine in rats with irritable bowel syndrome. *Chin Med J* 120:2069–2074.

97. Vogel, C., Mossner, R., Gerlach, M., Heinemann, T., Murphy, D.L., Riederer, P., Lesch, K.P., Sommer, C. (2003). Absence of thermal hyperalgesia in serotonin transporter-deficient mice. *J Neurosci* 23:708–715.

98. Coates, M.D., Johnson, A.C., Greenwood-Van Meerveld, B., Mawe, G.M. (2006). Effects of serotonin transporter inhibition on gastrointestinal motility and colonic sensitivity in the mouse. *Neurogastroenterol Motil* 18:464–471.

99. Coates, M.D., Mahoney, C.R., Linden, D.R., Sampson, J.E., Chen, J., Blaszyk, H., Crowell, M.D., Sharkey, K.A., Gershon, M.D., Mawe, G.M., Moses, P.L. (2004). Molecular defects in mucosal serotonin content and decreased serotonin reuptake transporter in ulcerative colitis and irritable bowel syndrome. *Gastroenterology* 126:1657–1664.

100. Suzuki, R., Rygh, L.J., Dickenson, A.H. (2004). Bad news from the brain: descending 5-HT pathways that control spinal pain processing. *Trends Pharmacol Sci* 25: 613–617.

101. Porreca, F., Ossipov, M.H., Gebhart, G.F. (2002). Chronic pain and medullary descending facilitation. *Trends Neurosci* 25:319–325.

102. Hains, B.C., Willis, W.D., Hulsebosch, C.E. (2003). Serotonin receptors 5-HT1A and 5-HT3 reduce hyperexcitability of dorsal horn neurons after chronic spinal cord hemisection injury in rat. *Exp Brain Res* 149:174–186.

103. Bardin, L., Tarayre, J.P., Koek, W., Colpaert, F.C. (2001). In the formalin model of tonic nociceptive pain, 8-OH-DPAT produces 5-HT1A receptor-mediated, behaviorally specific analgesia. *Eur J Pharmacol* 421:109–114.

104. Cervo, L., Rossi, C., Tatarczynska, E., Samanin, R. (1994). Role of 5-HT1A receptors in the antinociceptive action of 8-hydroxy-2-(di-n-propylamino)tetralin in the rat. *Eur J Pharmacol* 263:187–191.

105. Zhang, Y., Yang, Z., Gao, X., Wu, G. (2001). The role of 5-hydroxytryptamine1A and 5-hydroxytryptamine1B receptors in modulating spinal nociceptive transmission in normal and carrageenan-injected rats. *Pain* 92:201–211.

106. Millan, M.J., Seguin, L., Honore, P., Girardon, S., Bervoets, K. (1996). Pro- and antinociceptive actions of serotonin (5-HT)1A agonists and antagonists in rodents: relationship to algesiometric paradigm. *Behav Brain Res* 73:69–77.

107. Liu, Z.Y., Zhuang, D.B., Lunderberg, T., Yu, L.C. (2002). Involvement of 5-hydroxytryptamine(1A) receptors in the descending anti-nociceptive pathway

from periaqueductal gray to the spinal dorsal horn in intact rats, rats with nerve injury and rats with inflammation. *Neuroscience* 112:399–407.

108. Millan, M.J., Lejeune, F., Gobert, A. (2000). Reciprocal autoreceptor and heteroreceptor control of serotonergic, dopaminergic and noradrenergic transmission in the frontal cortex: relevance to the actions of antidepressant agents. *J Psychopharmacol* 14:114–138.
109. Ma, Q.P., Hill, R., Sirinathsinghji, D. (2001). Colocalization of CGRP with 5-HT1B/1D receptors and substance P in trigeminal ganglion neurons in rats. *Eur J Neurosci* 13:2099–2104.
110. el-Yassir, N., Fleetwood-Walker, S.M. (1990). A 5-HT1-type receptor mediates the antinociceptive effect of nucleus raphe magnus stimulation in the rat. *Brain Res* 523:92–99.
111. Zhang, X.F., McKenna, D.G., Briggs, C.A. (2001). Epibatidine, a nicotinic acetylcholine receptor agonist, inhibits the capsaicin response in dorsal root ganglion neurons. *Brain Research* 919:166–168.
112. Fonseca, M.I., Ni, Y.G., Dunning, D.D., Miledi, R. (2001). Distribution of serotonin 2A, 2C and 3 receptor mRNA in spinal cord and medulla oblongata. *Brain Res Mol Brain Res* 89:11–19.
113. Honda, M., Uchida, K., Tanabe, M., Ono, H. (2006). Fluvoxamine, a selective serotonin reuptake inhibitor, exerts its antiallodynic effects on neuropathic pain in mice via 5-HT2A/2C receptors. *Neuropharmacology* 51:866–872.
114. Bervoets, K., Millan, M.J., Colpaert, F.C. (1990). Agonist action at 5-HT1C receptors facilitates 5-HT1A receptor-mediated spontaneous tail-flicks in the rat. *Eur J Pharmacol* 191:185–195.
115. Sasaki, M., Ishizaki, K., Obata, H., Goto, F. (2001). Effects of 5-HT2 and 5-HT3 receptors on the modulation of nociceptive transmission in rat spinal cord according to the formalin test. *Eur J Pharmacol* 424:45–52.
116. Kia, H.K., Miquel, M.C., McKernan, R.M., Laporte, A.M., Lombard, M.C., Bourgoin, S., Hamon, M., Verge, D. (1995). Localization of 5-HT3 receptors in the rat spinal cord: immunohistochemistry and in situ hybridization. *Neuroreport* 6:257–261.
117. Kukushkin, M.L., Igon'kina, S.I. (2003). Role of 5-HT3 receptors in the mechanisms of central pain syndrome. *Bull Exp Biol Med* 135:552–555.
118. Giordano, J. (1991). Analgesic profile of centrally administered 2-methylserotonin against acute pain in rats. *Eur J Pharmacol* 199:233–236.
119. Kawamata, T., Omote, K., Toriyabe, M., Yamamoto, H., Namiki, A. (2003). The activation of 5-HT(3) receptors evokes GABA release in the spinal cord. *Brain Res* 978:250–255.
120. Oyama, T., Ueda, M., Kuraishi, Y., Akaike, A., Satoh, M. (1996). Dual effect of serotonin on formalin-induced nociception in the rat spinal cord. *Neurosci Res* 25:129–135.
121. Fone, K.C., Robinson, A.J., Marsden, C.A. (1991). Characterization of the 5-HT receptor subtypes involved in the motor behaviours produced by intrathecal administration of 5-HT agonists in rats. *Br J Pharmacol* 103:1547–1555.
122. Smith, M.I., Banner, S.E., Sanger, G.J. (1999). 5-HT4 receptor antagonism potentiates inhibition of intestinal allodynia by 5-HT3 receptor antagonism in conscious rats. *Neurosci Lett* 271:61–64.

123. Daher, J.B., de Melo, M.D., Tonussi, C.R. (2005). Evidence for a spinal serotonergic control of the peripheral inflammation in the rat. *Life Sci* 76:2349–2359.

124. Garraway, S.M., Hochman, S. (2001). Pharmacological characterization of serotonin receptor subtypes modulating primary afferent input to deep dorsal horn neurons in the neonatal rat. *Br J Pharmacol* 132:1789–1798.

125. Ribeiro, C.A., Cotrim, M.D., Morgadinho, M.T., Ramos, M.I., Santos, E.S., de Macedo Tdos, R. (1990). Migraine, serum serotonin and platelet 5-HT2 receptors. *Cephalalgia* 10:213–219.

126. Pichler, R., Maschek, W., Krieglsteiner, S., Raml, A., Schmekal, B., Berg, J. (2002). Pro-inflammatory role of serotonin and interleukin-6 in arthritis and spondyloarthropathies—measurement of disease activity by bone scan and effect of steroids. *Scand J Rheumatol* 31:41–43.

127. Russell, I.J., Vaeroy, H., Javors, M., Nyberg, F. (1992). Cerebrospinal fluid biogenic amine metabolites in fibromyalgia/fibrositis syndrome and rheumatoid arthritis [see comments]. *Arthritis Rheum* 35:550–556.

128. Legangneux, E., Mora, J.J., Spreux-Varoquaux, O., Thorin, I., Herrou, M., Alvado, G., Gomeni, C. (2001). Cerebrospinal fluid biogenic amine metabolites, plasma-rich platelet serotonin and [3H]imipramine reuptake in the primary fibromyalgia syndrome. *Rheumatology* 40:290–296.

129. Bianchi, M., Moser, C., Lazzarini, C., Vecchiato, E., Crespi, F. (2002). Forced swimming test and fluoxetine treatment: in vivo evidence that peripheral 5-HT in rat platelet-rich plasma mirrors cerebral extracellular 5-HT levels, whilst 5-HT in isolated platelets mirrors neuronal 5-HT changes. *Exp Brain Res* 143:191–197.

130. Russell, I.J., Michalek, J.E., Vipraio, G.A., Fletcher, E.M., Javors, M.A., Bowden, C.A. (1992). Platelet 3H-imipramine uptake receptor density and serum serotonin levels in patients with fibromyalgia/fibrositis syndrome [see comments]. *J Rheumatol* 19:104–109.

131. Stratz, T., Samborski, W., Hrycaj, P., Pap, T., Mackiewicz, S., Mennet, P., Müller, W. (1993). Die serotoninkonzentration im serum bei patienten mit generalisierter tendomyopathie (fibromyalgie) und chronischer polyarthritis. *Med Klin* 88:458–462.

132. Ernberg, M., Hedenberg-Magnusson, B., Alstergren, P., Lundeberg, T., Kopp, S. (1999). Pain, allodynia, and serum serotonin level in orofacial pain of muscular origin. *J Orofac Pain* 13:56–62.

133. Moldofsky, H., Warsh, J.J. (1978). Plasma tryptophan and musculoskeletal pain in non-articular rheumatism ("fibrositis syndrome"). *Pain* 5:65–71.

134. Yunus, M.B., Dailey, J.W., Aldag, J.C., Masi, A.T., Jobe, P.C. (1992). Plasma tryptophan and other amino acids in primary fibromyalgia: a controlled study. *J Rheumatol* 19:90–94.

135. Vaeroy, H., Helle, R., Førre, O., Kass, E., Terenius, L. (1988). Elevated CSF levels of substance P and high incidence of Raynaud phenomenon in patients with fibromyalgia: new features for diagnosis. *Pain* 32:21–26.

136. Russell, I.J., Orr, M.D., Littman, B., Vipraio, G.A., Alboukrek, D., Michalek, J.E., Lopez, Y., MacKillip, F. (1994). Elevated cerebrospinal fluid levels of substance P in patients with the fibromyalgia syndrome. *Arthritis Rheum* 37:1593–1601.

137. Jaschko, G., Hepp, U., Berkhoff, M., Schmet, M., Michel, B.A., Gay, S., Sprott, H. (2007). Serum serotonin levels are not useful in diagnosing fibromyalgia. *Ann Rheum Dis* 66:1267–1268.
138. Ernberg, M., Hedenberg-Magnusson, B., Alstergren, P., Kopp, S. (1999). The level of serotonin in the superficial masseter muscle in relation to local pain and allodynia. *Life Sci* 65:313–325.
139. Shah, J.P., Phillips, T.M., Danoff, J.V., Gerber, L.H. (2005). An in vivo microanalytical technique for measuring the local biochemical milieu of human skeletal muscle. *J Appl Physiol* 99:1977–1984.
140. Shah, J.P., Danoff, J.V., Desai, M.J., Parikh, S., Nakamura, L.Y., Phillips, T.M., Gerber, L.H. (2008). Biochemicals associated with pain and inflammation are elevated in sites near to and remote from active myofascial trigger points. *Arch Phys Med Rehabil* 89:16–23.
141. Rosendal, L., Larsson, B., Kristiansen, J., Peolsson, M., Søgaard, K., Kjær, M., Sørensen, J., Gerdle, B. (2004). Increase in muscle nociceptive substances and anaerobic metabolism in patients with trapezius myalgia: microdialysis in rest and during exercise. *Pain* 112:324–334.
142. Gerdle, B., Lemming, D., Kristiansen, J., Larsson, B., Peolsson, M., Rosendal, L. (2007). Biochemical alterations in the trapezius muscle of patients with chronic whiplash associated disorders (WAD)–a microdialysis study. *Eur J Pain* 12:82–93.
143. Kroeze, W.K., Roth, B.L. (1998). The molecular biology of serotonin receptors: therapeutic implications for the interface of mood and psychosis. *Biol Psychiatry* 44:1128–1142.
144. Dempsey, C.M., Mackenzie, S.M., Gargus, A., Blanco, G., Sze, J.Y. (2005). Serotonin (5HT), fluoxetine, imipramine and dopamine target distinct 5HT receptor signaling to modulate *Caenorhabditis elegans* egg-laying behavior. *Genetics* 169:1425–1436.
145. Aragona, M., Bancheri, L., Perinelli, D., Tarsitani, L., Pizzimenti, A., Conte, A., Inghilleri, M. (2005). Randomized double-blind comparison of serotonergic (Citalopram) versus noradrenergic (Reboxetine) reuptake inhibitors in outpatients with somatoform, DSM-IV-TR pain disorder. *Eur J Pain* 9:33–38.
146. van Zwieten, P.A., Blauw, G.J., van Brummelen, P. (1992). Serotonergic receptors and drugs in hypertension. *Pharmacol Toxicol* 70:S17–S22.
147. Moesker, A. (2000). Treatment of CRPS patients with ketanserin. *Thesis.* Erasmus University, Rotterdam, The Netherlands. 37–51.
148. Maura, G., Roccatagliata, E., Raiteri, M. (1986). Serotonin autoreceptor in rat hippocampus: pharmacological characterization as a subtype of the 5-HT1 receptor. *Naunyn Schmiedebergs Arch Pharmacol* 334:323–326.
149. Tack, J., Fried, M., Houghton, L.A., Spicak, J., Fisher, G. (2006). Systematic review: the efficacy of treatments for irritable bowel syndrome–a European perspective. *Aliment Pharmacol Ther* 24:183–205.
150. Gyermek, L. (1995). 5-HT3 receptors: pharmacologic and therapeutic aspects. *J Clin Pharmacol* 35:845–855.
151. Papadopoulos, I.A., Georgiou, P.E., Katsimbri, P.P., Drosos, A.A. (2000). Treatment of fibromyalgia with tropisetron, a 5HT3 serotonin antagonist: a pilot study. *Clin Rheumatol* 19:6–8.

152. Haus, U., Varga, B., Stratz, T., Späth, M., Müller, W. (2000). Oral treatment of fibromyalgia with tropisetron given over 28 days: influence on functional and vegetative symptoms, psychometric parameters and pain. *Scand J Rheumatol Suppl* 113:55–58.

153. Hrycaj, P., Stratz, T., Mennet, P., Müller, W. (1996). Pathogenetic aspects of responsiveness to ondansetron (5-hydroxytryptamine type 3 receptor antagonist) in patients with primary fibromyalgia syndrome—a preliminary study. *J Rheumatol* 23:1418–1423.

154. Höcherl, K., Färber, L., Ladenburger, S., Vosshage, D., Stratz, T., Müller, W., Grobecker, H. (2000). Effect of tropisetron on circulating catecholamines and other putative biochemical markers in serum of patients with fibromyalgia. *Scand J Rheumatol Suppl* 113:46–48.

155. Färber, L., Stratz, T., Brückle, W., Späth, M., Pongratz, D., Lautenschlager, J., Kötter, I., Zöller, B., Peter, H.H., Neeck, G., Alten, R., Müller, W. (2000). Efficacy and tolerability of tropisetron in primary fibromyalgia—a highly selective and competitive 5-HT3 receptor antagonist. German Fibromyalgia Study Group. *Scand J Rheumatol Suppl* 113:49–54.

156. Müller, W., Stratz, T. (2000). Results of the intravenous administration of tropisetron in fibromyalgia patients. *Scand J Rheumatol Suppl* 113:59–62.

157. Stratz, T., Fiebich, B., Haus, U., Müller, W. (2004). Influence of tropisetron on the serum substance P levels in fibromyalgia patients. *Scand J Rheumatol Suppl* 119:41–43.

158. Stratz, T., Müller, W. (2004). Treatment of chronic low back pain with tropisetron. *Scand J Rheumatol Suppl* 119:76–78.

159. Stratz, T., Varga, B., Müller, W. (2002). Treatment of tendopathies with tropisetron. *Rheumatol Int* 22:219–221.

160. Stratz, T., Färber, L., Müller, W. (2002). Local treatment of tendinopathies: a comparison between tropisetron and depot corticosteroids combined with local anesthetics. *Scand J Rheumatol* 31:366–370.

161. Ettlin, T. (2004). Trigger point injection treatment with the 5-HT3 receptor antagonist tropisetron in patients with late whiplash-associated disorder. First results of a multiple case study. *Scand J Rheumatol Suppl* 119:49–50.

162. Müller, W., Stratz, T. (2005). The use of the 5-HT_3 receptor antagonist tropisetron in trigger point therapy: a pilot study. *J Musculoskelet Pain* 13:43–48.

163. Voog, Ü, Alstergren, P., Leibur, E., Kallikorm, R., Kopp, S. (2000). Immediate effects of the serotonin antagonist granisetron on temporomandibular joint pain in patients with systemic inflammatory disorders. *Life Sci* 68:591–602.

164. Samborski, W., Stratz, T., Mackiewicz, S., Müller, W. (2004). Intra-articular treatment of arthritides and activated osteoarthritis with the 5-HT3 receptor antagonist tropisetron. A double-blind study compared with methylprednisolone. *Scand J Rheumatol Suppl* 119:51–54.

165. Stratz, T., Müller, W. (2004). Treatment of systemic sclerosis with the 5-HT3 receptor antagonist tropisetron. *Scand J Rheumatol Suppl* 119:59–62.

166. McCleane, G.J., Suzuki, R., Dickenson, A.H. (2003). Does a single intravenous injection of the 5HT3 receptor antagonist ondansetron have an analgesic effect in neuropathic pain? A double-blinded, placebo-controlled cross-over study. *Anesth Analg* 97:1474–1478.

CHAPTER 11

Adrenergic Receptors

ANTTI PERTOVAARA

Biomedicum Helsinki, Institute of Biomedicine/Physiology, University of Helsinki

Content

Peripheral Receptor Targets for Analgesia: Novel Approaches to Pain Management, Edited by Brian E. Cairns

11.1 OVERVIEW

Adrenoceptors are classified into various subtypes of α- and β-adrenoceptors. Peripheral adrenoceptors that potentially influence pain are located on sensory nerves, on postganglionic sympathetic nerve fibers, and on peripheral immune cells. Endogenous ligands of peripheral adrenoceptors are catecholamines norepinephrine and epinephrine, which are released from the postganglionic sympathetic nerve fibers and the adrenal medulla, respectively. Peripheral norepinephrine or epinephrine has little influence on pain in healthy tissues, whereas in injured tissues, they have variable effects, including aggravation of pain. The peripheral pronociceptive effect of norepinephrine has been associated with injury-induced expression of novel noradrenergic receptors, sprouting of sympathetic nerve fibers, and pronociceptive changes in the ionic channel properties of primary afferent nociceptors, while antinociceptive changes in the electrophysiological properties of sensory nerves and an interaction with the immune system may contribute to peripheral antinociception induced by norepinephrine. While there is a considerable amount of experimental evidence suggesting that peripheral α2-adrenoceptors activate various pain facilitatory mechanisms, clinical studies suggest that the net effect induced by activation of peripheral α2-adrenoceptors is pain suppression. Peripheral α1- and β-adrenoceptors may predominantly facilitate pain.

11.2 ADRENERGIC RECEPTORS

Catecholamine receptors are classically divided into two main categories: α- and β-adrenoceptors. α-Adrenoceptors are classified into subtypes 1A, 1B, 1D, 2A, 2B, and 2C, and β-adrenoceptors into subtypes 1, 2, and 3 [1,2]. In general, guanine nucleotide-binding regulatory proteins (G proteins) mediate the actions of adrenoceptors. α2-Adrenoceptors decrease intracellular adenylcyclase activity through G_i or directly modify the activity of ion channels such as the Na^+/H^+ transporter, Ca^{2+} channels, or K^+ channels [3]. β-adrenoceptors increase adenylcyclase activity through G_s. α1-Adrenoceptors are coupled to phospholipase C through G_q, or they are coupled directly to Ca^{2+} influx [3]. Adrenoceptors located on the catecholaminergic neurons are considered autoreceptors. α2-Adrenergic autoreceptors located in the somatodendritic area inhibit impulse discharge of adrenergic neurons, and those on axon terminals inhibit the release of the adrenergic neurotransmitter. Adrenoceptors located on nonadrenergic target cells are heteroreceptors that have varying effects depending on the target cell and the subtype of the adrenoceptor. α-Adrenoceptors have a key role in mediating pain regulatory effects of norepinephrine, whereas β-adrenoceptors may predominantly mediate epinephrine-induced modulation of pain.

The main sources of peripheral catecholamines are local release from postganglionic sympathetic nerve fibers and systemic release from the adrenal medulla. Postganglionic sympathetic nerve fibers release norepinephrine, whereas the adrenal medulla releases predominantly epinephrine. Assessments of mRNA in the dorsal root ganglion indicate that primary afferent neurons possess several types of α-adrenoceptors that potentially mediate peripheral actions of norepinephrine. All three subtypes of α1A, 1B, and 1D have been identified in the dorsal root ganglion [4,5], although mRNA for α1D-receptor has not been found in all studies [6]. Of these three subtypes of α1-adrenoceptors, subtype 1A is the most strongly expressed one in the dorsal root ganglion of intact animals [4]. The dorsal root ganglion also expresses α2-adrenoceptors. In intact animals, subtype α2C is the most common (80%) followed by α2A (20%), while α2B is rare in the dorsal root ganglion [7; however, see References 8 and 9]. While there are results suggesting that the dorsal root ganglion of an intact rat has no mRNA expression for β1- or β2-adrenoceptors [6], there are also results according to which the dorsal root ganglion neurons of an intact rat express mRNA for the β1-, β2-, and β3-adrenoceptors [5]. It is noteworthy that the immune system plays a significant role in pathophysiological pain conditions [10], and that the peripheral immune system expresses both α- and β-adrenoceptors [11]. Thus, adrenergic agents may modulate the excitability of primary afferent neurons not only through direct action on peripheral neurons but also indirectly through action on the immune system.

11.3 SENSORY EFFECTS BY CUTANEOUS ADMINISTRATION OF ENDOGENOUS ADRENERGIC LIGANDS

Administration of norepinephrine to the skin of healthy subjects does not evoke pain, although it may induce selective hyperalgesia to thermal stimulation [12]. However, in pathophysiological conditions, peripheral norepinephrine may have a significant influence on nerve endings mediating pain. This is shown by the finding that administration of norepinephrine or epinephrine to inflamed or neuropathic skin in humans aggravated pain and hyperalgesia [13–18], and plasma norepinephrine level was higher in patients with painful than nonpainful diabetic polyneuropathy [19]. In line with this, capsaicin-induced hypersensitivity [20,21], and in some conditions also spontaneous pain [21], was reduced by local administration of an α-adrenoceptor antagonist in humans. However, cutaneous administration of norepinephrine does not have a pronociceptive effect in all types of neuropathic conditions. This is shown by the findings that norepinephrine in the skin did not aggravate pain or hyperalgesia in a group of patients with painful sensory polyneuropathy [22] or complex regional pain syndrome [23], nor was capsaicin-induced pain or hyperalgesia influenced following physiological manipulations attenuating or increasing sympathetic activity in the skin [24]. In complex regional pain syndrome (see Chapter 2), pain relief induced by sympathectomy varied with time being stronger in the acute than in the chronic stage [25]. Curiously, in a subset of patients with complex regional pain syndrome, intradermal injection of an α1-adrenoceptor agonist produced pain in the intact, contralateral side, probably due to a central mechanism [26]. In inflamed conditions, peripheral injection of norepinephrine has had an antinociceptive [27] as well as a pronociceptive [28–31] action. Epinephrine may have a predominantly pronociceptive action in the skin as indicated by the finding that its intraplantar injection induced hypersensitivity in rats [32].

11.4 PLASTICITY IN PERIPHERAL ADRENERGIC SYSTEMS FOLLOWING INJURY OR INFLAMMATION

In line with psychophysical observations, neurophysiological studies in experimental animals indicate that intact nociceptive primary afferent fibers are only little, if at all, influenced by norepinephrine, by sympathetic stimulation, or by synthetic noradrenergic compounds [33,34]. Following peripheral nerve injury, however, myelinated and unmyelinated afferent nerve fibers innervating neuroma become sensitive to sympathetic stimulation and adrenergic compounds [35–39; however, see Reference 40]. Particularly injured nociceptive C-fibers, and to a lesser extent nociceptive Aδ-fibers, are excited by norepinephrine and by sympathetic stimulation [33,41–44]. Also inflammation or sensitization of the receptive field by heat or algogenic chemicals may lead to circumstances in which norepinephrine and sympathetic stimulation excite nociceptors [31,45–47; however, see Reference 48]. Norepinephrine-induced changes in nociceptor excitability may vary depending on the type of the stimulus used for eliciting the response. This is shown by the finding that after bradykinin treatment of the skin, norepinephrine alone excites C-fiber nociceptors, sensitizes C-nociceptors to subsequent bradykinin treatment, but suppresses their heat-evoked responses [49]. Peripheral nerve injury-induced sensitivity changes have been associated with sympathetic sprouting in the dorsal root ganglion [50–53] and in the skin [54–56]. Sympathetic sprouting of the dorsal root ganglion increased with age [57], and it was associated rather with mechanical than with thermal hypersensitivity [58].

In the dorsal root ganglion, the sprouting sympathetic fibers have contacts predominantly with large, neuropeptide-negative, presumably nonnociceptive neurons [51,53,59]. However, norepinephrine released from sympathetic sprouts may spread through volume transmission to small, nociceptive neurons. Moreover, if ectopic activity occurred in mechanoreceptive primary afferents, it might promote pain due to central convergence of inputs to wide dynamic range neurons of the spinal dorsal horn that are considered to have a role in mediation of pain [60]. Lidocaine treatment prevented the injury-induced sympathetic sprouting, suggesting that ectopic activity in the injured nerves has a role in the sprouting [61]. Nerve injury-induced mechanical hypersensitivity and sympathetic sprouting were reduced in mice with a knockout of cytokine interleukin-6 (see Chapter 4), indicating that that interleukin-6 has a facilitatory role in sympathetic sprouting [62].

Nerve injury influences expression of peripheral adrenoceptors as indicated by the finding that novel adrenoceptors, particularly α2A-adrenoceptors, develop in the peripheral terminals, perineurally at the injured site in the axon, and in the dorsal root ganglion [5,7,63–65] (Table 11.1). Injury may induce changes also in the expression of α2C-adrenoceptors in nociceptive peripheral nerve fibers. This is shown by the finding that following spinal nerve ligation, coexpression of α2C-adrenoceptors with immunoreactivity for transient receptor potential vanilloid 1 (TRPV1), an indicator of nociceptive functions, was increased in medium and large dorsal root ganglion cells [66], while some studies reported that peripheral nerve injury causes a decrease in the expression of peripheral α2C-adrenoceptors [7,64]. In contrast to nerve injury, peripheral inflammation produced little, if any, changes in the α2A- or α2C-adrenoceptor immunoreactivity or mRNA expression in the dorsal root ganglion [7,63]. Nerve injury also influences the expression of α1-adrenoceptors in the dorsal root ganglion: following nerve injury, the mRNA expression of the 1B subtype is increased, while that of 1A may decrease [4,5]. Curiously, although mRNA expression for the α1D-adrenoceptor was decreased in the dorsal root ganglion ipsilateral to the nerve injury, it was markedly increased in the contralateral, uninjured side [5]. In human patients with reflex sympathetic dystrophy (a form of chronic neuropathic pain), the density of cutaneous α1-adrenoceptors was significantly greater than in healthy control subjects, suggesting that α1-adrenoceptors might play a role in hyperalgesia associated with reflex sympathetic dystrophy [67]. Increased mRNA expression for the β2-adrenoceptor has also been described in the dorsal root ganglion following peripheral nerve injury [5]. Postganglionic sympathetic nerve fibers contain not only norepinephrine but also nonadrenergic substances. It should be noted that the release of nonadrenergic substances such as neuropeptide Y from the sympathetic nerves contributes to the modulation of responses in peripheral nerve fibers [68].

TABLE 11.1. The Change in the Expression of Adrenoceptors on Peripheral Somatosensory Neurons following Nerve Injury or Inflammation.

Adrenoceptor Type	Nerve Injury	Inflammation
α_{2A}	↑ [5,7,63–65]	↔ [7,63]
α_{2B}	↓ [5]	
α_{2C}	↑ [66] or ↔[5,63] or ↓ [7,64]	↔ [7,63]
α_{2D}	↑ [5]	
α_{1A}	↓ [4,5]	
α_{1B}	↑ [4,5]	
α_{1D}	↓ [5] and contralateral ↑ [5]	
β_1	↓ [5]	
β_2	↑ [5]	
β_3	↓ [5]	

11.5 PATHOPHYSIOLOGICAL CHANGES IN PERIPHERAL MECHANISMS CONTRIBUTING TO ADRENERGIC PAIN MODULATION

Genetically modified animals without N-type Ca^{2+} channels have reduced symptoms of inflammatory and neuropathic pain, indicating that the N-type Ca^{2+} channel is of importance for the development of neuropathic and inflammatory hypersensitivity [69]. Coupling of α2-adrenoceptors to N-type Ca^{2+} channels in injured nociceptive nerve fibers has been shown to be involved in noradrenergic generation of ectopic activity in injured peripheral nerve fibers that were presumably nociceptive ones [53,70] (Table 11.2). Norepinephrine-induced blockade of the N-type Ca^{2+} channels inhibits Ca^{2+}-activated K^+ channels (K_{Ca}). The consequent decrease of K^+ outflow from neurons has a depolarizing effect, and it provides a plausible explanation for the norepinephrine-induced increase in excitability and ectopic firing in dorsal root ganglion neurons of nerve-injured animals [53]. Nerve injury increases subthreshold membrane oscillation in dorsal root ganglion neurons. Subthreshold membrane oscillation depends on tetrodotoxin-sensitive Na^+ channels, and it is likely to contribute to neuropathic pain [71]. Norepinephrine, due to action on α2-adrenoceptors, increases subthreshold membrane oscillation in dorsal

TABLE 11.2. Adrenergic Mechanisms Influencing Peripheral Nociceptive Signals.

Action	Mediated by	Change in Nociception
Block of N-type calcium channel [70], leading to inhibition of K_{Ca} channel [53]	α2-AR	↑
Increase of subthreshold membrane oscillation [44]	α2-AR	↑
Enhanced response of $P2X_{2/3}$ receptors [5]	α1B-AR	↑
Enhancement of the stimulus-evoked increase of intracellular calcium [100,101]	α1- and β1-AR	↑
Activation of hyperpolarization-induced inward current (I_h) [95]	β-AR	↑
Decrease of subthreshold membrane oscillation [72]	α2-AR	↓
Reduction in the stimulus-evoked increase of intracellular calcium [98]	α2-AR	↓
Inhibition of hyperpolarization-induced inward current (I_h) [95]	α2-AR	↓
Opioid release from immune cells [27]	α1-, α2-, and β1-AR	↓
Reduced expression of proinflammatory cytokines [115]	α2A-AR	↓

AR, adrenoceptor.

root ganglion neurons, indicating that it is one of the pronociceptive noradrenergic mechanisms in the periphery [44]. In contrast to this finding, results of another intracellular recording study indicated that the nerve injury-induced membrane oscillation in dorsal root ganglion neurons was reduced following perineural administration of an α2-adrenoceptor agonist [72]. A recent whole-cell patch-clamp study indicated that following nerve injury, the slow type of ATP-evoked currents in dorsal root ganglion neurons, possibly mediated by $P2X_{2/3}$ receptors, was potentiated by norepinephrine, and this potentiation was reversed by a selective inhibitor of protein kinase C [5]. Based on this, it was proposed that norepinephrine released in association with noradrenergic sprouting into the dorsal root ganglion after peripheral nerve injury amplifies pain by enhancing $P2X_{2/3}$ receptor responses due to protein kinase C activation [5]. Furthermore, a parallel assessment of mRNA expression for various subtypes of adrenoceptors suggested that the norepinephrine-induced amplification of the sensory neuronal response in the dorsal root ganglion ipsilateral to nerve injury was mediated by the α1B-adrenoceptor and a consequent activation of G_q protein and protein kinase C [5]. A selective inhibitor of protein kinase A attenuated norepinephrine-induced subthreshold membrane oscillation, an underlying mechanism for the increased excitatory effect of norepinephrine in injured peripheral nerves [44]. This finding suggests that protein kinase A, possibly due to its action on voltage-gated Na^+ channels [73], is an intracellular messenger contributing to the excitation of nociceptors following the administration of norepinephrine into a neuropathic skin region.

Epinephrine-induced sensitization of primary afferent nociceptors has been shown to be mediated both by the protein kinase A and protein kinase C second messenger pathways [32]. It should be noted that noradrenergic modulation of somatosensory signals in primary afferent nerve fibers may not be a unique feature for nociceptors. Namely, five decades ago, it was shown that sympathomimetic agents and sympathetic stimulation modulate the activity of Pacinian corpuscles that mediate vibrotactile sensations [74].

11.6 FINDINGS SUPPORTING A PAIN FACILITATORY ROLE OF PERIPHERAL α2-ADRENOCEPTORS

The novel α2-adrenoceptors in the peripheral nerves may have a pronociceptive role as suggested by the electrophysiological findings that the excitatory effects induced by sympathetic stimulation and norepinephrine were attenuated by α2-adrenoceptor antagonists, and that the excitation of nociceptors induced by norepinephrine was mimicked by α2-adrenoceptor agonists [28,33,43,53,70,75,76]. The hypothesis that peripheral α2-adrenoceptors have a pain-inducing role in hyperalgesic skin is also supported by the following behavioral findings. Both the norepinephrine-induced and a nerve injury-induced hypersensitivity were attenuated by an α2-adrenoceptor antagonist but not by an α1-adrenoceptor antagonist [29,77–79]. Rekindling of mechanical hypersensitivity in nerve-injured animals by cutaneous administration of an α2-adrenoceptor agonist, but not by an α1-adrenoceptor agonist, supports the interpretation that peripheral α2-adrenoceptors mediate the norepinephrine-induced pain from the hyperalgesic skin [80]. In an experimental model of peripheral neuritis, intradermal injection of norepinephrine aggravated mechanical hyperalgesia [30]. This pronociceptive effect of norepinephrine was attenuated not only by an α2-adrenoceptor antagonist but also an α1-adrenoceptor antagonist suggesting that in neuritis, both the α2- and α1-adrenoceptors are mediating the peripheral pronociceptive effect of norepinephrine [30]. Cutaneous administration of norepinephrine aggravated nerve injury-induced hyperalgesia in an α2-adrenoceptor antagonist-reversible fashion, and this pronociceptive effect by norepinephrine was abolished following sympathectomy, suggesting that α2-adrenoceptors on postganglionic sympathetic terminals mediated the hyperalgesic effect [81]. The subtype A of the peripheral α2-adrenoceptor may have a selective role in mediating the norepinephrine-induced enhancement of pain. This is suggested by the finding that a peripherally acting α2-adrenoceptor antagonist selectively attenuated nerve injury-induced heat hyperalgesia in wild-type mice, and a knockout of α2A-adrenoceptors selectively attenuated the development of heat hyperalgesia after nerve injury [82].

11.7 BEHAVIORAL FINDINGS SUPPORTING A PAIN INHIBITORY ROLE OF PERIPHERAL α2-ADRENOCEPTORS AND PAIN FACILITATORY ROLE OF α1-ADRENOCEPTORS (AND β-ADRENOCEPTORS)

Although a number of studies suggest that the norepinephrine-induced pain response in the periphery is due to the activation of α2-adrenoceptors, there is a large amount of behavioral and neurophysiological evidence supporting the concept that it is the α1-adrenoceptor that mediates the norepinephrine-induced pain response, and that the peripheral α2-adrenoceptor has a pain-suppressive role. The following behavioral results support the hypothesis that peripheral α2-adrenoceptors have a pain inhibitory role. Peripheral administration of an α2-adrenoceptor agonist attenuated nociceptive responses in control animals [83] and hypersensitivity in inflammatory and neuropathic conditions [65,84–86]. In line with this, topical administration of norepinephrine increased pain, whereas an α2-adrenoceptor agonist relieved pain in human patients with a reflex sympathetic dystrophy [13]. Topical application of an α2-adrenoceptor agonist also attenuated pain in a subset of patients with diabetic neuropathy [87] or postherpetic neuralgia [88]. Moreover, intra-articular administration of a low dose of an α2-adrenoceptor agonist significantly attenuated postoperative pain by surgery of the knee joint in humans [89] and experimental arthritis in rats [90]. In arthritic mice, a knockout of the α2A-adrenoceptor or intra-articular, but not intrathecal, administration of an α2-adrenoceptor antagonist reversed the antihyperalgesic effect induced by transcutaneous electrical stimulation [91]. This finding suggests that the α2A-adrenoceptor is involved in mediating the peripheral pain-suppressive effect induced by transcutaneous electrical stimulation.

Pain-related behavior induced by intraplantar injection of norepinephrine and the selective serotonin (5-HT)2 receptor agonist α-methyl-5-HT was suppressed by an α1A-adrenoceptor antagonist but not by an α1B-adrenoceptor antagonist indicating that peripheral α1A-adrenoceptors promote pain [92]. Further evidence for the pronociceptive role of cutaneous α1-adrenoceptors is provided by a recent experimental human study showing that cutaneous administration of an α1-adrenoceptor agonist augmented thermal hyperalgesia in mildly burnt skin and that this pronociceptive effect was reversed by an α1-adrenoceptor antagonist [93]. The finding that mechanical hypersensitivity induced by intraplantar injection of epinephrine in rats was reversed by propranolol, an antagonist of β-adrenoceptors, suggests that peripheral β-adrenoceptors mediate epinephrine-induced hypersensitivity [32].

11.8 NEUROPHYSIOLOGICAL FINDINGS SUPPORTING A PAIN INHIBITORY ROLE OF PERIPHERAL α2-ADRENOCEPTORS AND PAIN FACILITATORY ROLE OF α1-ADRENOCEPTORS (AND β-ADRENOCEPTORS)

The hypothesis that the peripheral α2-adrenoceptor suppresses pain is supported by the neurophysiological findings indicating that the ectopic activity of injured nerve fibers is suppressed by an α1-adrenoceptor antagonist but not by an α2-adrenoceptor antagonist [79], and that following development of neurogenic inflammation, sympathectomy or an α1-adrenoceptor antagonist attenuates hypersensitivity of peripheral nociceptors [47]. In line with this, intracellular recording of dorsal root ganglion neurons indicated that perineural administration of an α2-adrenoceptor agonist attenuated axotomy-induced hyperexcitability [72]. A pain facilitatory role of α1-adrenoceptors is supported by the finding that an α1-adrenoceptor agonist more effectively activated C-fiber nociceptors innervating a partially denervated skin than an α2-adrenoceptor agonist [94]. A whole-cell patch-clamp study of dorsal root ganglion neurons indicated that an α2-adrenoceptor agonist inhibits and a β-adrenoceptor agonist increases a hyperpolarization-activated inward (excitatory) current [95]. Because the hyperpolarization-induced inward current (I_h) presumably facilitates the neuronal firing discharge, a plausible explanation for this *in vitro* electrophysiological finding is that α2-adrenoceptors have an antinociceptive effect on peripheral sensory neurons and β-adrenoceptors have a pronociceptive effect. This interpretation is supported by a behavioral study showing that perineural injection of a selective blocker of the hyperpolarization-activated cation current (I_h) reduced neuropathic and postoperative hypersensitivity [96]. Another whole-cell patch-clamp study showed that isoprenalin, a β-adrenoceptor agonist, reduced excitability of cultured dorsal root ganglion neurons, while phenylephrine, an α1-adrenoceptor agonist, had an opposite effect [97]. Intracellular Ca^{2+} response in dorsal root ganglion neurons, the key determinant of neurotransmitter release, was decreased by an α2, but not by an α1-adrenoceptor agonist, and this decrease was particularly strong in neurons obtained from nerve-injured animals [98].

Sustained activation of C-polymodal nociceptors by capsaicin produces tonic pain and neurogenic inflammation. It has been shown that a dorsal root reflex (i.e., centrifugal activation of primary afferent nerve nociceptors) contributes to the development of neurogenic inflammation in the skin and that sympathetic efferents acting on peripheral α1-adrenoceptors facilitate triggering of a dorsal root reflex in nociceptive nerve fibers [99]. This finding is in line with the evidence that norepinephrine acting on peripheral α1-adrenoceptors predominantly facilitates nociceptors. Cultured dorsal root ganglion neurons that were infected with varicella zoster virus gave significantly increased calcium responses to norepinephrine, phenylephrine (α1-adrenoceptor agonist), and isoproterenol (β1-adrenoceptor agonist) [100,101]. This finding suggests that peripheral α1- and β1-adrenoceptors contribute to pain and allodynia in shingles and in postherpetic neuralgia. On the other hand, hypersensitivity induced by herpes simplex virus inoculation in mice was not modulated by various α-adrenoceptor antagonists, suggesting that noradrenergic mechanisms are not involved in maintenance of hypersensitivity induced by herpetic infection [102].

11.9 ROLE OF THE IMMUNE SYSTEM IN MEDIATING ADRENERGIC PAIN MODULATION IN THE PERIPHERY

It has been suggested that release of opioidergic peptides from cutaneous immune cells may be mediating the pain-suppressive effect of norepinephrine in the inflamed skin of rats [27] (Table 11.2). This hypothesis is supported by findings that various types of adrenoceptors are found on immune cells and the antihyperalgesic effect induced by intraplantar or intra-articular administration of norepinephrine or an α2-adrenoceptor agonist was reversed not only by adrenoceptor antagonists but also by opioid receptor antagonists [27,84,90]. Interestingly, the norepinephrine-induced, opioid-mediated antihyperalgesia was reversed not only by an antagonist of α2-adrenoceptors but also by an antagonist of α1- or β1-adrenoceptors [27]. Thus, the immune cell-mediated pain-suppressive effect of peripheral norepinephrine seems to involve three different types of adrenoceptors.

A series of studies with experimental animal models of nerve injury and neuritis indicate that α2-adrenoceptors may modulate hypersensitivity not only due to action on inflammatory reaction in the tissues surrounding nociceptive terminals but also more proximally adjacent to the axon of the peripheral nerve. Following injury of the sciatic nerve, immunostaining for α2A-adrenoceptors was increased both in neurons and in immune cells, particularly macrophages and T lymphocytes, and perineural injection of an α2-adrenoceptor agonist at the injury site produced a long-lasting antihypersensitivity effect [65]. Long-lasting attenuation of neuropathic hypersensitivity by perineural injection of an α2-adrenoceptor agonist was accompanied by a reduction in the tissue content of proinflammatory cytokines interleukin-1 (IL-1)β and tumor necrosis factor α in the nerve injury site [103,104]. Perineural administration of an α2-adrenoceptor agonist also reduced p38 mitogen-activated protein kinase (MAPK) in injured primary afferent neurons [105]. Because p38 MAPK presumably drives sensitization of sensory neurons and it is increased by proinflammatory cytokines, its reduction probably explains the antihypersensitivity effect induced by perineural administration of an α2-adrenoceptor agonist. Neuritis-induced hypersensitivity and increase in proinflammatory cytokines were reduced by perineural injection of an α2-adrenoceptor agonist [106], and the antihypersensitive effect by a perineurally administered α2-adrenoceptor agonist was enhanced in persistent neuritis [107]. The slow onset and long duration of the α2-adrenergic antihypersensitivity effect by perineural treatment of neuritis were associated with a change in the balance of pro- and anti-inflammatory leukocytes that had a corresponding time course, indicating that the antihypersensitivity effect by perineural administration of an α2-adrenoceptor agonist may be explained by a local anti-inflammatory response [107].

11.10 ADRENERGIC PAIN MODULATION IN THE PERIPHERY: SUMMARY OF MIXED RESULTS

Peripheral norepinephrine has only little influence on pain in physiological conditions, but in inflamed and neuropathic conditions, it may aggravate pain [13–16], although not in all groups of patients [22]. A predominantly antinociceptive effect following peripheral administration of norepinephrine has also been described in inflammatory conditions [27]. Sympathetic sprouting and development of novel adrenoceptors accompany injury- and inflammation-induced changes in the function of peripheral norepinephrine (Table 11.1). It has been postulated that norepinephrine released from sympathetic sprouts and acting on novel adrenoceptors may contribute to maintenance of chronic pain and hyperalgesia [108]. It is still a matter of debate on which subtype of adrenoceptor in the periphery contributes to aggravation of pain and which one contributes to suppression of pain. Coexpression of multiple adrenoceptor types in the same peripheral neurons [8] is likely to contribute to the variability in norepinephrine-induced effects because different adrenoceptor types have at least partly different functions, and the expression of various adrenoceptor subtypes and their functional effects varies with the pathophysiological condition (e.g., see Reference 63), over time following injury [109], and with the strain of the experimental animals [29]. The net effect by a peripherally administered adrenoceptor agonist is a mixture of actions by the presynaptic adrenoceptor on the terminal of a postganglionic sympathetic nerve fiber, postsynaptic adrenoceptor on the nonadrenergic sensory neuron, and adrenoceptor on an adjacent immune cell; the same subtype of the adrenoceptor may have effects that vary widely between these different locations, which adds to the complexity of peripheral adrenergic actions. Both facilitatory (e.g., see References 53 and 70) and inhibitory (e.g., see Reference 95) neuronal mechanisms activated by noradrenergic compounds have been shown to exist in the dorsal root ganglion cells, a finding that is in line with the variability of the peripheral pain modulatory actions of norepinephrine (Table 11.2). Also, there is conflicting neurophysiological evidence on whether the excitatory effect of norepinephrine in the periphery is due to a direct action on peripheral nociceptors independent of the sympathetic nerve fibers [110–112], indirect action on nociceptors via the release of prostaglandins from the postganglionic sympathetic nerve fibers [113,114], or both. In inflamed tissues, opioid release from immune cells may be involved in mediating the pain-suppressive actions of norepinephrine on nociceptors [27]. Furthermore, perineural administration of α2-adrenoceptor agonists may reduce neuritis- or nerve injury-induced symptoms by suppressing proinflammatory cytokines and by promoting anti-inflammatory response [115].

11.11 POSTGANGLIONIC SYMPATHETIC NERVE FIBERS IN PAIN MODULATION

In healthy subjects, the sympathetic nervous system has only a small effect on pain, but following a nerve injury, it may have a significant and complex role in the regulation of pain [116]. In nerve-injured patients, the postganglionic sympathetic nerve fibers may interact with afferent neurons and may induce activity in nociceptors. This coupling between primary afferent nociceptive nerve fibers and postganglionic sympathetic nerve fibers may take place at the site of lesion or at a distant site, such as the dorsal root ganglion [117]. This pathologic interaction acts via norepinephrine released from sympathetic terminals and novel adrenoceptors on the nociceptive nerve fibers [108]. This pathological mechanism may contribute to the development of chronic allodynia, hyperalgesia, and spontaneous pain. One more hypothesis to explain the contribution of postganglionic sympathetic nerve fibers to chronic nerve injury-related pain is that cutaneous release of norepinephrine from the sympathetic nerves may produce pain by activating mechanoreceptive primary afferent nerve fibers with convergent inputs to pain-relay neurons in the spinal dorsal horn [118]. It should be noted that development of sympathetically maintained pain does not necessarily require higher than normal activity in the sympathetic nervous system, but due to nerve injury-induced hypersensitivity, even a low sympathetic tone may produce strong noradrenergic effects in peripheral target tissues. In some groups of patients, the nerve injury-induced symptoms are relieved by sympathectomy, indicating that the sympathetic system, indeed, contributes to maintenance of neuropathic pain in a subgroup of patients [116,119]. In line with this, surgical sympathectomy or depletion of sympathetic transmitters by guanethidine attenuated thermal hyperalgesia in nerve-injured animals [120,121], and activation of the sympathetic system by whole body cooling or iontophoresis of norepinephrine into the skin aggravated heat hyperalgesia in a subgroup of nerve entrapment patients with preexisting heat hyperalgesia [122]. Further evidence for the role of the sympathetic system in pain aggravation is given by the finding that activation of the sympathetic system by whole body cooling increased spontaneous pain and spatial distribution of mechanical hyperalgesia in a group of patients with complex regional pain syndrome [123].

Interestingly, while sympathectomy is used for the treatment of some chronic pain conditions (see above), sympathectomy per se may sensitize peripheral nociceptors to circulating norepinephrine [124], and this sensitization may lead to postsympathectomy neuralgia [125]. Sympathectomy per se also increased the peripheral antinociceptive action of a peripherally acting $\alpha 2$-adrenoceptor agonist, which may provide a possibility to relieve sympathectomy-induced hyperalgesia without central side effects [86].

11.12 POTENTIAL CONFOUNDING FACTORS IN THE ASSESSMENT OF PAIN MODULATION BY PERIPHERAL ADRENOCEPTORS

Postganglionic sympathetic nerve fibers and adrenergic receptors are involved in the regulation of cardiovascular, gastrointestinal, and respiratory systems [126]. Some of these adrenergic actions may provide confounding factors by indirectly influencing pain or pain measurements. For example, noradrenergic vasoconstriction of arteries may promote ischemia in peripheral tissues, and this may induce ischemic pain in some conditions.

When the latency of a radiant heat-induced sensory or withdrawal response is used as an index of pain sensitivity, it takes longer to reach the critical threshold temperature in cool than in warm skin. Therefore, an increased noradrenergic tone that causes vasoconstriction and a decrease of baseline skin temperature may produce an artifactual change in the index of pain sensitivity [127]. Decreased skin temperature caused by sympathetically induced vasoconstriction may also reduce inflammation, and this may lead to suppression of inflammation-related pain, without a change in the excitability of sensory neurons mediating pain sensation [127].

11.13 FUTURE IMPLICATIONS

Clinical studies suggest that peripheral administration of $\alpha 2$-adrenoceptor agonists might attenuate pain in some pathophysiological conditions

[13,87–89]. While central actions of α2-adrenoceptor agonists may induce analgesia [128], many of the side effects by α2-adrenoceptor agonists, such as sedation and blood pressure decrease, are also due to central actions. Therefore, topical administration of an α2-adrenoceptor agonist that only poorly spreads through the blood–brain barrier (e.g., see Reference 129) may provide a selective treatment, without central side effects, for some sympathetically maintained (e.g., see Reference 13) or inflammatory (e.g., References 27,84, and 115) pain conditions. Further studies are still needed to determine whether subtype-selective α2-adrenergic agents might prove more effective in the peripheral treatment of pain than those α2-adrenoceptor agonists that are currently available for clinical use. Peripheral analgesic actions by drugs acting on α1- or β-adrenoceptors have been only little studied in clinical settings, although experimental studies suggest that these receptors might contribute to pain in some pathophysiological conditions. Moreover, the dependence of peripheral α2-adrenergic antinociception on peripheral μ-opioid and adenosine A1 receptors [130] suggests that the interaction between adrenoceptors and other neurotransmitter receptors may provide a possibility to develop a combination therapy with enhanced peripheral analgesic action and reduced side effects.

ACKNOWLEDGMENTS

The author has been supported by grants from the Academy of Finland and from the Sigrid Jusélius Foundation, Helsinki, Finland. Some of the author's original studies on noradrenergic compounds were supported in part by Orion Pharma Inc., Turku, Finland.

REFERENCES

1. Ruffolo, R.R., Jr., Hieble, J.P. (1994). α-Adrenoceptors. *Pharmacol Ther* 61:1–64.
2. Bylund, D.B. (1995). Pharmacological characteristics of α_2 adrenergic subtypes. *Ann N Y Acad Sci* 763:1–7.
3. Summers, R.J., McMartin, L.R. (1993). Adrenoceptors and their second messenger systems. *J Neurochem* 60:10–23.
4. Xie, J., Lee Y.H., Wang, C., Chung J.M., Chung, K. (2001). Differential expression of α_1-adrenoceptor subtype mRNAs in the dorsal root ganglion after spinal nerve ligation. *Mol Brain Res* 93:164–172.
5. Maruo, K., Yamamoto, H., Yamamoto, S., Nagata, T., Fujikawa, H., Kanno, T., Yaguchi, T., Maruo, S., Yoshiya, S., Nishizaki, T. (2006). Modulation of P2X receptors via adrenergic pathways in rat dorsal root ganglion neurons after sciatic nerve injury. *Pain* 120:106–112.
6. Nicholson, R., Dixon, A.K., Spanswick, D., Lee, K. (2005). Noradrenergic receptor mRNA expression in adult rat superficial dorsal horn and dorsal root ganglion neurons. *Neurosci Lett* 380:316–321.

7. Shi, T.S., Winzer-Serhan, U., Leslie, F., Hökfelt, T. (2000). Distribution and regulation of α_2-adrenoceptors in rat dorsal root ganglia. *Pain* 84:319–330.
8. Gold, M.S., Dastmalchi, S., Levine, J.D. (1997). α2-Adrenergic receptor subtypes in rat dorsal root and superior cervical ganglion neurons. *Pain* 69:179–190.
9. Ongioco, R.R., Richardson, C.D., Rudner, X.L., Stafford-Smith, M., Schwinn, D.A. (2000). α_2-Adrenergic receptors in human dorsal root ganglia: predominance of α_{2b} and α_{2c} subtype mRNAs. *Anesthesiology* 92:968–976.
10. Moalem, G., Tracey, D.J. (2006). Immune and inflammatory mechanisms in neuropathic pain. *Brain Res Rev* 51:240–264.
11. Nance, D.M., Sanders, V.M. (2007). Autonomic innervation and regulation of the immune system (1987–2007). *Brain Behav Immun* 21:736–745.
12. Fuchs, P.N., Meyer, R.A., Raja, S.N. (2001). Heat, but not mechanical hyperalgesia, following adrenergic injections in normal human skin. *Pain* 90:15–23.
13. Davis, K.D., Treede, R.D., Raja, S.N., Meyer, R.A., Campbell, J.N. (1991). Topical application of clonidine relieves hyperalgesia in patients with sympathetically maintained pain. *Pain* 47:309–317.
14. Chabal, C., Jacobson, L., Russell, L.C., Burchiel, K.J. (1992). Pain response to perineuromal injection of normal saline, epinephrine, and lidocaine in humans. *Pain* 49:9–12.
15. Drummond, P.D. (1995). Noradrenaline increases hyperalgesia to heat in skin sensitized by capsaicin. *Pain* 60:311–315.
16. Torebjörk, H.E., Wahren, L., Wallin, G., Hallin, R., Koltzenburg, M. (1995). Noradrenaline-evoked pain in neuralgia. *Pain* 63:11–20.
17. Choi, B., Rowbotham, M.C. (1997). Effect of adrenergic receptor activation on post-herpetic neuralgia pain and sensory disturbances. *Pain* 69:55–63.
18. Ali, Z., Raja, S.N., Wesselmann, U., Fuchs, P.N., Meyer, R.A., Campbell, J.N. (2000). Intradermal injection of norepinephrine evokes pain in patients with sympathetically maintained pain. *Pain* 88:161–168.
19. Tsigos, C., Reed, P., Weinkove, C., White, A., Young, R.J. (1993). Plasma norepinephrine in sensory diabetic polyneuropathy. *Diabetes Care* 16:722–727.
20. Liu, M., Max, M.B., Parada, S., Rowan, J.S., Bennett, G.J. (1996). The sympathetic nervous system contributes to capsaicin-evoked mechanical allodynia but not pinprick hyperalgesia in humans. *J Neurosci* 16:7331–7335.
21. Kinnman, E., Nygårds, B.E., Hansson, P. (1997). Peripheral α-adrenoceptors are involved in the development of capsaicin induced ongoing and stimulus evoked pain in humans. *Pain* 69:79–85.
22. Schattschneider, J., Uphoff, J., Binder, A., Wasner, G., Baron, R. (2006). No adrenergic sensitization of afferent neurons in painful sensory polyneuropathy. *J Neurol* 253:280–286.
23. Birklein, F., Riedl, B., Claus, D., Neundorfer, B, Handwerker, H.O. (1997). Cutaneous norepinephrine application in complex regional pain syndrome. *Eur J Pain* 1:123–132.
24. Baron, R., Wasner, G., Borgstedt, R., Hastedt, E., Schulte, H., Binder, A., Kopper, F., Rowbotham, M., Levine, J.D., Fields, H.L. (1999). Effect of sympathetic activity on capsaicin-evoked pain, hyperalgesia, and vasodilatation. *Neurology* 52: 923–932.

25. Schattschneider, J., Binder, A., Siebrecht, D., Wasner, G., Baron, R. (2006). Complex regional pain syndromes: the influence of cutaneous and deep somatic sympathetic innervation on pain. *Clin J Pain* 22:240–244.

26. Mailis-Gagnon, A., Bennett, G.J. (2005). Abnormal contralateral pain responses from an intradermal injection of phenylephrine in a subset of patients with complex regional pain syndrome (CRPS). *Pain* 115:213–214.

27. Binder, W., Mousa, S.A., Sitte, N., Kaiser, M., Stein, C., Schäfer, M. (2004). Sympathetic activation triggers endogenous opioid release and analgesia within peripheral inflamed tissue. *Eur J Neurosci* 20:92–100.

28. Sato, J., Suzuki, S., Iseki, T., Kumazawa, T. (1993). Adrenergic excitation of cutaneous nociceptors in chronically inflamed rats. *Neurosci Lett* 164:225–228.

29. Banik, R.K., Sato, J., Yajima, H., Mizumura, K. (2001). Differences between the Lewis and Sprague-Dawley rats in chronic inflammation induced norepinephrine sensitivity of cutaneous C-fiber nociceptors. *Neurosci Lett* 299:21–24.

30. Baik, E., Chung, J.M., Chung, K. (2003). Peripheral norepinephrine exacerbates neuritis-induced hyperalgesia. *J Pain* 4:212–221.

31. Banik, R.K., Sato, J., Giron, R., Yajima, H., Mizumura, K. (2004). Interactions of bradykinin and norepinephrine on rat cutaneous nociceptors in both normal and inflamed conditions in vitro. *Neurosci Res* 49:421–425.

32. Khasar, S.G., McCarter, G., Levine, J.D. (1999). Epinephrine produces a β-adrenergic receptor-mediated mechanical hyperalgesia and *in vitro* sensitization of rat nociceptors. *J Neurosci* 81:1104–1112.

33. Sato, J., Perl, E.R. (1991). Adrenergic excitation of cutaneous pain receptors induced by peripheral nerve injury. *Science* 251:1608–1610.

34. Hämäläinen, M.M., Jyväsjärvi, E., Pertovaara, A. (1995). Can the α-2-adrenoceptor agonist-mediated suppression of nocifensive reflex responses be due to action on motoneurons or peripheral nociceptors? *Neurosci Lett* 196:29–32.

35. Wall, P.D., Gutnick, M. (1974). Ongoing activity in peripheral nerves: the physiology and pharmacology of impulses originating from a neuroma. *Exp Neurol* 43: 580–593.

36. Devor, M., Jänig, W. (1981). Activation of myelinated afferents ending in a neuroma by stimulation of the sympathetic supply in the rat. *Neurosci Lett* 24: 43–47.

37. Korenman, E.M., Devor, M. (1981). Ectopic adrenergic sensitivity in damaged peripheral nerve axons in the rat. *Exp Neurol* 72:63–81.

38. Scadding, J.W. (1981). Development of ongoing activity, mechanosensitivity, and adrenaline sensitivity in severed peripheral nerve axons. *Exp Neurol* 73:345–364.

39. Zhang, J.M., Song, X.J., LaMotte, R.H. (1997). An in vitro study of ectopic discharge generation and adrenergic sensitivity in the intact, nerve-injured rat dorsal root ganglion. *Pain* 72:51–57.

40. De Armentia, M.L., Leeson, A.H., Stebbing, M.J., Urban, L., McLachlan, E.M. (2003). Responses to sympathomimetics in rat sensory neurones after nerve transaction. *Neuroreport* 14:9–13.

41. Bossut, D.F., Perl, E.R. (1995). Effects of nerve injury on sympathetic excitation of A-delta mechanical nociceptors. *J Neurophysiol* 73:1721–1723.

42. Petersen, M., Zhang, J., Zhang, J.M., LaMotte, R.H. (1996). Abnormal spontaneous activity and response to norepinephrine in dissociated dorsal root ganglion cells after chronic nerve constriction. *Pain* 67:391–397.

43. Leem, J.W., Gwak, Y.S., Nam, T.S., Paik, K.S. (1997). Involvement of α_2-adrenoceptors in mediating sympathetic excitation of injured dorsal root ganglion neurons in rats with spinal nerve ligation. *Neurosci Lett* 234:39–42.

44. Xing, J.L., Hu, S.J., Jian, Z., Duan, J.H. (2003). Subthreshold membrane potential oscillation mediates the excitatory effect of norepinephrine in chronically compressed dorsal root ganglion neurons in the rat. *Pain* 105:177–183.

45. Roberts, W.J., Elardo, S.M. (1985). Sympathetic activation of Aδ nociceptors. *Somatosens Res* 3:33–44.

46. Hu, S.J., Zhu, J. (1989). Sympathetic facilitation of sustained discharges of polymodal nociceptors. *Pain* 38:85–90.

47. Ren, Y., Zou, X., Fang, L., Lin, Q. (2005). Sympathetic modulation of activity in Aδ- and C-primary nociceptive afferents after intradermal injection of capsaicin in rats. *J Neurophysiol* 93:365–377.

48. Shea, V.K., Perl, E.R. (1985). Failure of sympathetic stimulation to affect responsiveness of rabbit polymodal nociceptors. *J Neurophysiol* 54:513–519.

49. Sato, J., Yajima, H., Banik, R.K., Kumazawa, T., Mizumura, K. (2005). Norepinephrine reduces heat responses of cutaneous C-fiber nociceptors in Sprague-Dawley rats *in vitro*. *Neurosci Lett* 378:111–116.

50. Chung, K., Kim, H.J., Na, H.S., Park, M.J., Chung, J.M. (1993). Abnormalities of sympathetic innervation in the area of an injured spinal nerve in a rat neuropathic model. *Neurosci Lett* 162:85–88.

51. McLachlan, E.M., Jänig, W., Devor, M., Michaelis, M. (1993). Peripheral nerve injury triggers noradrenergic sprouting within dorsal root ganglia. *Nature* 363:543–546.

52. Ramer, M.S., Bisby, M.A. (1997). Rapid sprouting of sympathetic axons in dorsal root ganglia of rats with a chronic constriction injury. *Pain* 70:237–244.

53. Honma, Y., Yamakage, M., Ninomiya, T. (1999). Effects of adrenergic stimulus on the activities of Ca^{2+} and K^+ channels of dorsal root ganglion neurons in a neuropathic pain model. *Brain Res* 832:195–206.

54. Ruocco, I., Cuello, A.C., Ribeiro-da-Silva, A. (2000). Peripheral nerve injury leads to the establishment of a novel pattern of sympathetic fiber innervation in the rat skin. *J Comp Neurol* 422:287–296.

55. Grelik, C., Bennett, G.J., Ribeiro-da-Silva, A. (2005). Autonomic fibre sprouting and changes in nociceptive sensory innervation in the rat lower lip skin following chronic constriction injury. *Eur J Neurosci* 21:2475–2487.

56. Yen, L.D., Bennett, G.J., Ribeiro-da-Silva, A. (2006). Sympathetic sprouting and changes in nociceptive sensory innervation in the glabrous skin of the rat hind paw following partial peripheral nerve injury. *J Comp Neurol* 495:679–690.

57. Ramer, M.S., Bisby, M.A. (1998). Normal and injury-induced sympathetic innervation of rat dorsal root ganglia increases with age. *J Comp Neurol* 394:38–47.

58. Ramer, M.S., Bisby, M.A. (1998). Differences in sympathetic innervation of mouse DRG following proximal or distal nerve lesions. *Exp Neurol* 152:197–207.

59. Ramer, M.S., Bisby, M.A. (1998). Sympathetic axons surround neuropeptide-negative axotomized sensory neurons. *Neuroreport* 9:3109–3113.

60. Willis, W.D, Jr., Coggeshall, R.E. (1991). *Sensory Mechanisms of the Spinal Cord*, 2nd ed. New York: Plenum Press.

61. Zhang, J.M., Li, H., Munir, M.A. (2004). Decreasing sympathetic sprouting in pathologic sensory ganglia: a new mechanism for treating neuropathic pain using lidocaine. *Pain* 109:143–149.

62. Ramer, M.S., Murphy, P.G., Richardson, P.M., Bisby, M.A. (1998). Spinal nerve lesion-induced mechanoallodynia and adrenergic sprouting in sensory ganglia are attenuated in interleukin-6 knockout mice. *Pain* 78:115–121.

63. Birder, L.A., Perl, E.R. (1999). Expression of α_2-adrenergic receptors in rat primary afferent neurones after peripheral nerve injury or inflammation. *J Physiol* 515.2:533–542.

64. Cho, H.J., Kim, D.S., Lee, N.H., Kim, J.K., Lee, K.M., Han, K.S., Kang, Y.N., Kim, K.J. (1999). Changes in the α_2-adrenergic receptor subtypes gene expression in rat dorsal ganglion in an experimental model of neuropathic pain. *Neuroreport* 8:3119–3122.

65. Lavand'homme, P.M., Ma, W., De Kock, M., Eisenach, J.C. (2002). Perineural α_{2A}-adrenoceptor inhibits spinal cord neuroplasticity and tactile allodynia after nerve injury. *Anesthesiology* 97:972–980.

66. Ma, W., Zhang, Y., Bantel, C., Eisenach, J.C. (2005). Medium and large injured dorsal root ganglion cells increase TRPV-1, accompanied by increased α_{2C}-adrenoceptor co-expression and functional inhibition by clonidine. *Pain* 113: 386–394.

67. Drummond, P.D., Skipworth, S., Finch, P.M. (1996). α1-adrenoceptors in normal and hyperalgesic human skin. *Clin Sci (Lond)* 91:73–77.

68. Lin, Q., Zou, X., Ren, Y., Wang, J., Fang, L., Willis, W.D. (2004). Involvement of peripheral neuropeptide Y receptors in sympathetic modulation of acute cutaneous flare induced by intradermal capsaicin. *Neuroscience* 123:337–347.

69. Saegusa, H., Kurihara, T., Zong, S., Kazuno, A., Matsuda, Y., Nonaka, T., Han, W., Toriyama, H., Tanabe, T. (2001). Suppression of inflammatory and neuropathic pain symptoms in mice lacking the N-type Ca^{2+} channel. *EMBO J* 20:2349–2356.

70. Abdulla, F.A., Smith, P.A. (1997). Ectopic α_2-adrenoceptors couple to N-type Ca^{2+} channels in axotomized rat sensory neurons. *J Neurosci* 17:1633–1641.

71. Amir, R., Michaelis, M., Devor, M. (1999). Membrane oscillations in dorsal root ganglion neurons: role in normal electrogenesis and neuropathic pain. *J Neurosci* 19:8589–8596.

72. Liu, B., Eisenach, J.C. (2005) Hyperexcitability of axotomized and neighboring unaxotomized sensory neurons is reduced days after perineural clonidine at the site of injury. *J Neurophysiol* 94:3159–3167.

73. Costa, M.R., Catterall, W.A. (1984). Cyclic AMP-dependent phosphorylation of the α subunit of the sodium channel in synaptic nerve ending particles. *J Biol Chem* 259:8210–8218.

74. Loewenstein, W.R., Altamirano-Orrego, R. (1956). Enhancement of activity in a Pacinian corpuscle by sympathomimetic agents. *Nature* 178:1292–1293.

75. Chen, Y., Michaelis, M., Jänig, W., Devor, M. (1996). Adrenoceptor subtype mediating sympathetic-sensory coupling in injured neurons. *J Neurophysiol* 76:3721–3730.
76. O'Halloran, K.D., Perl, E.R. (1997). Effects of partial nerve injury on the resposes of C-fiber polymodal nociceptors to adrenergic agonists. *Brain Res* 759:233–240.
77. Khasar, S.G., Green, P.G., Levine, J.D. (1995). Peripheral nociceptive effects of α 2-adrenergic receptor agonists in the rat. *Neuroscience* 66:427–432.
78. Tracey, D.J., Cunningham, J.E., Romm, M.A. (1995). Peripheral hyperalgesia in experimental neuropathy: mediation by α-2-adrenoceptors on post-ganglionic sympathetic terminals. *Pain* 60:317–327.
79. Lee, D.H., Liu, X., Kim, H.T., Chung, K., Chung, J.M. (1999). Receptor subtype mediating the adrenergic sensitivity of pain behavior and ectopic discharges in neuropathic Lewis rats. *J Neurophysiol* 81:2226–2233.
80. Moon, D.E., Lee, D.H., Han, H.C., Xie, J., Coggeshall, R.E., Chung, J.M. (1999). Adrenergic sensitivity of the sensory receptors modulating mechanical allodynia in a rat neuropathic pain model. *Pain* 80:589–595.
81. Tracey, D.J., Cunningham, J.E., Romm, M.A. (1995). Peripheral hyperalgesia in experimental neuropathy: mediation by α 2-adrenoceptors on post-ganglionic sympathetic terminals. *Pain* 60:317–325.
82. Kingery, W.S., Guo, T.Z., Davies, M.F., Limbird, L., Maze, M. (2000). The α_{2A} adrenoceptor and the sympathetic postganglionic neuron contribute to the development of neuropathic heat hyperalgesia in mice. *Pain* 85:345–358.
83. Dogrul, A., Uzbay, I.T. (2004). Topical clonidine antinociception. *Pain* 111:385–391.
84. Nakamura, M., Ferreira, S.H. (1988). Peripheral analgesic action of clonidine: mediation by release of endogenous enkephalin-like substances. *Eur J Pharmacol* 146:223–228.
85. Wei, H., Pertovaara, A. (1997). Peripherally administered α_2-adrenoceptor agonist in the modulation of chronic allodynia induced by spinal nerve ligation in the rat. *Anesth Analg* 85:1122–1127.
86. Wei, H., Jyväsjärvi, E., Niissalo, S., Hukkanen, M., Waris, E., Konttinen, Y.T., Pertovaara, A. (2002). The influence of chemical sympathectomy on pain responsivity and α_2-adrenergic antinociception in neuropathic animals. *Neuroscience* 114:655–668.
87. Zeigler, D., Lynch, S.A., Muir, J., Benjamin, J., Max, M.B. (1992). Transdermal clonidine versus placebo in painful diabetic neuropathy. *Pain* 48, 403–408.
88. Kirkpatrick, A.F., Derasari, M., Glodek, J.A., Piazza, P.A. (1992). Postherpetic neuralgia: a possible application for topical clonidine. *Anesthesiology* 76:1065–1066.
89. Gentili, M., Juhel, A., Bonnet, F. (1996). Peripheral analgesic effect of intra-articular clonidine. *Pain* 64:593–596.
90. Ansah, O.B., Pertovaara, A. (2007). Peripheral suppression of arthritic pain by intraarticular fadolmidine, an α_2-adrenoceptor agonist, in the rat. *Anesth Analg* 105:245–250.
91. King, E.W., Audette, K., Athman, G.A., Nguyen, H.O., Sluka, K.A., Fairbanks, C.A. (2005). Transcutaneous electrical nerve stimulation activates peripherally located α-2A adrenergic receptors. *Pain* 115:364–373.

92. Hong, Y., Abbott, F.V. (1996). Contribution of peripheral α_{1A}-adrenoceptors to pain induced by formalin or by α-methyl-5-hydroxytryptamine plus noradrenaline. *Eur J Pharmacol* 301:41–48.

93. Drummond, P.D. (2009). α_1-Adrenoceptors augment thermal hyperalgesia in mildly burnt skin. *Eur J Pain* 13:273–279.

94. Ali, Z., Ringkamp, M., Hartke, T.V., Chien, H.F., Flavahan, N.A., Campbell, J.N., Meyer, R.A. (1999). Uninjured C-fiber nociceptors develop spontaneous activity and α-adrenergic sensitivity following L6 spinal nerve ligation in monkey. *J Neurophysiol* 81:455–466.

95. Yagi, J., Sumino, R. (1998). Inhibition of a hyperpolarization-activated current by clonidine in rat dorsal root ganglion neurons. *J Neurophysiol* 80:1094–1104.

96. Dalle, C., Eisenach, J.C. (1995). Peripheral block of of the hyperpolarization-activated cation current (I_h) reduces mechanical allodynia in animal models of postoperative and neuropathic pain. *Reg Anesth Pain Med* 30:243–248.

97. Pluteanu, F., Ristoiu, V., Flonta, M.L., Reid, G. (2002). α_1-Adrenoceptor-mediated depolarization and β-mediated hyperpolarization in cultured dorsal root ganglion neurones. *Neurosci Lett* 329:277–280.

98. Eisenach, J.C., Zhang, Y., Duflo, F. (2005). α_2-Adrenoceptors inhibit the intracellular Ca^{2+} response to electrical stimulation in normal and injured sensory neurons, with increased inhibition of calcitonin gene-related peptide expressing neurons after injury. *Neuroscience* 131:189–197.

99. Wang, J., Ren, Y., Zou, X.J., Fang, L., Willis, W.D., Lin, Q. (2004). Sympathetic influence on capsaicin-evoked enhancement of dorsal root reflexes in rats. *J Neurophysiol* 92:2017–2026.

100. Kress, M., Fickenscher, H. (2001). Infection by human varicella-zoster virus confers norepinephrine sensitivity to sensory neurons from rat dorsal root ganglia. *FASEB J* 15:1037–1043.

101. Schmidt, M., Kress, M., Heinemann, S., Fickenscher, H. (2003). Varicella-zoster virus isolates, but not the vaccine strain OKA, induce sensitivity to α_1 and β_1 adrenergic stimulation of sensory neurones in culture. *J Med Virol* 70(Suppl. 1): S82–S89.

102. Sasaki, A., Takasaki, I., Andoh, T., Nojima, H., Shiraki, K., Kuraishi, Y. (2003). Roles of α-adrenoceptors and sympathetic nerve in acute herpetic pain induced by herpes simplex virus inoculation in mice. *J Pharmacol Sci* 92:329–336.

103. Lavand'homme, P.M., Eisenach, J.C. (2003). Perioperative administration of the α_2-adrenoceptor agonist clonidine at the site of nerve injury reduces the development of mechanical hypersensitivity and modulates local cytokine expression. *Pain* 105:247–254.

104. Romero-Sandoval, A., Eisenach, J.C. (2006). Perineural clonidine reduces mechanical hypersensitivity and cytokine production in established nerve injury. *Anesthesiology* 104:351–355.

105. Liu, B., Eisenach, J.C. (2006) Perineural clonidine reduces p38 mitogen-activated protein kinase activation in sensory neurons. *Neuroreport* 17:1313–1317.

106. Romero-Sandoval, A., McCall, C., Eisenach, J.C. (2005). α_2-Adrenoceptor stimulation transforms immune responses in neuritis and blocks neuritis-induced pain. *J Neurosci* 25:8988–8994.

107. Romero-Sandoval, A., Bynum, T., Eisenach, J.C. (2007) Analgesia induced by perineural clonidine is enhanced in persistent neuritis. *Neuroreport* 18:67–71.

108. Baron, R. (2000). Peripheral neuropathic pain: from mechanisms to symptoms. *Clin J Pain* 16(Suppl. 2):S12–S20.

109. Michaelis, M., Devor, M., Jänig, W. (1996). Sympathetic modulation of activity in rat dorsal root ganglion neurons changes over time following peripheral nerve injury. *J Neurophysiol* 76:753–763.

110. Koltzenburg, M., Kress, M., Reeh, P. (1992). The nociceptor sensitization by bradykinin does not depend on sympathetic neurons. *Neuroscience* 46:465–473.

111. Sato, J., Suzuki, S., Tamura, R., Kumazawa, T. (1994). Norepinephrine excitation of cutaneous nociceptors in adjuvant-induced inflamed rats does not depend on sympathetic neurons. *Neurosci Lett* 177:135–138.

112. Rubin, G., Kaspi, T., Rappaport, Z.H., Cohen, S., Ravikovitch, M., Lomazov, P., Devor, M. (1997). Adrenosensitivity of injured afferent neurons does not require the presence of postganglionic sympathetic terminals. *Pain* 72:183–191.

113. Levine, J.D., Taiwo, Y.O., Collins, S.D., Tam, J.K. (1986). Noradrenaline hyperalgesia is mediated through interaction with sympathetic postganglionic neurone terminals rather than activation of primary afferent nociceptors. *Nature* 323:158–160.

114. Gold, M.S., White, D.M., Ahlgren, S.C., Guo, M., Levine, J.D. (1994). Catecholamine-induced mechanical sensitization of cutaneous nociceptors in the rat. *Neurosci Lett* 175:166–170.

115. Romero-Sandoval, A., Eisenach, J.C. (2007) Clonidine reduces hypersensitivity and alters the balance of pro- and anti-inflammatory leukocytes after local injection at the site of inflammatory neuritis. *Brain Behav Immun* 21:569–580.

116. Jänig, W., Häbler, H.J. (2000). Sympathetic nervous system: contribution to neuropathic pain. *Prog Brain Res* 129:451–468.

117. Devor, M., Jänig, W., Michaelis, M. (1994). Modulation of activity in dorsal root ganglion neurons by sympathetic activation in nerve-injured rats. *J Neurophysiol* 71:38–47.

118. Roberts, W.J., Foglesong, M.E. (1988). Identification of afferents contributing to sympathetically evoked activity in wide-dynamic range neurons. *Pain* 34:305–314.

119. Wahren, L.K., Gordh, T., Jr., Torebjörk, K. (1995). Effects of regional intravenous guanethidine in patients with neuralgia in the hand: a follow-up study over a decade. *Pain* 62:379–385.

120. Neil, A., Attal, N., Guilbaud, G. (1991). Effects of guanethidine on sensitization to natural stimuli and self-mutilation behaviour in rats with a peripheral neuropathy. *Brain Res* 565:237–246.

121. Desmeules, J.A., Kayser, V., WeilFugazza, J., Bertrand, A., Guilbaud, G. (1995). Influence of the sympathetic nervous system in the development of abnormal pain-related behaviours in a rat model of neuropathic pain. *Neuroscience* 67:941–951.

122. Schattschneider, J., Scarano, M., Binder, A., Wasner, G., Baron, R. (2008). Modulation of sensitized C-fibers by adrenergic stimulation in human neuropathic pain. *Eur J Pain* 12:517–524.

123. Baron, R., Schattschneider, J., Binder, A., Siebrecht, D., Wasner, G. (2002). Relation between sympathetic vasoconstrictor activity and pain and hyperalgesia in complex regional pain syndromes: a case-control study. *Lancet* 359:1655–1660.

124. Bossut, D.F., Shea, V.K., Perl, E.R. (1996). Sympathectomy induces adrenergic excitability of cutaneous C-fiber nociceptors. *J Neurophysiol* 75:514–517.

125. Raskin, N.H., Levinson, S., Hoffman, P.M., Pickett, J.B., Fields, H.L. (1974). Postsympathectomy neuralgia. Amelioration with diphenylhydantoin and carbamazepine. *Am J Surg* 128:75–78.

126. Jänig, W. (2006). *The integrative action of the autonomic nervous system.* Cambridge: Cambridge University Press.

127. Hole, K., Tjølsen, A. (1993). The tail-flick and formalin test in rodents: changes in skin temperature as a confounding factor. *Pain* 53:247–254.

128. Pertovaara, A. (2006). Noradrenergic pain modulation. *Prog Neurobiol* 80:53–83.

129. Pertovaara, A. (2004). Antinociceptive properties of fadolmidine (MPV-2426), a novel α_2-adrenoceptor agonist. *CNS Drug Rev* 10:117–126.

130. Aley, K.O., Levine, J.D. (1997). Multiple receptors involved in peripheral α_2, μ, and A1 antinociception, tolerance, and withdrawal. *J Neurosci* 17:735–744.

CHAPTER 12

Cholinergic Receptors and Botulinum Toxin

PARISA GAZERANI

Faculty of Pharmaceutical Sciences, The University of British Columbia
Center for Sensory-Motor Interaction (SMI), Aalborg University

Content

Peripheral Receptor Targets for Analgesia: Novel Approaches to Pain Management, Edited by Brian E. Cairns

This chapter provides a brief overview of targeting cholinergic receptors with a focus on potential peripheral sites toward pain treatment. Botulinum toxin serotype A, an inhibitor of acetylcholine (ACh) release at the neuromuscular junction (NMJ), will be discussed further with a focus on its potential antinociceptive/analgesic efficacy for targeting pain.

12.1 CHOLINERGIC RECEPTORS

ACh mediates its broad spectrum effects through binding and activating of G protein-coupled muscarinic acetylcholine receptors (mAChRs) and ligand-gated channel nicotinic acetylcholine receptors (nAChRs) [1].

12.1.1 G Protein-Coupled mAChRs

Molecular cloning studies have shown five (M_1–M_5) distinct mAChRs. They are subdivided into two main functional classes: the M_1, M_3, and M_5 receptors selectively couple to G proteins of the G_q/G_{11} family, whereas the M_2 and M_4 receptors preferentially activate G_i/G_o-type G proteins. Muscarinic receptors are present in neurons in the central and peripheral nervous systems, cardiac and smooth muscles, secretory glands, and in many other cell types and tissues [2]. Central mAChRs are involved in cognitive, behavioral, sensory, motor, and autonomic processes, and changes in mAChR levels and activity have been implicated in the pathophysiology of Alzheimer's disease, Parkinson's disease, depression, and schizophrenia. Peripheral mAChRs mediate the actions of ACh on tissues that are innervated by parasympathetic nerves, for instance, decrease in heart rate (M_2 mAChRs), increases in smooth muscle contractility, and glandular secretion (M_3 mAChRs) [3].

12.1.2 Targeting mAChRs for the Treatment of Pain

Centrally acting muscarinic agonists are known to induce analgesic effects via the activation of spinal and supraspinal mAChRs [1,4]. The M_2 is the predominant mAChR-mediating antinociception at these levels; however, the M_4 receptors also contribute to the analgesic activity of muscarinic agonists [5].

The precise mechanisms by which spinal and supraspinal M_2 and M_4 receptors mediate their analgesic effects remain to be fully clarified.

In addition to the central effects, evidence is also accumulating for a peripheral site of action for mAChRs in analgesia. The activity of M_2 receptors located on peripheral nociceptors of the skin has been reported [6,7]. In an *in vitro* skin nerve preparation taken from both M_2 and M_4 knockout mice and their wild-type littermates, electrical activity was recorded from mechanical and heat-sensitive C-fibers following tactile and thermal stimulation. In both sets of wild-type controls, muscarine increased the threshold for heat-induced neuronal firing and also decreased mechanical sensitivity to von Frey filaments. In knockout mice, the response of M_4 knockout mice samples was not significantly different from wild-type controls; however, an increase in neuronal firing thresholds was absent in M_2 knockout mice samples [7]. Stimulation of the peripheral mAChRs also reduced the release of calcitonin gene-related peptide (CGRP) due to heat stimulation in control groups, an effect not seen in M_2 knockout samples [8]. M_2 agonists also inhibit nociceptive responses in an animal model of orofacial pain through peripheral M_2 receptors, which may open a view toward the treatment of orofacial pain and inflammation [9]. Taken together, peripheral mAChRs may be a potential target for peripherally acting agents for the treatment of pain.

Under normal physiological conditions, there might be several possible sources of peripheral endogenous ACh. It has been shown that sensory neurons synthesize ACh [10]. Nonneural cells also release ACh. For example, keratinocytes in human skin release ACh [11] adjacent to epidermal nerve endings expressing M_2 [6,12]. It could be hypothesized that nociceptor sensitivity is under inhibitory control through tonic activation of M_2 receptors under normal physiological conditions. This concept may be worth investigating under pathological conditions.

Taken together, electrophysiological and neurochemical studies, together with the immunocytochemical data, have demonstrated that M_2 and M_4 receptors play a major role in muscarinic-induced peripheral antinociception [6]. Although there is a potential therapeutic option using selective muscarinic agonists for M_2 receptors to treat pain, the participation of this receptor subtype in vagal nerve stimulation and decrease in heart rate may be a major limiting factor [2,13]. Such limitations may be overcome with local application, such as a topical administration of M_2 agonists. Selective M_4 agonists seem more attractive as analgesic drugs to treat pain in the future because the activation of M_4 receptors does not seem to alter critical peripheral physiological functions.

12.1.3 Ligand-Gated Nicotinic Receptors (nAChRs)

The nAChRs belong to the family of ligand-gated ion channels that includes γ-aminobutyric acid ($GABA_A$), glycine, and $5\text{-}HT_3$ (5-hydroxytriptamine 3) receptors [14]. To date, genes encoding 17 different subunits of the vertebrate nicotinic receptors have been cloned. These subunits are identified as α1–α10, β1–β4, γ, δ, and ε. The nAChRs are classified into muscle-type and neuronal-type receptors. Muscle-type nAChRs consist of five receptor subunits (α1, β1, δ, ε, and γ) and mediate ion permeation at the end plate of the NMJ. Neuronal-type nAChRs are also pentameric ion channels (α2–α6 and β2–β4) and regulate the release of neurotransmitters [15]. The nAChR subunits are also expressed in lymphocytes, skin, epithelial cells [16], and microglia [17].

12.1.4 Targeting nAChRs for the Treatment of Pain

12.1.4.1 nAChR Agonists. Nicotinic transmission is involved in pain processing [18]. Nicotine has long been known to have antinociceptive properties [19] and nicotinic receptors are present on sensory afferent neurons [20,21]. Thus, targeting nAChRs provides insights for the treatment of pain.

nAChR agonists such as epibatidine, ABT-594, A-85380, and DBO-83 have shown antinociceptive activity [22]. Epibatidine, a compound isolated from the skin of an Ecuadorian tree frog, *Epipedobates tricolor* [23], is a potent nAChR agonist and produces antinociceptive effects in rodents, which can be blocked by the noncompetitive nAChR antagonist mecamylamine. The compound produces hypothermia, ataxia, and seizures at doses only slightly higher than those required for antinociception. Epibatidine also has marked effects on the cardiovascular system in dogs [24]. A more selective compound is ABT-594, which exhibited epibatidine-like potency in preclinical pain models with decreased side effects. ABT-594 also attenuates capsaicin-induced CGRP release from primary afferents [25]. Selective nAChR-targeted compounds may be efficacious as analgesics in the future.

12.1.4.2 nAChR Antagonists. Although efforts to discover nAChR-targeted analgesics have focused on agonists, the use of nAChR antagonists has also been proposed [26]. An nAChR antagonist, Vc1.1 α-conotoxin, has been shown to have antinociceptive properties [27]. α-conotoxin has been shown to suppress the vascular response to unmyelinated sensory nerve C-fiber activation in rats [28]. It has also been effective in an acute pain model of capsaicin to the conjunctiva and in the application of substance P to the eye in rats [27]. A study has identified neuronal-type nAChR subunits α3, α5, and β4 present in the human sural nerve (a peripheral sensory nerve) [29,30]. Such nAChRs can be blocked by Vc1.1 toward the attenuation of pain and hyperalgesia for several types of chronic pain including diabetic neuropathy.

Although antagonists might avoid the multiple adverse events of agonists, such as gastrointestinal effects and abuse liability, they might induce cognitive deficits by blocking central nAChRs or decreases in blood pressure by blocking ganglionic nAChRs. Taken together, based on the available data, development of nAChR-targeted compounds as analgesics represents an emerging area of research in pain.

12.2 NICOTINIC RECEPTORS AT NMJs

Muscle-type nAChRs are expressed in the postsynaptic membranes of skeletal NMJs [31]. The NMJ consists of the presynaptic nerve terminal and the postsynaptic muscle. The action potential conducted along the motor nerve causes depolarization, and an influx of calcium consequently stimulates the release of ACh from storage vesicles into the synapse. ACh then binds through the α-subunit to the nicotinic receptors on the motor end plate. Stimulation of the ACh receptor results in the opening of sodium and some potassium channels and depolarization. If the depolarization is sufficient, an action potential is produced and muscle contraction occurs. One of the methods to alter the transmission at the NMJ is the inhibition of ACh release. Botulinum toxin, which is produced by *Clostridium botulinum*, inhibits the release of ACh, which will be discussed further in the next section.

12.3 BOTULINUM TOXIN

12.3.1 History

The anaerobic gram-positive spore-forming bacterium *C. botulinum* was first identified as a causative agent in food poisoning back in 1895 in Belgium, by Emile Pierre van Ermengem [32]. In 1919, Burke proposed an alphabetic classification system for the different botulinum toxins and named the two serotypes identified in his own experiments types A and B [33]. Subsequent studies led to the identification of five more neurotoxin serotypes, each with unique properties named C_1, D, E, F, and G [34]. Edward Schantz and his colleagues were working on purifying the toxin in 1944, and crystalline form was isolated in 1946 [35,36]. The first insights into the mechanism of action of botulinum toxin A came in the 1950s when Vernon Brook showed that it blocked the release of ACh from motor nerve endings [35,36]. In the 1960s and 1970s, Alan Scott began testing botulinum toxin A in monkeys as a possible therapy for strabismus. The paper that first showed the safety and efficacy of botulinum toxin A in the treatment of human disease came in 1980 [37,38]. The benefits Scott documented in the treatment of strabismus led to the prediction that botulinum toxin A would eventually be useful in a wide range of other conditions characterized by muscle spasms or hyperactivity [38].

Currently, botulinum toxin A is in use for the treatment of a variety of conditions in addition to the traditional use of botulinum toxin A for hyperactive skeletal muscles [39,40]. The ability of botulinum toxin A to block the release of ACh from autonomic nerve endings innervating smooth muscle or glandular tissue has led to its use in the treatment of hyperhidrosis, detrusor hyperreflexia, and several gastrointestinal conditions [41]. Some promising results have also been obtained from botulinum toxin A in different pain syndromes [42].

12.3.2 Structure

Botulinum neurotoxins are complex protein structures produced by different clostridial bacterial species, for example, *C. botulinum*, *Clostridium butyricum* and *Clostridium baratii* [43]. The neurotoxins are synthesized as macromolecular complexes containing the neurotoxin molecule and nontoxin proteins that may include a hemagglutinin. The role of the nontoxin proteins is most likely stabilization and protection of the neurotoxin molecule from degradation. The size and composition of the nontoxin protein depends on the serotype and the clostridial strain. The progenitor toxin is found in three forms with molecular masses of 900kDa (LL toxin for type A), 500kDa (L toxin for types A–D and G), and 300kDa (M toxin for types A–F) [44,45].

Botulinum toxin exists in eight immunologically distinct serotypes synthesized as A, B, C_1, C_2, D, E, F, and G. They differ in biosynthesis, size, and mechanism of action. All subtypes, except C_2, are capable of inhibiting ACh release at the peripheral nerve endings and cause muscle relaxation. C_2 appears to be a lethal vasodilating toxin [46,47]. All neurotoxins in this family are synthesized as a single-chain polypeptide of molecular mass approximately 150kDa associated with nontoxic proteins [45,48]. When the 150-kDa toxin polypeptide is cleaved by proteases into a 100-kDa heavy chain (HC) and a 50-kDa light chain (LC), the toxin gains the maximum biological activity. Some clostridial strains contain endogenous proteases that cleave the neurotoxin, for example, type A; however, type E must be exposed to exogenous proteases such as trypsin in order to be activated. The two chains produced by peptidases remain connected via a disulfide bond and noncovalent interactions (Figure 12.1) [45,48]. The integrity of this disulfide bridge is essential for biological activity [49]. Botulinum toxin type A is readily denatured by heat at temperatures above 40°C, particularly at alkaline pH.

The HC consists of two domains, each of ~50kDa. The C-terminal domain (H_C) is required for high-affinity neuronal binding. The N-terminal domain (H_N), however, is assumed to be involved in membrane translocation. The LC is a zinc-dependent metalloprotease responsible for the cleavage of specific proteins called soluble N-ethylmaleimide-sensitive factor attachment protein receptor (SNARE) (soluble N-ethylmaleimide-sensitive fusion [NSF] attachment protein receptors) complex [50]. Figure 12.2 illustrates the botulinum neurotoxin domain structure. The activity of the toxin at the NMJ is believed to occur in a four-stage process: binding, internalization, translocation, and blockade of vesicle exocytosis.

12.3.3 Binding, Internalization, Translocation, and Blockade of Exocytosis

The C-terminal region (H_C) of botulinum neurotoxins binds to specific external high-affinity acceptors, for example, presynaptic motor nerve endings [45]. Botulinum toxin receptors/acceptors are identified and localized. It has been

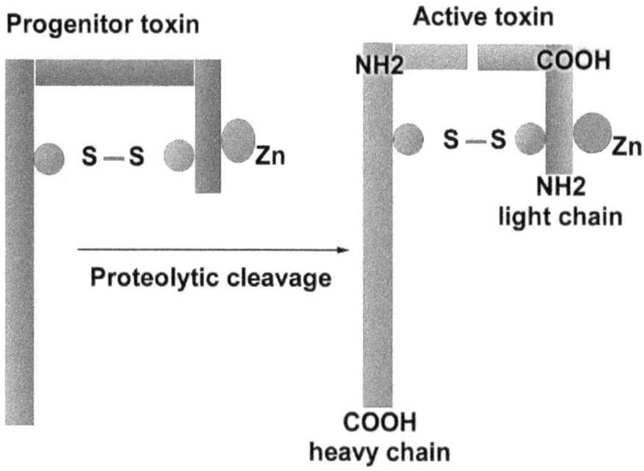

FIGURE 12.1. Botulinum toxin structure (schematic diagram) (image reprinted with permission from eMedicine.com. (2008). http://www.emedicine.com/pmr/topic216.htm (accessed January 2009)). See color insert.

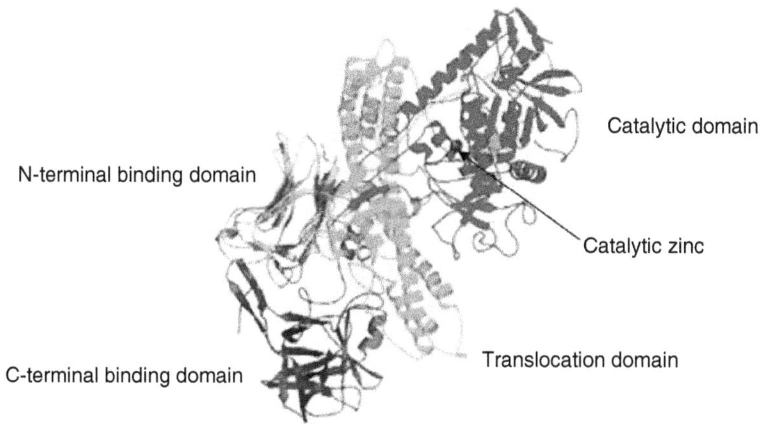

FIGURE 12.2. Domain structure of botulinum neurotoxin type A: The catalytic domain is colored blue; the translocation domain is green; the N-terminal binding subdomain is yellow, and the C-terminal binding subdomain is red. The catalytic zinc is depicted as a ball in gray (image reprinted with permission from Nature Publishing Group. (2008); available at Lacy, D.B., Tepp, W., Cohen, A.C., DasGupta, B.R., Stevens, R.C. (1998). Crystal structure of botulinum neurotoxin type A and implications for toxicity. *Nat Struct Biol* 10:898–902). See color insert.

reported that the membrane receptor protein for botulinum toxin A is synaptic vesicle protein 2 (SV2), which is localized to synaptic vesicles and large dense core vesicles [51,52]. Botulinum toxin A binds to C isoform of SV (SV2C) [51] or to all three isoforms (SV2A, SV2B, SV2C) [52]. SV2 distribution is not restricted to cholinergic and primary sensory neurons. Another candidate protein receptor for botulinum toxin A is fibroblast growth factor receptor 3 (FGFR3). The relationship between SV2 and FGFR3 binding is unknown [53].

After binding, toxin is taken up into the motor neuron via endocytosis process. Following internalization, the LC is translocated into the cytoplasm of the motor neuron. The LC has a zinc-dependent protease activity and specifically targets SNARE proteins involved in mediating neurotransmitter release from the motor nerve ending. The LC of the different botulinum toxin serotypes disables different SNARE components. For example, botulinum toxin serotype A cleaves synaptosome-associated protein of 25-kDa molecular weight (SNAP-25) by removing nine amino acids from the C-terminus, whereas serotype E cleaves 26 amino acids from the C-terminus of SNAP-25. The LCs of the other botulinum toxin serotypes cleave syntaxin (C_1) and synaptobrevin (B, D, F, and G) at various locations. Proteolytic cleavage of the SNARE components serves to inactivate the individual proteins and to disrupt the functioning of the SNARE complex, resulting in the prevention of exocytosis (Figure 12.3) [45,48]. Because various serotypes act on different sites of SNAREs and neurotransmitter inhibition profile, the duration of the blockade and consequently the mode of clinical application would be different.

Botulinum toxin A proteolytic activity persists for over 31 days [54], while other serotypes have shorter duration of action, for instance, 25 days for C_1, 10 days for B, 2 days for F, and 0.8 days for E [55,56]. Long-term properties of the serotype A activity make it a suitable option for clinical use because short-acting neurotoxins may require more frequent administration to maintain therapeutic effect. An increased number of injections contribute to more visits, higher costs, and higher protein load in patients, which can be linked to antibody formation.

12.3.4 Sprouting

Blockade of the cholinergic nerve by botulinum toxin leads to the formation of functional neuronal sprouts. This process is known as sprouting [57–59]. It became clear that sprouting is only a temporary recovery process and original synapses are eventually regenerated while the sprouts are being removed [60]. Therefore, botulinum toxin temporarily interrupts synaptic transmission. Depending on the target tissue, botulinum toxin can block the ACh release at the NMJ and at the autonomic neuroeffector junction of sweat glands, tear glands, salivary glands, and smooth muscles, which make it applicable for clinical conditions related to those tissues and organs.

12.4 ANTINOCICEPTIVE/ANALGESIC ACTIVITY OF BOTULINUM TOXIN

Interestingly, dystonic patients who received botulinum toxin A injections experienced pain relief, which was found to exceed improvement from muscle

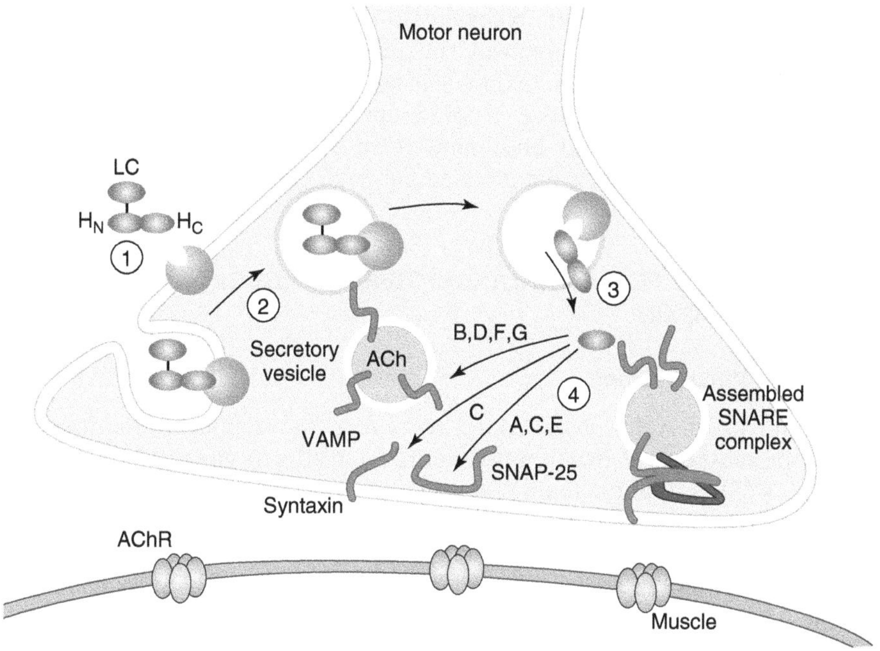

FIGURE 12.3. Biological activity of botulinum toxins at the neuromuscular junction. The heavy-chain domain of the botulinum neurotoxin complex binds to the plasma membrane receptor (1) and the complex is internalized (2). The LC fragment is then released into the cytoplasm (3), where it cleaves the soluble N-ethylmaleimide-sensitive factor attachment protein receptor (SNARE) protein complex at a site determined by the neurotoxin serotype (4). This disruption of the SNARE complex prevents exocytosis of acetylcholine (ACh) into the synaptic space of the neuromuscular junction. A through G, neurotoxin serotypes; AChR, acetylcholine receptor; LC, light chain; H_C, heavy-chain C-terminus; H_N, heavy-chain N-terminus; SNAP-25, synaptosome-associated protein of 25-kDa molecular weight; VAMP, vesicle-associated membrane protein (image reprinted with permission from Wolff, K., Goldsmith, L.A., Katz, S.I., Gilchrest, B.A., Paller, A.S., Leffell, D.J., eds. *Fitzpatrick's Dermatology in General Medicine*, 7th ed. New York: The McGraw-Hill Companies, 2008. http://www.accessmedicine.com/ (accessed January 2009)). See color insert.

hyperactivity and to extend beyond the region of neuromuscular effects [61]. Subsequently, Binder et al. [62] reported relief of migraine pain after botulinum toxin A injections to reduce facial hyperfunctional lines.

As mentioned earlier, the efficacy of botulinum toxin A in most of the treated disorders appears to be due to inhibition of ACh release from nerve terminals at neuromuscular and/or autonomic neuroeffector junctions. Inhibition of ACh release at the NMJ leads to muscle relaxation [63]. Botulinum toxin A also produces localized chemical denervation when injected in the vicinity of parasympathetic postganglionic cholinergic fibers, making it useful for hyperhidrosis and hypersalivation [41]. In terms of pain reduction, however, it seems that in addition to the blockade of ACh secretion, other mechanisms and/or transmitters must be involved. The possibility of such additional mechanisms of action for botulinum toxin A has led to new, exciting discoveries and the expansion of the clinical use of botulinum toxin A. Evidence for antinociceptive/analgesic actions of botulinum toxin A and possible mechanisms involved in such an effect are addressed below in greater detail.

12.5 EVIDENCE FOR ANTINOCICEPTIVE/ANALGESIC ACTIVITY OF BOTULINUM TOXIN

12.5.1 *In Vitro* Studies

Botulinum toxin A has been found to reduce the depolarization-induced release of substance P from embryonic rat dorsal root ganglion neurons in culture [64,65]. Botulinum toxin A also inhibits substance P-mediated contractions of the rabbit iris sphincter muscle induced by electrical field stimulation (EFS) without affecting the adrenergic-mediated contractions of the iris dilator muscle [66]. In addition, botulinum toxin A inhibits the stimulated but not the basal release of CGRP from cultured trigeminal ganglion neurons and from bladder afferent nerve terminals in a preclinical model of bladder pain [67]. Botulinum toxin A also inhibits surface expression of transient receptor potential vanilloid 1 (TRPV1) in dorsal root ganglion cells [68]. It has been shown that an increased level of TRPV1 expression is involved in the maintenance of hyperalgesia [69].

12.5.2 Experimental Animal Studies

Animal investigations have demonstrated the antinociceptive action of botulinum toxin A [70–74]. Subcutaneous injection of formalin into the rat footpad elicits behavioral responses such as licking the treated paw, which can be quantified as pain indicators. In this model, the pain response occurs as an initial acute phase (I) following a prolonged second phase (II) characterized by local inflammatory responses and signs of central sensitization. Pretreatment of the footpad with botulinum toxin A [70] dose dependently reduced pain responses without muscle weakness. The effect was only seen during phase II, which the authors suggested was evidence that the toxin was not exerting a local anesthetic effect on the nociceptors. Microdialysis indicated that botulinum toxin A exerted an inhibitory effect on formalin-induced glutamate release in the footpad during the phase II. Botulinum toxin A also blocked the phase II increased activity in the spinal wide dynamic range neurons. In addition, pretreatment of botulinum toxin A indicated a reduction in *c-fos* gene expression, which is a marker of second-order neuronal expression [70]. It is then hypothesized that botulinum toxin A inhibits peripheral sensitization directly via blocking the release of a variety of neurotransmitters that would be secreted upon nociceptive stimulation or peripheral nerve injury. Consequently, the central sensitization would be prevented indirectly [75,76].

In another model, capsaicin was applied to the rat footpad and the pain was assessed according to the magnitude of pressure stimulus or temperature elevation required to induce a paw-withdrawal response [71]. Pretreatment of the footpad with botulinum toxin A blocked the capsaicin-induced expansion of wide dynamic range neuron-receptive field, which was correlated with a reduced frequency of foot withdrawal in response to pressure and with an increased latency period in response to elevated temperature. A reduction in blood flow in the capsaicin-treated footpad [47] was also seen following pretreatment with botulinum toxin A.

One of the proposed mechanisms for pain reduction in the capsaicin model is the effect of botulinum toxin A on TRPV1 receptors, which are located on sensory nerve endings and modulate noxious chemical and thermal stimuli [77]. The peripheral sensitization mediated by capsaicin involves upregulation of the number of TRPV1 receptors on the surface of sensory neurons. TRPV1 receptors are transferred to the plasma membrane via a SNARE-dependent exocytosis. Thus, the ability of botulinum toxin A to block exocytosis may contribute to the observed effect [47]. Such a phenomenon is supported by the results obtained from patients with intractable detrusor (bladder) muscle overactivity, which shows reduced levels of TRPV1 in bladder biopsy samples after botulinum toxin A treatment [78].

Botulinum toxin A also inhibits pain in rat models of neuropathic pain [72–74]. It has been demonstrated that the peripheral injection of botulinum toxin A significantly reduces thermal and mechanical hyperalgesia after peripheral nerve damage. The significant analgesic activity of botulinum toxin A appeared 5 days after the toxin peripheral application and lasted for more than 10 days [72]. Reduction of cold allodynia in a rat model of neuropathic pain has also been shown [73]. Botulinum toxin A was also able to relieve neuropathic pain symptoms (allodynia) in a mouse model of neuropathic pain, which lasted for at least 3 weeks after a single injection [74].

12.5.3 Experimental Human Studies

Several human volunteer studies have examined the analgesic effects of botulinum toxin A. Some paradigms have supported the analgesic efficacy of botulinum toxin A, while others have not. Blersch et al. [79] and Voller et al. [80] found no effect of botulinum toxin A on electrical and heat pain thresholds in human skin. A study by Krämer et al. [81] showed a small reduction of pain (10%) at day 7 in an electrically induced pain model. A reduction of the neurogenic flare was also observed in this model. In an experimental burn pain model, no analgesic or anti-inflammatory effect of botulinum toxin A was seen [82]. Recent results indicate that subcutaneous and intramuscular injection of botulinum toxin A inhibits the intradermal capsaicin-evoked pain and neurogenic vasodilation in forehead skin [83,84]. A similar effect was seen in the forearm skin [85]; however, this result could not be repeated by others [86]. Such a diversity of results may be explained by a different timing of botulinum toxin A administration versus the pain stimulus, different botulinum toxin A doses, or differential effects of botulinum toxin A in various body regions (e.g., due to different number or sensitivity of receptors/acceptors). The type of pain model may also be relevant.

12.5.4 Clinical Studies

The use of botulinum toxin A has been increasingly reported in many conditions of pathological pain syndromes [42,87]. Botulinum toxin A is not considered a first-line treatment for pain; however, it may offer a chance for pain relief in uncontrolled cases. The specific conditions for which botulinum toxin has been approved by the Food and Drug Administration are listed below:

(1) blepharospasm associated with dystonia in adults and children age ≥12 years,
(2) strabismus associated with dystonia in adults and children age ≥12 years,
(3) primary axillary hyperhidrosis,
(4) reduction of glabellar lines in adults ≤65 years, and
(5) cervical dystonia in adults.

Botulinum toxin A has not been approved for any pain condition yet, which appears to be due to the lack of enough supportive data or clinical evidence from randomized clinical trials.

Botulinum toxin has been considered a potential treatment for a number of different types of headache. At present, there is only limited clinical data that appear to support the use of botulinum toxin A for this indication. A double-blind, placebo-controlled study assessed the efficacy of botulinum toxin A in cervicogenic headache and reported improvement in pain score and range of motion in a treatment group compared with placebo; however, more randomized clinical trials are required to draw any firm conclusions about the efficacy of botulinum toxin A for this indication [88]. A recent multicenter, double-blind, randomized, placebo-controlled study for the prophylaxis of episodic migraine by botulinum toxin A did not result in significantly greater improvement than placebo [89]. It has been suggested that responders to botulinum toxin A treatment for migraine headache differ from nonresponders in their subjective description of headache pain [90]. Most responders described their pain as a crushing or clamping headache pain labeled "imploding" pain, while nonresponders described their pain as building up from the inside of the head out, labeled as "exploding" pain. Similarly, a recent multicenter, double-blind, randomized, placebo-controlled study for tension-type headache found no significant improvement in the primary efficacy parameter (number of headache-free days), although secondary efficacy variables (mean headache intensity) improved after botulinum toxin A injections [91]. No randomized clinical trials support the use of botulinum toxin A in cluster headache, although an open-label study suggested that botulinum toxin A may be beneficial as an add-on prophylactic therapy for a limited number of patients with chronic cluster headache [92]. Taken together, the present research does not offer strong support for the treatment of headache with botulinum toxin A.

Botulinum toxin A has also been studied as a potential treatment for musculoskeletal pain conditions. A small double-blind study appeared to show efficacy of botulinum toxin A for treatment of low back pain; however, investigators suggested caution because of the small study sample size [93]. In a more recent double-blind, randomized, placebo-controlled study, administration of botulinum toxin A produced significant pain relief in 60% of patients with chronic, refractory low back pain [94]. Thus, it may prove to be effective for this pain condition. Chronic neck pain studies have not revealed significant efficacy [95], but a small number of studies on temporomandibular disorders pain have shown an improved pain score after botulinum toxin A injection into jaw or masticatory muscles [96,97].

Animal studies (above) also suggest that botulinum A toxin might be effective for neuropathic pain. Preliminary data from human case studies suggest that botulinum toxin A may provide analgesic effects in this condition [98,99]. Several investigators have also described the effects of botulinum toxin injections on trigeminal neuralgia in open-label studies [100–102]. Although the results from open-label and case studies are interesting, they do not provide enough quality data to make any recommendation about the efficacy of botulinum toxin in trigeminal neuralgia. In the absence of reports of botulinum toxin A being used to treat other craniofacial neuropathic pain conditions, it is impossible to formulate an opinion on whether botulinum toxin A will be helpful in treating these problems [96]. Controlled randomized trials are required to better elucidate the role of botulinum toxin A in the management of neuropathic pain as well as a myriad of other painful and nonpainful conditions where its use is being advocated [39,40].

12.6 POSSIBLE MECHANISMS OF THE ANTINOCICEPTIVE EFFECT OF BOTULINUM TOXIN A

12.6.1 Effect on Muscle

ACh is released by alpha motor neurons that innervate extrafusal muscle fibers and gamma motor neurons that innervate intrafusal fibers of the muscle spindle. Botulinum toxin A affects both extrafusal and intrafusal fibers [103]. Electrophysiological evidence also supports the effect of botulinum toxin A on muscle spindle output [104]. It is then suggested that botulinum toxin A may change the muscle spindle activity that could lead to altered sensory input [47].

Activation of muscle nociceptors is not only due to normal contractions of muscle fibers but also by the presence of sensitizing agents; that is, muscle pain can result from ischemic, thermal, or mechanical stimulation. Chemicals known to sensitize muscle nociceptors include bradykinins, serotonin, potassium, prostaglandin E_2, substance P, and glutamate [105]. Adenosine triphosphate (ATP) has also been considered as a peripheral pain mediator. This molecule is present in large amounts in muscle [106]. The effect of botulinum toxin A on muscle sensitization pathways, which may consequently lead to pain reduction, needs further clarification.

12.6.2 Effect on Central Nervous System (CNS)

12.6.2.1 Direct Effect on CNS. Although many neurons in the CNS are cholinergic, the targeted administration of botulinum toxin A and the relatively low doses used make it unlikely that there is any direct blockade. The observed CNS effect most likely reflects neuroplasticity, probably driven by botulinum toxin A-induced alterations in peripheral sensorimotor patterns [107].

12.6.2.2 Indirect Effects on CNS. Botulinum toxin A may alter the sensory input from intrafusal fibers, which may lead to indirect changes in the CNS [108]. Inhibition of ACh release may alter the gain of sensory organs leading to changes in the information traveling to central parts. Such changes may influence how pain is processed or perceived. Thus, indirect changes in the CNS are possible from peripheral delivery of botulinum toxin A [47].

12.6.3 Effects on Autonomic Function

The effect of botulinum toxin A on pain may be due to the suppression of neurogenic inflammation [107]. It has been hypothesized that botulinum toxin can reduce pain in many inflammatory conditions by blocking early events in the cascade, such as the release of autacoids (e.g., histamine) [109].

Regional blood flow patterns are also affected by botulinum toxin A, and these may be potentially linked to pain. Botulinum toxin A may block some of the autonomic vascular control functions through an alteration in the release of ACh and non-ACh neurotransmitter substances. The relationship between regional blood flow and pain is controversial, especially in the area of headache, but blood flow is clearly altered in both inflammation and ischemic pain, and is probably involved in the sensitization of nociceptors. For example, CGRP, a potent vasodilator that is released under conditions of inflammation, may have its release altered by the administration of botulinum toxin A [107].

12.6.4 Effect on Peripheral Neurotransmitter Release

Botulinum toxin A may inhibit the release of neurotransmitters besides ACh, including those proposed to play a role in pain (see above) [46]. In an *in vitro* preparation of the rabbit eye, the iris sphincter specimen and eye dilator muscle specimen were exposed to EFS. In the sphincter muscle, EFS produced biphasic contractions containing fast (cholinergic mediated) and slow (substance P mediated) components. Botulinum toxin A inhibited the fast cholinergic component of the twitch contraction, which suggests its inhibitory effect on ACh release from the parasympathetic nerve terminals of the iris sphincter. In addition, botulinum toxin A inhibited the slow substance P-ergic response to exogenously applied substance P, which indicates that botulinum toxin also binds to trigeminal nerve endings in the iris sphincter and inhibits the release of substance P. On the other hand, no effect of botulinum toxin was seen on the EFS-induced contraction in the iris dilator muscle. Therefore, botulinum toxin A has an inhibitory effect on cholinergic and substance P-ergic neurotransmission and has little or no effect on adrenergic neurotransmission in this tissue in rabbits [66]. In addition, certain noncholinergic cells may be also affected by botulinum toxin A. For instance, *in vitro* studies have shown that botulinum toxin A inhibits the release of substance P from embryonic dorsal root ganglion neurons [65]. Botulinum toxin A has also been shown to suppress the release of glutamate [70], which is involved in nociception both in the periphery and in the CNS [110]. The release of noradrenaline in PC12 cells (the pheochromocytoma cell line, which secretes both ACh and noradrenaline in a calcium-dependent manner) [111] and CGRP in autonomic vascular nerve terminals [112] is also reduced by botulinum toxin A.

12.6.5 Other Mechanisms

Several other mechanisms have been described for botulinum toxin A, which need further investigation. One of these mechanisms is the effect of botulinum toxin A on the surface expression of TRPV1 in dorsal ganglion cells. As noted before, botulinum toxin A inhibits the TRPV1 expression via vesicle- and SNAP-25-dependent processes [68]. In certain tissues, such as the suburethelium, botulinum toxin A also suppresses the expression of purinergic P2X3 receptors as well as TRPV1 receptors [78]. Another mechanism of botulinum toxin A may involve suppression of the nerve growth factor (NGF) release. It has been reported that the NGF in bladder tissue is significantly and persistently decreased by botulinum toxin A, perhaps through an action of botulinum toxin A on the SNARE proteins SNAP-25 and syntaxin [113–115]. It is not unlikely that botulinum toxin A could also exert its effects on pain via as yet unknown mechanisms.

12.7 THERAPEUTIC BOTULINUM TOXIN PREPARATIONS

The botulinum toxin A products currently available for clinical use are BOTOX® (Allergan, Inc., Irvine, CA, USA), Dysport® (Ipsen Limited, Slough, Berks, UK), and Xeomin® (Merz Pharmaceuticals, Frankfurt am Main,

Germany). A botulinum toxin B preparation, NeuroBloc®/Myobloc® (Solstice Neurosciences, Inc., Malvern, PA, USA), is also available [50]. All therapeutic botulinum toxin A preparations are powders and are required to be reconstituted before application. NeuroBloc/Myobloc is available as a ready-to-use solution. BOTOX and Dysport need to be stored under special temperature conditions as recommended by the manufacturer. Xeomin (NT 201), a highly purified formulation containing pure neurotoxin, would be expected to reduce the likelihood of antibody formation and treatment failure due to immunogenicity. Intradermal testing in rabbits has shown that there is no formation of neutralizing antibodies [50]. Xeomin can be stored at room temperature. This product also has a long shelf life.

Table 12.1 summarizes the properties of therapeutic botulinum toxin preparations [50]. The pharmacological and side-effect profiles vary between these products. For instance, the migration of the toxin is different. The migration differences may be related to neurotoxin complex size because smaller complexes migrate faster [116,117]. Botulinum toxin A products are not equivalent, even when they contain the same serotype and/or the same number of labeled units; each product must be dosed based on data generated with that specific product, and the units should not be converted [50].

12.8 THE FUTURE OF BOTULINUM TOXIN A

As described earlier, the structures of botulinum toxin A (and B) have been identified. There are three distinct domains responsible for binding, translocation, and catalytic activity. The binding domain is located in the C-terminal of the HC; the translocation domain is in the N-terminal of the HC, and the catalytic domain is in the LC. The catalytic domain is responsible for the cleavage of SNARE protein and, consequently, inhibition of neurotransmitter release. Botulinum toxin A has neuronal selectivity, which is due to the binding characteristics of its binding domain, H_C. Therefore, it is possible to reengineer the toxin molecule and to replace the binding domain with other binding ligands to target the cells of interest [118]. The reengineered molecule should contain both the L_C catalytic and the H_N translocation functions. This strategy is being explored in relation to different target cells relevant to clinical use, for example, pain. The rational is to target peripheral nociceptive afferents and thereby to develop analgesics for the treatment of pain and consequently, to avoid the undesirable effects on muscle function through blockade of ACh release at the NMJ. To achieve such goal, the ligands that can specifically target nociceptive afferents are being identified. Galactose-containing carbohydrates have been reported to be present selectively on nociceptive afferents in the central and in the periphery. Lectins from *Erythrina* species have been identified to bind such galactose-containing carbohydrates [119,120]. Therefore, a reengineered botulinum toxin A molecule containing *Erythrina crista-galli* lectin has been examined for the selectivity of the retargeted toxin to nociceptive

TABLE 12.1. Properties of Different Therapeutic Botulinum Toxin Preparations.

	BOTOX	Dysport	Xeomin	NeuroBloc/Myobloc
Manufacturer	Allergan, Inc., Irvine, CA, USA	Ipsen Limited, Slough, Berks, UK	Merz Pharmaceuticals, Frankfurt am Main, Germany	Solstice Neurosciences, Inc., Malvern, PA, USA
Pharmaceutical preparation	Powder	Powder	Powder	Ready-to-use solution
Storage conditions	Below 8 °C	Below 8 °C	Below 25 °C	Below 8 °C
Shelf life, months	24	15	36	24
Botulinum toxin type	A	A	A	B
Clostridium botulinum strain	Hall A	Ipsen strain	Hall A	Bean B
SNARE target	SNAP-25	SNAP-25	SNAP-25	VAMP
Purification process	Precipitation and chromatography	Precipitation and chromatography	Precipitation and chromatography	Precipitation and chromatography
pH value of the reconstituted preparation	7.4	7.4	7.4	5.6
Stabilization	Vacuum drying	Freeze drying (lyophilisate)	Vacuum drying	pH reduction
Excipients	Human serum albumin 500 µg/vial NaCl 900 µg/vial	Human serum albumin 125 µg/vial Lactose 2500 µg/vial	Human serum albumin 1 mg/vial Sucrose 5 mg/vial	?
Biological activity	100MU-A/vial	500MU-I/vial	100MU-M/vial	1.0/2.5/10.0kMU-E/vial
Biological activity in relation to BOTOX	1	1/3	1	1/40
Specific biological activity	60MU-EV/ngBNT	100MU-EV/ngBNT	167MU-EV/ngBNT	5MU-EV/ngBNT

Source: Reprinted with permission from Dressler, D., and Benecke, R. (2007). Pharmacology of therapeutic botulinum toxin preparations. *Disabil Rehabil* 29(23):1761–1768.

BNT, botulinum neurotoxin; MU-A, mouse unit in the Allergan mouse lethality assay; MU-E, mouse unit in the Solstice mouse lethality assay; MU-I, mouse unit in the Ipsen mouse lethality assay; MU-M, mouse unit in the Merz mouse lethality assay; MU-EV, equivalence mouse unit; 1MU-EV = 1MU-A = 1MU-M = 3MU-I = 40MU-E.

afferents. This conjugate could inhibit the release of both substance P and glutamate from embryonic dorsal root ganglion neurons in culture. The properties of this conjugate were also tested in an electrophysiological model [119] and in *in vivo* analgesia models [120]. The antinociceptive benefits of reengineered botulinum toxin molecules are worth exploring in humans.

In addition to pain, this concept is also being explored in a wide range of conditions, for example, chronic obstructive pulmonary disorder, diabetes, and inflammatory and immune disorders [121,122]. For instance, by modifying the HC while coupling the molecule to the epidermal growth factor, it is possible to target the molecule to epithelial cells and to inhibit mucus secretion to treat, for example, cystic fibrosis. By altering the binding domain while coupling the molecule to a cytotoxin, it is possible to target the drug to a specific type of cancer cell [121].

Although challenging, the future of botulinum toxin appears to contain new opportunities for this interesting compound. It will likely include novel products (engineered toxins with higher specificity for novel targets) and new applications (through elucidation of novel mechanisms of action, e.g., P2X3 receptors and NGF release) [54,122]. Desirable properties of new products in the future would be efficacy, specificity, safety, tolerability, low antigenicity, and long duration of action.

12.8.1 Adverse Effects

Botulinum toxin A has provided relatively safe and effective therapy for thousands of patients worldwide [123]. At the injection site of botulinum toxin A, localized pain, edema, erythema, ecchymosis, tenderness, and short-term hyperesthesia may occur. In addition, due to the migration of the toxin to the adjacent muscles, muscle weakness can be present, although this is generally mild and lasts for a limited duration. Clinical experience, optimal dose, and muscle targeting can minimize the migration of the toxin from the site of application. In addition to localized adverse effects, systemic adverse reaction may also occur including nausea, fatigue, malaise, flu-like symptoms and rash. Other side effects reported are dysphagia, upper respiratory infection, neck pain, headache, and dry mouth [45,48].

Neutralizing antibody formation has been linked to high neurotoxin complex protein loads. This phenomenon is important when botulinum toxin is used for disorders that require its repeated injection [124]. Formation of neutralizing antibodies can impact the long-term efficacy of botulinum toxin. There are several factors that promote antibody formation: short interval between injections, the administration of booster injection, the use of increasing doses of botulinum toxin, high dose of the toxin, and early onset of botulinum toxin therapy [125]. The development of new botulinum toxin A formulations can reduce the risk of neutralizing antibody formation. The minimum dose and injection schedule that induces antibodies is not yet known.

12.8.2 Contraindications/Precautions/Drug Interactions

Botulinum toxin A is contraindicated in the presence of infection at the proposed injection site and in individuals with known hypersensitivity to any ingredients in the commercially available formulations. Furthermore, individuals with peripheral motor neuropathic diseases (e.g., amyotrophic lateral sclerosis or motor neuropathy) or neuromuscular junction disorders (e.g., myasthenia gravis or Lambert–Eaton syndrome) should not receive botulinum toxin A [125,126]. Epinephrine, antihistamine, and prednisolone should be kept available. Trained personnel should also be on hand who can set an infusion and maintain first aid in the case of an anaphylactic reaction. The safe and effective use of botulinum toxin A depends upon the proper storage of the product, the selection of the correct dose, and proper reconstitution and administration techniques.

The drug types in question are aminoglycosides, aminoquinolines, cyclosporine, d-penicillamine, tubocurarine, pancuronium, gallamine, and succinylcholine. These drugs can either increase muscle weakness or antagonize the onset of paralysis from botulinum toxin A [127]. Botulinum toxin A belongs to "pregnancy category C," meaning that there are no adequate, well-controlled studies available in pregnant women. It is not known whether this agent can pass into human milk. Therefore, the use of botulinum toxin A in pregnant or nursing women is contraindicated [127].

12.9 SUMMARY

Botulinum toxins inhibit the exocytosis of ACh on cholinergic nerve endings of motor nerves [128]. Autonomic nerves are also affected by the inhibition of ACh release at the neuroeffector junction in glands and in smooth muscles [129]. Botulinum toxin achieves this effect by its endopeptidase activity against SNARE proteins, which are required for the docking of the ACh vesicle to the presynaptic membrane. A marked analgesic benefit has been noted when botulinum toxin A was used for the treatment of dystonia [61]. Initially, this benefit was believed to be due to the direct muscle relaxation effect of botulinum toxin A. Various recent observations now suggest that botulinum toxin A may exert an independent action on peripheral nociceptors by blocking the exocytosis of several neurotransmitters. Botulinum toxin A has been demonstrated to inhibit the release of substance P and CGRP (implicated in the genesis of pain) from cultured embryonic dorsal ganglion and trigeminal ganglion neurons, respectively [65, 130]. These findings have been supported *in vivo* by data showing that CGRP release from afferent nerve terminals is inhibited by botulinum toxin A in a preclinical model of bladder pain [67]. Botulinum toxin A has also been demonstrated to inhibit the release of glutamate [70], which stimulates local nociceptive neurons through the activation of receptors on peripheral cutaneous afferent fibers [131], and to inhibit expression of the vanilloid receptor TRPV1 [68], which plays a key role in the perception of cutaneous thermal and inflammatory pain. In addition, reports indicate that botulinum toxin A inhibits firing of wide dynamic range neurons in the dorsal horn, suggesting that indirect inhibition of central sensitization plays a part in the antinociceptive effect of botolinum toxin A [75]. Because botulinum toxin A does not cross the blood–brain barrier, and because it is inactivated during its retrograde axonal transport, the effect is believed to be in the first-order sensory nerve and not centrally [63]. The chemical composition of botulinum toxin A presents unique opportunities to reengineer the molecule. By altering the binding characteristics of botulinum toxin A, it may be possible to target the drug to specifically inhibit pain without motor effects.

REFERENCES

1. Jones, P.G., Dunlop, J. (2007). Targeting the cholinergic system as a therapeutic strategy for the treatment of pain. *Neuropharmacology* 53:197–206.
2. Nathanson, N.M. (2008). Synthesis, trafficking, and localization of muscarinic acetylcholine receptors. *Pharmacol Ther* 119:33–43.
3. Eglen, R.M. (2005). Muscarinic receptor subtype pharmacology and physiology. *Prog Med Chem* 43:105–136.
4. Iwamoto, E.T., Marion, L. (1993). Characterization of the antinociception produced by intrathecally administered muscarinic agonists in rats. *J Pharmacol Exp Ther* 266:329–338.
5. Duttaroy, A., Gomeza, J., Gan, J.W., Siddiqui, N., Basile, A.S., Harman, W.D., Smith, P.L., Felder, C.C., Levey, A.I., Wess, J. (2002). Evaluation of muscarinic agonist-induced analgesia in muscarinic acetylcholine receptor knockout mice. *Mol Pharmacol* 62:1084–1093.
6. Bernardini, N., Sauer, S.K., Haberberger, R., Fischer, M.J., Reeh, P.W. (2001). Excitatory nicotinic and desensitizing muscarinic (M2) effects on C-nociceptors in isolated rat skin. *J Neurosci* 21:3295–3302.
7. Bernardini, N., Roza, C., Sauer, S.K., Gomeza, J., Wess, J., Reeh, P.W. (2002). Muscarinic M2 receptors on peripheral nerve endings: a molecular target of antinociception. *J Neurosci* 22:RC229.
8. Bernardini, N., Reeh, P.W., Sauer, S.K. (2001). Muscarinic M2 receptors inhibit heat-induced CGRP release from isolated rat skin. *Neuroreport* 12:2457–2460.
9. Dussor, G.O., Helesic, G., Hargreaves, K.M., Flores, C.M. (2004). Cholinergic modulation of nociceptive responses in vivo and neuropeptide release *in vitro* at the level of the primary sensory neuron. *Pain* 107:22–32.
10. Tata, A.M., Plateroti, M., Cibati, M., Biagioni, S., Augusti-Tocco, G. (1994). Cholinergic markers are expressed in developing and mature neurons of chick dorsal root ganglia. *J Neurosci Res* 37:247–255.
11. Grando, S.A., Kist, D.A., Qi, M., Dahl, M.V. (1993). Human keratinocytes synthesize, secrete, and degrade acetylcholine. *J Invest Dermatol* 101:32–36.
12. Tata, A.M., Vilaró, M.T., Mengod, G. (2000). Muscarinic receptor subtypes expression in rat and chick dorsal root ganglia. *Brain Res Mol Brain Res* 82:1–10.

13. Fisher, J.T., Vincent, S.G., Gomeza, J., Yamada, M., Wess, J. (2004). Loss of vagally mediated bradycardia and bronchoconstriction in mice lacking M2 or M3 muscarinic acetylcholine receptors. *FASEB J* 8:711–713.
14. Lindstrom, J., Anand, R., Gerzanich, V., Peng, X., Wang, F., Wells, G. (1996). Structure and function of neuronal nicotinic acetylcholine receptors. *Prog Brain Res* 109:125–137.
15. Colquhoun, L.M., Patrick, J.W. (1997). Pharmacology of neuronal nicotinic acetylcholine receptor subtypes. *Adv Pharmacol* 39:191–220.
16. Gotti, C., Fornasari, D., Clementi, F. (1997). Human neuronal nicotinic receptors. *Prog Neurobiol* 53:199–237.
17. Shytle, R.D., Mori, T., Townsend, K., Vendrame, M., Sun, N., Zeng, J., Ehrhart, J., Silver, A.A., Sanberg, P.R., Tan, J. (2004). Cholinergic modulation of microglial activation by alpha 7 nicotinic receptors. *J Neurochem* 89:337–343.
18. Decker, M.W., Rueter, L.E., Bitner, R.S. (2004). Nicotinic acetylcholine receptor agonists: a potential new class of analgesics. *Curr Top Med Chem* 4:369–384.
19. Aceto, M.D., Awaya, H., Martin, B.R., May, E.L. (1983). Antinociceptive action of nicotine and its methiodide derivatives in mice and rats. *Br J Pharmacol* 79: 869–876.
20. Boyd, R.T., Jacob, M.H., McEachern, A.E., Caron, S., Berg, D.K. (1991). Nicotinic acetylcholine receptor mRNA in dorsal root ganglion neurons. *J Neurobiol* 22:1–14.
21. Roberts, R.G., Stevenson, J.E., Westerman, R.A., Pennefather, J. (1995). Nicotinic acetylcholine receptors on capsaicin-sensitive nerves. *Neuroreport* 6:1578–1582.
22. Decker, M.W. (1999). The analgesic potential of compounds acting at acetylcholine receptors. *Curr Opin Anaesthesiol* 12:597–601.
23. Badio, B., Daly, J.W. (1994). Epibatidine, a potent analgetic and nicotinic agonist. *Mol Pharmacol* 45:563–569.
24. Decker, M.W., Meyer, M.D. (1999). Therapeutic potential of neuronal nicotinic acetylcholine receptor agonists as novel analgesics. *Biochem Pharmacol* 58: 917–923.
25. Holladay, M.W., Wasicak, J.T., Lin, N.H., He, Y., Ryther, K.B., Bannon, A.W., Buckley, M.J., Kim, D.J., Decker, M.W., Anderson, D.J., Campbell, J.E., Kuntzweiler, T.A., Donnelly-Roberts, D.L., Piattoni-Kaplan, M., Briggs, C.A., Williams, M., Arneric, S.P. (1998). Identification and initial structure-activity relationships of (R)-5-(2-azetidinylmethoxy)-2-chloropyridine (ABT-594), a potent, orally active, non-opiate analgesic agent acting via neuronal nicotinic acetylcholine receptors. *J Med Chem* 41:407–412.
26. Rueter, L.E., Decker, M.W., Bitner, R.S. (2004). Improving the therapeutic window in the treatment of pain with nicotinic ligands. *Drug Discov Today* 1:89–96.
27. Livett, B.G., Sandall, D.W., Keays, D., Down, J., Gayler, K.R., Satkunanathan, N., Khalil, Z. (2006). Therapeutic applications of conotoxins that target the neuronal nicotinic acetylcholine receptor. *Toxicon* 48:810–829.
28. Sandall, D.W., Satkunanathan, N., Keays, D.A., Polidano, M.A., Liping, X., Pham, V., Down, J.G., Khalil, Z., Livett, B.G., Gayler, K.R. (2003). A novel alpha-conotoxin identified by gene sequencing is active in suppressing the vascular response to selective stimulation of sensory nerves in vivo. *Biochemistry* 42:6904–6911.

29. Lang, P.M., Burgstahler, R., Sippel, W, Irnich, D, Schlotter-Weigel, B, Grafe, P. (2003). Characterization of neuronal nicotinic acetylcholine receptors in the membrane of unmyelinated human C-fiber axons by in vitro studies. *J Neurophysiol* 90:3295–3303.
30. Lang, P.M., Burgstahler, R., Haberberger, R.V., Sippel, W., Grafe, P. (2005). A conus peptide blocks nicotinic receptors of unmyelinated axons in human nerves. *Neuroreport* 16:479–483.
31. Apel, E.D., Merlie, J.P. (1995). Assembly of the postsynaptic apparatus. *Curr Opin Neurobiol* 5:62–67.
32. DasGupta, B.R. (1994). Structures of botulinum neurotoxin, its functional domains, and perspectives on the crystalline type A toxin. In: Jankovic, J., Hallet, M. (eds.). *Therapy with Botulinum Toxin*. New York: Marcel Dekker, pp. 15–39.
33. Burke, G.S. (1919). Notes on *Bacillus botulinus*. *J Bacteriol* 4:555–565.
34. Jankovic, J., Hallett, M. (1994). *Therapy with Botulinum Toxin*. New York: Marcel Dekker.
35. Schantz, E.J. (1994). Historical perspective. In: Jankovic, J., Hallet, M. (eds.). *Therapy with Botulinum Toxin*. New York: Marcel Dekker, pp. xxiii–xxvi.
36. Schantz, E.J., Johnson, E.A. (1997). Botulinum toxin: the story of its development for the treatment of human disease. *Perspect Biol Med* 40:317–327.
37. Scott, A.B., Rosenbaum, A., Collins, C.C. (1973). Pharmacologic weakening of extraocular muscles. *Invest Ophthalmol* 12:924–927.
38. Scott, A.B. (1980). Botulinum toxin injection into extraocular muscles as an alternative to strabismus surgery. *Ophthalmology* 87:1044–1049.
39. Cheng, C.M., Chen, J.S., Patel, R.P. (2006). Unlabeled uses of botulinum toxins: a review, part 1. *Am J Health Syst Pharm* 63:145–152.
40. Cheng, C.M., Chen, J.S., Patel, R.P. (2006). Unlabeled uses of botulinum toxins: a review, part 2. *Am J Health Syst Pharm* 63:225–232.
41. Jost, W.H. (2006). Other indications of botulinum toxin therapy. *Eur J Neurol* 13:65–69.
42. Casale, R., Tugnoli, V. (2008). Botulinum toxin for pain. *Drugs R D* 9:11–27.
43. Hatheway, C.L. (1990). Toxigenic clostridia. *Clin Microbiol Rev* 3:66–98.
44. Sakaguchi, G., Kozaki, S., Ohishi, I. (1984). Structure and function of botulinum toxins. In: Alouf, J.E. (ed.). *Bacterial Protein Toxins*. London: Academic Press, pp. 435–443.
45. Aoki, K.R. (2005). Pharmacology and immunology of botulinum neurotoxins. *Int Ophthalmol Clin* 45:25–37.
46. Aoki, K.R. (2003). Pharmacology and immunology of botulinum toxin type A. *Clin Dermatol* 21:476–480.
47. Dolly, J.O., Aoki, K.R. (2006). The structure and mode of action of different botulinum toxins. *Eur J Neurol* 13:1–9.
48. Gonnering, R.S. (1993). Pharmacology of botulinum toxin. *Int Ophthalmol Clin* 33:203–226.
49. Aoki, K.R., Guyer, B. (2001). Botulinum toxin type A and other botulinum toxin serotypes: a comparative review of biochemical and pharmacological actions. *Eur J Neurol* 8:21–29.

50. Dressler, D., Benecke, R. (2007). Pharmacology of therapeutic botulinum toxin preparations. *Disabil Rehabil* 29:1761–1768.
51. Foster, K.A. (2005). A new wrinkle on pain relief: re-engineering clostridial neurotoxins for analgesics. *Drug Discov Today* 10:563–569.
52. Mahrhold, S., Rummel, A., Bigalke, H., Davletov, B., Binz, T. (2006). The synaptic vesicle protein 2C mediates the uptake of botulinum neurotoxin A into phrenic nerves. *FEBS Lett* 580:2011–2014.
53. Dong, M., Yeh, F., Tepp, W.H., Dean, C., Johnson, E.A., Janz, R., Chapman, E.R. (2006). SV2 is the protein receptor for botulinum neurotoxin A. *Science* 312:592–596.
54. Aoki, K.R. (2008). Future aspects of botulinum neurotoxins. *J Neural Transm* 115:567–573.
55. Foran, P.G., Mohammed, N., Lisk, G.O., Nagwaney, S., Lawrence, G.W., Johnson, E., Smith, L., Aoki, K.R., Dolly, J.O. (2003). Evaluation of the therapeutic usefulness of botulinum neurotoxin B, C1, E, and F compared with the long lasting type A. Basis for distinct durations of inhibition of exocytosis in central neurons. *J Biol Chem* 278:1363–1371.
56. Fernández-Salas, E., Ho, H., Garay, P., Steward, L.E., Aoki, K.R. (2004). Is the light chain subcellular localization an important factor in botulinum toxin duration of action? *Mov Disord* 19:S23–S34.
57. Fernández-Salas, E., Steward, L.E., Ho, H., Garay, P.E., Sun, S.W., Gilmore, M.A., Ordas, J.V., Wang, J., Francis, J., Aoki, K.R. (2004). Plasma membrane localization signals in the light chain of botulinum neurotoxin. *Proc Natl Acad Sci U S A* 101:3208–3213.
58. Duchen, L.W. (1971). Changes in the electron microscopic structure of slow and fast skeletal muscle fibres of the mouse after the local injection of botulinum toxin. *J Neurol Sci* 14:61–74.
59. Duchen, L.W. (1971). An electron microscopic study of the changes induced by botulinum toxin in the motor end-plates of slow and fast skeletal muscle fibres of the mouse. *J Neurol Sci* 14:47–60.
60. de Paiva, A., Meunier, F.A., Molgó, J., Aoki, K.R., Dolly, J.O. (1999). Functional repair of motor endplates after botulinum neurotoxin type A poisoning: biphasic switch of synaptic activity between nerve sprouts and their parent terminals. *Proc Natl Acad Sci U S A* 96:3200–3205.
61. Brin, M.F., Fahn, S., Moskowitz, C., Friedman, A., Shale, H.M., Greene, P.E., Blitzer, A., List, T., Lange, D., Lovelace, R.E. (1987). Localized injections of botulinum toxin for the treatment of focal dystonia and hemifacial spasm. *Mov Disord* 2:237–254.
62. Binder, W.J., Blitzer, A., Brin, M.F. (1998). Treatment of hyperfunctional lines of the face with botulinum toxin A. *Dermatol Surg* 24:1198–1205.
63. Dressler, D., Adib Saberi, F. (2005). Botulinum toxin: mechanisms of action. *Eur Neurol* 53:3–9.
64. McMahon, H.T., Foran, P., Dolly, J.O., Verhage, M., Wiegant, V.M., Nicholls, D.G. (1992). Tetanus toxin and botulinum toxins type A and B inhibit glutamate, gamma-aminobutyric acid, aspartate, and met-enkephalin release from synaptosomes. Clues to the locus of action. *J Biol Chem* 267:21338–21343.

65. Welch, M.J., Purkiss, J.R., Foster, K.A. (2000). Sensitivity of embryonic rat dorsal root ganglia neurons to *Clostridium botulinum* neurotoxins. *Toxicon* 38:245–258.

66. Ishikawa, H., Mitsui, Y., Yoshitomi, T., Mashimo, K., Aoki, S., Mukuno, K., Shimizu, K. (2000). Presynaptic effects of botulinum toxin type A on the neuronally evoked response of albino and pigmented rabbit iris sphincter and dilator muscles. *Jpn J Ophthalmol* 44:106–109.

67. Chiang, Y.C., Yoshimura, N., Huang, C.C., Chiang, P.H., Chancellor, M.B. (2004). Intravesical botulinum toxin a administration produces analgesia against acetic acid induced bladder pain responses in rats. *J Urol* 172:1529–1532.

68. Morenilla-Palao, C., Planells-Cases, R., García-Sanz, N., Ferrer-Montiel, A. (2004). Regulated exocytosis contributes to protein kinase C potentiation of vanilloid receptor activity. *J Biol Chem* 279:25665–25672.

69. Ji, R.R., Samad, T.A., Jin, S.X., Schmoll, R., Woolf, C.J. (2002). p38 MAPK activation by NGF in primary sensory neurons after inflammation increases TRPV1 levels and maintains heat hyperalgesia. *Neuron* 36:57–68.

70. Cui, M., Khanijou, S., Rubino, J., Aoki, K.R. (2004). Subcutaneous administration of botulinum toxin A reduces formalin-induced pain. *Pain* 107:125–133.

71. Bach-Rojecky, L., Lacković, Z. (2005). Antinociceptive effect of botulinum toxin type a in rat model of carrageenan and capsaicin induced pain. *Croat Med J* 46: 201–208.

72. Bach-Rojecky, L., Relja, M., Lacković, Z. (2005). Botulinum toxin type A in experimental neuropathic pain. *J Neural Transm* 112:215–219.

73. Park, H.J., Lee, Y., Lee, J., Park, C., Moon, D.E. (2006). The effects of botulinum toxin A on mechanical and cold allodynia in a rat model of neuropathic pain. *Can J Anaesth* 53:470–477.

74. Luvisetto, S., Marinelli, S., Cobianchi, S., Pavone, F. (2007). Anti-allodynic efficacy of botulinum neurotoxin A in a model of neuropathic pain. *Neuroscience* 145: 1–4.

75. Aoki, K.R. (2003). Evidence for antinociceptive activity of botulinum toxin type A in pain management. *Headache* 43:S9–S15.

76. Aoki, K.R. (2005). Review of a proposed mechanism for the antinociceptive action of botulinum toxin type A. *Neurotoxicology* 26:785–793.

77. Gunthorpe, M.J., Szallasi, A. (2008). Peripheral TRPV1 receptors as targets for drug development: new molecules and mechanisms. *Curr Pharm Des* 14:32–41.

78. Apostolidis, A., Popat, R., Yiangou, Y., Cockayne, D., Ford, A.P., Davis, J.B., Dasgupta, P., Fowler, C.J., Anand, P. (2005). Decreased sensory receptors P2X3 and TRPV1 in suburothelial nerve fibers following intradetrusor injections of botulinum toxin for human detrusor overactivity. *J Urol* 174:977–982.

79. Blersch, W., Schulte-Mattler, W.J., Przywara, S., May, A., Bigalke, H., Wohlfarth, K. (2002). Botulinum toxin A and the cutaneous nociception in humans: a prospective, double-blind, placebo-controlled, randomized study. *J Neurol Sci* 205:59–63.

80. Voller, B., Sycha, T., Gustorff, B., Schmetterer, L., Lehr, S., Eichler, H.G., Auff, E., Schnider, P. (2003). A randomized, double-blind, placebo controlled study on analgesic effects of botulinum toxin A. *Neurology* 61:940–944.

81. Krämer, H.H., Angerer, C., Erbguth, F., Schmelz, M., Birklein, F. (2003). Botulinum toxin A reduces neurogenic flare but has almost no effect on pain and hyperalgesia in human skin. *J Neurol* 250:188–193.

82. Sycha, T., Samal, D., Chizh, B., Lehr, S., Gustorff, B., Schnider, P., Auff, E. (2006). A lack of antinociceptive or antiinflammatory effect of botulinum toxin A in an inflammatory human pain model. *Anesth Analg* 102:509–516.

83. Gazerani, P., Pedersen, N.S., Staahl, C., Drewes, A.M., Arendt-Nielsen, L. (2009). Subcutaneous botulinum toxin type A reduces capsaicin-induced trigeminal pain and vasomotor reactions in human skin. *Pain* 141:60–69.

84. Gazerani, P., Staahl, C., Drewes, A.M., Arendt-Nielsen, L. (2006). The effects of Botulinum toxin type A on capsaicin-evoked pain, flare, and secondary hyperalgesia in an experimental human model of trigeminal sensitization. *Pain* 122: 315–325.

85. Tugnoli, V., Capone, J.G., Eleopra, R., Quatrale, R., Sensi, M., Gastaldo, E., Tola, M.R., Geppetti, P. (2007). Botulinum toxin type A reduces capsaicin-evoked pain and neurogenic vasodilatation in human skin. *Pain* 130:76–83.

86. Schulte-Mattler, W.J., Opatz, O., Blersch, W., May, A., Bigalke, H., Wohlfahrt, K. (2007). Botulinum toxin A does not alter capsaicin-induced pain perception in human skin. *J Neurol Sci* 260:38–42.

87. Jeynes, L.C., Gauci, C.A. (2008). Evidence for the use of botulinum toxin in the chronic pain setting–a review of the literature. *Pain Pract* 8:269–276.

88. Freund, B.J., Schwartz, M. (2000). Treatment of chronic cervical-associated headache with botulinum toxin A: a pilot study. *Headache* 40:231–236.

89. Relja, M., Poole, A.C., Schoenen, J., Pascual, J., Lei, X., Thompson, C.; European BoNTA Headache Study Group. (2007). A multicentre, double-blind, randomized, placebo-controlled, parallel group study of multiple treatments of botulinum toxin type A (BoNTA) for the prophylaxis of episodic migraine headaches. *Cephalalgia* 27:492–503.

90. Jakubowski, M., McAllister, P.J., Bajwa, Z.H., Ward, T.N., Smith, P., Burstein, R. (2006). Exploding vs. imploding headache in migraine prophylaxis with Botulinum Toxin A. *Pain* 125:286–295.

91. Straube, A., Empl, M., Ceballos-Baumann, A., Tölle, T., Stefenelli, U., Pfaffenrath, V. (2008). Dysport Tension-Type Headache Study Group. Pericranial injection of botulinum toxin type A (Dysport) for tension-type headache—a multicentre, double-blind, randomized, placebo-controlled study. *Eur J Neurol* 15:205–213.

92. Sostak, P., Krause, P., Förderreuther, S., Reinisch, V., Straube, A. (2007). Botulinum toxin type-A therapy in cluster headache: an open study. *J Headache Pain* 8: 236–241.

93. Foster, L., Clapp, L., Erickson, M., Jabbari, B. (2001). Botulinum toxin A and chronic low back pain: a randomized, double-blind study. *Neurology* 56: 1290–1293.

94. Jabbari, B. (2007). Treatment of chronic low back pain with botulinum neurotoxins. *Curr Pain Headache Rep* 11:352–358.

95. Wheeler, A.H., Goolkasian, P., Gretz, S.S. (2001). Botulinum toxin A for the treatment of chronic neck pain. *Pain* 94:255–260.

96. Clark, G.T., Stiles, A., Lockerman, L.Z., Gross, S.G. (2007). A critical review of the use of botulinum toxin in orofacial pain disorders. *Dent Clin North Am* 51:245–261, ix.

97. Song, P.C., Schwartz, J., Blitzer, A. (2007). The emerging role of botulinum toxin in the treatment of temporomandibular disorders. *Oral Dis* 13:253–260.

98. Liu, H.T., Tsai, S.K., Kao, M.C., Hu, J.S. (2006). Botulinum toxin A relieved neuropathic pain in a case of post-herpetic neuralgia. *Pain Med* 7, 89–91.

99. Ranoux, D., Attal, N., Morain, F., Bouhassira, D. (2008). Botulinum toxin type A induces direct analgesic effects in chronic neuropathic pain. *Ann Neurol* 64: 274–283.

100. Zakrzewska, J.M., Cohen, J., Brown, J., Alksne, J., Gemillion, H., Linskey, M., Sirois, D., Pollock, B. (2006). An open study of botulinum-A toxin treatment of trigeminal neuralgia. *Neurology* 66:1458–1459.

101. Voller, B., Sycha, T., Gustorff, B., Kranz, G., Auff, E. (2006). An open study of botulinum-A toxin treatment of trigeminal neuralgia. *Neurology* 66: 1458–1459.

102. Brenner, S.R. (2006). An open study of botulinum-A toxin treatment of trigeminal neuralgia. *Neurology* 66:1458–1459.

103. Rosales, R.L., Arimura, K., Takenaga, S., Osame, M. (1996). Extrafusal and intrafusal muscle effects in experimental botulinum toxin-A injection. *Muscle Nerve* 19:488–496.

104. Filippi, G.M., Errico, P., Santarelli, R., Bagolini, B., Manni, E. (1993). Botulinum A toxin effects on rat jaw muscle spindles. *Acta Otolaryngol* 113:400–404.

105. Graven-Nielsen, T., Mense, S. (2001). The peripheral apparatus of muscle pain: evidence from animal and human studies. *Clin J Pain* 17:2–10.

106. Hamilton, S.G., McMahon, SB. (2000). ATP as a peripheral mediator of pain. *J Auton Nerv Syst* 81:187–194.

107. Arezzo, J.C. (2002). Possible mechanisms for the effects of botulinum toxin on pain. *Clin J Pain* 18:S125–S132.

108. Giladi, N. (1997). The mechanism of action of botulinum toxin type A in focal dystonia is most probably through its dual effect on efferent (motor) and afferent pathways at the injected site. *J Neurol Sci* 152:132–135.

109. Borodic, G.E., Acquadro, M., Johnson, E.A. (2001). Botulinum toxin therapy for pain and inflammatory disorders: mechanisms and therapeutic effects. *Expert Opin Investig Drugs* 10:1531–1544.

110. Bleakman, D., Alt, A., Nisenbaum, E.S. (2006). Glutamate receptors and pain. *Semin Cell Dev Biol* 17:592–604.

111. Shone, C.C., Melling, J. (1992). Inhibition of calcium-dependent release of noradrenaline from PC12 cells by botulinum type-A neurotoxin. Long-term effects of the neurotoxin on intact cells. *Eur J Biochem* 207:1009–1016.

112. Morris, J.L., Jobling, P., Gibbins, I.L. (2001). Differential inhibition by botulinum neurotoxin A of cotransmitters released from autonomic vasodilator neurons. *Am J Physiol Heart Circ Physiol* 281:H2124–H2132.

113. Blöchl, A. (1998). SNAP-25 and syntaxin, but not synaptobrevin 2, cooperate in the regulated release of nerve growth factor. *Neuroreport* 9:1701–1705.

114. Liu, H.T., Kuo, H.C. (2007). Intravesical botulinum toxin A injections plus hydrodistension can reduce nerve growth factor production and control bladder pain in interstitial cystitis. *Urology* 70:463–8.

115. Giannantoni, A., Di, Stasi, S.M., Nardicchi, V., Zucchi, A., Macchioni, L., Bini, V., Goracci, G., Porena, M. (2006). Botulinum-A toxin injections into the detrusor muscle decrease nerve growth factor bladder tissue levels in patients with neurogenic detrusor overactivity. *J Urol* 175:2341–2344.

116. Aoki, K.R. (2001). A comparison of the safety margins of botulinum neurotoxin serotypes A, B, and F in mice. *Toxicon* 39:1815–1820.

117. Aoki, K.R. (2002). Physiology and pharmacology of therapeutic botulinum neurotoxins. *Curr Probl Dermatol* 30:107–116.

118. Foster, K.A., Adams, E.J., Durose, L., Cruttwell, C.J., Marks, E., Shone, C.C., Chaddock, J.A., Cox, C.L., Heaton, C., Sutton, J.M., Wayne, J., Alexander, F.C., Rogers, D.F. (2006). Re-engineering the target specificity of Clostridial neurotoxins—a route to novel therapeutics. *Neurotox Res* 9:101–107.

119. Duggan, M.J., Quinn, C.P., Chaddock, J.A., Purkiss, J.R., Alexander, F.C., Doward, S., Fooks, S.J., Friis, L.M., Hall, Y.H., Kirby, E.R., Leeds, N., Moulsdale, H.J., Dickenson, A., Green, G.M., Rahman, W., Suzuki, R., Shone, C.C., Foster, K.A. (2002). Inhibition of release of neurotransmitters from rat dorsal root ganglia by a novel conjugate of a *Clostridium botulinum* toxin A endopeptidase fragment and *Erythrina cristagalli* lectin. *J Biol Chem* 277:34846–34852.

120. Chaddock, J.A., Purkiss, J.R., Alexander, F.C., Doward, S., Fooks, S.J., Friis, L.M., Hall, Y.H., Kirby, E.R., Leeds, N., Moulsdale, H.J., Dickenson, A., Green, G.M., Rahman, W., Suzuki, R., Duggan, M.J., Quinn, C.P., Shone, C.C., Foster, K.A. (2004). Retargeted clostridial endopeptidases: inhibition of nociceptive neurotransmitter release in vitro, and antinociceptive activity in in vivo models of pain. *Mov Disord* 19:S42–S47.

121. Kostrzewa, R.M., Segura-Aguilar, J. (2007). Botulinum neurotoxin: evolution from poison, to research tool–onto medicinal therapeutic and future pharmaceutical panacea. *Neurotox Res* 12:275–290.

122. Chaddock, J.A., Marks, PM. (2006). Clostridial neurotoxins: structure-function led design of new therapeutics. *Cell Mol Life Sci* 63:540–551.

123. Naumann, M., Albanese, A., Heinen, F., Molenaers, G., Relja, M. (2006). Safety and efficacy of botulinum toxin type A following long-term use. *Eur J Neurol* 13:35–40.

124. Dressler, D., Hallett, M. (2006). Immunological aspects of BOTOX, Dysport and Myobloc/NeuroBloc. *Eur J Neurol* 13:11–15.

125. Borodic, G. (1998). Myasthenic crisis after botulinum toxin. *Lancet* 352:1832.

126. Erbguth, F., Claus, D., Engelhardt, A., Dressler, D. (1993). Systemic effect of local botulinum toxin injections unmasks subclinical Lambert-Eaton myasthenic syndrome. *J Neurol Neurosurg Psychiatry* 56:1235–1236.

127. Prescribing information for BOTOX® neurotoxin. http://www.botoxmedical.com/images/pdfs/BOTOX_prescribing_information.pdf (accessed January 2009).

128. Meunier, F.A., Schiavo, G., Molgó, J. (2002). Botulinum neurotoxins: from paralysis to recovery of functional neuromuscular transmission. *J Physiol (Paris)* 96:105–113.

129. Bhidayasiri, R., Truong, D.D. (2005). Expanding use of botulinum toxin. *J Neurol Sci* 235:1–9.

130. Durham, P.L., Cady, R., Cady, R. (2004). Regulation of calcitonin gene-related peptide secretion from trigeminal nerve cells by botulinum toxin type A: implications for migraine therapy. *Headache* 44:35–42.

131. Coggeshall, R.E., Carlton, S.M. (1998). Ultrastructural analysis of NMDA, AMPA, and kainate receptors on unmyelinated and myelinated axons in the periphery. *J Comp Neurol* 391:78–86.

CHAPTER 13

Cannabinoids and Pain Control in the Periphery

JASON J. McDOUGALL

Department of Physiology and Biophysics, University of Calgary

Content

13.1 INTRODUCTION

Never has there been a drug that has been so reviled, revered, and rebuked than that of cannabis. Often referred to as a medicinal "cure all," a political hot potato and a social mischief, cannabis permeates all levels of society, provoking greater discussion than any other herbage. The history and biology of cannabis is a curious tale that is worth reflecting upon before judging the merits of cannabis as a pain therapeutic. The stigma associated with medicinal cannabis use is astonishing in light of the sanctioned use of other, arguably

Peripheral Receptor Targets for Analgesia: Novel Approaches to Pain Management, Edited by Brian E. Cairns

more risky medicines such as opioids, antidepressants, and sleeping pills. So why should a drug that has been used as a restorative by our ancestors throughout the ages be so vilified and shunned? The emerging scientific evidence clearly demonstrates that cannabis derivatives have huge medical value and are likely to become mainstay drugs in the pharmacopoeial armory of the clinician. The discovery and sequencing of cannabinoid receptors and the recent identification of a natural endogenous cannabinoid system have greatly enhanced our understanding of the biology of this drug and its physiological effects. Before we examine the checkered history of cannabis and cannabis use, let us first grasp the weed.

13.1.1 A Botanical Perspective

Cannabis is derived from the hemp plant *Cannabis sativa*, which was originally farmed in Asia and in the Middle East where it was used for both its textile and medicinal properties. While hemp cultivation existed in these areas for millennia, commercial production in Western countries did not take off until the eighteenth century. In addition to *C. sativa*, at least two other strains of cannabis are known, viz, *Cannabis indica* and *Cannabis ruderalis*. Years of selective breeding have produced multiple strains of cannabis, which have properties that make them suitable for the manufacture of textiles, paper, biodegradable plastics, or fuel. Other strains of cannabis have also been preferentially cultivated for their nutritional and medicinal benefits as well as for their psychoactive properties. It is this latter mood-altering effect of cannabis consumption that makes the drug so controversial. The main psychoactive ingredient of cannabis is Δ^9-tetrahydrocannabinol (Δ^9-THC), which is present in the leaves, stems, roots, and flowers of the cannabis plant. An oily resin produced by glands (trichomes) at the base of the hairs found on the leaves and on the female flower head is particularly rich in Δ^9-THC. Drying of these resin glands results in a potent substance called *kief*, which may then be compressed into blocks of *hashish*. The presence of seeds in the cannabis flower reduces Δ^9-THC concentration by up to 500% so that during cannabis cultivation, male plants are often removed from the crop prior to flowering. The resultant sterile female flower heads (*sinsemilla*) are rich in cannabis resin, which, when dried and compressed, produce the Δ^9-THC-loaded commodity known as *ganja*. Supercritical fluid extraction of the cannabis plant with an alcohol solvent produces a yellow, viscous oil (*honey oil*) that has particularly strong psychoactive effects.

Cultivation of cannabis requires rich, fertile soil that retains moisture. The plant flourishes in warm, sunny climates with long daylight hours. In order to optimize Δ^9-THC levels, the cannabis plant is usually grown indoors where environmental factors and nutrients can be carefully monitored and controlled. Advanced horticultural techniques such as hydroponics, aeroponics, cloning, and intensive artificial lighting can all alter the Δ^9-THC content of individual plants. While cannabis cultivation is usually viewed in the context of producing favorable Δ^9-THC concentration, similar techniques are used commercially to produce plants with excellent fiber content for use in the textile industry. Cannabis and associated hemp plants are therefore extremely versatile flora that will forever play an important role in agriculture, industry, medicine, and culture.

13.1.2 Cannabis through the Ages

Evidence of hemp use in the manufacture of ropes and clothing dates back about 10,000 years when in Asia imprints of a hemplike material were identified on ancient shards of pottery. Medicinal use of cannabis, however, appears to be relatively more recent. As the myth goes, around 2700 BC, the Chinese emperor and revered god Shennong took about sampling 365 herbs to test for their medicinal and poisonous properties. During this incredible journey of chemical discovery, Shennong consumed cannabis, called *ma*, which caused mild narcosis and hallucinations. The extraordinary descriptions of these self-medications earned Shennong the moniker "Emperor of the Five Grains" as well as the deific title of "The Father of Traditional Chinese Medicine." Other texts describe mixing ma with wine, and this combination was lauded for its pain-relieving qualities.

In Marco Polo's alleged account of his visit to Alamut in 1273, he retells the story of an order of "Holy Killers" who were drugged with hashish and, while in a stupefied state, swore allegiance to the cult's leader, Hasan-i Sabbah. When they awoke from the psychoactive effects of the cannabis, they found themselves in a paradisiacal garden being served wine and food by beautiful virgins. Unsurprisingly, the brainwashed minions were convinced that they were in heaven, and when instructed by Hasan-i Sabbah to go out and kill a defined target, they were told that they would return to this paradise dead or alive. This mythical narrative is probably false because it would be unlikely for a stoned assassin to be capable of sneaking up on an unsuspecting victim and successfully carrying out unspeakable acts of violence. In fact, cannabis use typically leads to sluggishness and indolence with no evidence that the drug incites brutality. In addition, the city of Alamut, in which Marco Polo learned of the assassins, was raised by the Mongols in 1256—13 years before Marco Polo's alleged visit. Nevertheless, the menacing image of these clandestine, drug-crazed maniacs being deployed to kill and rampage has served to propagate antidrug feelings and to fuel propaganda. An advocate of this superstition was Harry Jacob Anslinger, the first commissioner of the Federal Bureau of Narcotics in the United States. In *The American Magazine*, Anslinger wrote:

> In the year 1090, there was founded in Persia the religious and military order of the Assassins, whose history is one of cruelty, barbarity and murder, and for good reason. The members were confirmed users of hashish and marijuana, and it is from the Arab 'hashishin' that we have the English word 'assassin'.

Between 1930 and 1937, Harry J. Anslinger waged a ferocious war on marijuana, using all political means at his disposal and manipulating the media to help support his puritanical cause. Writing a regular column called "Gore File" in *The American Magazine*, Anslinger trundled out quote after quote from police reports, which graphically highlighted the dangers and criminal consequences associated with cannabis use. Although Anslinger likely believed that cannabis was the root of all that was evil in American society, he was also an astute government bureaucrat who used the marijuana debate as a means of furthering his political and professional ambitions. To put into context the persuasiveness of his preaching, in the mid-1930s, American doctors had at their disposal 28 different therapeutic agents that contained cannabis for use in the clinic. Furthermore, the pharmaceutical industry had multiple research programs investigating the medicinal benefits of cannabis in different disease states and psychiatric disorders. By 1937, Anslinger had pushed through the controversial Cannabis Tax Act and all cannabis-related research was forthwith deemed untenable. It is unnerving to think that one man's single-handed crusade to abolish cannabis use in any form set American cannabinoid research back 30 years.

13.2 CANNABINOIDS AND CANNABINOID RECEPTORS

C. sativa is composed of at least 66 distinct alkaloid compounds called phytocannabinoids; the human body naturally produces several forms of its own cannabis termed endocannabinoids, and there are an ever-growing number of manufactured agents with cannabis-like properties called synthetocannabinoids. Collectively, these chemicals are simply called cannabinoids. While Δ^9-THC is the most commonly known cannabinoid due to its potent psychoactive effects, cannabinol was in fact the first phytocannabinoid to be isolated from cannabis. This was closely followed by the identification of a second phytocannabinoid called cannabidiol, and then in 1942, Wollner and colleagues successfully extracted tetrahydrocannabinol (THC) (for review, see Reference 1). During the 1960s, Raphael Mechoulam used nuclear magnetic resonance imaging to elucidate the structure of cannabidiol [2] and then set about searching for the other chemical constituents of cannabis. Grunfeld and Edery extracted and then administered various different fractions of cannabis to monkeys and dogs before finally discovering an active compound that caused ataxia and somnolescence [3]. The structure of this phytocannabinoid was Δ^1-THC, later to be renamed Δ^9-THC.

The first endocannabinoid was isolated from porcine brain where it was found to inhibit electrically evoked contractions of mouse vas deferens [4]. The active agent in the brain material was then synthesized and identified as arachidonyl ethanolamide and was named anandamide after *ananda*, the ancient Sanskrit word for "supreme joy." The other main endocannabinoid that has been studied in recent years is 2-arachidonylglycerol (2-AG), although other endocannabinoids have been described (i.e., virodhamine, noladin ether, and N-arachadonyl-dopamine [NADA]). Both anandamide and 2-AG are synthesized from phospholipid precursors found in cell membranes. Endocannabinoids are not preformed and stored in tissue vesicles; rather, they are produced "on demand" in response to an external stimulus. Indeed, anandamide and 2-AG are synthesized in response to increased intracellular Ca^{2+}, which may occur by either membrane depolarization or by mobilization of intracellular Ca^{2+} stores following $G_{q/11}$ protein-coupled receptor activation. The fate of the endocannabinoids is relatively short-lived as they are removed from the site of action by a facilitated, carrier-mediated transport system that actively transports the endocannabinoids back into the cell. The endocannabinoid is then hydrolyzed by a specific enzyme, which, in the case of anandamide, is fatty acid amide hydrolase (FAAH); 2-AG is broken down by monoacylglycerol lipase (MAGL). An overview of the biosynthetic pathway and inactivation of anandamide and 2-AG is illustrated in Figures 13.1 and 13.2.

Because cannabinoids produce such profound physiological and psychophysical effects in the human body, it stands to reason that there must be receptors to which these chemicals are able to bind. Currently, there are two prominent cannabinoid receptors (CB_1 and CB_2) with a putative third cannabinoid receptor (GPR55) having recently been described [5]. The CB_1 receptor was originally cloned and expressed in the mammalian central nervous system [6]. Three years later, a second cannabinoid receptor was cloned (CB_2), which did not appear to be expressed in the brain, but rather on peripherally circulating macrophages and in the spleen [7]. Later research would redress this observation by showing that CB_2 receptors are functionally expressed in the brain stem where their activation inhibits emetic activity [8]. Both CB_1 and CB_2 receptors are $G_{i/o}$ protein-coupled receptors that inhibit adenylate cyclase activity and stimulate mitogen-activated protein kinase activity. CB_1 receptors are also positively coupled to inwardly rectifying potassium channels and are negatively coupled to N-type and P/Q-type calcium channels [9,10]. Activation of CB_1 receptors on neurons therefore leads to neuronal hyperpolarization and inhibition of calcium-dependent neurotransmitter release. CB_1 receptors have been identified at all levels of the pain pathway including peripheral nerves, spinal neurons, and in pain processing areas of the brain [11–14]. In fact, it is believed that CB_1 receptors are the most prevalent of all G protein-coupled receptors in the brain [6,15,16]. Although there is a high abundance of CB_1 receptors in the nervous system, they typically reside presynaptically and are therefore seen as synaptic modulators. This presynaptic localization of CB_1 receptors was originally described for hippocampal gamma-aminobutyric acid (GABA)ergic neurons [17,18], but they have also been identified on cholinergic [19], noradrenergic [20], and serotonergic [21] neurons of the brain.

In contrast to CB_1 receptors, CB_2 receptors do not couple to Q-type calcium channels or to inwardly rectifying potassium channels [22]. There are relatively few CB_2 receptors in the central nervous system with the preponderance of the receptors being expressed by immunocytes [7,23,24]. These differences in

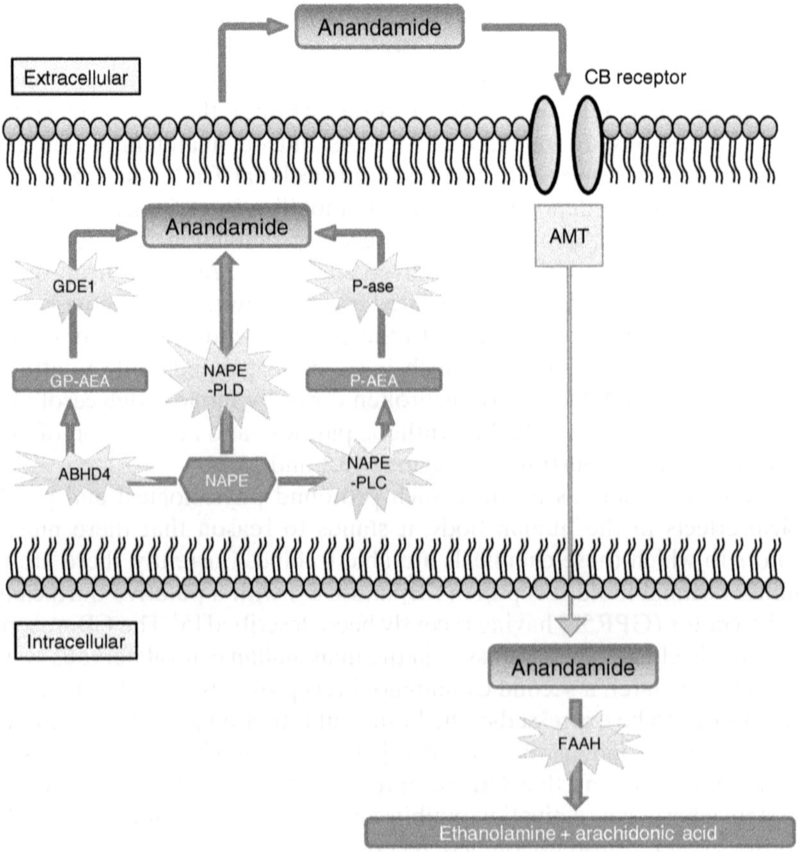

FIGURE 13.1. Biosynthesis and degradation of anandamide. N-arachidonoyl-phosphatidylethanolamine (NAPE) is hydrolyzed by phospholipase type D (NAPE-PLD) to produce anandamide. Alternatively, NAPE may be cleaved by α,β-hydrolase 4 (ABHD4) and phospholipase C (NAPE-PLC) to produce glycerophosphoanandamide (GP-AEA) and phosphoanandamide (P-AEA) intermediaries, respectively. GP-AEA is then hydrolyzed by glycerophosphodiesterase-1 (GDE1) to produce anandamide, while P-AEA is hydrolyzed by phosphatase (P-ase) to produce anandamide. Following signaling via cannabinoid receptors, anandamide undergoes active reuptake by the cell and is carried intracellularly by an anandamide membrane transporter (AMT). Once inside the cell, anandamide is broken down by a fatty acid amide hydrolase (FAAH) to produce ethanolamine and arachidonic acid. CB, cannabinoid. See color insert.

receptor distribution and second messenger signaling pathways suggest that ligands directed toward CB_2 receptors may be beneficial for the control of pain while circumventing centrally mediated side effects. Indeed, the CB_2 receptor agonists HU308 and AM1241 show antinociceptive properties without causing central effects such as catalepsy and hypomobility [25,26]. Thus, CB_2 receptor agonists may be an attractive target for the control of chronic pain syndromes.

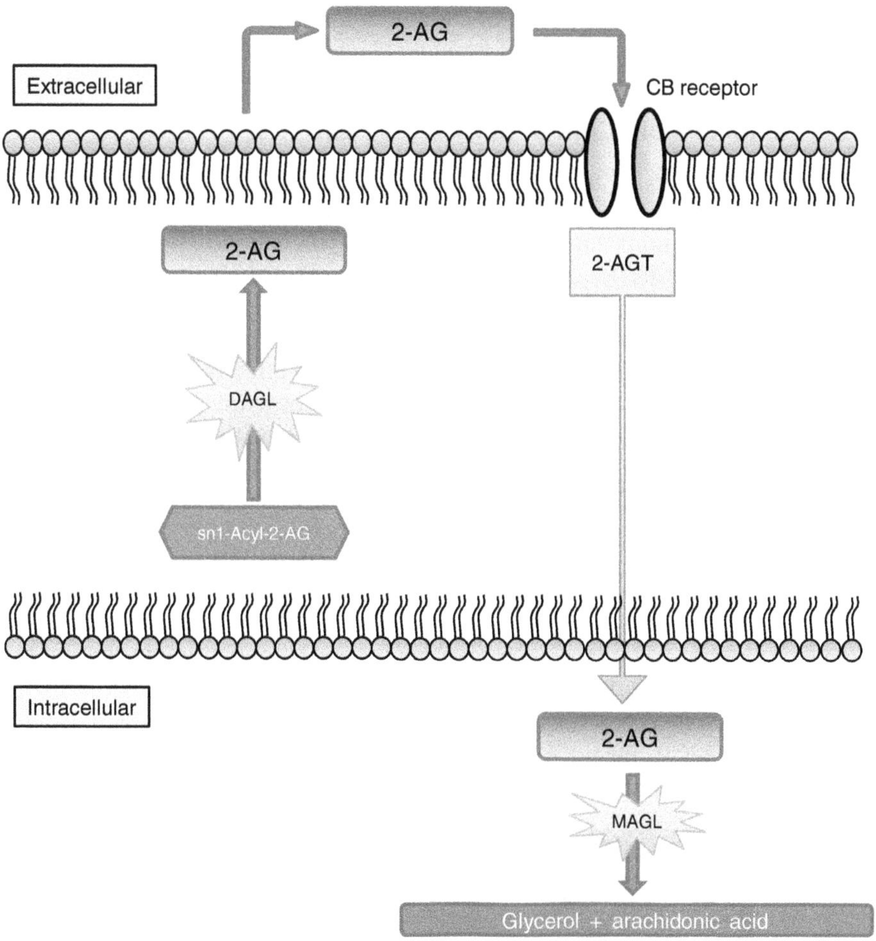

FIGURE 13.2. Biosynthesis and degradation of 2-acyl-glycerol (2-AG). Initially, sn1-acyl-2-arachidonoylglycerol (sn1-acyl-2-AG) is converted to 2-AG by diacylglycerol lipase (DAGL). Following cannabinoid receptor signaling, 2-AG is transported intracellularly by a 2-AG transporter (2-AGT) and is then broken down by monoacylglycerol lipase (MAGL) to produce glycerol and arachidonic acid. See color insert.

13.3 CANNABINOIDS AND PAIN

Phytocannabinoids have been used to treat painful conditions for thousands of years. The reluctance of modern medicine to embrace this family of agents for their analgesic properties is mostly embedded in political misinformation and in an unproven fear of addiction. There are also concerns that cannabis may be a "gateway" drug where patients fear that taking a cannabinoid will lead to harder drug use in the future [27]. There is, however, no empirical evidence of this being the case. What follows here is an appraisal of current scientific knowledge of the effect of cannabinoids on pain control in different pain conditions as documented in preclinical and clinical studies.

13.3.1 Cannabinoid Control of Arthritis Pain

Arthritis is a group of over a hundred different diseases with a common symptom: pain. Patients suffering from arthritis typically do not request therapies to heal their joint cartilage or to improve their bone structure, but all patients share a desire for a life free of pain. The World Health Organization recently estimated that about a third of the world's adult population is afflicted with some form of musculoskeletal disease [28]. This equates to millions of people in chronic pain for which there is currently no effective long-term relief. The underlying causes of arthritis pain are also obscure in these patients, making targeted analgesia problematic [29,30]. Arthritis pain is currently managed by nonsteroidal anti-inflammatory drugs, high-dose steroids, cytokine blockers, or opioids. These approaches can be prohibitively expensive or can produce major side effects such as gastric bleeding, kidney failure, respiratory depression, and severe constipation. Clearly, there is a pressing need for safe and effective drugs to alleviate joint pain.

Using immunohistochemistry, we have found that CB_1 receptors are present on nerve terminals in the synovium of rodent knee joints (Figure 13.3). Preclinical work found that a CB_1-selective agonist (arachidonyl-2-chloroethylamide [ACEA]) could reduce joint nociceptor activity in a rat model of osteoarthritis, while a CB_1 receptor antagonist sensitized joint afferents [31]. These findings suggest that endocannabinoids are tonically released in osteoarthritic

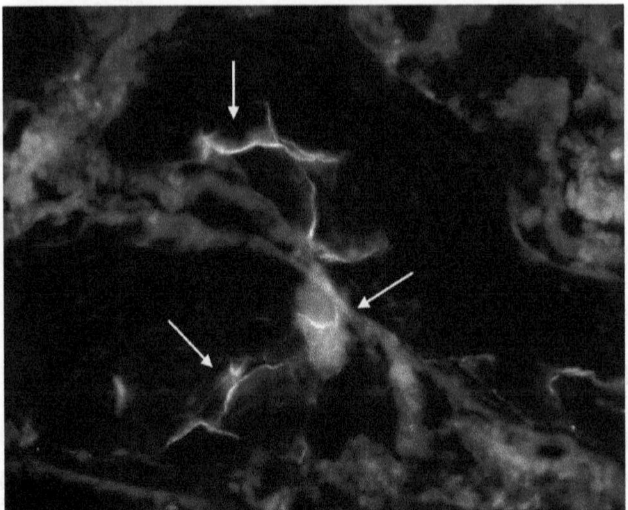

FIGURE 13.3. Immunolocalization of CB_1 receptors in the synovium of rat knee joints. Arrows point to positive staining on synovial nerve terminals (magnification = ×400).

joints and that CB_1 receptor activation could reduce joint pain. Pain behavior studies corroborate an analgesic effect of cannabinoids in arthritic animals with both CB_1 and CB_2 receptors being implicated [32–34]. Further mechanistic studies showed that the capsaicin-sensitive transient receptor potential vanilloid 1 (TRPV1) ion channel is involved in cannabinoid-mediated responses in joints [31,35,36]. TRPV1 is a nonselective cation channel with six transmembrane-spanning domains. The channel is typically activated by noxious heat (>43 °C), low pH, and the naturally occurring vanilloids capsaicin and resiniferatoxin [37–39]. Recently, however, it has been found that anandamide can bind to and activate TRPV1 channels [40–43]. So how can we reconcile the dichotomy of analgesic cannabinoids activating pronociceptive TRPV1 channels in arthritic joints? In order to answer this puzzle, a number of factors need to be taken into consideration. First, during inflammation and heightened pain states, TRPV1 expression is significantly enhanced [44,45], while TRPV1 and CB_1 receptor coexpression is also increased [46]. This increase in the receptor reserve promotes anandamide from the ranks of partial agonist to a full agonist at the TRPV1 ion channel. Second, phosphorylation of TRPV1 by protein kinase C and protein kinase A sensitizes the ion channel to anandamide [47–49]. It has been suggested that TRPV1 phosphorylation occurs during tissue inflammation [50]. Finally, stimulation of adenylyl cyclase activity to cause cyclic adenosine monophosphate production causes CB_1 receptor agonists to desensitize TRPV1 channels [51]. Taken together, it appears that during inflammation, endocannabinoids bind either directly to TRPV1 channels at a discrete receptor domain or bind to TRPV1/CB_1 receptor dimers to deactivate the TRPV1 channel component. Electrophysiological recordings from knee joint afferents support this hypothesis because a CB_1 receptor agonist was found to elicit an initial burst response from the sensory nerve followed by nociceptor desensitization in a TRPV1-dependent manner [31]. Thus, the antinociceptive action of cannabinoids not only occurs directly through a cannabinoid receptor-mediated mechanism but also by silencing TRPV1 channel activity.

A clinical role for cannabinoids in arthritis pain management is also looking promising. A preliminary study examining synovial fluid extracted from patients with either osteoarthritis or rheumatoid arthritis discovered significant levels of anandamide and 2-AG [52]. Furthermore, both CB_1 and CB_2 receptors were also identified in synovial tissue indicating the existence of an endocannabinoid system in human joints. Both the preclinical and clinical data pave the way for future trials to test the effectiveness of cannabinoids in controlling arthritis pain. The advantages of peripherally restricted cannabinoids are clear, and further research may finally allow us to address the social quandary as to whether it is acceptable to put cannabis in our joints.

13.3.2 Cannabinoid Control of Neuropathic Pain

Neuropathic pain typically develops in response to nerve damage as a consequence of neuronal injury, metabolic factors, viral infections, surgical transection, or chemical destruction. The nerve lesions can occur in the peripheral and central nervous systems, and the resulting excruciating pain may be episodic or constant. It is estimated that between 2% and 3% of the developed world's population suffer from neuropathic pain, and the pharmacological management of the disorder is limited. The first lines of defense against neuropathic pain are tricyclic antidepressants (e.g., amitryptiline) or anticonvulsants (e.g., gabapentin). Second-line treatments are serotonin and noradrenaline reuptake inhibitors or topical lidocaine. Third-level neuropathic pain medications for moderate to severe pain include opioids. All of these treatment strategies are fraught with adverse side effects such as dizziness, nausea, renal failure, constipation, and weight gain. Once again, better therapeutics are required to control neuropathic pain.

The potential for cannabinoids to modulate neuropathic pain is highlighted in studies that report an increase in cannabinoid receptor expression both centrally and peripherally following nerve injury [53–57]. Pain behavioral studies using animal models of neuropathic pain show that cannabinoids are efficacious in the alleviation of this type of pain. For example, the nonselective CB_1/CB_2 receptor agonist CP55,940 was effective in reducing tactile allodynia in the rat spinal nerve ligation model of neuropathic pain [58]. Similarly, systemic administration of the nonselective cannabinoid agonist WIN55,212-2 reduced the nociceptive responses associated with sciatic nerve chronic constriction-induced peripheral neuropathy [59] and with the spinal nerve ligation model [60]. Because these nonselective drugs were given systemically, it is impossible to determine which cannabinoid receptor is mediating the analgesia or whether the cannabinoid is acting centrally or peripherally. Intraplantar injection of WIN55,212-2 into the hindpaw of rats revealed an antinociceptive effect which could be blocked by a CB_1 antagonist [61]. The effect of selective CB_1 and CB_2 receptor agonists and antagonists on neuropathic pain behavior and calcium mobilization suggests that cannabinoids act peripherally via both receptor subtypes, while only CB_2 receptors show functional relevance centrally [62]. The use of CB_1 knockout mice has also uncovered some interesting albeit contrasting observations as to the role of cannabinoids in neuropathic pain control. Castane et al. found that mice lacking CB_1 receptors developed mechanical and thermal pain responses in a similar manner to wild-type control animals, suggesting that CB_1 receptors are superfluous for neuropathic pain generation [63]. Similarly, sciatic nerve injury induced comparable increases in *cfos* expression in the lumbar and sacral regions of the spinal cords taken from CB_1 knockout and wild-type mice [64]. In contrast, an intriguing model in which CB_1 receptors were deleted from peripheral nociceptors but were preserved on central neuronal terminals showed a reduced analgesic response to local and systemic cannabinoid administration; intrathecally injected cannabinoids retained their analgesic action [65]. This study indicates that peripheral CB_1 receptors are crucial for cannabinoid-mediated analgesia, and the authors suggest that peripherally restricted CB_1 agonists could be useful for the treatment of neuropathic pain while obviating centrally mediated side effects.

The ability of CB_2 receptor ligands to attenuate neuropathic pain was first described in the L5-L6 spinal nerve ligation model [66]. Systemic administration of the CB_2 receptor agonist AM1241 reduced thermal and mechanical hypersensitivity in the model, which could be inhibited by the CB_2 receptor antagonist AM630. Furthermore, this antinociceptive effect of AM1241 was still apparent in CB_1 receptor knockout animals, confirming that this drug acts purely via CB_2 receptors. Electrophysiological studies found that peripheral administration of another selective CB_2 receptor agonist JWH133 reduced neuronal activity in response to noxious mechanical stimuli in spinally ligated rats [67]. The pain caused by sciatic nerve ligation could also be ameliorated by treatment with GW405833, although the specificity of this drug was not tested [68,69]. It should also be noted, however, that extremely high levels of GW405833 (100 mg/kg intraperitoneal) were required to elicit an antinociceptive response in these animals.

In addition to these nerve injury models, cannabinoids have been shown to be effective in alleviating other types of neuropathic pain. In rats with diabetic neuropathy, for example, WIN55,212-2 was able to reduce mechanical and thermal nociception in a dose-dependent manner [70,71]. Elsewhere, neuropathic pain produced by chemotherapeutic agents could be partially suppressed by AM1241, but was fully blocked by WIN55,212-2 [72].

The data emerging from clinical trials are very encouraging, with a number of reports recommending the cannabinoid class of medications as potential therapies for neuropathic pain control [73]. Karst et al. found that 20 mg of ajulemic acid twice daily for 4 days followed by 40 mg twice daily for 4 days significantly reduced pain levels compared to placebo, although this analgesic effect was short-lived [74]. In a couple of randomized, controlled crossover trials, neuropathic pain patients receiving either THC, THC/cannabidiol, or placebo as a sublingual spray reported an improvement in pain severity and overall quality of life [75,76]. The most common side effects associated with cannabinoid treatment in these patients were dry mouth, fatigue, and transient hypotension. A major limitation of these studies is that the number of participants in these trials was small. Nevertheless, the findings of these and other studies were compelling enough for Health Canada to approve the use of synthetic cannabinoids for the treatment of neuropathic pain in multiple sclerosis patients. The synthetic cannabinoid Sativex is available in the United Kingdom as an unlicensed medicine, while the Federal Drug Administration in the United States has allowed Sativex to enter into late-stage phase III trials for neuropathic pain management.

13.3.3 Cannabinoids and Cancer Pain

Cannabis has been used to great effect as an adjunct to cancer treatments primarily from the standpoint of its antiemetic properties. With the advent of more effective chemotherapeutic agents to limit tumor growth came the distressing side effects of nausea and vomiting. A plethora of basic science studies and clinical trials consistently shows that cannabis and cannabinomimetic compounds successfully reduce nausea and vomiting in cancer patients undergoing chemotherapy [77–79]. Writing about his battle with abdominal cancer, the renowned science writer Stephen Jay Gould lauded the antiemetic effects of cannabis use:

> ... when I started intravenous chemotherapy (Adriamycin), absolutely nothing in the available arsenal of antiemetics worked at all ... marijuana worked like a charm ... the sheer bliss of not experiencing nausea—and then not having to fear it for all the days intervening between treatments—was the greatest boost I received in all my year of treatment, and surely had a most important effect upon my eventual cure.

Because recreational cannabis is usually taken in the form of smoking a joint, a number of investigations have looked at the possibility of cannabis causing lung cancer. Multiple confounding factors are associated with these types of studies, however, not least of which is that cannabis is often mixed with tobacco in a joint prior to smoking. Also, joint smokers tend to inhale more deeply and longer than cigarette smokers, thereby allowing cannabis particles to reach and interact with terminal alveoli for a more protracted period of time. One key study looked at the effect of high-dose Δ^9-THC taken over a 2-year period on primary tumor growth in rats [80]. What they found was that Δ^9-THC treatment significantly improved survival rate and lowered the number of primary tumors in these animals. Elsewhere, it has been shown that cannabinoids are antiangiogenic agents and possess the ability to inhibit tumor metastasis [81]. Thus, cannabinoids appear to have anticancer effects, but what about their analgesic properties in this disease? Unfortunately, very little experimental work has been carried out to test the role of cannabinoids in altering cancer pain severity. Anecdotal evidence seems to suggest that cannabis has multiple palliative properties, but this may be associated with cannabis' ability to improve mood rather than with any direct analgesic effect. Nevertheless, it has been observed in pancreatic cancer patients that peripheral cannabinoid receptor number was inversely proportional to clinical pain scores, suggesting that cannabinoids may be involved in cancer pain modulation [82]. One of the earliest studies into the possible analgesic action of cannabis in cancer pain patients found that Δ^9-THC produced analgesia equivalent to that of codeine [83]. More recently, in a phase III clinical trial, it was found that Sativex reduced the degree of intractable cancer pain in patients who were unresponsive to opioids [84]. Studies in preclinical animal models also indicate a potential analgesic effect of cannabinoids on cancer pain. In a bone cancer pain model, systemic treatment with the nonselective cannabinoids WIN55,212-2 or CP55,940 reduced deep tissue hyperalgesia, which could be blocked by a CB_1 antagonist but not by CB_2 antagonism [85,86]. Similarly, cancer pain produced by intraplantar injection of human oral squamous carcinoma cells was attenuated by peripheral injection of WIN55,212-2 [87]. Interestingly in these experiments, local administration of the CB_2 receptor agonist AM1241 also reduced mechanonociception, suggesting that both cannabinoid receptors could be involved in cancer pain modulation in the periphery. This hypothesis is supported by the observation that the peripheral antinociceptive effect of WIN55,212-2 in a rodent cancer model could be blocked by both a CB_1 and a CB_2 antagonist [88]. It is clear, therefore, that in addition to their antiemetic and antitumorogenic effects, cannabinoids can also ameliorate cancer pain, making them a powerful pharmacological weapon in the fight against cancer.

13.3.4 Cannabinoids and Gastrointestinal Pain

In addition to the antiemetic responses previously described, cannabinoids exert a number of other physiological effects on the mammalian gastrointestinal system. For example, cannabinoids are able to alter gastrointestinal motility, to control digestive enzyme secretion, and to stimulate appetite. Immunohistochemical and ligand binding experiments identified CB_1 receptors in the smooth muscle of the gastrointestinal tract as well as in the enteric nervous system [89–92], corroborating the suggestions that cannabinoids can modulate gastrointestinal function. More importantly from the standpoint of gastrointestinal pain control, CB_1 receptors were later found to be colocalized with TRPV1 channels on gut perivascular nerves indicating an extrinsic source of cannabinoid receptors on primary afferent nerves [93].

Pain behavioral studies indicate that cannabinoids can act peripherally to alleviate gastrointestinal nociception. One of the earliest studies to examine the role of cannabinoids in controlling gastrointestinal pain was performed by Welburn et al., who found that the writhing response to intraluminal injection of formic acid could be dose dependently attenuated by oral administration of either Δ^9-THC or cannabinol [94]. More recently, a colorectal distension model has been used to assess cannabinoid effectiveness in controlling gastrointestinal pain. In these investigations, a small balloon was placed into the terminal portion of the digestive tract and then was inflated up to 60 mmHg, thereby producing intense abdominal pain. The severity of this pain was then quantified by recording the frequency of evoked abdominal contractions. Local administration of the CB_1 receptor agonist WIN55,212-2 (1 mg/kg) or the CB_2 receptor agonist JWH015 (1 mg/kg) reduced the number of contractile responses to colorectal distension [95]. This antinociceptive effect of the cannabinoids could be blocked by a CB_1 (rimonabant) and a CB_2 (SR144528) receptor antagonist, respectively (10 mg/kg, i.p.). Furthermore, the authors also reported that WIN55,212-2 and JWH015 could reduce mechanical hyperalgesia in a model of inflammatory colitis, thereby confirming the analgesic value of cannabinoids in treating digestive diseases. Abdominal pain resulting from acute pancreatitis was also found to be ameliorated by synthetocannabinoids acting on peripheral CB_1 and CB_2 receptors [96]. The analgesia produced by these agonists occurred in the absence of any centrally mediated side effects, affirming the therapeutic benefit of cannabinoids in managing visceral pain.

13.4 THE FUTURE OF CANNABINOIDS: MORE THAN A PIPE DREAM

For all that has been written and debated about cannabis, it is evident that the drug has its benefits while at the same time being somewhat misunderstood. The majority of public and political inquiries have tended to conclude that cannabis is a safe and effective therapeutic that, pending further investigation, should be accepted into the general practitioner's pharmacopoeia. Yet still the sniggers of derision and disapproval persist. Science is making huge strides in trying to understand the pharmacology of cannabinoids and thereby to assuage the fears of a concerned public. What is clear is that cannabinoids relieve pain in a host of acute and chronic illnesses. How we go about tapping into this powerful analgesic system is not yet apparent, but further research will help to guide us. The vision of using CB_2 receptor ligands to control pain in the periphery has been blurred somewhat by the realization that these receptors are also found in the central nervous system, albeit at a lower level. Nevertheless, cannabinoids that do not cross the blood–brain barrier could have an enormous impact on how we manage pain clinically. Peripherally restricted CB_1 and/or CB_2 receptor agonists, for example, could alleviate tissue pain at the site of injury while avoiding centrally mediated side effects.

The lipophilic nature of cannabinoids and their dose-limiting psychotropic effects mean that other pharmacological approaches that exploit the body's natural endocannabinoid system may be advantageous. Inhibitors of FAAH and MAGL enzymes would promote a buildup of endocannabinoids in the damaged tissue, which could then exert their analgesic effects while circumventing undesirable central responses. Similarly, peripheral delivery of endocannabinoid transport inhibitors would prevent the cellular reuptake of endocannabinoids, thereby prolonging their analgesic effect locally in the tissue. By physiologically manipulating the endocannabinoid system in these ways, it should be possible to enhance endocannabinoid levels in the periphery, allowing us to control pain at the source and to avoid muddling the brain.

Further research and clinical assessment of cannabinoids is of course still needed. The widespread health benefits of cannabinoids are evident; however, we should still be vigilant with respect to known side effects and other possible safety issues associated with long-term cannabinoid use heretofore unknown. In order for patients, physicians, and policy makers to be better informed regarding cannabinoids, we must shun the idea that cannabis is an enfant terrible. Rather, cannabinoids should be seen as viable treatment strategies that could provide much needed relief to millions of chronic pain sufferers.

REFERENCES

1. Pertwee, R.G. (2006). Cannabinoid pharmacology: the first 66 years. *Brit J Pharmacol* 147(Suppl. 1):S163–S171.

2. Mechoulam, R., Shvo, Y. (1963). The structure of cannabidiol. *Tetrahedron* 19: 2073–2078.
3. Grunfeld, Y., Edery, H. (1969). Psychopharmacological activity of the active constituents of hashish and some related cannabinoids. *Psychopharmacologia* 14:200–210.
4. Devane, W.A., Hanus, L., Breuer, A., Pertwee, R.G., Stevenson, L.A., Griffin, G., Gibson, D., Mandelbaum, A., Etinger, A., Mechoulam, R. (1992). Isolation and structure of a brain constituent that binds to the cannabinoid receptor. *Science* 258:1946–1949.
5. Ryberg, E., Larsson, N., Sjogren, S., Hjorth, S., Hermansson, N.O., Leonova, J., Elebring, T., Nilsson, K., Drmota, T., Greasley, P.J. (2007). The orphan receptor GPR55 is a novel cannabinoid receptor. *Brit J Pharmacol* 152:1092–1101.
6. Matsuda, L.A., Lolait, S.J., Brownstein, M.J., Young, A.C., Bonner, T.I. (1990). Structure of a cannabinoid receptor and functional expression of the cloned cDNA. *Nature* 346:561–564.
7. Munro, S., Thomas, K.L., Abu-Shaar, M. (1993). Molecular characterization of a peripheral receptor for cannabinoids. *Nature* 365:61–65.
8. Van Sickle, M.D., Duncan, M., Kingsley, P.J., Mouihate, A., Urbani, P., Mackie, K., Stella, N., Makriyannis, A., Piomelli, D., Davison, J.S., Marnett, L.J., Di Marzo, V., Pittman, Q.J., Patel, K.D., Sharkey, K.A. (2005). Identification and functional characterization of brainstem cannabinoid CB2 receptors. *Science* 310:329–332.
9. Mackie, K., Devane, W.A., Hille, B. (1993). Anandamide, an endogenous cannabinoid, inhibits calcium currents as a partial agonist in N18 neuroblastoma cells. *Mol Pharmacol* 44:498–503.
10. Mackie, K., Lai, Y., Westenbroek, R., Mitchell, R. (1995). Cannabinoids activate an inwardly rectifying potassium conductance and inhibit Q-type calcium currents in AtT20 cells transfected with rat brain cannabinoid receptor. *J Neurosci* 15: 6552–6561.
11. Hohmann, A.G. (2002). Spinal and peripheral mechanisms of cannabinoid antinociception: behavioral, neurophysiological and neuroanatomical perspectives. *Chem Phys Lipids* 121:173–190.
12. Pertwee, R.G. (1999). Evidence for the presence of CB1 cannabinoid receptors on peripheral neurones and for the existence of neuronal non-CB1 cannabinoid receptors. *Life Sci* 65:597–605.
13. Pertwee, R.G. (2001). Cannabinoid receptors and pain. *Prog Neurobiol* 63: 569–611.
14. Tsou, K., Brown, S., Sanudo-Pena, M.C., Mackie, K., Walker, J.M. (1998). Immunohistochemical distribution of cannabinoid CB1 receptors in the rat central nervous system. *Neuroscience* 83:393–411.
15. Devane, W.A., Dysarz, F.A., III, Johnson, M.R., Melvin, L.S., Howlett, A.C. (1988). Determination and characterization of a cannabinoid receptor in rat brain. *Mol Pharmacol* 34:605–613.
16. Piomelli, D. (2003). The molecular logic of endocannabinoid signalling. *Nat Rev Neurosci* 4:873–884.
17. Katona, I., Sperlagh, B., Sik, A., Kafalvi, A., Vizi, E.S., Mackie, K., Freund, T.F. (1999). Presynaptically located CB1 cannabinoid receptors regulate GABA release from axon terminals of specific hippocampal interneurons. *J Neurosci* 19: 4544–4558.

18. Nyiri, G., Cserep, C., Szabadits, E., Mackie, K., Freund, T.F. (2005). CB1 cannabinoid receptors are enriched in the perisynaptic annulus and on preterminal segments of hippocampal GABAergic axons. *Neuroscience* 136:811–822.
19. Degroot, A., Kofalvi, A., Wade, M.R., Davis, R.J., Rodrigues, R.J., Rebola, N., Cunha, R.A., Nomikos, G.G. (2006). CB1 receptor antagonism increases hippocampal acetylcholine release: site and mechanism of action. *Mol Pharmacol* 70: 1236–1245.
20. Oropeza, V.C., Mackie, K., Van Bockstaele, E.J. (2007). Cannabinoid receptors are localized to noradrenergic axon terminals in the rat frontal cortex. *Brain Res* 1127:36–44.
21. Balazsa, T., Biro, J., Gullai, N., Ledent, C., Sperlagh, B. (2008). CB1-cannabinoid receptors are involved in the modulation of non-synaptic [3H]serotonin release from the rat hippocampus. *Neurochem Int* 52:95–102.
22. Felder, C.C., Joyce, K.E., Briley, E.M., Mansouri, J., Mackie, K., Blond, O., Lai, Y., Ma, A.L., Mitchell, R.L. (1995). Comparison of the pharmacology and signal transduction of the human cannabinoid CB1 and CB2 receptors. *Mol Pharmacol* 48:443–450.
23. Facci, L., Dal Toso, R., Romanello, S., Buriani, A., Skaper, S.D., Leon, A. (1995). Mast cells express a peripheral cannabinoid receptor with differential sensitivity to anandamide and palmitoylethanolamide. *Proc Natl Acad Sci U S A* 92: 3376–3380.
24. Pertwee, R.G. (1999). Pharmacology of cannabinoid receptor ligands. *Curr Med Chem* 6:635–664.
25. Hanus, L., Breuer, A., Tchilibon, S., Shiloah, S., Goldenberg, D., Horowitz, M., Pertwee, R.G., Ross, R.A., Mechoulam, R., Fride, E. (1999). HU-308: a specific agonist for CB(2), a peripheral cannabinoid receptor. *Proc Natl Acad Sci U S A* 96:14228–14233.
26. Malan, T.P., Jr., Ibrahim, M.M., Deng, H., Liu, Q., Mata, H.P., Vanderah, T., Porreca, F., Makriyannis, A. (2001). CB2 cannabinoid receptor-mediated peripheral antinociception. *Pain* 93:239–245.
27. Kandel, D.B. (2003). Does marijuana use cause the use of other drugs? *J Am Med Assoc* 289:482–483.
28. Anon. (2003). The burden of musculoskeletal conditions at the start of the new millennium. *World Health Organ Tech Rep Ser* 919:1–218.
29. Hunter, D.J., McDougall, J.J., Keefe, F.J. (2008). The symptoms of osteoarthritis and the genesis of pain. *Rheum Dis Clin North Am* 34:623–643.
30. McDougall, J.J. (2006). Arthritis and pain. Neurogenic origin of joint pain. *Arthritis Res Ther* 8:220–229.
31. Schuelert, N., McDougall, J.J. (2008). Cannabinoid-mediated antinociception is enhanced in rat osteoarthritic knees. *Arthritis Rheum* 58:145–153.
32. Cox, M.L., Haller, V.L., Welch, S.P. (2007). The antinociceptive effect of Δ9-tetrahydrocannabinol in the arthritic rat involves the CB_2 cannabinoid receptor. *Eur J Pharmacol* 570:50–56.
33. Croci, T., Zarini, E. (2007). Effect of the cannabinoid CB(1) receptor antagonist rimonabant on nociceptive responses and adjuvant-induced arthritis in obese and lean rats. *Brit J Pharmacol* 150:559–566.

34. Smith, F.L., Fujimori, K., Lowe, J., Welch, S.P. (1998). Characterization of Δ9-tetrahydrocannabinol and anandamide antinociception in nonarthritic and arthritic rats. *Pharmacol Biochem Behav* 60:183–191.

35. Baker, C.L., McDougall, J.J. (2004). The cannabinomimetic arachidonyl-2-chloroethylamide (ACEA) acts on capsaicin-sensitive TRPV1 receptors but not cannabinoid receptors in rat joints. *Brit J Pharmacol* 142:1361–1367.

36. McDougall, J.J., Yu, V., Thomson, J. (2008). In vivo effects of CB2 receptor-selective cannabinoids on the vasculature of normal and arthritic rat knee joints. *Brit J Pharmacol* 153:358–366.

37. Szallasi, A. (2002). Vanilloid (capsaicin) receptors in health and disease. *Am J Clin Pathol* 118:110–121.

38. Szolcsanji, J. (1987). Capsaicin and nociception. *Acta Physiol Hung* 69:323–332.

39. Szolcsanyi, J. (2002). Capsaicin receptors as target molecules on nociceptors for development of novel analgesic agents. In: Keri, G., Toth, I. (eds.). *Molecular Pathomechanisms and New Trends in Drug Research.* London and New York: Taylor & Francis, pp. 319–333.

40. Costa, B., Giagnoni, G., Franke, C., Trovato, A.E., Colleoni, M. (2004). Vanilloid TRPV1 receptor mediates the antihyperalgesic effect of the nonpsychoactive cannabinoid, cannabidiol, in a rat model of acute inflammation. *Brit J Pharmacol* 143:247–250.

41. Gauldie, S.D., McQueen, D.S., Pertwee, R., Chessell, I.P. (2001). Anandamide activates peripheral nociceptors in normal and arthritic rat knee joints. *Brit J Pharmacol* 132:617–621.

42. Smart, D., Gunthorpe, M.J., Jerman, J.C., Nasir, S., Gray, J., Muir, A.I., Chambers, J.K., Randall, A.D., Davis, J.B. (2000). The endogenous lipid anandamide is a full agonist at the human vanilloid receptor (hVR1). *Brit J Pharmacol* 129:227–230.

43. Zygmunt, P.M., Petersson, J., Andersson, D.A., Chuang, H., Sorgard, M., Di Marzo, V., Julius, D., Hogestatt, E.D. (1999). Vanilloid receptors on sensory nerves mediate the vasodilator action of anandamide. *Nature* 400:452–457.

44. Hudson, L.J., Bevan, S., Wotherspoon, G., Gentry, C., Fox, A., Winter, J. (2001). VR1 protein expression increases in undamaged DRG neurons after partial nerve injury. *Eur J Neurosci* 13:2105–2114.

45. Yiangou, Y., Facer, P., Dyer, N.H., Chan, C.L., Knowles, C., Williams, N.S., Anand, P. (2001). Vanilloid receptor 1 immunoreactivity in inflamed human bowel. *Lancet* 357:1338–1339.

46. Amaya, F., Shimosato, G., Kawasaki, Y., Hashimoto, S., Tanaka, Y., Ji, R.R., Tanaka, M. (2006). Induction of CB1 cannabinoid receptor by inflammation in primary afferent neurons facilitates antihyperalgesic effect of peripheral CB1 agonist. *Pain* 124:175–183.

47. Di Marzo, V., Blumberg, P.M., Szallasi, A. (2002). Endovanilloid signaling in pain. *Curr Opin Neurobiol* 12:372–379.

48. Hong, S., Wiley, J.W. (2005). Early painful diabetic neuropathy is associated with differential changes in the expression and function of vanilloid receptor 1. *J Biol Chem* 280:618–627.

49. Premkumar, L.S., Ahern, G.P. (2000). Induction of vanilloid receptor channel activity by protein kinase C. *Nature* 408:985–990.

50. Cesare, P., Dekker, L.V., Sardini, A., Parker, P.J., McNaughton, P.A. (1999). Specific involvement of PKC-epsilon in sensitization of the neuronal response to painful heat. *Neuron* 23:617–624.

51. Hermann, H., De Petrocellis, L., Bisogno, T., Schiano Moriello, A., Lutz, B., Di Marzo, V. (2003). Dual effect of cannabinoid CB1 receptor stimulation on a vanilloid VR1 receptor-mediated response. *Cell Mol Life Sci* 60:607–616.

52. Richardson, D., Pearson, R.G., Kurian, N., Latif, M.L., Garle, M.J., Barrett, D.A., Kendall, D.A., Scammell, B.E., Reeve, A.J., Chapman, V. (2008). Characterisation of the cannabinoid receptor system in synovial tissue and fluid in patients with osteoarthritis and rheumatoid arthritis. *Arthritis Res Ther* 10:R43.

53. Lim, G., Sung, B., Ji, R.R., Mao, J. (2003). Upregulation of spinal cannabinoid-1-receptors following nerve injury enhances the effects of Win 55,212-2 on neuropathic pain behaviors in rats. *Pain* 105:275–283.

54. Siegling, A., Hofmann, H.A., Denzer, D., Mauler, F., De Vry, J. (2001). Cannabinoid CB(1) receptor upregulation in a rat model of chronic neuropathic pain. *Eur J Pharmacol* 415:R5–R7.

55. Walczak, J.S., Pichette, V., Leblond, F., Desbiens, K., Beaulieu, P. (2006). Characterization of chronic constriction of the saphenous nerve, a model of neuropathic pain in mice showing rapid molecular and electrophysiological changes. *J Neurosci Res* 83:1310–1322.

56. Wotherspoon, G., Fox, A., McIntyre, P., Colley, S., Bevan, S., Winter, J. (2005). Peripheral nerve injury induces cannabinoid receptor 2 protein expression in rat sensory neurons. *Neuroscience* 135:235–245.

57. Zhang, J., Hoffert, C., Vu, H.K., Groblewski, T., Ahmad, S., O'Donnell, D. (2003). Induction of CB2 receptor expression in the rat spinal cord of neuropathic but not inflammatory chronic pain models. *Eur J Neurosci* 17:2750–2754.

58. Scott, D.A., Wright, C.E., Angus, J.A. (2004). Evidence that CB-1 and CB-2 cannabinoid receptors mediate antinociception in neuropathic pain in the rat. *Pain* 109:124–131.

59. Herzberg, U., Eliav, E., Bennett, G.J., Kopin, I.J. (1997). The analgesic effects of R(+)-WIN 55,212-2 mesylate, a high affinity cannabinoid agonist, in a rat model of neuropathic pain. *Neurosci Lett* 221:157–160.

60. Bridges, D., Ahmad, K., Rice, A.S. (2001). The synthetic cannabinoid WIN55,212-2 attenuates hyperalgesia and allodynia in a rat model of neuropathic pain. *Brit J Pharmacol* 133:586–594.

61. Fox, A., Kesingland, A., Gentry, C., McNair, K., Patel, S., Urban, L., James, I. (2001). The role of central and peripheral Cannabinoid$_1$ receptors in the antihyperalgesic activity of cannabinoids in a model of neuropathic pain. *Pain* 92: 91–100.

62. Sagar, D.R., Kelly, S., Millns, P.J., O'Shaughnessey, C.T., Kendall, D.A., Chapman, V. (2005). Inhibitory effects of CB1 and CB2 receptor agonists on responses of DRG neurons and dorsal horn neurons in neuropathic rats. *Eur J Neurosci* 22:371–379.

63. Castane, A., Celerier, E., Martin, M., Ledent, C., Parmentier, M., Maldonado, R., Valverde, O. (2006). Development and expression of neuropathic pain in CB1 knockout mice. *Neuropharmacology* 50:111–122.

64. Pol, O., Murtra, P., Caracuel, L., Valverde, O., Puig, M.M., Maldonado, R. (2006). Expression of opioid receptors and c-fos in CB1 knockout mice exposed to neuropathic pain. *Neuropharmacology* 50:123–132.

65. Agarwal, N., Pacher, P., Tegeder, I., Amaya, F., Constantin, C.E., Brenner, G.J., Rubino, T., Michalski, C.W., Marsicano, G., Monory, K., Mackie, K., Marian, C., Batkai, S., Parolaro, D., Fischer, M.J., Reeh, P., Kunos, G., Kress, M., Lutz, B., Woolf, C.J., Kuner, R. (2007). Cannabinoids mediate analgesia largely via peripheral type 1 cannabinoid receptors in nociceptors. *Nature Neurosci* 10:870–879.

66. Ibrahim, M.M., Deng, H., Zvonok, A., Cockayne, D.A., Kwan, J., Mata, H.P., Vanderah, T.W., Lai, J., Porreca, F., Makriyannis, A., Malan, T.P., Jr. (2003). Activation of CB2 cannabinoid receptors by AM1241 inhibits experimental neuropathic pain: pain inhibition by receptors not present in the CNS. *Proc Natl Acad Sci U S A* 100:10529–10533.

67. Elmes, S.J., Jhaveri, M.D., Smart, D., Kendall, D.A., Chapman, V. (2004). Cannabinoid CB2 receptor activation inhibits mechanically evoked responses of wide dynamic range dorsal horn neurons in naive rats and in rat models of inflammatory and neuropathic pain. *Eur J Neurosci* 20:2311–2320.

68. Valenzano, K.J., Tafesse, L., Lee, G., Harrison, J.E., Boulet, J.M., Gottshall, S.L., Mark, L., Pearson, M.S., Miller, W., Shan, S., Rabadi, L., Rotshteyn, Y., Chaffer, S.M., Turchin, P.I., Elsemore, D.A., Toth, M., Koetzner, L., Whiteside, G.T. (2005). Pharmacological and pharmacokinetic characterization of the cannabinoid receptor 2 agonist, GW405833, utilizing rodent models of acute and chronic pain, anxiety, ataxia and catalepsy. *Neuropharmacology* 48:658–672.

69. Whiteside, G.T., Gottshall, S.L., Boulet, J.M., Chaffer, S.M., Harrison, J.E., Pearson, M.S., Turchin, P.I., Mark, L., Garrison, A.E., Valenzano, K.J. (2005). A role for cannabinoid receptors, but not endogenous opioids, in the antinociceptive activity of the CB2-selective agonist, GW405833. *Eur J Pharmacol* 528:65–72.

70. Dogrul, A., Gul, H., Yildiz, O., Bilgin, F., Guzeldemir, M.E. (2004). Cannabinoids blocks tactile allodynia in diabetic mice without attenuation of its antinociceptive effect. *Neurosci Lett* 368:82–86.

71. Ulugol, A., Karadag, H.C., Ipci, Y., Tamer, M., Dokmeci, I. (2004). The effect of WIN 55,212-2, a cannabinoid agonist, on tactile allodynia in diabetic rats. *Neurosci Lett* 371:167–170.

72. Rahn, E.J., Makriyannis, A., Hohmann, A.G. (2007). Activation of cannabinoid CB1 and CB2 receptors suppresses neuropathic nociception evoked by the chemotherapeutic agent vincristine in rats. *Brit J Pharmacol* 152:765–777.

73. Ware, M., Beaulieu, P. (2005). Cannabinoids for the treatment of pain: an update on recent clinical trials. *Pain Res Manag* 10(Suppl. A):27A–30A.

74. Karst, M., Salim, K., Burstein, S., Conrad, I., Hoy, L., Schneider, U. (2003). Analgesic effect of the synthetic cannabinoid CT-3 on chronic neuropathic pain: a randomized controlled trial. *J Am Med Assoc* 290:1757–1762.

75. Berman, J.S., Symonds, C., Birch, R. (2004). Efficacy of two cannabis based medicinal extracts for relief of central neuropathic pain from brachial plexus avulsion: results of a randomised controlled trial. *Pain* 112:299–306.

76. Wade, D.T., Robson, P., House, H., Makela, P., Aram, J. (2003). A preliminary controlled study to determine whether whole-plant cannabis extracts can improve intractable neurogenic symptoms. *Clin Rehabil* 17:21–29.

77. Einhorn, L.H., Nagy, C., Furnas, B., Williams, S.D. (1981). Nabilone: an effective antiemetic in patients receiving cancer chemotherapy. *J Clin Pharmacol* 21:64S–69S.

78. Slatkin, N.E. (2007). Cannabinoids in the treatment of chemotherapy-induced nausea and vomiting: beyond prevention of acute emesis. *J Support Oncol* 5:1–9.

79. Tramer, M.R. (2001). A rational approach to the control of postoperative nausea and vomiting: evidence from systematic reviews. Part I. Efficacy and harm of antiemetic interventions, and methodological issues. *Acta Anaesthesiol Scand* 45:4–13.

80. Chan, P.C., Sills, R.C., Braun, A.G., Haseman, J.K., Bucher, J.R. (1996). Toxicity and carcinogenicity of delta 9-tetrahydrocannabinol in Fischer rats and B6C3F1 mice. *Fundam Appl Toxicol* 30:109–117.

81. Guzman, M. (2003). Cannabinoids: potential anticancer agents. *Nat Rev Cancer* 3:745–755.

82. Michalski, C.W., Oti, F.E., Erkan, M., Sauliunaite, D., Bergmann, F., Pacher, P., Batkai, S., Muller, M.W., Giese, N.A., Friess, H., Kleeff, J. (2008). Cannabinoids in pancreatic cancer: correlation with survival and pain. *Int J Cancer* 122:742–750.

83. Noyes, R., Jr., Brunk, S.F., Avery, D.A., Canter, A.C. (1975). The analgesic properties of delta-9-tetrahydrocannabinol and codeine. *Clin Pharmacol Ther* 18:84–89.

84. Johnson, J.R., Potts, R. (2005). Paper presented at the 38th British Pain Society Annual Scientific Meeting. Edinburgh, Scotland.

85. Hamamoto, D.T., Giridharagopalan, S., Simone, D.A. (2007). Acute and chronic administration of the cannabinoid receptor agonist CP 55,940 attenuates tumor-evoked hyperalgesia. *Eur J Pharmacol* 558:73–87.

86. Kehl, L.J., Hamamoto, D.T., Wacnik, P.W., Croft, D.L., Norsted, B.D., Wilcox, G.L., Simone, D.A. (2003). A cannabinoid agonist differentially attenuates deep tissue hyperalgesia in animal models of cancer and inflammatory muscle pain. *Pain* 103:175–186.

87. Guerrero, A.V., Quang, P., Dekker, N., Jordan, R.C., Schmidt, B.L. (2008). Peripheral cannabinoids attenuate carcinoma-induced nociception in mice. *Neurosci Lett* 433:77–81.

88. Potenzieri, C., Harding-Rose, C., Simone, D.A. (2008). The cannabinoid receptor agonist, WIN 55, 212-2, attenuates tumor-evoked hyperalgesia through peripheral mechanisms. *Brain Res* 1215:69–75.

89. Adami, M., Frati, P., Bertini, S., Kulkarni-Narla, A., Brown, D.R., de Caro, G., Coruzzi, G., Soldani, G. (2002). Gastric antisecretory role and immunohistochemical localization of cannabinoid receptors in the rat stomach. *Brit J Pharmacol* 135:1598–1606.

90. Casu, M.A., Porcella, A., Ruiu, S., Saba, P., Marchese, G., Carai, M.A., Reali, R., Gessa, G.L., Pani, L. (2003). Differential distribution of functional cannabinoid CB1 receptors in the mouse gastroenteric tract. *Eur J Pharmacol* 459:97–105.

91. Kulkarni-Narla, A., Brown, D.R. (2000). Localization of CB1-cannabinoid receptor immunoreactivity in the porcine enteric nervous system. *Cell Tissue Res* 302: 73–80.

92. Ross, R.A., Brockie, H.C., Fernando, S.R., Saha, B., Razdan, R.K., Pertwee, R.G. (1998). Comparison of cannabinoid binding sites in guinea-pig forebrain and small intestine. *Brit J Pharmacol* 125:1345–1351.

93. MacNaughton, W.K., Van Sickle, M.D., Keenan, C.M., Cushing, K., Mackie, K., Sharkey, K.A. (2004). Distribution and function of the cannabinoid-1 receptor in the modulation of ion transport in the guinea pig ileum: relationship to capsaicin-sensitive nerves. *Am J Physiol Gastrointest Liver Physiol* 286:G863–G871.

94. Welburn, P.J., Starmer, G.A., Chesher, G.B., Jackson, D.M. (1976). Effect of cannabinoids on the abdominal constriction response in mice: within cannabinoid interactions. *Psychopharmacologia* 46:83–85.

95. Sanson, M., Bueno, L., Fioramonti, J. (2006). Involvement of cannabinoid receptors in inflammatory hypersensitivity to colonic distension in rats. *Neurogastroenterol Motil* 18:949–956.

96. Michalski, C.W., Laukert, T., Sauliunaite, D., Pacher, P., Bergmann, F., Agarwal, N., Su, Y., Giese, T., Giese, N.A., Batkai, S., Friess, H., Kuner, R. (2007). Cannabinoids ameliorate pain and reduce disease pathology in cerulein-induced acute pancreatitis. *Gastroenterology* 132:1968–1978.

CHAPTER 14

Opioid Receptors

CLAUDIA HERRERA TAMBELI,[1] LUANA FISCHER,[2] and
CARLOS AMILCAR PARADA[3]

[1]Department of Physiology, Piracicaba Dental School, University of Campinas
[2]Laboratory of Pain Physiology, Division of Biological Sciences, Department of Physiology, Federal University of Parana
[3]Department of Physiology and Biophysics, Institute of Biological Sciences, University of Campinas

Content

14.1 HISTORICAL OVERVIEW ON OPIOID RECEPTORS AND PEPTIDES

Pain-relieving and euphorigenic properties of opium and its extracts have been known for centuries, but it was only in the twentieth century that there were substantial advances made in our understanding of how opiates produced their selective effects on the body. Morphine was isolated from raw opium in 1805 by a German pharmacologist, Friedrich Wilhelm Adam Serturner [1], and is one of the most widely used analgesics today. The name morphine comes from the Greek "god of dreams," Morpheus.

Peripheral Receptor Targets for Analgesia: Novel Approaches to Pain Management, Edited by Brian E. Cairns

The proposal that morphine and related opioids cause analgesia by interacting with a specific receptor was favored by the extraordinary potency of some opiates, the availability of selective antagonists, and the stereospecificity of opiate actions. In 1973, opioid receptors were first demonstrated within the central nervous system (CNS) using a binding assay [2–5]. The idea of multiple opioid receptors evolved from clinical trials with morphine/nalorphine combinations [6] and from pharmacological approaches *in vivo* that led Martin and coworkers in 1976 [7] to propose that opioids activated μ-opioid receptor (MOR) and κ-opioid receptor (KOR) for which the prototypical agonists were morphine and ketocyclazocine, respectively. The identification of the δ-opioid receptor (DOR) followed the discovery of the first endogenous opioid receptor ligands, Met- and Leu-enkephalin [8], when it was shown that their pattern of agonist activity *in vitro* differed from that of the prototypical opioid ligands [9]. Although pharmacological studies were consistent with the existence of multiple opioid receptors, definitive demonstration of the three major families of receptors came afterward from ligand binding studies [10–14].

The genes encoding the MOR, DOR, and KOR were cloned in early 1990s, starting with the DOR-1 [15–18], which was followed shortly afterward by the MOR-1 [19–22] and KOR-1 receptors [23–26]. Although the presence of subdivisions of these three subtype receptors such as μ1 and μ2 [14], δ1 and δ2 [27], and κ1, κ2, and κ3 [28] has been proposed, only three opioid receptor genes have been characterized so far. These subdivisions may result from splice variants [29–32] and receptor dimerization to form a homomeric and heteromeric complex [33].

By the early 1970s, the idea had arisen that the opioid receptors in the brain should have a physiological function. The observation that the properties of opioid receptors resembled those of receptors for neurotransmitters motivated researchers to start the search for endogenous opioid agonists fulfilling a physiological function. The isolation of sufficient material from porcine brain for analysis took about 2 years and resulted in the identification of the enkephalins Met-enkephalin (Tyr-Gly-Gly-Phe-Met; [Met(5)]enkephalin) and Leu-enkephalin (Tyr-Gly-Gly-Phe-Leu; [Leu(5)]enkephalin) [8]; the name is derived from the Greek meaning "in the head." Soon after the discovery of enkephalins, a fragment of the pituitary protein β-lipoprotein [34] that was found to contain the sequence of Met-enkephalin [35] was named β-endorphin, meaning endogenous morphine. Another fragment, which was found to contain the sequence of Leu-enkephalin, was named dynorphin, meaning "power" from the Greek [36–38].

The endogenous opioid peptides are derived from protein precursors through hydrolysis by proteases that recognize basic amino acid sequences positioned just before and after the opioid peptide sequences [39]. The precursors of Leu- and Met-enkephalins, β-endorphin, and dynorphins are proenkephalin [40,41], pro-opiomelanocortin [42], and prodynorphin [43], respectively. Opioid peptides vary in their affinity for MOR, DOR, and KOR, that is, Leu- and Met-enkephalins have a high affinity for DOR and MOR;

β-endorphin has a high affinity for MOR and DOR, and dynorphin has a high affinity for the KOR [39].

Opioid analgesia is mediated by modulation of ascending [44–46] and descending pain pathways [47,48]. Accordingly, the MOR, DOR, and KOR are expressed in dorsal root ganglia, in the spinal cord, and in the trigeminal nucleus of the ascending pain pathway as well as in several areas of the CNS including those involved in pain modulation such as the periaqueductal gray nuclei, raphe magnus nuclei, gigantocellular reticular nuclei, and nucleus accumbens [49,50]. The functional consequences arising from expression patterns of opioid receptors may affect many physiological systems, which can have important implications for the clinical use of opioids, particularly in the adverse side effects of systemically administered opioid receptor agonists. Many dose-limiting side effects of systemic treatment with opioids, such as respiratory depression and sedation, are due to activation of central opioid receptors. However, in addition to the central opioid receptors, opioid receptors expressed on peripheral neurons can also contribute to antinociception. This important finding opened up the development of an entirely novel generation of peripherally active opioid analgesics devoid of centrally mediated side effects.

14.2 PERIPHERAL OPIOID RECEPTORS

The first functional evidence of peripheral opioid receptors dates from the end of the 1970s [51], and almost a decade after their central characterization, the peripheral localization of opioid receptors was demonstrated [52]. Recent saturation and competition experiments indicate that the pharmacology of these peripheral receptors is very similar to that of those in the brain [53,54].

14.2.1 Subtypes, Synthesis, and Localization

The three opioid receptor subtypes MOR, DOR, and KOR are expressed in primary sensory neurons [55], and it has been previously demonstrated that an equal proportion of small and large dorsal root ganglion neurons expresses opioid receptor mRNAs [56]. Colocalization studies confirmed their presence on nociceptive C-fibers [55,57], where they mediate the peripheral analgesic effect of opioids, as demonstrated by the blockade of peripheral opioid analgesia by pretreatment with capsaicin, a neurotoxin selective for C-fibers [58]. These peripheral opioid receptors are synthesized in the cell body, in the dorsal root, or in the trigeminal ganglion, and are transported along intra-axonal microtubules to central and peripheral nerve terminals of the primary afferents, where they are incorporated into the neuronal membrane and become functional receptors [59]. Some functional studies have suggested that peripheral opioid receptors are located on sympathetic postganglionic terminals [60,61]. However, studies attempting the direct demonstration of opioid receptor expression in sympathetic ganglia have produced negative results [62,63]. Furthermore, a functional study demonstrated that sympathetic neurons do not mediate peripheral analgesia induced by exogenous opioids [58].

In addition to their role in peripheral nociceptive mechanisms, opioid receptors expressed on neurons innervating peripheral organs, such as the skin and gastrointestinal tract [64,65], mediate, in whole or in part, some of the side effects attributed to opioids, such as constipation, cough suppression, pruritus, and decreased ventilatory response to hypoxia [66]. While these peripheral mediated side effects are of some clinical importance, especially in patients undergoing chronic opioid therapy [66], they are undoubtedly less relevant than those that are centrally mediated such as sedation, dysphoria, respiratory depression, tolerance, and addiction. Opioid receptors have also been described in several nonneuronal tissues not traditionally assigned a primarily nociceptive function, such as vascular and cardiac epithelia [67], keratinocytes [64], and endothelial [68] and immune [69] cells. Although the significance of opioid receptor expression in the majority of these non-nociceptive tissues is not clear, it is well known that opioid receptors expressed in immune cells mediate important physiological and pathological functions of the immune system [69], including the macrophage oxidative burst and cytokine production [70]. However, whether the activation of opioid receptors expressed in immune cells and other nonneuronal sites contributes, in any way, to endogenous or exogenous opioid mediated analgesia has yet to be determined. Therefore, according to our present knowledge, the peripheral antinociceptive effect induced by endogenous and exogenous opioid ligands is believed to be mediated by opioid receptors located in primary nociceptive afferents [58,59,71].

14.2.2 Molecular Structure and Signaling Mechanisms

Opioid receptors belong to the G protein-coupled receptor family. As shown in Figure 14.1, they consist of seven transmembrane hydrophobic domains (I–VII), with the amino group terminal at the extracellular side and the carboxyl tail inside the cytoplasm of the cell (Figure 14.1). The extracellular region consists of the N-terminal and the first, second, and third loops (first extracellular loop [EL-I], second extracellular loop [EL-II], and third extracellular loop [EL-III]), while the intracellular region consists of the first, second, and third loops (first intracellular loop [IL-I], second intracellular loop [IL-II], and third intracellular loop [IL-III]) and the C-terminal. MOR, DOR, and KOR have approximately 60% of homology. Amino acid residues are conserved particularly in the transmembrane regions (73–76%) and in the intracellular regions (63–63%). On the other hand, the extracellular regions of MOR, DOR, and KOR have only 34–40% of homology. Specific binding domains are located in specific regions of MOR, DOR, and KOR. Transmembrane domains V–VII are selectively involved with DOR binding [72]. EL-I is essential for MOR binding [72], while EL-II and half of transmembrane region IV are particularly important to KOR binding [73]. IL-I and

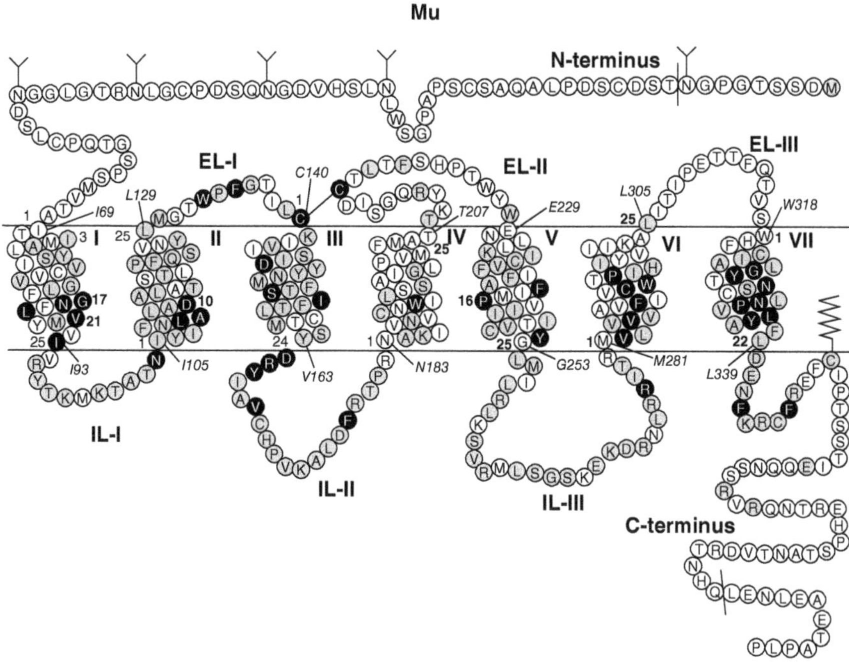

FIGURE 14.1. Serpentine model of the of μ-opioid receptor (MOR) molecular structure. EL, extracellular loop; IL, intracellular loop (from Portoghese, P.S., http://www.opioid.umn.edu (accessed May 15, 2009)).

IL-III, the V transmembrane, and the C-terminal domains of opioid receptors are responsible for G protein-coupled intracellular signaling [73,74]. The opioid receptors are coupled with G_i or G_o proteins, sensitive to pertussis toxin (PTX). The binding of an opioid to its receptor activates the coupled G protein resulting in the dissociation of $G\alpha_i$ from inhibitory $G\beta\gamma$ dimer [75]. The dissociation between $G\alpha_i$- and $G\beta\gamma$-subunits initiates a cascade of downstream intracellular effector events that mediate the antinociceptive effect of opioids on primary afferent neurons. These intracellular effector events include inhibition of adenylate cyclase (AC) activity [76–78] as well as of N- and L-type Ca^{2+} channel [79,80] and activation of the L-arginine/nitric oxide (NO)/cyclic guanosine monophosphate (cGMP) pathway in the subcutaneous tissue [81,82], the ATP-sensitive K^+ channel (KATP) [83], and the phosphotidylinositol 3-kinase (PI3K)/akt pathway [84], as illustrated in Figure 14.2.

14.2.3 Endogenous Ligands

Immune cells are the most extensively examined source of endogenous opioids interacting with peripheral opioid receptors [85]. The prevailing peptides are endorphins and enkephalins [86]. Small amounts of dynorphins are detectable [86] and, recently, endomorphins have been also identified in immune cells. The subpopulation of leukocytes expressing opioid peptides includes lympho-

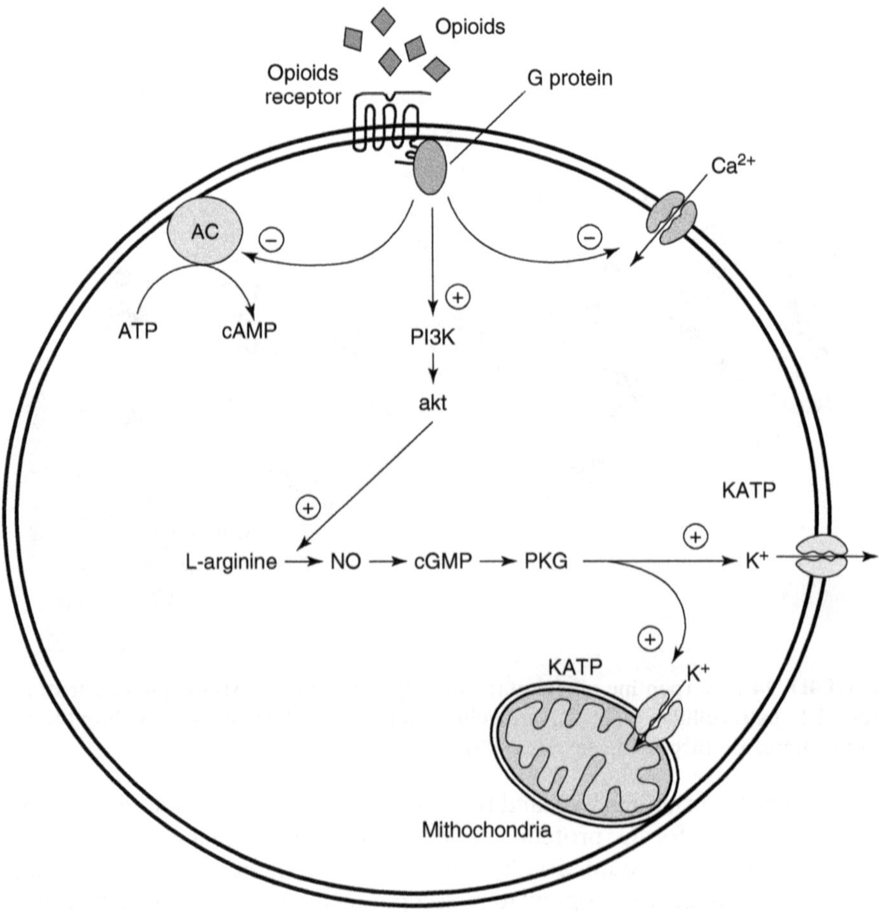

FIGURE 14.2. Proposed model for opioid receptor-mediated analgesia in the peripheral terminal of primary sensory neurons. Activation of opioid receptor by endogenous or exogenous opioid promotes G protein coupling. Opioid receptors coupled G protein directly inhibit Voltage-dependent Ca^{2+} channel and adenylate cyclase (AC) and consequently inhibit cyclic AMP (cAMP). Activation of opioid receptors activate the L-arginine/NO/cGMP/PKG pathway that, in turn, opens ATP-sensitive K^+ channel (KATP). The activation of NO synthase enzyme by opioid receptor-coupled G protein may utilize PI3Kinase/akt as intermediary messenger system. AMP, adenosine 5′-monophosphate; PKG, protein kinase G. See color insert.

cytes, monocytes, and granulocytes in the peripheral blood, lymph nodes, and mainly, at the site of inflammation [86–89], where they are released upon certain types of stimulation. Originally, the role of these opioid peptides was thought to be the regulation of local immune function through the neuroendocrine axis [90–92]. This was supported by the observation that immune cells express opioid receptors [93] and by functional evidence that opioids can modulate immune function [94]. An additional role for these peptides emerged with the observation that opioid peptides released locally from immune cells can act on opioid receptors expressed on peripheral neurons to exert an anti-hyperalgesic effect in inflamed tissue [95]. Recent findings have also demonstrated that in addition to immune cells, keratinocytes also express opioid peptides and release them to induce analgesia after stimulation [96].

14.3 PERIPHERAL EXOGENOUS OPIOID ANALGESIA

In the late 1970s and during the 1980s, reports about the peripheral analgesic effects of opiates began to accumulate [51,97–100]. Peripheral opioid analgesia has been reported in nociceptive pain [101,102] and in neurophatic pain [103–106], although it is reduced in the latter condition. However, there is no consensus about the peripheral analgesic effects of opiates on noninflammatory pain. It was suggested that the preexistent neuronal opioid receptors are inactive [107] and are not available due to the perineurium barrier [108] in normal tissue, which is consistent with many studies that found no opioid analgesia mediated by these receptors under normal tissue conditions [109–114].

The analgesic efficacy of opiates is greatly enhanced under conditions of inflammation as demonstrated in many tissues such as the subcutaneous [101,115,116], articular [117,118], and muscular [119]. Many events contribute to this. First, inflammation of peripheral tissue leads to increased synthesis and axonal transport of opioid receptors in neurons of the dorsal root ganglia, resulting in their upregulation [53,120,121]. Second, the low pH of the inflamed tissue increases opioid agonist efficacy by enhancing the interaction of opioid receptors with G proteins at peripheral nerve terminals [122]. Third, the number of nociceptor endings increases in inflamed tissue [123]. Finally, the perineural barrier is disrupted, which facilitates the access of opioid agonists to their receptors on sensory neurons [108]. This latter event contributes to the enhanced antinociceptive effects of peripheral opioids during the early stages of inflammation and helps to explain why this effect is more difficult to detect in noninflamed tissue.

Under conditions of inflammation, in addition to the finding that the analgesic efficacy of opiates is greatly enhanced, chronic morphine treatment does not seem to result in antinociceptive tolerance (decreased opioid analgesia after prolonged administration of a constant dose of opioids). For example, in animals with persistent inflammation, no tolerance to the acute intraplantar injection of fentanyl is seen after chronic morphine application [124]. Persistent painful inflammation prevents the development of tolerance to peripheral opioid receptors by enhancing MOR endocytosis, recycling, and recovery of opioid responsiveness. The ability of exogenous opioids to stimulate μ-receptor endocytosis in sensory neurons and thereby to reduce the development of morphine tolerance is facilitated by the release of endogenous opioid peptides from leucocytes in inflammation. Consistent with this, when endogenous ligands of these receptors are removed by antibodies or by depleting opioid-producing granulocytes, monocytes, and lymphocytes with cyclophosphamide, decreased MOR endocytosis/function and tolerance ensue [124].

Previous studies [125,126] have shown that in animals without tissue injury, chronic opioid treatment can induce tolerance to peripheral opioid receptors. However, this is not clinically relevant because patients usually do not consume opioids in the absence of painful tissue injury.

14.4 PERIPHERAL ENDOGENOUS OPIOID ANALGESIA

The first direct evidence that endogenous opioids modulate pain in humans dates from the end of the 1970s [127] and for many years, this intrinsic mechanism of pain control has been thought to be mediated exclusively within the CNS. However, the observation that intra-articular naloxone exacerbates pain and increases medication consumption after knee surgery [95] began to introduce the idea that an intrinsic peripheral opioid mechanism may also contribute to pain control. It is now becoming clear that recruitment of opioid peptide-containing immune cells to the site of inflammation may counteract inflammatory pain under certain conditions. During inflammation, both precursor proteins as well as opioid peptide expression appear to be increased in leukocytes from inflamed tissue [88,128,129]. Opioid peptide-containing immune cells migrate to injured tissues directed by cytokines, chemokines, and adhesion molecules and by neuropeptides, such as substance P via NK1 receptors [130–132].

The migration of leukocytes to the site of inflammation is enabled by the interaction of adhesion molecules expressed on leukocytes and on the vascular endothelium (Figure 14.3). These adhesion molecules comprise the selectins, immunoglobulin-like family members such as intercellular adhesion molecule (ICAM) and platelet–endothelial cell adhesion molecule (PECAM), and the integrin family of α- and β-subunit heterodimers [133]. Initially, leukocytes roll along the inflamed endothelium. This process is mediated predominantly by L-, P-, and E-selectins. L-selectins are constitutively expressed on leukocytes, and P- and E-selectins are expressed on vascular endothelium [134]. Then, leukocytes are activated by chemokines and cytokines released from inflammatory cells and presented on the endothelium. This leads to the upregulation of integrins, which mediate the firm adhesion of leukocytes to endothelial cells via ICAM-1. Finally, leukocytes transmigrate through the relaxed endothelial junctions and into the inflamed tissue, a process mediated by PECAM-1 [135; reviewed in Reference 136]. Afterward, these cells travel to the regional lymph nodes, depleted of peptides.

In early inflammation, granulocytes are the major source of opioid peptides [137] that are stored in primary granules and are released together with bactericidal enzymes such as myeloperoxidase [138]. In contrast, at later stages, monocytes and macrophages are the predominant suppliers of opioid peptides [137].

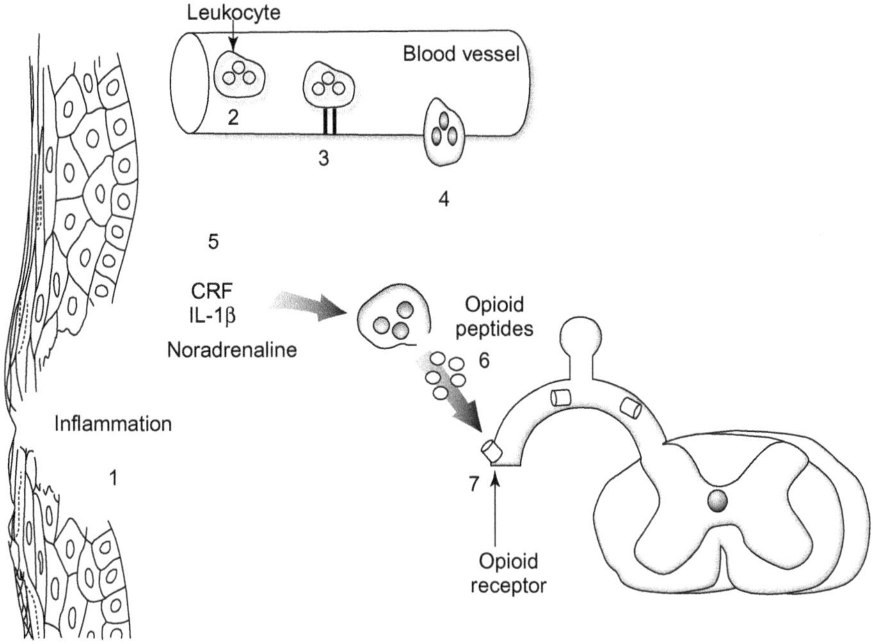

FIGURE 14.3. During inflammation (1), opioid-containing leukocytes (2), via adhesion molecules (3), migrate (4) into inflamed tissue. Then, noradrenaline and inflammatory mediators such as corticotropin-releasing factor (CRF) and interleukin-1β (IL-1β) (5) stimulate these cells to secrete opioid peptides (6). These peptides activate opioid receptors (7) expressed in the primary afferent nociceptors and reduce inflammatory pain.

Endogenous peripheral opioid analgesia was demonstrated experimentally in a model of stress-induced analgesia [95,100,107,131,137,139,140]. Classically, the analgesia induced by stressful stimulation was described as a central mediated opioid mechanism (first reviewed in Reference 141). The response to stress is characterized by stimulation of the hypothalamic–pituitary–adrenocortical axis and by activation of the sympathetic nervous system. Then, epinephrine and noradrenaline, respectively, are released from the adrenal medulla and sympathetic nerve endings, and the subsequent analgesia is mediated by the activation of the endogenous central opioid system [141]. In rats with inflammation of the hind paw, however, stress-induced analgesia is mediated predominantly by endogenous opioids released from immune cells that bind to peripheral opioid receptors in primary nociceptive neurons [140]. This analgesia may also be induced by pretreatment with releasing agents corticotropin-releasing factor [CRF] [128], noradrenaline [142], and interleukin-1 [128] and is blocked by opioid receptor antagonists locally administered [140] as well as by antibodies against opioid peptides [142]. The relevance of immune cells for the generation of endogenous peripheral opioid analgesia is supported by studies showing that it is abolished by treatments that decrease immune cell function, such as selectin blockers and immunosuppressant drugs [86,88,143,144]. These important findings expand the concept that leukocytes are only members of the frontline defense mechanism; they are now also known to produce and secrete opioid peptides to counteract inflammatory pain. These findings may also lead to the idea that therapeutic strategies that decrease immune cell recruitment to the site of inflammation may, in fact, exacerbate pain. However, a cautious analysis of the literature data is crucial to understand the role of immune cells in inflammatory pain based on our present knowledge. First, in addition to opioids, leukocytes release a large body of hyperalgesic mediators (such as cytokines, prostaglandin, and chemokines). Second, it was demonstrated that only 16–20% of immune cells that infiltrate the inflamed tissue contain endogenous opioid peptides [139]. Third, analgesia induced by the release of opioid peptides from these cells may be experimentally demonstrated only under specific stimulation (stress or pretreatment with releasing agents) [95,100,107,131,137,139,140]. Fourth, treatments that impair immune cell function abolish endogenous peripheral opioid analgesia but do not affect the hyperalgesic threshold in animals not submitted to stress or pretreated with releasing agents [86,88,143,144]. This latter finding suggests that endogenous peripheral opioid analgesia is not tonically activated during inflammation, which is consistent with numerous studies using opioid receptor antagonists or mice lacking either opioid receptors or opioid peptides, which have shown no changes in inflammatory pain [145–147]. Finally, there is a large body of evidence demonstrating that decreased recruitment of inflammatory cells to the site of inflammation is associated with decreased hyperalgesia and nociception [148–152] Therefore, further studies are necessary to determine the pronociceptive and antinociceptive role of immune cells in inflammatory conditions and, therefore, to determine the clinical significance of immune-derived peripheral antinociception.

Undoubtedly, the finding that an intrinsic peripheral opioid mechanism may effectively control pain opens exciting possibilities for pain research and therapy. Of major importance is the identification of a possible differential characteristic of opioid peptide-containing immune cells as well as strategies to stimulate more specifically their migration. Studies in this field have recently been conducted [139,153]; however, the results do not show any specific strategy to stimulate exclusively the mechanisms mediated by opioid peptide-containing immune cells.

14.5 CLINICAL STUDIES ON PERIPHERAL OPIOID ANALGESIA

Traditionally, opioids were considered the prototype of centrally acting analgesics. This idea begun to be changed by evidences that peripherally administered opioids decreased prostaglandin-induced hyperalgesia [51]. The first evidence of a peripheral effect of opioids in humans came some years later, by data showing that an opioid administered prior to the painful stimulation of the nasal mucosa decreased the electrophysiological response evoked from the nasal nociceptors [154]. In the last two decades, substantial literature has emerged demonstrating that opioids can induce potent and clinically measurable analgesia by acting on peripheral opioid receptors. Among the unquestionable advantages of targeting peripheral opioid receptors are the avoidance of central opioid side effects such as respiratory depression, nausea, dysphoria, addiction, and high rate of analgesic tolerance. To evaluate the effect of a therapeutic strategy in clinical pain studies, it is necessary to use standardized and validated tools to measure pain, which is essentially a subjective experience. In these studies, pain relief is commonly measured (i) by reductions in subjective pain intensity scores, (ii) by extended time intervals to the patient's first request for additional pain medication, (iii) by a decreased number of patients asking for supplemental analgesic drugs, (iv) by diminished total consumption of supplemental analgesics, or (v) by the ability of the patient to resume normal functioning. The majority of controlled trials in peripheral opioid analgesia have used MOR agonists, and although a growing number of studies have demonstrated successful results with the use of KOR-agonists, the utility of DOR agonists in the peripheral setting has to be investigated in clinical pain studies.

Consistent with experimental studies, evidence from clinical studies points to a critical role of inflammation for the occurrence of peripheral analgesic effects of opioids [155–157]. In fact, some studies that have compared the efficacy of peripheral opioid analgesia under inflammatory and noninflammatory conditions support the important role of inflammation in this kind of analgesia. For example, human inflammatory, but not noninflammatory experimental pain is significantly reduced by a peripherally acting morphine metabolite [156]. In addition, in patients undergoing dental surgery, the local injection of 1 mg of morphine into inflamed, but not into noninflamed tissue results in significant and prolonged postoperative analgesia with reduced supplementary analgesic intake [157]. As discussed above, peripheral opioid analgesia may be dependent on the enhanced perineurium permeability and of structural changes in opioid receptors in the terminal nerve endings exposed to an acidic environment of inflammation. In fact, even in the presence of long-lasting inflammation, morphine is ineffective when it is administered around the mandibular nerve instead of at the site of the inflamed tooth [157]. This suggests that intra-axonal opioid receptors may be "in transit" and not functional, and that the perineural barrier of peripheral nerves may hinder the access of opioids to their receptors. In fact, the majority of studies that have found no peripheral analgesic effects of opioids examined the injection of agonists along nerve trunks [158–160] or in the noninflamed tissues [109–114].

Initially, the strategies to induce clinical significant analgesia by targeting peripheral opioid receptors have involved the local administration of conventional opioids, and its great advantage probably relays on the lack of not only central but also peripheral side effects related to the conventional use of opioids. From the end of the 1980s until the present, a large number of studies have demonstrated significant analgesic effects following local application of systemically inactive doses of opioids in various clinical settings [157,161–167]. The most extensively studied clinical situation is the intra-articular administration of morphine in patients undergoing knee surgery. A review of 33 randomized and controlled trials concluded that 5 mg is effective to reduce postoperative pain for up to 24 hours [168]. In contrast, after temporomandibular joint surgery, intra-articular morphine has been associated with mild or no analgesic effects [169–171]; however, these negative results are probably related to low doses used (1 or 2 mg).

Chronic inflammatory diseases, such as rheumatoid and osteoarthritis, have been also effectively controlled by intra-articular morphine, and its effect is surprisingly long lasting (up to 7 days) [165,172]. However, this effect cannot solely be explained by a direct action of morphine on opioid receptors on the peripheral nociceptive neurons, decreasing their excitability [173]. In addition to that, it may also result from morphine's anti-inflammatory activity. As evidenced in numerous animal studies, opioids have a potent anti-inflammatory effect (reviewed in Reference 174). Therefore, in addition to their action on sensory neurons, local opioids can also act on resident immune cells to decrease inflammation. This is supported by the findings that local opioids can decrease cytokine secretion, can downregulate the expression of adhesion molecules, and can reduce the migration of immune cells into the injured tissue [175]. The combination of analgesic and anti-inflammatory effects of local opioids may result in therapeutic effects comparable or even better than those induced by standard treatments for arthritis (nonsteroidal anti-inflammatory drugs and steroids). However, a serious limitation of local opioid treatment is the requirement of repeated intra-articular injections, which carry a risk of infection and cannot be easily applied to more than one joint. To avoid these problems, the major goal of pharmaceutical companies is to develop novel opioid compounds that do not pass the blood–brain barrier and, therefore, act selectively on peripheral opioid receptors when systemically administered. A common approach is the use of hydrophilic compounds; however, penetration of the blood–brain barrier may not be entirely precluded at high doses, and the polarizing residues may interfere with the affinity at opioid receptors [176,177]. The great advantage of these peripherally restricted opioids is the oral or intravenous administration avoiding some or all central side effects. However, some peripherally mediated side effects may remain problematic [177]. For this reason, the development of peripherally acting κ-opioid agonists is of special interest because they are not associated with visceral side effects, such as spasm and constipation [178]. Some of these new opioids have already been tested in human studies, either in experimental or in clinical conditions. Fedotozine was the first peripheral κ-opioid agonist to be studied clinically [179]. Despite initial positive outcomes in visceral pain states [180,181], in additional studies, it was apparently less effective, and subsequent clinical development of the drug was suspended [182]. Asimadoline is a peripheral κ-opioid agonist with positive results in animal models [183–185]; however, it was not effective in reducing experimental pain in humans [186] and in patients undergoing knee surgery [187]. A second generation of peripherally restricted κ-agonist markedly reduced visceral pain in patients with chronic pancreatitis without severe side effects [178]. A metabolite of morphine, known to cross the blood–brain barrier with difficulty [188], was effective in reducing experimental inflammatory pain in humans by a peripheral mechanism [156].

The findings from the literature clearly show a high efficacy of peripheral acting opioids for inflammatory pain control. A possible contribution of peripheral opioid receptors in neuropathic pain states remains to be investigated. This apparent disinterest may result from the inconsistencies among animal studies [61,189,190]. In contrast, animal studies about sex differences in peripheral analgesic sensitivity have produced more consistent results, showing a greater sensitivity of males to μ-opioid agonists [191] and a greater sensitivity of females to κ-opioid agonists [118]. In view of these preclinical results, any sex differences in clinical peripheral opioid analgesia should be investigated, and opioid agonists and doses should be fit adapted to these differences.

While our understanding of peripheral opioid mechanisms has expanded considerably in recent years, highly effective strategies to obtain peripheral opioid analgesia without side effects are still lacking. Strategies could be developed that improve analgesia through selective enhancement of endogenous analgesia, for example, by enhancing the availability of endogenous opioids within injured tissue and the expression or signal transduction of peripheral opioid receptors. Some initial experimental studies have shown exciting results in this field. For example, a recent human study has shown that the increase in endogenous peripherally released opioids significantly reduces postoperative pain [192]. In the same way, recent animal studies have demonstrated that the overexpression of opioid receptors or peptides, induced by their gene transfection in dorsal root or trigeminal ganglion, ameliorates pain in inflammatory and neuropathic pain models [103,193–195].

REFERENCES

1. Schmitz, R. (1985). Friedrich Wilhelm Serturner and the discovery of morphine. *Pharm Hist* 27:61–74.
2. Pert, C.B., Snyder, S.H. (1973). Opiate receptor: demonstration in nervous tissue. *Science* 179:1011–1014.
3. Simon, E.J., Hiller, J.M., Edelman, I. (1973). Stereospecific binding of the potent narcotic analgesic (3H) etorphine to rat-brain homogenate. *Proc Natl Acad Sci U S A* 70:1947–1949.

4. Terenius, L. (1973). Stereospecific interaction between narcotic analgesics and a synaptic plasm a membrane fraction of rat cerebral cortex. *Acta Pharmacol Toxicol (Copenh)* 32:317–320.

5. Terenius, L. (1973). Characteristics of the "receptor" for narcotic analgesics in synaptic plasma membrane fraction from rat brain. *Acta Pharmacol Toxicol (Copenh)* 33:377–384.

6. Martin, W.R. (1967). Opioid antagonists. *Pharmacol Rev* 19:463–521.

7. Martin, W.R., Eades, C.G., Thompson, J.A., Huppler, R.E., Gilbert, P.E. (1976). The effects of morphine- and nalorphine- like drugs in the nondependent and morphine-dependent chronic spinal dog. *J Pharmacol Exp Ther* 197:517–532.

8. Hughes, J., Smith, T.W., Kosterlitz, H.W., Fothergill, L.A., Morgan, B.A., Morris, H.R. (1975). Identification of two related pentapeptides from the brain with potent opiate agonist activity. *Nature* 258:577–580.

9. Lord, J.A., Waterfield, A.A., Hughes, J., Kosterlitz, H.W. (1977). Endogenous opioid peptides: multiple agonists and receptors. *Nature* 267:495–499.

10. Chang, K.J., Cooper, B.R., Hazum, E., Cuatrecasas, P. (1979). Multiple opiate receptors: different regional distribution in the brain and differential binding of opiates and opioid peptides. *Mol Pharmacol* 16:91–104.

11. Kosterlitz, H.W., Paterson, S.J., Robson, L.E. (1981). Characterization of the kappa-subtype of the opiate receptor in the guinea-pig brain. *Br J Pharmacol* 73: 939–949.

12. Leslie, F.M., Kosterlitz, H.W. (1979). Comparison of binding of [3H]-methionine-enkephalin, [3H]-naltrexone and [3H]-dihydromorphine in the mouse vas deferens and the myenteric plexus and brain of the ginea pig. *Eur J Pharmacol* 56:379–383.

13. Pasternak, G.W., Snyder, S.H. (1975). Identification of novel high affinity opiate receptor binding in rat brain. *Nature* 253:563–565.

14. Wolozin, B.L., Nishimura, S., Pasternak, G.W. (1982). The binding of kappa- and sigma-opiates in rat brain. *J Neurosci* 2:708–713.

15. Evans, C.J., Keith, D.E., Jr., Morrison, H., Magendzo, K., Edwards, R.H. (1992). Cloning of a delta opioid receptor by functional expression. *Science* 258: 1952–1955.

16. Kieffer, B.L., Befort, K., Gaveriaux-Ruff, C., Hirth, C.G. (1992). The delta-opioid receptor: isolation of a cDNA by expression cloning and pharmacological characterization. *Proc Natl Acad Sci U S A* 89:12048–12052.

17. Knapp, R.J., Malatynska, E., Fang, L., Li, X., Babin, E., Nguyen, M., Santoro, G., Varga, E.V., Hruby, V.J., Roeske, W.R., et al. (1994). Identification of a human delta opioid receptor: cloning and expression. *Life Sci* 54:PL463–PL469.

18. Simonin, F., Befort, K., Gaveriaux-Ruff, C., Matthes, H., Nappey, V., Lannes, B., Micheletti, G., Kieffer, B. (1994). The human delta-opioid receptor: genomic organization, cDNA cloning, functional expression, and distribution in human brain. *Mol Pharmacol* 46:1015–1021.

19. Chen, Y., Mestek, A., Liu, J., Hurley, J.A., Yu, L. (1993). Molecular cloning and functional expression of a mu-opioid receptor from rat brain. *Mol Pharmacol* 44:8–12.

20. Thompson, R.C., Mansour, A., Akil, H., Watson, S.J. (1993). Cloning and pharmacological characterization of a rat mu opioid receptor. *Neuron* 11:903–913.
21. Wang, J.B., Imai, Y., Eppler, C.M., Gregor, P., Spivak, C.E., Uhl, G.R. (1993). Mu opiate receptor: cDNA cloning and expression. *Proc Natl Acad Sci U S A* 90: 10230–10234.
22. Wang, J.B., Johnson, P.S., Persico, A.M., Hawkins, A.L., Griffin, C.A., Uhl, G.R. (1994). Human mu opiate receptor. cDNA and genomic clones, pharmacologic characterization and chromosomal assignment. *FEBS Lett* 338:217–222.
23. Chen, Y., Mestek, A., Liu, J., Yu, L. (1993). Molecular cloning of a rat kappa opioid receptor reveals sequence similarities to the mu and delta opioid receptors. *Biochem J* 295(Pt 3):625–628.
24. Meng, F., Xie, G.X., Thompson, R.C., Mansour, A., Goldstein, A., Watson, S.J., Akil, H. (1993). Cloning and pharmacological characterization of a rat kappa opioid receptor. *Proc Natl Acad Sci U S A* 90:9954–9958.
25. Simonin, F., Gaveriaux-Ruff, C., Befort, K., Matthes, H., Lannes, B., Micheletti, G., Mattei, M.G., Charron, G., Bloch, B., Kieffer, B. (1995). Kappa-opioid receptor in humans: cDNA and genomic cloning, chromosomal assignment, functional expression, pharmacology, and expression pattern in the central nervous system. *Proc Natl Acad Sci U S A* 92:7006–7010.
26. Zhu, J., Chen, C., Xue, J.C., Kunapuli, S., DeRiel, J.K., Liu-Chen, L.Y. (1995). Cloning of a human kappa opioid receptor from the brain. *Life Sci* 56: PL201–PL207.
27. Mattia, A., Vanderah, T., Mosberg, H.I., Porreca, F. (1991). Lack of antinociceptive cross-tolerance between [D-Pen2, D-Pen5]enkephalin and [D-Ala2]deltorphin II in mice: evidence for delta receptor subtypes. *J Pharmacol Exp Ther* 258: 583–587.
28. Attali, B., Gouarderes, C., Mazarguil, H., Audigier, Y., Cros, J. (1982). Evidence for multiple "kappa" binding sites by use of opioid peptides in the guinea-pig lumbo-sacral spinal cord. *Neuropeptides* 3:53–64.
29. Gaveriaux-Ruff, C., Peluso, J., Befort, K., Simonin, F., Zilliox, C., Kieffer, B.L. (1997). Detection of opioid receptor mRNA by RT-PCR reveals alternative splicing for the delta- and kappa-opioid receptors. *Brain Res Mol Brain Res* 48:298–304.
30. Pan, Y.X., Xu, J., Bolan, E., Abbadie, C., Chang, A., Zuckerman, A., Rossi, G., Pasternak, G.W. (1999). Identification and characterization of three new alternatively spliced mu-opioid receptor isoforms. *Mol Pharmacol* 56:396–403.
31. Pasternak, G.W. (2004). Multiple opiate receptors: deja vu all over again. *Neuropharmacology* 47(Suppl. 1):312–323.
32. Schuller, A.G., King, M.A., Zhang, J., Bolan, E., Pan, Y.X., Morgan, D.J., Chang, A., Czick, M.E., Unterwald, E.M., Pasternak, G.W., Pintar, J.E. (1999). Retention of heroin and morphine-6 beta-glucuronide analgesia in a new line of mice lacking exon 1 of MOR-1. *Nat Neurosci* 2:151–156.
33. Gaveriaux-Ruff, C., Kieffer, B.L. (1999). Opioid receptors: gene structutre and function. In: Stein, C. (ed.). *Opioids in Pain Control.* Cambridge: Cambridge University Press, pp. 1–20.
34. Li, C.H., Chung, D. (1976). Primary structure of human beta-lipotropin. *Nature* 260:622–624.

35. Li, C.H., Chung, D., Doneen, B.A. (1976). Isolation, characterization and opiate activity of beta-endorphin from human pituitary glands. *Biochem Biophys Res Commun* 72:1542–1547.

36. Cox, B.M., Opheim, K.E., Teschemacher, H., Goldstein, A. (1975). A peptide-like substance from pituitary that acts like morphine. 2. Purification and properties. *Life Sci* 16:1777–1782.

37. Goldstein, A., Tachibana, S., Lowney, L.I., Hunkapiller, M., Hood, L. (1979). Dynorphin-(1-13), an extraordinarily potent opioid peptide. *Proc Natl Acad Sci U S A* 76:6666–6670.

38. Teschemacher, H., Opheim, K.E., Cox, B.M., Goldstein, A. (1975). A peptide-like substance from pituitary that acts like morphine. I. Isolation. *Life Sci* 16: 1771–1775.

39. Akil, H., Watson, S.J., Young, E., Lewis, M.E., Khachaturian, H., Walker, J.M. (1984). Endogenous opioids: biology and function. *Annu Rev Neurosci* 7:223–255.

40. Comb, M., Seeburg, P.H., Adelman, J., Eiden, L., Herbert, E. (1982). Primary structure of the human Met- and Leu-enkephalin precursor and its mRNA. *Nature* 295:663–666.

41. Gubler, U., Seeburg, P., Hoffman, B.J., Gage, L.P., Udenfriend, S. (1982). Molecular cloning establishes proenkephalin as precursor of enkephalin-containing peptides. *Nature* 295:206–208.

42. Nakanishi, S., Inoue, A., Kita, T., Nakamura, M., Chang, A.C., Cohen, S.N., Numa, S. (1979). Nucleotide sequence of cloned cDNA for bovine corticotropin-beta-lipotropin precursor. *Nature* 278:423–427.

43. Kakidani, H., Furutani, Y., Takahashi, H., Noda, M., Morimoto, Y., Hirose, T., Asai, M., Inayama, S., Nakanishi, S., Numa, S. (1982). Cloning and sequence analysis of cDNA for porcine beta-neo-endorphin/dynorphin precursor. *Nature* 298:245–249.

44. Gear, R.W., Levine, J.D. (1995). Antinociception produced by an ascending spino-supraspinal pathway. *J Neurosci* 15:3154–3161.

45. Schmidt, B.L., Tambeli, C.H., Levine, J.D., Gear, R.W. (2002). Mu/delta cooperativity and opposing kappa-opioid effects in nucleus accumbens-mediated antinociception in the rat. *Eur J Neurosci* 15:861–868.

46. Tambeli, C.H., Parada, C.A., Levine, J.D., Gear, R.W. (2002). Inhibition of tonic spinal glutamatergic activity induces antinociception in the rat. *Eur J Neurosci* 16:1547–1553.

47. Tambeli, C.H., Seo, K., Sessle, B.J., Hu, J.W. (2001). Central mu opioid receptor mechanisms modulate mustard oil-evoked jaw muscle activity. *Brain Res* 913:90–94.

48. Fields, H. (2004). State-dependent opioid control of pain. *Nat Rev Neurosci* 5: 565–575.

49. Mansour, A., Fox, C.A., Akil, H., Watson, S.J. (1995). Opioid-receptor mRNA expression in the rat CNS: anatomical and functional implications. *Trends Neurosci* 18:22–29.

50. Mansour, A., Khachaturian, H., Lewis, M.E., Akil, H., Watson, S.J. (1988). Anatomy of CNS opioid receptors. *Trends Neurosci* 11:308–314.

51. Ferreira, S.H., Nakamura, M. (1979). II - Prostaglandin hyperalgesia: the peripheral analgesic activity of morphine, enkephalins and opioid antagonists. *Prostaglandins* 18:191–200.

52. Wuster, M., Schulz, R., Herz, A. (1981). Multiple opiate receptors in peripheral tissue preparations. *Biochem Pharmacol* 30:1883–1887.

53. Hassan, A.H., Ableitner, A., Stein, C., Herz, A. (1993). Inflammation of the rat paw enhances axonal transport of opioid receptors in the sciatic nerve and increases their density in the inflamed tissue. *Neuroscience* 55:185–195.

54. Zollner, C., Shaqura, M.A., Bopaiah, C.P., Mousa, S., Stein, C., Schafer, M. (2003). Painful inflammation-induced increase in mu-opioid receptor binding and G-protein coupling in primary afferent neurons. *Mol Pharmacol* 64:202–210.

55. Minami, M., Maekawa, K., Yabuuchi, K., Satoh, M. (1995). Double in situ hybridization study on coexistence of mu-, delta- and kappa-opioid receptor mRNAs with preprotachykinin A mRNA in the rat dorsal root ganglia. *Brain Res Mol Brain Res* 30:203–210.

56. Wang, H., Wessendorf, M.W. (2001). Equal proportions of small and large DRG neurons express opioid receptor mRNAs. *J Comp Neurol* 429:590–600.

57. Poonyachoti, S., Kulkarni-Narla, A., Brown, D.R. (2002). Chemical coding of neurons expressing delta- and kappa-opioid receptor and type I vanilloid receptor immunoreactivities in the porcine ileum. *Cell Tissue Res* 307:23–33.

58. Zhou, L., Zhang, Q., Stein, C., Schafer, M. (1998). Contribution of opioid receptors on primary afferent versus sympathetic neurons to peripheral opioid analgesia. *J Pharmacol Exp Ther* 286:1000–1006.

59. Stein, C., Schafer, M., Machelska, H. (2003). Attacking pain at its source: new perspectives on opioids. *Nat Med* 9:1003–1008.

60. Taiwo, Y.O., Levine, J.D. (1991). Kappa- and delta-opioids block sympathetically dependent hyperalgesia. *J Neurosci* 11:928–932.

61. Pertovaara, A., Wei, H. (2001). Peripheral effects of morphine in neuropathic rats: role of sympathetic postganglionic nerve fibers. *Eur J Pharmacol* 429:139–145.

62. Schafer, M.K., Bette, M., Romeo, H., Schwaeble, W., Weihe, E. (1994). Localization of kappa-opioid receptor mRNA in neuronal subpopulations of rat sensory ganglia and spinal cord. *Neurosci Lett* 167:137–140.

63. Wenk, H.N., Honda, C.N. (1999). Immunohistochemical localization of delta opioid receptors in peripheral tissues. *J Comp Neurol* 408:567–579.

64. Bigliardi-Qi, M., Sumanovski, L.T., Buchner, S., Rufli, T., Bigliardi, P.L. (2004). Mu-opiate receptor and beta-endorphin expression in nerve endings and keratinocytes in human skin. *Dermatology* 209:183–189.

65. Bagnol, D., Mansour, A., Akil, H., Watson, S.J. (1997). Cellular localization and distribution of the cloned mu and kappa opioid receptors in rat gastrointestinal tract. *Neuroscience* 81:579–591.

66. Bates, J.J., Foss, J.F., Murphy, D.B. (2004). Are peripheral opioid antagonists the solution to opioid side effects? *Anesth Analg* 98:116–122.

67. Cadet, P., Bilfinger, T.V., Fimiani, C., Peter, D., Stefano, G.B. (2000). Human vascular and cardiac endothelia express mu opiate receptor transcripts. *Endothelium* 7:185–191.

68. Vidal, E.L., Patel, N.A., Wu, G., Fiala, M., Chang, S.L. (1998). Interleukin-1 induces the expression of mu opioid receptors in endothelial cells. *Immunopharmacology* 38:261–266.

69. Bidlack, J.M., Khimich, M., Parkhill, A.L., Sumagin, S., Sun, B., Tipton, C.M. (2006). Opioid receptors and signaling on cells from the immune system. *J Neuroimmune Pharmacol* 1:260–269.

70. Bidlack, J.M. (2000). Detection and function of opioid receptors on cells from the immune system. *Clin Diagn Lab Immunol* 7:719–723.

71. Kapitzke, D., Vetter, I., Cabot, P.J. (2005). Endogenous opioid analgesia in peripheral tissues and the clinical implications for pain control. *Ther Clin Risk Manag* 1:279–297.

72. Chaturvedi, K., Christoffers, K.H., Singh, K., Howells, R.D. (2000). Structure and regulation of opioid receptors. *Biopolymers* 55:334–346.

73. Meng, F., Hoversten, M.T., Thompson, R.C., Taylor, L., Watson, S.J., Akil, H. (1995). A chimeric study of the molecular basis of affinity and selectivity of the kappa and the delta opioid receptors. Potential role of extracellular domains. *J Biol Chem* 270:12730–12736.

74. Minami, M., Satoh, M. (1995). Molecular biology of the opioid receptors: structures, functions and distributions. *Neurosci Res* 23:121–145.

75. Standifer, K.M., Pasternak, G.W. (1997). G proteins and opioid receptor-mediated signalling. *Cell Signal* 9:237–248.

76. Ozawa, T., Nakagawa, T., Minami, M., Satoh, M. (1999). Supersensitization of the adenylyl cyclase system in Chinese hamster ovary cells co-expressing cloned opioid receptors and Gz, a PTX-insensitive G protein. *Neurosci Lett* 267: 117–120.

77. Prather, P.L., Loh, H.H., Law, P.Y. (1994). Interaction of delta-opioid receptors with multiple G proteins: a non-relationship between agonist potency to inhibit adenylyl cyclase and to activate G proteins. *Mol Pharmacol* 45:997–1003.

78. Smart, D., Hirst, R.A., Hirota, K., Grandy, D.K., Lambert, D.G. (1997). The effects of recombinant rat mu-opioid receptor activation in CHO cells on phospholipase C, [Ca2+]i and adenylyl cyclase. *Br J Pharmacol* 120:1165–1171.

79. Piros, E.T., Prather, P.L., Loh, H.H., Law, P.Y., Evans, C.J., Hales, T.G. (1995). Ca2+ channel and adenylyl cyclase modulation by cloned mu-opioid receptors in GH3 cells. *Mol Pharmacol* 47:1041–1049.

80. Tallent, M., Dichter, M.A., Bell, G.I., Reisine, T. (1994). The cloned kappa opioid receptor couples to an N-type calcium current in undifferentiated PC-12 cells. *Neuroscience* 63:1033–1040.

81. Duarte, I.D., Ferreira, S.H. (1992). The molecular mechanism of central analgesia induced by morphine or carbachol and the L-arginine-nitric oxide-cGMP pathway. *Eur J Pharmacol* 221:171–174.

82. Ferreira, S.H., Duarte, I.D., Lorenzetti, B.B. (1991). The molecular mechanism of action of peripheral morphine analgesia: stimulation of the cGMP system via nitric oxide release. *Eur J Pharmacol* 201:121–122.

83. Rodrigues, A.R., Duarte, I.D. (2000). The peripheral antinociceptive effect induced by morphine is associated with ATP-sensitive K(+) channels. *Br J Pharmacol* 129:110–114.

84. Polakiewicz, R.D., Schieferl, S.M., Gingras, A.C., Sonenberg, N., Comb, M.J. (1998). Mu-opioid receptor activates signaling pathways implicated in cell survival and translational control. *J Biol Chem* 273:23534–23541.
85. Machelska, H., Stein, C. (2002). Immune mechanisms in pain control. *Anesth Analg* 95:1002–1008.
86. Przewlocki, R., Hassan, A.H., Lason, W., Epplen, C., Herz, A., Stein, C. (1992). Gene expression and localization of opioid peptides in immune cells of inflamed tissue: functional role in antinociception. *Neuroscience* 48:491–500.
87. Cabot, P.J., Carter, L., Gaiddon, C., Zhang, Q., Schafer, M., Loeffler, J.P., Stein, C. (1997). Immune cell-derived beta-endorphin. Production, release, and control of inflammatory pain in rats. *J Clin Invest* 100:142–148.
88. Mousa, S.A., Machelska, H., Schafer, M., Stein, C. (2002). Immunohistochemical localization of endomorphin-1 and endomorphin-2 in immune cells and spinal cord in a model of inflammatory pain. *J Neuroimmunol* 126:5–15.
89. Rittner, H.L., Brack, A., Stein, C. (2008). Pain and the immune system. *Br J Anaesth* 101:40–44.
90. Lolait, S.J., Clements, J.A., Markwick, A.J., Cheng, C., McNally, M., Smith, A.I., Funder, J.W. (1986). Pro-opiomelanocortin messenger ribonucleic acid and post-translational processing of beta endorphin in spleen macrophages. *J Clin Invest* 77:1776–1779.
91. Oates, E.L., Allaway, G.P., Armstrong, G.R., Boyajian, R.A., Kehrl, J.H., Prabhakar, B.S. (1988). Human lymphocytes produce pro-opiomelanocortin gene-related transcripts. Effects of lymphotropic viruses. *J Biol Chem* 263: 10041–10044.
92. Rosen, H., Behar, O., Abramsky, O., Ovadia, H. (1989). Regulated expression of proenkephalin A in normal lymphocytes. *J Immunol* 143:3703–3707.
93. Carr, D.J., DeCosta, B.R., Kim, C.H., Jacobson, A.E., Guarcello, V., Rice, K.C., Blalock, J.E. (1989). Opioid receptors on cells of the immune system: evidence for delta- and kappa-classes. *J Endocrinol* 122:161–168.
94. Manfredi, B., Clementi, E., Sacerdote, P., Bassetti, M., Panerai, A.E. (1995). Age-related changes in mitogen-induced beta-endorphin release from human peripheral blood mononuclear cells. *Peptides* 16:699–706.
95. Stein, C., Hassan, A.H., Lehrberger, K., Giefing, J., Yassouridis, A. (1993). Local analgesic effect of endogenous opioid peptides. *Lancet* 342:321–324.
96. Khodorova, A., Navarro, B., Jouaville, L.S., Murphy, J.E., Rice, F.L., Mazurkiewicz, J.E., Long-Woodward, D., Stoffel, M., Strichartz, G.R., Yukhananov, R., Davar, G. (2003). Endothelin-B receptor activation triggers an endogenous analgesic cascade at sites of peripheral injury. *Nat Med* 9:1055–1061.
97. Smith, T.W., Buchan, P., Parsons, D.N., Wilkinson, S. (1982). Peripheral antinociceptive effects of N-methyl morphine. *Life Sci* 31:1205–1208.
98. Joris, J.L., Dubner, R., Hargreaves, K.M. (1987). Opioid analgesia at peripheral sites: a target for opioids released during stress and inflammation? *Anesth Analg* 66:1277–1281.
99. Levine, J.D., Taiwo, Y.O. (1989). Involvement of the mu-opiate receptor in peripheral analgesia. *Neuroscience* 32:571–575.
100. Stein, C., Millan, M.J., Shippenberg, T.S., Peter, K., Herz, A. (1989). Peripheral opioid receptors mediating antinociception in inflammation. Evidence for involvement of mu, delta and kappa receptors. *J Pharmacol Exp Ther* 248:1269–1275.

101. Furst, S., Riba, P., Friedmann, T., Timar, J., Al-Khrasani, M., Obara, I., Makuch, W., Spetea, M., Schutz, J., Przewlocki, R., Przewlocka, B., Schmidhammer, H. (2005). Peripheral versus central antinociceptive actions of 6-amino acid-substituted derivatives of 14-O-methyloxymorphone in acute and inflammatory pain in the rat. *J Pharmacol Exp Ther* 312:609–618.

102. Sandner-Kiesling, A., Pan, H.L., Chen, S.R., James, R.L., DeHaven-Hudkins, D.L., Dewan, D.M., Eisenach, J.C. (2002). Effect of kappa opioid agonists on visceral nociception induced by uterine cervical distension in rats. *Pain* 96:13–22.

103. Guan, Y., Johanek, L.M., Hartke, T.V., Shim, B., Tao, Y.X., Ringkamp, M., Meyer, R.A., Raja, S.N. (2008). Peripherally acting mu-opioid receptor agonist attenuates neuropathic pain in rats after L5 spinal nerve injury. *Pain* 138:318–329.

104. Kolesnikov, Y., El-Maarouf, A., Rutishauser, U., Pasternak, G. (2007). Reorganization of dorsal root ganglion neurons following chronic sciatic nerve constriction injury: correlation with morphine and lidocaine analgesia. *Eur J Pharmacol* 568:124–133.

105. Meunier, A., Latremoliere, A., Mauborgne, A., Bourgoin, S., Kayser, V., Cesselin, F., Hamon, M., Pohl, M. (2005). Attenuation of pain-related behavior in a rat model of trigeminal neuropathic pain by viral-driven enkephalin overproduction in trigeminal ganglion neurons. *Mol Ther* 11:608–616.

106. Obara, I., Makuch, W., Spetea, M., Schutz, J., Schmidhammer, H., Przewlocki, R., Przewlocka, B. (2007). Local peripheral antinociceptive effects of 14-O-methyloxymorphone derivatives in inflammatory and neuropathic pain in the rat. *Eur J Pharmacol* 558:60–67.

107. Machelska, H., Stein, C. (2000). Pain control by immune-derived opioids. *Clin Exp Pharmacol Physiol* 27:533–536.

108. Antonijevic, I., Mousa, S.A., Schafer, M., Stein, C. (1995). Perineurial defect and peripheral opioid analgesia in inflammation. *J Neurosci* 15:165–172.

109. Atanassoff, P.G., Brull, S.J., Printsev, Y., Silverman, D.G. (1997). The effect of intradermal administration of lidocaine and morphine on the response to thermal stimulation. *Anesth Analg* 84:1340–1343.

110. Bullingham, R.E., McQuay, H.J., Moore, R.A. (1984). Studies on the peripheral action of opioids in postoperative pain in man. *Acta Anaesthesiol Belg* 35(Suppl. 35):285–290.

111. Malo, J.L., Inouye, T., Hawkins, R., Simon, G., Turner-Warwick, M., Pepys, J. (1977). Studies in chronic allergic bronchopulmonary aspergillosis. 4. Comparison with a group of asthmatics. *Thorax* 32:275–280.

112. Schulte-Steinberg, H., Weninger, E., Jokisch, D., Hofstetter, B., Misera, A., Lange, V., Stein, C. (1995). Intraperitoneal versus interpleural morphine or bupivacaine for pain after laparoscopic cholecystectomy. *Anesthesiology* 82:634–640.

113. Worrich, S., Schuler, G., Janicki, P.K. (2007). Effect of local administration of transdermal fentanyl on peripheral opioid analgesia. *Pain Med* 8:41–47.

114. Yarussi, A., Sands, R., Edge, S., Lema, M.J., de Leon-Casasola, O.A. (1999). Evaluation of peripheral morphine analgesia for lumpectomy and axillary node dissection: a randomized, double-blind, placebo-controlled study. *Reg Anesth Pain Med* 24:142–145.

115. Binder, W., Machelska, H., Mousa, S., Schmitt, T., Riviere, P.J., Junien, J.L., Stein, C., Schafer, M. (2001). Analgesic and antiinflammatory effects of two novel kappa-opioid peptides. *Anesthesiology* 94:1034–1044.
116. Pacheco, D.F., Reis, G.M., Francischi, J.N., Castro, M.S., Perez, A.C., Duarte, I.D. (2005). Delta-opioid receptor agonist SNC80 elicits peripheral antinociception via delta(1) and delta(2) receptors and activation of the l-arginine/nitric oxide/cyclic GMP pathway. *Life Sci* 78:54–60.
117. Bakke, M., Hu, J.W., Sessle, B.J. (1998). Morphine application to peripheral tissues modulates nociceptive jaw reflex. *Neuroreport* 9:3315–3319.
118. Clemente, J.T., Parada, C.A., Veiga, M.C., Gear, R.W., Tambeli, C.H. (2004). Sexual dimorphism in the antinociception mediated by kappa opioid receptors in the rat temporomandibular joint. *Neurosci Lett* 372:250–255.
119. Nunez, S., Lee, J.S., Zhang, Y., Bai, G., Ro, J.Y. (2007). Role of peripheral mu-opioid receptors in inflammatory orofacial muscle pain. *Neuroscience* 146: 1346–1354.
120. Jeanjean, A.P., Moussaoui, S.M., Maloteaux, J.M., Laduron, P.M. (1995). Interleukin-1 beta induces long-term increase of axonally transported opiate receptors and substance P. *Neuroscience* 68:151–157.
121. Ji, R.R., Zhang, Q., Law, P.Y., Low, H.H., Elde, R., Hokfelt, T. (1995). Expression of mu-, delta-, and kappa-opioid receptor-like immunoreactivities in rat dorsal root ganglia after carrageenan-induced inflammation. *J Neurosci* 15:8156–8166.
122. Selley, D.E., Breivogel, C.S., Childers, S.R. (1993). Modification of G protein-coupled functions by low-pH pretreatment of membranes from NG108-15 cells: increase in opioid agonist efficacy by decreased inactivation of G proteins. *Mol Pharmacol* 44:731–741.
123. Woolf, C.J. (1996). Phenotypic modification of primary sensory neurons: the role of nerve growth factor in the production of persistent pain. *Philos Trans R Soc Lond B Biol Sci* 351:441–448.
124. Zollner, C., Mousa, S.A., Fischer, O., Rittner, H.L., Shaqura, M., Brack, A., Shakibaei, M., Binder, W., Urban, F., Stein, C., Schafer, M. (2008). Chronic morphine use does not induce peripheral tolerance in a rat model of inflammatory pain. *J Clin Invest* 118:1065–1073.
125. Aley, K.O., Green, P.G., Levine, J.D. (1995). Opioid and adenosine peripheral antinociception are subject to tolerance and withdrawal. *J Neurosci* 15: 8031–8038.
126. Kolesnikov, Y., Pasternak, G.W. (1999). Topical opioids in mice: analgesia and reversal of tolerance by a topical N-methyl-D-aspartate antagonist. *J Pharmacol Exp Ther* 290:247–252.
127. Levine, J.D., Gordon, N.C., Fields, H.L. (1979). Naloxone dose dependently produces analgesia and hyperalgesia in postoperative pain. *Nature* 278:740–741.
128. Cabot, P.J., Carter, L., Schafer, M., Stein, C. (2001). Methionine-enkephalin- and dynorphin A-release from immune cells and control of inflammatory pain. *Pain* 93:207–212.
129. Mousa, S.A., Shakibaei, M., Sitte, N., Schafer, M., Stein, C. (2004). Subcellular pathways of beta-endorphin synthesis, processing, and release from immunocytes in inflammatory pain. *Endocrinology* 145:1331–1341.
130. Cao, T., Pinter, E., Al-Rashed, S., Gerard, N., Hoult, J.R., Brain, S.D. (2000). Neurokinin-1 receptor agonists are involved in mediating neutrophil accumula-

tion in the inflamed, but not normal, cutaneous microvasculature: an in vivo study using neurokinin-1 receptor knockout mice. *J Immunol* 164:5424–5429.

131. Rittner, H.L., Stein, C. (2005). Involvement of cytokines, chemokines and adhesion molecules in opioid analgesia. *Eur J Pain* 9:109–112.

132. Rittner, H.L., Brack, A., Stein, C. (2008). The other side of the medal: how chemokines promote analgesia. *Neurosci Lett* 437:203–208.

133. Wahl, S.M., Feldman, G.M., McCarthy, J.B. (1996). Regulation of leukocyte adhesion and signaling in inflammation and disease. *J Leukoc Biol* 59:789–796.

134. Brown, E. (1997). Neutrophil adhesion and the therapy of inflammation. *Semin Hematol* 34:319–326.

135. von Andrian, U.H., Mackay, C.R. (2000). T-cell function and migration. Two sides of the same coin. *N Engl J Med* 343:1020–1034.

136. Machelska, H., Stein, C. (2006). Leukocyte-derived opioid peptides and inhibition of pain. *J Neuroimmune Pharmacol* 1:90–97.

137. Rittner, H.L., Brack, A., Machelska, H., Mousa, S.A., Bauer, M., Schafer, M., Stein, C. (2001). Opioid peptide-expressing leukocytes: identification, recruitment, and simultaneously increasing inhibition of inflammatory pain. *Anesthesiology* 95:500–508.

138. Rittner, H.L., Labuz, D., Richter, J.F., Brack, A., Schafer, M., Stein, C., Mousa, S.A. (2007). CXCR1/2 ligands induce p38 MAPK-dependent translocation and release of opioid peptides from primary granules in vitro and in vivo. *Brain Behav Immun* 21:1021–1032.

139. Machelska, H., Mousa, S.A., Brack, A., Schopohl, J.K., Rittner, H.L., Schafer, M., Stein, C. (2002). Opioid control of inflammatory pain regulated by intercellular adhesion molecule-1. *J Neurosci* 22:5588–5596.

140. Stein, C., Gramsch, C., Herz, A. (1990). Intrinsic mechanisms of antinociception in inflammation: local opioid receptors and beta-endorphin. *J Neurosci* 10: 1292–1298.

141. Bodnar, R.J., Kelly, D.D., Brutus, M., Glusman, M. (1980). Stress-induced analgesia: neural and hormonal determinants. *Neurosci Biobehav Rev* 4:87–100.

142. Binder, W., Mousa, S.A., Sitte, N., Kaiser, M., Stein, C., Schafer, M. (2004). Sympathetic activation triggers endogenous opioid release and analgesia within peripheral inflamed tissue. *Eur J Neurosci* 20:92–100.

143. Schafer, M., Carter, L., Stein, C. (1994). Interleukin 1 beta and corticotropin-releasing factor inhibit pain by releasing opioids from immune cells in inflamed tissue. *Proc Natl Acad Sci U S A* 91:4219–4223.

144. Machelska, H., Cabot, P.J., Mousa, S.A., Zhang, Q., Stein, C. (1998). Pain control in inflammation governed by selectins. *Nat Med* 4:1425–1428.

145. Mogil, J.S., Grisel, J.E. (1998). Transgenic studies of pain. *Pain* 77:107–128.

146. Qiu, C., Sora, I., Ren, K., Uhl, G., Dubner, R. (2000). Enhanced delta-opioid receptor-mediated antinociception in mu-opioid receptor-deficient mice. *Eur J Pharmacol* 387:163–169.

147. Roques, B.P., Noble, F., Dauge, V., Fournie-Zaluski, M.C., Beaumont, A. (1993). Neutral endopeptidase 24.11: structure, inhibition, and experimental and clinical pharmacology. *Pharmacol Rev* 45:87–146.

148. Oliveira, M.C., Pelegrini-da-Silva, A., Parada, C.A., Tambeli, C.H. (2007). 5-HT acts on nociceptive primary afferents through an indirect mechanism to induce hyperalgesia in the subcutaneous tissue. *Neuroscience* 145:708–714.

149. Tambeli, C.H., Oliveira, M.C., Clemente, J.T., Pelegrini-da-Silva, A., Parada, C.A. (2006). A novel mechanism involved in 5-hydroxytryptamine-induced nociception: the indirect activation of primary afferents. *Neuroscience* 141:1517–1524.

150. Cunha, T.M., Verri, W.A., Jr., Schivo, I.R., Napimoga, M.H., Parada, C.A., Poole, S., Teixeira, M.M., Ferreira, S.H., Cunha, F.Q. (2008). Crucial role of neutrophils in the development of mechanical inflammatory hypernociception. *J Leukoc Biol* 83:824–832.

151. Guerrero, A.T., Verri, W.A., Jr., Cunha, T.M., Silva, T.A., Schivo, I.R., Dal-Secco, D., Canetti, C., Rocha, F.A., Parada, C.A., Cunha, F.Q., Ferreira, S.H. (2008). Involvement of LTB4 in zymosan-induced joint nociception in mice: participation of neutrophils and PGE2. *J Leukoc Biol* 83:122–130.

152. Bennett, G., al-Rashed, S., Hoult, J.R., Brain, S.D. (1998). Nerve growth factor induced hyperalgesia in the rat hind paw is dependent on circulating neutrophils. *Pain* 77:315–322.

153. Brack, A., Rittner, H.L., Machelska, H., Shaqura, M., Mousa, S.A., Labuz, D., Zollner, C., Schafer, M., Stein, C. (2004). Endogenous peripheral antinociception in early inflammation is not limited by the number of opioid-containing leukocytes but by opioid receptor expression. *Pain* 108:67–75.

154. Kobal, G. (1985). Pain-related electrical potentials of the human nasal mucosa elicited by chemical stimulation. *Pain* 22:151–163.

155. Koppert, W., Likar, R., Geisslinger, G., Zeck, S., Schmelz, M., Sittl, R. (1999). Peripheral antihyperalgesic effect of morphine to heat, but not mechanical, stimulation in healthy volunteers after ultraviolet-B irradiation. *Anesth Analg* 88:117–122.

156. Tegeder, I., Meier, S., Burian, M., Schmidt, H., Geisslinger, G., Lotsch, J. (2003). Peripheral opioid analgesia in experimental human pain models. *Brain* 126: 1092–1102.

157. Likar, R., Koppert, W., Blatnig, H., Chiari, F., Sittl, R., Stein, C., Schafer, M. (2001). Efficacy of peripheral morphine analgesia in inflamed, non-inflamed and perineural tissue of dental surgery patients. *J Pain Symptom Manage* 21:330–337.

158. Bullingham, R., O'Sullivan, G., McQuay, H., Poppleton, P., Rolfe, M., Evans, P., Moore, A. (1983). Perineural injection of morphine fails to relieve postoperative pain in humans. *Anesth Analg* 62:164–167.

159. Murphy, D.B., McCartney, C.J., Chan, V.W. (2000). Novel analgesic adjuncts for brachial plexus block: a systematic review. *Anesth Analg* 90:1122–1128.

160. Picard, P.R., Tramer, M.R., McQuay, H.J., Moore, R.A. (1997). Analgesic efficacy of peripheral opioids (all except intra-articular): a qualitative systematic review of randomised controlled trials. *Pain* 72:309–318.

161. Cerchietti, L.C., Navigante, A.H., Korte, M.W., Cohen, A.M., Quiroga, P.N., Villaamil, E.C., Bonomi, M.R., Roth, B.M. (2003). Potential utility of the peripheral analgesic properties of morphine in stomatitis-related pain: a pilot study. *Pain* 105:265–273.

162. Duckett, J.W., Cangiano, T., Cubina, M., Howe, C., Cohen, D. (1997). Intravesical morphine analgesia after bladder surgery. *J Urol* 157:1407–1409.

163. Kaczmarzyk, T., Stypulkowska, J. (2005). Assessment of the effectiveness of peripheral administration of morphine with local articaine anaesthesia for surgery in inflamed oral and maxillofacial tissues. *Pain* 115:348–354.

164. Likar, R., Sittl, R., Gragger, K., Pipam, W., Blatnig, H., Breschan, C., Schalk, H.V., Stein, C., Schafer, M. (1998). Peripheral morphine analgesia in dental surgery. *Pain* 76:145–150.

165. Stein, A., Yassouridis, A., Szopko, C., Helmke, K., Stein, C. (1999). Intraarticular morphine versus dexamethasone in chronic arthritis. *Pain* 83:525–532.

166. Uhle, R.A., Reader, A., Nist, R., Weaver, J., Beck, M., Meyers, W.J. (1997). Peripheral opioid analgesia in teeth with symptomatic inflamed pulps. *Anesth Prog* 44:90–95.

167. Zajaczkowska, R., Wnek, W., Wordliczek, J., Dobrogowski, J. (2004). Peripheral opioid analgesia in laparoscopic cholecystectomy. *Reg Anesth Pain Med* 29:424–429.

168. Kalso, E., Smith, L., McQuay, H.J., Andrew Moore, R. (2002). No pain, no gain: clinical excellence and scientific rigour–lessons learned from IA morphine. *Pain* 98:269–275.

169. Bryant, C.J., Harrison, S.D., Hopper, C., Harris, M. (1999). Use of intra-articular morphine for postoperative analgesia following TMJ arthroscopy. *Br J Oral Maxillofac Surg* 37:391–396.

170. Furst, I.M., Kryshtalskyj, B., Weinberg, S. (2001). The use of intra-articular opioids and bupivacaine for analgesia following temporomandibular joint arthroscopy: a prospective, randomized trial. *J Oral Maxillofac Surg* 59:979–983; discussion 983–974.

171. Zuniga, J.R., Ibanez, C., Kozacko, M. (2007). The analgesic efficacy and safety of intra-articular morphine and mepivicaine following temporomandibular joint arthroplasty. *J Oral Maxillofac Surg* 65:1477–1485.

172. Likar, R., Schafer, M., Paulak, F., Sittl, R., Pipam, W., Schalk, H., Geissler, D., Bernatzky, G. (1997). Intraarticular morphine analgesia in chronic pain patients with osteoarthritis. *Anesth Analg* 84:1313–1317.

173. Schafer, M. (1999). Peripheral opioid analgesia: from experimental to clinical studies. *Curr Opin Anaesthesiol* 12:603–607.

174. Walker, J.S. (2003). Anti-inflammatory effects of opioids. *Adv Exp Med Biol* 521: 148–160.

175. Wilson, J.L., Walker, J.S., Antoon, J.S., Perry, M.A. (1998). Intercellular adhesion molecule-1 expression in adjuvant arthritis in rats: inhibition by kappa-opioid agonist but not by NSAID. *J Rheumatol* 25:499–505.

176. Barber, A., Bartoszyk, G.D., Bender, H.M., Gottschlich, R., Greiner, H.E., Harting, J., Mauler, F., Minck, K.O., Murray, R.D., Simon, M., et al. (1994). A pharmacological profile of the novel, peripherally-selective kappa-opioid receptor agonist, EMD 61753. *Br J Pharmacol* 113:1317–1327.

177. DeHaven-Hudkins, D.L. (2003). Peripherally restricted opioid drugs: advances and retreats. *Curr Opin Anaesthesiol* 16:541–545.

178. Eisenach, J.C., Carpenter, R., Curry, R. (2003). Analgesia from a peripherally active kappa-opioid receptor agonist in patients with chronic pancreatitis. *Pain* 101:89–95.

179. Fraitag, B., Homerin, M., Hecketsweiler, P. (1994). Double-blind dose-response multicenter comparison of fedotozine and placebo in treatment of nonulcer dyspepsia. *Dig Dis Sci* 39:1072–1077.

180. Dapoigny, M., Abitbol, J.L., Fraitag, B. (1995). Efficacy of peripheral kappa agonist fedotozine versus placebo in treatment of irritable bowel syndrome. A multicenter dose-response study. *Dig Dis Sci* 40:2244–2249.

181. Read, N.W., Abitbol, J.L., Bardhan, K.D., Whorwell, P.J., Fraitag, B. (1997). Efficacy and safety of the peripheral kappa agonist fedotozine versus placebo in the treatment of functional dyspepsia. *Gut* 41:664–668.

182. Callahan, M.J. (2002). Irritable bowel syndrome neuropharmacology. A review of approved and investigational compounds. *J Clin Gastroenterol* 35:S58–S67.

183. Walker, J., Catheline, G., Guilbaud, G., Kayser, V. (1999). Lack of cross-tolerance between the antinociceptive effects of systemic morphine and asimadoline, a peripherally-selective kappa-opioid agonist, in CCI-neuropathic rats. *Pain* 83:509–516.

184. Binder, W., Walker, J.S. (1998). Effect of the peripherally selective kappa-opioid agonist, asimadoline, on adjuvant arthritis. *Br J Pharmacol* 124:647–654.

185. Caram-Salas, N.L., Reyes-Garcia, G., Bartoszyk, G.D., Araiza-Saldana, C.I., Ambriz-Tututi, M., Rocha-Gonzalez, H.I., Arreola-Espino, R., Cruz, S.L., Granados-Soto, V. (2007). Subcutaneous, intrathecal and periaqueductal grey administration of asimadoline and ICI-204448 reduces tactile allodynia in the rat. *Eur J Pharmacol* 573:75–83.

186. Bickel, A., Dorfs, S., Schmelz, M., Forster, C., Uhl, W., Handwerker, H.O. (1998). Effects of antihyperalgesic drugs on experimentally induced hyperalgesia in man. *Pain* 76:317–325.

187. Machelska, H., Pfluger, M., Weber, W., Piranvisseh-Volk, M., Daubert, J.D., Dehaven, R., Stein, C. (1999). Peripheral effects of the kappa-opioid agonist EMD 61753 on pain and inflammation in rats and humans. *J Pharmacol Exp Ther* 290:354–361.

188. Lotsch, J., Geisslinger, G. (2001). Morphine-6-glucuronide: an analgesic of the future? *Clin Pharmacokinet* 40:485–499.

189. Obara, I., Przewlocki, R., Przewlocka, B. (2004). Local peripheral effects of mu-opioid receptor agonists in neuropathic pain in rats. *Neurosci Lett* 360:85–89.

190. Rashid, M.H., Inoue, M., Toda, K., Ueda, H. (2004). Loss of peripheral morphine analgesia contributes to the reduced effectiveness of systemic morphine in neuropathic pain. *J Pharmacol Exp Ther* 309:380–387.

191. Cai, B.B., Cairns, B.E., Sessle, B.J., Hu, J.W. (2001). Sex-related suppression of reflex jaw muscle activity by peripheral morphine but not GABA. *Neuroreport* 12:3457–3460.

192. Likar, R., Mousa, S.A., Steinkellner, H., Koppert, W., Philippitsch, G., Stein, C., Schafer, M. (2007). Involvement of intra-articular corticotropin-releasing hormone in postoperative pain modulation. *Clin J Pain* 23:136–142.

193. Braz, J., Beaufour, C., Coutaux, A., Epstein, A.L., Cesselin, F., Hamon, M., Pohl, M. (2001). Therapeutic efficacy in experimental polyarthritis of viral-driven enkephalin overproduction in sensory neurons. *J Neurosci* 21:7881–7888.

194. Kyrkanides, S., Fiorentino, P.M., Miller, J.N., Gan, Y., Lai, Y.C., Shaftel, S.S., Puzas, J.E., Piancino, M.G., O'Banion, M.K., Tallents, R.H. (2007). Amelioration of pain and histopathologic joint abnormalities in the Col1-IL-1beta(XAT) mouse model of arthritis by intraarticular induction of mu-opioid receptor into the temporomandibular joint. *Arthritis Rheum* 56:2038–2048.

195. Lu, C.Y., Chou, A.K., Wu, C.L., Yang, C.H., Chen, J.T., Wu, P.C., Lin, S.H., Muhammad, R., Yang, L.C. (2002). Gene-gun particle with pro-opiomelanocortin cDNA produces analgesia against formalin-induced pain in rats. *Gene Ther* 9:1008–1014.

CHAPTER 15

Calcitonin Gene-Related Peptide and Substance P

RANJINIDEVI AMBALAVANAR and DEAN DESSEM

Department of Neural and Pain Sciences and Program in Neuroscience, University of Maryland

Contents

Peripheral Receptor Targets for Analgesia: Novel Approaches to Pain Management, Edited by Brian E. Cairns

15.1 INTRODUCTION

Promising recent developments in the therapeutic value of neuropeptide antagonists have generated renewed importance in understanding the functional role of neuropeptides in nociception and inflammation. Calcitonin gene-related peptide (CGRP) and substance P (SP) are two neuropeptides expressed primarily in unmyelinated C-fibers and in small myelinated Aδ-fibers. Because 73% of C-fiber primary afferent neurons are nociceptors [1], CGRP- and SP-containing neurons constitute a subpopulation mostly of nociceptive primary afferents. Following synthesis in the cell bodies of these neurons, neuropeptides such as CGRP and SP are transported to peripheral and central terminals [2]. Previous studies have demonstrated correlations between the neurochemical content of primary afferent neurons and their function [3,4]. For example, CGRP is present in high-threshold mechanoreceptors [3] and comprises about 50% of the nociceptive neurons [5] in the dorsal root ganglion (DRG). Several *in vivo* animal studies have also implicated CGRP and SP in the relay of nociceptive information from both cutaneous [6] and deep tissues including muscle [3,7] and joint [8–10]. In this chapter, we discuss the role of CGRP and SP in the pathophysiology of nociception and pain and their receptor antagonists as potential therapeutics in the treatment of pain.

15.2 GENERAL OVERVIEW

15.2.1 CGRP

CGRP is a 37-amino acid peptide produced by alternative RNA processing of calcitonin gene-generated mRNAs [11]. Two isoforms of CGRP, αCGRP and βCGRP exist with >90% structural similarity. While αCGRP is a product of the calcitonin gene and is expressed in neuronal tissues in a tissue-specific manner [12], βCGRP is generated from a discrete gene and is found in enteric nerves. For this review, we will limit our discussion to αCGRP, which has been implicated in nociception and pain. The amino acid sequence of αCGRP is given below:

Ala-Cys-Asp-Thr-Ala-Thr-Cys-Val-Thr-His-Arg-Leu-Ala-Gly-Leu-Leu-Ser-Arg-Ser-Gly-Gly-Val-Val-Lys-Asn-Asn-Phe-Val-Pro-Thr-Asn-Val-Gly-Ser-Lys-Ala-Phe-NH2

Of the various neuropeptides identified in subpopulations of primary afferent neurons, CGRP is the most prevalent, found in 40–50% of the DRG [13–17] and the trigeminal ganglion (TG) [18] neurons of different species. CGRP is expressed in capsaicin-sensitive primary afferent neurons comprising 50% of C-fiber neurons and 30% of Aδ-fiber neurons [19]. Not only can CGRP be released from peripheral and central terminals [20] but also from within the ganglion [21] following noxious stimulation. CGRP is a potent vasodilator in skin [22] and in skeletal muscles [23] and is involved in the transmission of nociceptive information [7]. Because CGRP can depolarize peripheral [24] and dorsal horn neurons [25], it likely plays a role in both peripheral as well as central sensitization. For instance, the release of CGRP from the central terminals of primary afferent neurons enhances thermal and mechanical nociceptive sensitivity [25]. CGRP-evoked allodynia and hyperalgesia are mediated by protein kinase A and protein kinase C (PKC) second messenger systems [25].

Intrathecal administration of anti-CGRP serum increases the nociceptive threshold in normal rats and reduces hyperalgesia following adjuvant-induced arthritis [26] and thermal injury to the hind paw [27]. Spinal superfusion of CGRP (8-37) also prevents and reverses sensitization of dorsal horn neurons [25]. Recent studies on different strains of mice reveal that differences in pain sensitivity are linked to strain-dependent CGRP expression [28], further supporting a role for CGRP in nociception.

15.2.2 SP

In 1931, von Euler and Gaddum named the "substance" capable of reducing blood pressure, extracted into a "powder" form as "substance P" (SP). SP is an 11-amino acid peptide [29]. SP belongs to the tachykinin family of proteins, also known as neurokinins. SP and neurokinin A are derived from a common precursor β-preprotachykinin (PPT-1) and are primarily present in sensory neurons. The amino acid sequence of SP is given below:

Arg-Pro-Lys-Pro-Gln-Gln-Phe-Phe-Gly-Leu-Met-NH2

SP is expressed in small sensory neurons [2,17,23,30], being 20–25% of total DRG and TG neurons [30]. SP-containing neurons constitute 50% of C-fiber neurons and 30% of Aδ-fiber neurons [31] with their central terminals in laminae I and II of the spinal cord [2].

SP plays a major role in the processing of nociceptive information [32]. For example, peripheral noxious stimuli evoke the release of SP from the central and peripheral terminals of primary afferent neurons, and this release is increased following inflammation [33,34]. For example, in normal animals, SP is released from the central terminals of primary afferent neurons only following noxious stimulation and not non-noxious stimulation [32]. After sensitization of primary afferent neurons, however, both noxious as well as non-noxious stimuli induce the release of SP [32,35]. Several studies have implicated SP-mediated events in the development and maintenance of inflammation-induced central sensitization [35–37]. Spinal injection of SP elicits hyperalgesia [38] and skin scratching behavior, which can be blocked by intrathecal administration of SP receptor antagonists [39]. Moreover, mice lacking either the PPT-1 gene [40] or the SP receptor neurokinin-1 (NK-1) [41] display a reduced response to painful stimuli. Selective ablation of NK-1-expressing cells with SP–saporin conjugate causes loss of hyperalgesia in rats [42] and loss of windup in NK-1 knockout mice [41]. These observations strongly support a role for SP in nociception and pain.

It is interesting to note that the amount of SP transported to peripheral terminals is fourfold higher than that transported to the central terminals [43], suggesting that SP released from peripheral terminals plays an important role in nociception and in neurogenic inflammation [44]. SP is a potent mediator of microvascular permeability [45] and edema formation [46] either by mast cell degranulation or by acting directly on specific vascular receptors [47]. Thus, NK-1 receptor antagonists CP-96,345 [45] and RP-67,580 [48] completely abolish edema formation, while the selective NK-1 receptor agonist GR73632 does not increase blood flow in rat skin. Blockade of NK-1 receptors by RP-67,580, aprepitant, LY30380, and CP-99,994 also prevents extravasation in the dura mater [49].

15.3 COEXPRESSION AND COTRANSMISSION OF CGRP AND SP

SP is found in a subpopulation of CGRP-containing primary afferent neurons [14,15,18]. Both SP and CGRP are also colocalized in many nerve fibers in peripheral tissues including skin [50] and in the central terminals of primary afferent neurons [6,20,51]. More importantly, ultrastructural studies demonstrate the presence of both CGRP and SP in single secretory granules of primary afferent neurons [52]. This observation supports the notion that these peptides are coreleased following electrical stimulation of TG neurons [51] and act as cotransmitters in pain transmission. Experimental evidence further suggests that simultaneous application of CGRP and SP potentiates nociceptive behaviors in rodents [15]. CGRP augments SP-induced nociception by facilitating the release of SP within the spinal cord [6] and by spreading the released SP in the dorsal horn [53] while inhibiting the degradation of SP [54,55]. Furthermore, CGRP increases the expression of the SP receptor NK-1 in spinal neurons [37]. In human subjects, injection of CGRP [56] or SP [57] alone into the temporal muscles does not evoke pain, but when coinjected with SP or neurokinin A, CGRP induces pain sensation [56].

Edema-inducing effects of SP are potentiated by CGRP via increasing blood flow. In peripheral cutaneous tissue, CGRP produces little or no plasma extravasation [22] but acts as a potent vasodilator [46] and potentiates extravasation evoked by SP [22,46,58]. These studies support the concept that CGRP and SP act synergistically in inflammation and nociception.

15.4 TISSUE-SPECIFIC DISTRIBUTION

By maintaining a variety of transmitter types in primary afferent neurons, information relevant to a peripheral tissue type may be sent to the central nervous system (CNS) [59,60]. For example, the characteristics of cutaneous and deep somatic pain are different and probably indicate differences in the processing of nociceptive information [61,62]. Neuropeptide expression within primary afferent neurons that innervate different target tissues such as skin, muscle, and viscera has typically been examined at the level of the DRG [8,50,63–69] and TG [70]. Although these studies found somewhat differing data about the proportion of CGRP- and SP-containing neurons that innervate different targets (summarized in Table 15.1), they support the supposition that the neurochemical phenotype of primary afferent neurons differs with the target they innervate. Hence, redirection of cutaneous afferents to muscle reduces the number of SP-containing nerve fibers, while redirection of muscle afferents to skin increases the percentage of SP-containing nerve fibers [59].

15.4.1 Cutaneous Tissue

Neuropeptides CGRP and SP are present in primary afferent nerve fibers that innervate cutaneous tissue [6,50,58,64–68,71] (see Table 15.1). As these neuropeptides control cutaneous blood flow and vascular permeability, they play a major role in neurogenic inflammation and plasma extravasation [72]. Injection of small amounts of CGRP into human skin increases blood flow to the skin for several hours [46]. Hence, the increased blood flow induced by capsaicin injection into the skin can be inhibited by coinjection with the CGRP receptor antagonist CGRP (8-37) [73]. While CGRP acting via CGRP1 receptors causes arteriolar vasodilation, SP acting via NK-1 receptors mediates venular permeability [46,72].

TABLE 15.1. Percentage of Cutaneous and Deep Tissue Primary Afferent Neurons Positive for CGRP and SP.

Tissue	CGRP, %	SP, %	Ganglion	Reference
Skin	20	10	DRG	[63]
	49	29	DRG	[64]
	19	—	DRG	[65]
	51	—	DRG	[67]
	51	21	DRG	[66]
	41	—	DRG	[68]
	27	7	TG	[70]
Muscle	30	15	DRG	[63]
	66	35	DRG	[64]
	70	51	DRG	[66]
	37	5	TG	[70]
Joint (wrist)	45	—	DRG	[69]
Joint (lumbar facet)	25–50	—	DRG	[8]
Lumbar disk	55	—	DRG	[68]

DRG, dorsal root ganglion; TG, trigeminal ganglion.

Many studies demonstrate change in the expression of SP and CGRP in primary afferent neurons following cutaneous inflammation and nociception [9,10,74]. For example, increased expression of CGRP and SP [36] occurs in the DRG following inflammation of the skin. In addition, larger primary afferent neurons such as Aβ neurons that normally do not express SP and CGRP begin to express these neuropeptides following peripheral cutaneous inflammation [75]. Increases of CGRP mRNA have also been reported following hind paw inflammation [36,76]. It has been suggested that the increased expression of neuropeptides and phenotypic switch in primary afferent neurons contribute to the increased nociceptive sensitivity following cutaneous inflammation.

15.4.2 Muscle Tissue

In the DRG, about 50–60% of muscle sensory afferent neurons contain CGRP (see Table 15.1) [63,64,66]. These CGRP-containing muscle afferents include high-threshold muscle mechanoreceptors [3]. In the TG, about 37% of muscle afferent neurons contain CGRP, and these neurons are restricted to a smaller-size range [70].

In the human temporalis muscle, peptidergic nerve fibers are perivascular and are involved in vasoregulation [77,78]. This morphological relationship makes it likely that CGRP released from axons in close association with arterioles can modulate local muscle blood flow and plasma extravasation. This supposition is supported by the observation that CGRP is released when peripheral muscle nerves are stimulated [79], and this stimulation produces plasma extravasation in muscle [80]. These events can be abolished by a CGRP antagonist [81,82] (see Figure 15.1f). While plasma extravasation may be initiated by SP, it can be dramatically amplified by CGRP [56]. Thus, one potential function of CGRP in peripheral afferent axons is to modulate muscle blood flow and hence to amplify plasma extravasation in muscle. Studies on both craniofacial and limb muscles also implicate CGRP [81,83,84] and SP [7] in muscle nociception. Myositis induced in extracranial muscles increases the number of peripheral fibers expressing SP [83]. This increased innervation density may represent a mechanism leading to enhanced muscle pain [85]. While it is currently unknown what the effects of CGRP are on muscle afferent neurons, antagonists directed against CGRP could be particularly efficient because they attenuate plasma extravasation and inflammation and could potentially also reduce nociceptor activity [81].

Activation of the NK-1 receptor increases the blood flow in human temporal muscle [78]. In addition, levels of CGRP and SP are elevated in patients with chronic muscle pain [86] including myofascial pain syndrome [87]. Moreover, SP and CGRP may be integrally related to fibromyalgia symptoms because the concentration of SP and CGRP is elevated two- to threefold in the cerebrospinal fluid (CSF) of these patients and the increase is correlated with the severity of pain [88]. Animal studies also support a role for CGRP

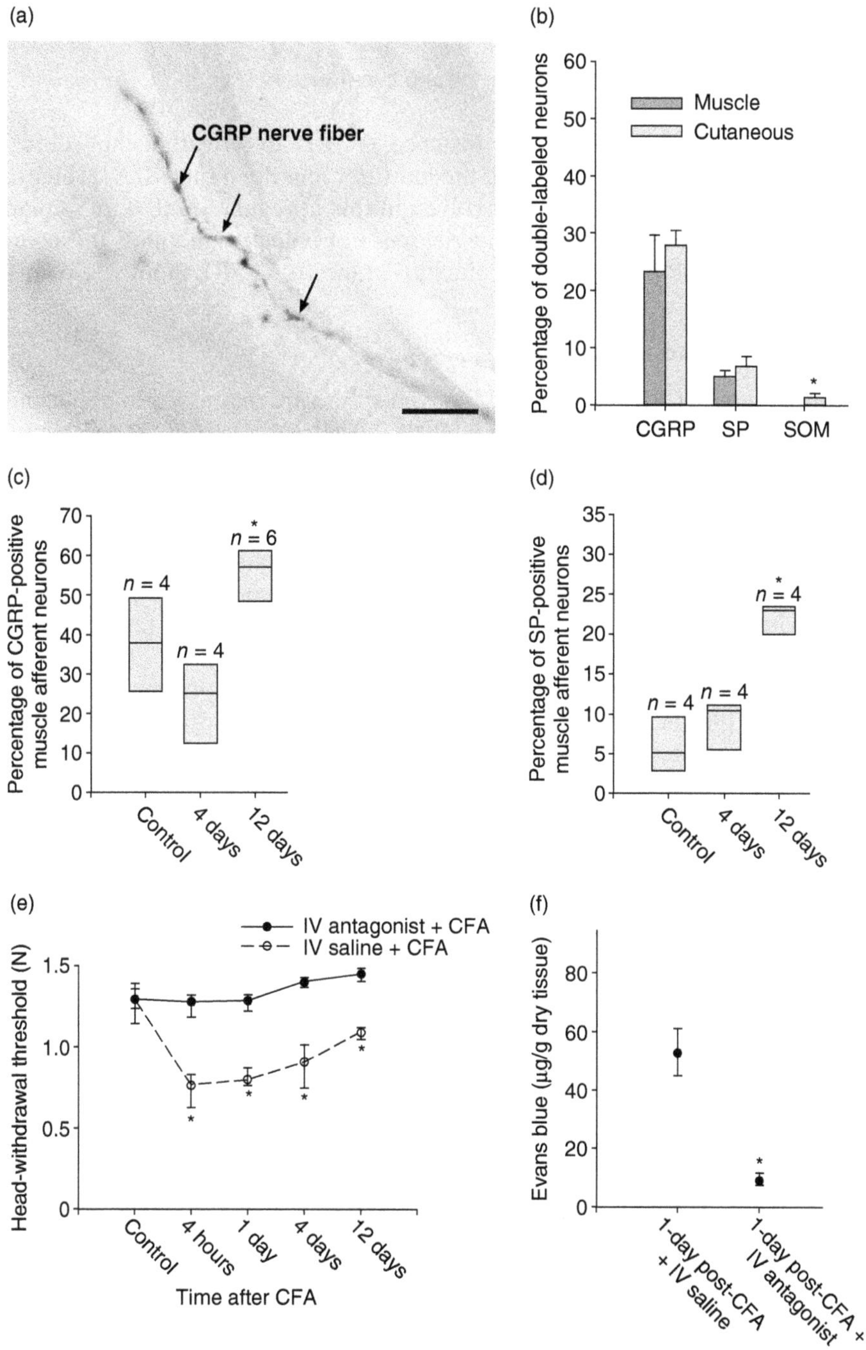

FIGURE 15.1. (a) Histological section of masseter muscle showing a nerve fiber immunoreactive to CGRP (arrows). Scale bar = 20 µm. (b) Percentage of retrogradely labeled muscle and cutaneous primary afferent neurons positive for CGRP, SP, and somatostatin (SOM) in the trigeminal ganglion (TG). (c,d) Following muscle inflammation, the percentage of (c) CGRP- and (d) SP-positive muscle afferent neurons increases at 12 days. (e) Intravenous (IV) injection of CGRP antagonist CGRP (8-37) but not saline before muscle inflammation eliminates the inflammation-induced allodynia. (f) Intravenous injection of CGRP antagonist CGRP (8-37) before muscle inflammation eliminates the inflammation-induced plasma extravasation in masseter muscle. Asterisks indicate significant differences from baseline. CFA, complete Freud's adjuvant.

in muscle pain (Figure 15.1). For instance, CGRP levels within the TG are elevated following inflammation of the masseter muscle in rats [81,84] (Figure 15.1c), and gene transcription is involved in this upregulation [89]. In human subjects, injection of SP into the muscle does not induce pain unless it is coinjected with CGRP [57], indicating the importance of CGRP in muscle pain.

15.4.3 Joint and Bone

Neuropeptides CGRP and SP and their receptors are expressed in joints and play a role in arthritis and joint pain [68,69,90–94]. CGRP- and SP-containing DRG neurons innervate the lumbar facet joints [8], suggesting that these neuropeptides play a role in pain pathologies associated with the vertebral column. Following joint inflammation, there is a change in the expression of CGRP and SP at various joints [95] as well as in neuronal somata innervating the joint [8,91]. The increase in these neuropeptides may result from a phenotypic switch in primary afferent neurons as reported for lumbar facet joints in rats [8].

In humans, CGRP- and SP-containing nerve fibers are present in the sacroiliac joint [96] and in normal and arthritic hip joints [93], suggesting that these neuropeptides play a role in human joint pathologies. In fact, the expression of CGRP and SP appears to be closely related to joint pain because a positive correlation exists between the levels of CGRP in the temporomandibular joint and the severity of joint pain in patients with arthritic temporomandibular disorders [94] and arthritic hip joints [93].

15.4.4 Meninges

Cerebral blood vessels are densely innervated by CGRP- and SP-containing sensory nerve fibers, and the release of these neuropeptides results in neurogenic inflammation and activation of nociceptive primary afferent neurons [49,97]. Thus, considerable interest is focused on the therapeutic potential of peptide and nonpeptide CGRP antagonists for the treatment of migraine [98–100], a subject that has been reviewed extensively [101–107].

15.5 INTRAGANGLIONIC RELEASE OF CGRP AND SP

It has been reported that the neuropeptides CGRP and SP can be released within the TG [21,108] and that this release is enhanced following inflammation [33]. Thus, peptidergic primary afferents can be functionally linked to neighboring neurons within the ganglia via nonsynaptic, paracrine-like signaling [109,110], whereby they develop a change in their excitability or spontaneous firing without any peripheral stimuli.

Radioimmunoassay studies report that the TG contains considerable amounts of CGRP as well as detectable levels of $CGRP^{125}$ binding sites. A recent study further confirms the presence of CGRP receptors in TG neurons

[111]. Because the application of CGRP enhances tetrodotoxin (TTX)-resistant sodium channels in DRG neurons [112], it is possible that CGRP released from primary afferent neurons contributes to this neuronal activity. CGRP receptor activation regulates gene transcription in primary afferent neurons through a cyclic adenosine monophosphate (cAMP)-dependent pathway [113], suggesting that CGRP receptors may regulate protein expression in primary afferent neurons in response to tissue-damaging stimuli leading to plastic changes in primary afferent neurons. In cultured TG neurons, for instance, application of CGRP induces an upregulation of $P2X_3$ receptor expression and function [114]. Studies from our laboratory have shown that the ATP receptor $P2X_3$ is found in TG muscle afferent neurons and is colocalized with 75% of CGRP-containing muscle afferent neurons [115]. Following masseter muscle inflammation, there is an increased expression not only of CGRP [81] but also of $P2X_3$ [115,116] in rat TG muscle afferent neurons. Taken together, it is tempting to speculate that increased CGRP expression and release following muscle inflammation upregulate $P2X_3$, resulting in peripheral sensitization. Because CGRP (8-37) blocks CGRP-induced upregulation and the potentiation of $P2X_3$ receptors in cultured TG neurons [114], CGRP antagonists are likely to reduce the sensitization of $P2X_3$ receptors and thus may be highly efficacious for treating deep tissue pain.

SP is also released within the ganglion following inflammation [33,108], and functional tachykinin receptors are present on primary afferent neuron somata [71,117]. SP-induced depolarization of DRG neurons was first reported in 1982 [118]. The presence of the SP receptor NK-1 has been demonstrated in TG as well as in DRG neurons using electrophysiological [109] and morphological studies [37,117]. Because NK-1 is also present in SP-containing primary afferent neurons [109,110], autocrine activation of SP-containing neurons is possible in ganglion neurons. NK-1 receptor expression is increased following tissue inflammation [109]. Interestingly, inflammation of the jaw joint increases not only the number of NK-1 immunoreactive skin afferent neurons but also the excitability of Aβ neurons that innervate the facial skin. This increase in expression and function is mediated by a paracrine mechanism in which SP is released from other neurons in the TG [109]. These observations suggest that NK-1 receptor activation in primary afferent neurons contributes to the neuronal excitability following injury or inflammation [109,110] and may explain the mechanical allodynia in facial skin following temporomandibular joint inflammation [110].

15.6 RECEPTORS: ANTAGONISTS AND CLINICAL STUDIES

15.6.1 CGRP Receptors

Two classes of CGRP receptors have been characterized: CGRP1 and CGRP2. CGRP1 receptors are widely distributed, while CGRP2 receptors have only been described in rat vas deferens and are considered to lack selectivity [119]. Thus, CGRP appears to act mainly on CGRP1 receptors [120].

The CGRP1 receptor belongs to the large family of G protein-coupled receptors (GPCRs) [121], and the receptor complex is made up of three main components. The first component, a seven-transmembrane protein, the calcitonin receptor-like receptor (CLR), is responsible for the ligand binding site for CGRP [122,123]. The second component, a single-transmembrane domain, the receptor activity-modifying protein-1 (RAMP1), is involved in receptor trafficking and is responsible for receptor phenotype and species selectivity [123,124]. For example, RAMP1 forms a complex with CLR to convert it to a more specific receptor for CGRP. Thus, coexpression of CLR with RAMP1 forms the CGRP receptor [123], which has little affinity for related peptides including adrenomodulin. Furthermore, RAMP1 can be functionally rate limiting for CGRP receptor activity in TG neurons [125]. The third component, the intracellular component, the receptor-modifying protein (RCP), couples the receptor to the intracellular signaling pathway, including cAMP production [126].

Immunohistochemical distribution of the different components of CGRP1 receptor has recently been reported [111,127]. The CGRP receptor components are not only present in peripheral and central neurons but also in peripheral tissues including blood vessels and Schwann cells in the dura mater [111]. CGRP receptors are also present in axon terminals and on dorsal horn neurons [128]. Studies also suggest that the CGRP receptors are postsynaptic in the trigeminocervical complex [97].

15.6.2 CGRP Receptor Antagonists

A selective competitive receptor antagonist, CGRP (8-37) inhibits the actions of CGRP at the CGRP1 receptor [120] with a 10-fold greater affinity than for CGRP2 receptors [119]. CGRP (8-37) reduces capsaicin-induced vasodilation in human skin [129]. Peptide antagonists including CGRP (8-37), however, have a short half-life and therefore have not been clinically effective. A selective nonpeptide CGRP receptor antagonist, BIBN4096BS [102,106], displays a 10-fold higher affinity for CGRP1 than for CGRP2 receptors [130] and is valuable in the treatment of migraine headache in humans [98]. The major drawback of BIBN4096 is its low oral bioavailability (<1%). Consequently, another orally active potent CGRP antagonist, MK-0974, has recently been tested for the treatment of migraine headache [99].

Species differences in the affinity of CGRP receptors must be taken into consideration when choosing the receptor antagonists for animal studies. Although BIBN4096BS exhibits high affinity for the human CGRP receptor, it displays a >100-fold lower affinity for the rat CGRP receptor [124] than for the human CGRP receptor. Orally active MK-0974 shows more than 1500 times lower affinity for nonprimate CGRP receptors than for human CGRP receptors [131]. Therefore, compounds such as CGRP (8-37) play an important role in studying CGRP-related mechanisms in animal models of neurogenic inflammation and nociception.

Available data suggest several potential sites of action for CGRP receptor antagonists. Blockade of CGRP receptors reduces or blocks neurogenic inflammation and plasma extravasation in peripheral tissues [73,81] and blocks the activation of nociceptive pathways at different levels. Studies show that local injection of CGRP (8-37) into the skin [46] or muscle [81] is less effective, though intravenous injection eliminates muscle allodynia [81] (Figure 15.1e). Similarly, topical application of BIBN4096BS onto meningeal primary afferent terminals does not change the neuronal activity in spinal trigeminal nucleus, while an intravenous injection of BIBN4096BS results in a profound and long-lasting lowering of spinal trigeminal neuronal activity [132]. Furthermore, microiontophoretic injection of BIBN4096BS and CGRP (8-37) [97] or direct application [132] effectively lowers the activity of neurons with nociceptive input to the spinal cord and brain stem. Intrathecal administration of CGRP antagonist (8-37) attenuates nocifensive behaviors evoked by inflammation [26] and prevents and reverses the sensitization of dorsal horn neurons [25]. Thus, a central site of action may contribute to the effects of CGRP receptor antagonists despite the unfavorable brain penetration properties of these compounds, and may explain why relatively high plasma levels of an orally active antagonist, MK-0974, are required to alleviate headache in migraine patients [99].

15.6.3 Therapeutic Potential of CGRP Antagonists

Two recent clinical trials using CGRP antagonists [98,99] have provided a promising new direction in the treatment of migraine headache. Intravenous injection of the CGRP antagonist BIBN4096 and an orally active nonpeptide antagonist, MK-0974 [99], has shown tremendous promise in the treatment of migraine headache. These studies indicate that neuropeptide antagonists can be formulated to be efficacious and safe for human use, and that these antagonists could perhaps be utilized to treat other deep tissue pain disorders where CGRP levels are increased, including temporomandibular disorders and fibromyalgia [81,84,86,89,94,133].

15.6.4 SP Receptor

Release of SP from nerve terminals and subsequent activation of its receptor, NK-1, are important effector mechanisms involved in nociception [35,37,110]. The NK-1 receptor is present in primary afferent cell bodies and their peripheral [71] and central processes [117]. In addition to the presence and plasticity of NK-1 receptors in primary afferent neurons [109,110], NK-1-expressing dorsal horn neurons also undergo receptor internalization and upregulation following peripheral tissue inflammation [35]. Thus, a range of studies relating to inflammation and nociception in NK-1 receptor knockout mice [41] gives similar responses to those observed in mice lacking the PPT-1 gene that encodes SP [40].

NK-1 is a GPCR expressed in peripheral tissues [92] including vascular endothelium and mast cells as well as central neurons in the superficial and deep laminae of the spinal dorsal horn [134]. NK-1-expressing neurons in the spinal and medullary dorsal horn receive input from SP-containing primary afferents [134]. Upon release of SP from the central terminals of primary afferent neurons, SP binds to NK-1 receptors in central neurons, and both SP and NK-1 undergo internalization into endosomes [35,135]. This effect can be blocked by NK-1 antagonists [135]. Because nearly all NK-1-positive neurons project to the parabrachial nucleus or thalamus [136], these neurons are involved in ascending nociceptive pathways.

15.6.5 SP Receptor Antagonists

Animal experiments using several highly selective compounds have demonstrated that antagonists to NK-1 receptors possess antinociceptive properties [137–144]. The first nonpeptide antagonist, CP-96,345, has been demonstrated as a potent inhibitor of neuronal excitation in cat dorsal horn neurons following peripheral noxious stimulation [139]. Intrathecal injection of CP-96,345 [140] and LY303870 [143] also attenuates the late phase of formalin test response in rats, suggesting a central role for NK-1 receptors in the development of the late phase. Due to the limited selectivity and oral bioavailability of these compounds, many new NK-1 receptor compounds have been developed. For example, L-733,060 is a highly selective NK-1 antagonist that readily penetrates the CNS with a long duration of action. Following intravenous injection, L-733,060 inhibits the late phase of nociceptive responses to formalin injection in gerbil hind paw [141] and reverses carrageenan-induced mechanical hyperalgesia in guinea pigs. These observations further confirm a role for central NK-1 receptors in the development of the late phase of nociceptive behavior and suggest that these antagonists can be of therapeutic use as centrally acting analgesics. Orally active NK-1 antagonists CP-99,994 and SDZ NKT 343 or LY303870 were effective in reducing mechanical hyperalgesia induced by carrageenan or by sciatic nerve ligation in guinea pigs [142]. Antagonist LY30380 is effective in inhibiting neurogenic dural inflammation in guinea pigs when administered via oral, intravenous, or inhalation routes [145]. Local NK-1 receptors play a role in the induction of arthritic pain because a local injection of NK-1 antagonist L-703,606 was effective in reducing nociception when given before but not after the induction of knee joint inflammation [92]. In addition, local subcutaneous injections of NK-1 receptor antagonist L-760,735 daily for 21 days reduced the thermal and mechanical hyperalgesia and paw edema in arthritic guinea pigs, further suggesting a role for local NK-1 receptors in nociception.

15.6.6 Therapeutic Potential of SP Receptor Antagonists

Although many studies show antinociceptive effects when NK-1 receptor antagonists are administered in animals, several clinical trials have failed to demonstrate the analgesic efficacy of these compounds in humans [146–148; reviewed by References 106,146–150]. For example, an orally administered NK-1 antagonist lanepitant (LY303870) failed to show a significant effect over placebo in patients with migraine headache [147], osteoarthritis [146], or diabetic neuropathy [151]. Moreover, aprepitant L-754,030 (MK-0869), a selective NK-1 antagonist with good CNS permeability, failed not only to reduce pain intensity in patients with postherpetic neuralgia [150,152] but also to attenuate measures of central sensitization in human volunteers [153]. In patients with painful diabetic polyneuropathy, daily dose of a nonpeptide NK-1 receptor antagonist TK731 failed to relieve pain after 2 weeks of treatment [148]. While the outcome of these recent clinical trials supports the earlier observations that the currently available NK-1 receptor antagonists are ineffective as analgesics, it is important to note that these antagonists have been successful in the treatment of diverse conditions. Particularly, aprepitant (MK-0869) [154] effectively reduces depression, chemotherapy-induced emesis [137,155,156] and inflammatory bowel disease [137].

15.7 SUMMARY

One construct that readily emerges from the studies reviewed here is that CGRP and SP play a pivotal role in the processing of nociceptive information arising from various peripheral tissues. It is essential therefore to thoroughly understand neuropeptide mechanisms so that a scientific rationale for safe and efficacious pain therapies can be developed. For instance, growing evidence suggests that CGRP and SP are released from ganglionic neuronal cell bodies and act on neighboring neurons. This cross talk involves nonsynaptic paracrine signaling via CGRP and NK-1 receptors, suggesting that not only primary afferent peripheral and central terminals but also neuronal somata may be productive therapeutic targets. It is encouraging that receptor antagonists for both CGRP and SP reduce nociceptive behaviors in animal models and do not appear to have deleterious side effects in human studies. Although NK-1 receptor antagonists have not been successful as analgesics in humans, to date, CGRP receptor antagonists have shown clinical effectiveness in the treatment of pain, specifically migraine pain. We propose that neuropeptide antagonists such as these may have much broader clinical applications especially as therapeutics for deep tissue pain disorders such as temporomandibular disorders.

ACKNOWLEDGMENT

This work was supported by the National Institute of Dental and Craniofacial Research grants DE10132, DE1538, and DE16795.

REFERENCES

1. Lynn, B., Carpenter, S.E. (1982). Primary afferent units from the hairy skin of the rat hind limb. *Brain Res* 238(1):29–43.
2. Cuello, A.C., Del, F.M., Paxinos, G. (1978). The central and peripheral ends of the substance P-containing sensory neurones in the rat trigeminal system. *Brain Res* 152(3):499–500.
3. Hoheisel, U., Mense, S., Scherotzke, R. (1994). Calcitonin gene-related peptide-immunoreactivity in functionally identified primary afferent neurones in the rat. *Anat Embryol (Berl)* 189(1):41–49.
4. Fang, X., McMullan, S., Lawson, S.N., Djouhri, L. (2005). Electrophysiological differences between nociceptive and non-nociceptive dorsal root ganglion neurones in the rat in vivo. *J Physiol* 565(Pt 3):927–943.
5. Lawson, S.N., Crepps, B., Perl, E.R. (2002). Calcitonin gene-related peptide immunoreactivity and afferent receptive properties of dorsal root ganglion neurones in guinea-pigs. *J Physiol* 540(Pt 3):989–1002.
6. Oku, R., Satoh, M., Fujii, N., Otaka, A., Yajima, H., Takagi, H. (1987). Calcitonin gene-related peptide promotes mechanical nociception by potentiating release of substance P from the spinal dorsal horn in rats. *Brain Res* 403(2):350–354.
7. Mense, S., Hoheisel, U., Reinert, A. (1996). The possible role of substance P in eliciting and modulating deep somatic pain. *Prog Brain Res* 110:125–135.
8. Ohtori, S., Takahashi, K., Chiba, T., Yamagata, M., Sameda, H., Moriya, H. (2001). Phenotypic inflammation switch in rats shown by calcitonin gene-related peptide immunoreactive dorsal root ganglion neurons innervating the lumbar facet joints. *Spine* 26(9):1009–1013.
9. Ruscheweyh, R., Forsthuber, L., Schoffnegger, D., Sandkuhler, J. (2007). Modification of classical neurochemical markers in identified primary afferent neurons with Abeta-, Adelta-, and C-fibers after chronic constriction injury in mice. *J Comp Neurol* 502(2):325–336.
10. Greco, R., Tassorelli, C., Sandrini, G., Di, B.P., Buscone, S., Nappi, G. (2008). Role of calcitonin gene-related peptide and substance P in different models of pain. *Cephalalgia* 28(2):114–126.
11. Amara, S.G., Jonas, V., Rosenfeld, M.G., Ong, E.S., Evans, R.M. (1982). Alternative RNA processing in calcitonin gene expression generates mRNAs encoding different polypeptide products. *Nature* 298(5871):240–244.
12. Brain, S.D., Grant, A.D. (2004). Vascular actions of calcitonin gene-related peptide and adrenomedullin. *Physiol Rev* 84(3):903–934.
13. Skofitsch, G., Jacobowitz, D.M. (1985). Calcitonin gene-related peptide: detailed immunohistochemical distribution in the central nervous system. *Peptides* 6(4)721–745.
14. Skofitsch, G., Jacobowitz, D.M. (1985). Calcitonin gene-related peptide coexists with substance P in capsaicin sensitive neurons and sensory ganglia of the rat. *Peptides* 6(4):747–754.
15. Wiesenfeld-Hallin, Z., Hokfelt, T., Lundberg, J.M., Forssmann, W.G., Reinecke, M., Tschopp, F.A., Fischer, J.A. (1984). Immunoreactive calcitonin gene-related peptide and substance P coexist in sensory neurons to the spinal cord and interact in spinal behavioral responses of the rat. *Neurosci Lett* 52(1-2):199–204.

16. Hokfelt, T., Arvidsson, U., Ceccatelli, S., Cortes, R., Cullheim, S., Dagerlind, A., Johnson, H., Orazzo, C., Piehl, F., Pieribone, V. (1992). Calcitonin gene-related peptide in the brain, spinal cord, and some peripheral systems. *Ann N Y Acad Sci* 657:119–134.

17. Ju, G., Hokfelt, T., Brodin, E., Fahrenkrug, J., Fischer, J.A., Frey, P., Elde, R.P., Brown, J.C. (1987). Primary sensory neurons of the rat showing calcitonin gene-related peptide immunoreactivity and their relation to substance P-, somatostatin-, galanin-, vasoactive intestinal polypeptide- and cholecystokinin-immunoreactive ganglion cells. *Cell Tissue Res* 247(2):417–431.

18. Lee, Y., Kawai, Y., Shiosaka, S., Takami, K., Kiyama, H., Hillyard, C.J., Girgis, S., MacIntyre, I., Emson, P.C., Tohyama, M. (1985). Coexistence of calcitonin gene-related peptide and substance P-like peptide in single cells of the trigeminal ganglion of the rat: immunocytochemical analysis. *Brain Res* 330:194–196.

19. McCarthy, P.W., Lawson, S.N. (1990). Cell type and conduction velocity of rat primary sensory neurons with calcitonin gene-related peptide-like immunoreactivity. *Neuroscience* 34(3):623–632.

20. Saria, A., Gamse, R., Petermann, J., Fischer, J.A., Theodorsson-Norheim, E., Lundberg, J.M. (1986). Simultaneous release of several tachykinins and calcitonin gene-related peptide from rat spinal cord slices. *Neurosci Lett* 63(3):310–314.

21. Ulrich-Lai, Y.M., Flores, C.M., Harding-Rose, C.A., Goodis, H.E., Hargreaves, K.M. (2001). Capsaicin-evoked release of immunoreactive calcitonin gene-related peptide from rat trigeminal ganglion: evidence for intraganglionic neurotransmission. *Pain* 91(3):219–226.

22. Gamse, R., Posch, M., Saria, A., Jancso, G. (1987). Several mediators appear to interact in neurogenic inflammation. *Acta Physiol Hung* 69(3-4):343–354.

23. Ohlen, A., Wiklund, N.P., Persson, M.G., Hedqvist, P. (1988). Calcitonin gene-related peptide desensitizes skeletal muscle arterioles to substance P in vivo. *Br J Pharmacol* 95(3):673–674.

24. Ryu, P.D., Murase, K., Gerber, G., Randic, M. (1988). Actions of calcitonin gene-related peptide on rat sensory ganglion neurones. *Physiol Bohemoslov* 37(3): 259–265.

25. Sun, R.Q., Tu, Y.J., Lawand, N.B., Yan, J.Y., Lin, Q., Willis, W.D. (2004). Calcitonin gene-related peptide receptor activation produces PKA- and PKC-dependent mechanical hyperalgesia and central sensitization. *J Neurophysiol* 92(5): 2859–2866.

26. Yu, L.C., Hansson, P., Lundeberg, S., Lundeberg, T. (1998). Effects of calcitonin gene-related peptide-(8-37) on withdrawal responses in rats with inflammation. *Eur J Pharmacol* 347(2-3):275–282.

27. Lofgren, O., Yu, L.C., Theodorsson, E., Hansson, P., Lundeberg, T. (1997). Intrathecal CGRP(8-37) results in a bilateral increase in hindpaw withdrawal latency in rats with a unilateral thermal injury. *Neuropeptides* 31(6):601–607.

28. Mogil, J.S., Breese, N.M., Witty, M.F., Ritchie, J., Rainville, M.L., Ase, A., Abbadi, N., Stucky, C.L., Seguela, P. (2005). Transgenic expression of a dominant-negative ASIC3 subunit leads to increased sensitivity to mechanical and inflammatory stimuli. *J Neurosci* 25(43):9893–9901.

29. Chang, M.M., Leeman, S.E., Niall, H.D. (1971). Amino-acid sequence of substance P. *Nat.New Biol.*, 232(29), 86–87.

30. Hokfelt, T., Kellerth, J.O., Nilsson, G., Pernow, B. (1975). Experimental immunohistochemical studies on the localization and distribution of substance P in cat primary sensory neurons. *Brain Res* 100(2):235–252.

31. McCarthy, P.W., Lawson, S.N. (1989). Cell type and conduction velocity of rat primary sensory neurons with substance P-like immunoreactivity. *Neuroscience* 28(3):745–753.

32. Duggan, A.W., Hendry, I.A., Morton, C.R., Hutchison, W.D., Zhao, Z.Q. (1988). Cutaneous stimuli releasing immunoreactive substance P in the dorsal horn of the cat. *Brain Res* 451(1-2):261–273.

33. Neubert, J.K., Maidment, N.T., Matsuka, Y., Adelson, D.W., Kruger, L., Spigelman, I. (2000). Inflammation-induced changes in primary afferent-evoked release of substance P within the trigeminal ganglia in vivo. *Brain Res* 871:181–191.

34. Oku, R., Satoh, M., Takagi, H. (1987). Release of substance P from the spinal dorsal horn is enhanced in polyarthritic rats. *Neurosci Lett* 74(3):315–319.

35. Abbadie, C., Trafton, J., Liu, H., Mantyh, P.W., Basbaum, A.I. (1997). Inflammation increases the distribution of dorsal horn neurons that internalize the neurokinin-1 receptor in response to noxious and non-noxious stimulation. *J Neurosci* 17(20): 8049–8060.

36. Galeazza, M.T., Garry, M.G., Yost, H.J., Strait, K.A., Hargreaves, K.M., Seybold, V.S. (1995). Plasticity in the synthesis and storage of substance P and calcitonin gene-related peptide in primary afferent neurons during peripheral inflammation. *Neuroscience* 66(2):443–458.

37. Seybold, V.S., McCarson, K.E., Mermelstein, P.G., Groth, R.D., Abrahams, L.G. (2003). Calcitonin gene-related peptide regulates expression of neurokinin1 receptors by rat spinal neurons. *J Neurosci* 23(5):1816–1824.

38. Yasphal, K., Wright, D.M., Henry, J.L. (1982). Substance P reduces tail-flick latency: implications for chronic pain syndromes. *Pain* 14(2):155–167.

39. Piercey, M.F., Moon, M.W., Blinn, J.R., Dobry-Schreur, P.J. (1986). Analgesic activities of spinal cord substance P antagonists implicate substance P as a neurotransmitter of pain sensation. *Brain Res* 385(1):74–85.

40. Cao, Y.Q., Mantyh, P.W., Carlson, E.J., Gillespie, A.M., Epstein, C.J., Basbaum, A.I. (1998). Primary afferent tachykinins are required to experience moderate to intense pain. *Nature* 392(6674):390–394.

41. De Felipe, C., Herrero, J.F., O'Brien, J.A., Palmer, J.A., Doyle, C.A., Smith, A.J., Laird, J.M., Belmonte, C., Cervero, F., Hunt, S.P. (1998). Altered nociception, analgesia and aggression in mice lacking the receptor for substance P. *Nature* 392(6674):394–397.

42. Mantyh, P.W., Rogers, S.D., Honore, P., Allen, B.J., Ghilardi, J.R., Li, J., Daughters, R.S., Lappi, D.A., Wiley, R.G., Simone, D.A. (1997). Inhibition of hyperalgesia by ablation of lamina I spinal neurons expressing the substance P receptor. *Science* 278(5336):275–279.

43. Keen, P., Harmar, A.J., Spears, F., Winter, E. (1982). Biosynthesis, axonal transport and turnover of neuronal substance P. *Ciba Found Symp* (91):145–164.

44. Richardson, J.D., Vasko, M.R. (2002). Cellular mechanisms of neurogenic inflammation. *J Pharmacol Exp Ther* 302(3):839–845.

45. Lembeck, F., Donnerer, J., Tsuchiya, M., Nagahisa, A. (1992). The non-peptide tachykinin antagonist, CP-96,345, is a potent inhibitor of neurogenic inflammation. *Br J Pharmacol* 105(3):527–530.

46. Brain, S.D., Williams, T.J. (1989). Interactions between the tachykinins and calcitonin gene-related peptide lead to the modulation of oedema formation and blood flow in rat skin. *Br J Pharmacol* 97(1):77–82.

47. Foreman, J., Jordan, C. (1983). Histamine release and vascular changes induced by neuropeptides. *Agents Actions* 13(2-3):105–116.

48. Garret, C., Carruette, A., Fardin, V., Moussaoui, S., Peyronel, J.F., Blanchard, J.C., Laduron, P.M. (1991). Pharmacological properties of a potent and selective non-peptide substance P antagonist. *Proc Natl Acad Sci U S A* 88(22):10208–10212.

49. Shepheard, S.L., Williamson, D.J., Williams, J., Hill, R.G., Hargreaves, R.J. (1995). Comparison of the effects of sumatriptan and the NK1 antagonist CP-99,994 on plasma extravasation in dura mater and c-fos mRNA expression in trigeminal nucleus caudalis of rats. *Neuropharmacology* 34(3):255–261.

50. Gibbins, I.L., Furness, J.B., Costa, M., MacIntyre, I., Hillyard, C.J., Girgis, S. (1985). Co-localization of calcitonin gene-related peptide-like immunoreactivity with substance P in cutaneous, vascular and visceral sensory neurons of guinea pigs. *Neurosci Lett* 57(2):125–130.

51. Samsam, M., Covenas, R., Ahangari, R., Yajeya, J., Narvaez, J.A., Tramu, G. (2000). Simultaneous depletion of neurokinin A, substance P and calcitonin gene-related peptide from the caudal trigeminal nucleus of the rat during electrical stimulation of the trigeminal ganglion. *Pain* 84(2-3):389–395.

52. Merighi, A., Polak, J.M., Gibson, S.J., Gulbenkian, S., Valentino, K.L., Peirone, S.M. (1988). Ultrastructural studies on calcitonin gene-related peptide-, tachykinins- and somatostatin-immunoreactive neurones in rat dorsal root ganglia: evidence for the colocalization of different peptides in single secretory granules. *Cell Tissue Res* 254(1):101–109.

53. Schaible, H.G., Hope, P.J., Lang, C.W., Duggan, A.W. (1992). Calcitonin gene-related peptide causes intraspinal spreading of substance P released by peripheral stimulation. *Eur J Neurosci* 4(8):750–757.

54. Le, G.P., Nyberg, F., Terenius, L., Hokfelt, T. (1985). Calcitonin gene-related peptide is a potent inhibitor of substance P degradation. *Eur J Pharmacol* 115(2-3): 309–311.

55. Nyberg, F., Le, G.P., Terenius, L. (1988). Modulation of endopeptidase activity by calcitonin gene related peptide: a mechanism affecting substance P action? *Biochimie* 70(1):65–68.

56. Pedersen-Bjergaard, U., Nielsen, L.B., Jensen, K., Edvinsson, L., Jansen, I., Olesen, J. (1991). Calcitonin gene-related peptide, neurokinin A and substance P: effects on nociception and neurogenic inflammation in human skin and temporal muscle. *Peptides* 12(2):333–337.

57. Pedersen-Bjergaard, U., Nielsen, L.B., Jensen, K., Edvinsson, L., Jansen, I., Olesen, J. (1989). Algesia and local responses induced by neurokinin A and substance P in human skin and temporal muscle. *Peptides* 10(6):1147–1152.

58. Gamse, R., Saria, A. (1985). Potentiation of tachykinin-induced plasma protein extravasation by calcitonin gene-related peptide. *Eur J Pharmacol* 114(1):61–66.

59. McMahon, S.B., Gibson, S. (1987). Peptide expression is altered when afferent nerves reinnervate inappropriate tissue. *Neurosci Lett* 73(1):9–15.
60. McMahon, S.B., Lewin, G.R., Anand, P., Ghatei, M.A., Bloom, S.R. (1989). Quantitative analysis of peptide levels and neurogenic extravasation following regeneration of afferents to appropriate and inappropriate targets. *Neuroscience* 33(1):67–73.
61. Mense, S. (1993). Nocicpeption from skeletal muscle in relation to clinical muscle pain. *Pain* 54:241–289.
62. Dubner, R. (1991). Basic mechanisms of pain associated with deep tissues. *Can J Physiol Pharmacol* 69(5):607–609.
63. Molander, C., Ygge, J., Dalsgaard, C.J. (1987). Substance P-, somatostatin- and calcitonin gene-related peptide-like immunoreactivity and fluoride resistant acid phosphatase-activity in relation to retrogradely labeled cutaneous, muscular and visceral primary sensory neurons in the rat. *Neurosci Lett* 74(1):37–42.
64. O'Brien, C., Woolf, C.J., Fitzgerald, M., Lindsay, R.M., Molander, C. (1989). Differences in the chemical expression of rat primary afferent neurons which innervate skin, muscle or joint. *Neuroscience* 32(2):493–502.
65. Kashiba, H., Senba, E., Ueda, Y., Tohyama, M. (1991). Cell size and cell type analysis of calcitonin gene-related peptide-containing cutaneous and splanchnic sensory neurons in the rat. *Peptides* 12(1):101–106.
66. Perry, M.J., Lawson, S.N. (1998). Differences in expression of oligosaccharides, neuropeptides, carbonic anhydrase and neurofilament in rat primary afferent neurons retrogradely labelled via skin, muscle or visceral nerves. *Neuroscience* 85(1):293–310.
67. Bennett, D.L., Dmietrieva, N., Priestley, J.V., Clary, D., McMahon, S.B. (1996). trkA, CGRP and IB4 expression in retrogradely labelled cutaneous and visceral primary sensory neurones in the rat. *Neurosci Lett* 206(1):33–36.
68. Aoki, Y., Ohtori, S., Takahashi, K., Ino, H., Douya, H., Ozawa, T., Saito, T., Moriya, H. (2005). Expression and co-expression of VR1, CGRP, and IB4-binding glycoprotein in dorsal root ganglion neurons in rats: differences between the disc afferents and the cutaneous afferents. *Spine* 30(13):1496–1500.
69. Kuniyoshi, K., Ohtori, S., Ochiai, N., Murata, R., Matsudo, T., Yamada, T., Ochiai, S.S., Moriya, H., Takahashi, K. (2007). Characteristics of sensory DRG neurons innervating the wrist joint in rats. *Eur J Pain* 11(3):323–328.
70. Ambalavanar, R., Moritani, M., Haines, A., Hilton, T., Dessem, D. (2003). Chemical phenotypes of muscle and cutaneous afferent neurons in the rat trigeminal ganglion. *J Comp Neurol* 460(2):167–179.
71. Carlton, S.M., Zhou, S., Coggeshall, R.E. (1996). Localization and activation of substance P receptors in unmyelinated axons of rat glabrous skin. *Brain Res* 734:103–108.
72. Holzer, P. (1998). Neurogenic vasodilatation and plasma leakage in the skin. *Gen Pharmacol* 30(1):5–11.
73. Chiba, T., Yamaguchi, A., Yamatani, T., Nakamura, A., Morishita, T., Inui, T., Fukase, M., Noda, T., Fujita, T. (1989). Calcitonin gene-related peptide receptor antagonist human CGRP-(8-37). *Am J Physiol* 256(2 Pt 1):E331–E335.
74. Woolf, C.J., Ma, Q. (2007). Nociceptors–noxious stimulus detectors. *Neuron* 55(3):353–364.

75. Neumann, S., Doubell, T.P., Leslie, T., Woolf, C.J. (1996). Inflammatory pain hypersensitivity mediated by phenotypic switch in myelinated primary sensory neurons. *Nature* 384(6607):360–364.
76. Bulling, D.G.S., Kelly, D., Bond, S., McQueen, D.S., Seckl, J.R. (2001). Adjuvant-induced joint inflammation causes very rapid transcription of beta-preprotachykinin and alpha-CGRP genes in innervating sensory ganglia. *J Neurochem* 77:372–382.
77. Uddman, R., Edvinsson, L., Jansen, I., Stiernholm, P., Jensen, K., Olesen, J., Sundler, F. (1986). Peptide-containing nerve fibres in human extracranial tissue: a morphological basis for neuropeptide involvement in extracranial pain? *Pain* 27(3): 391–399.
78. Tuxen, C., Jensen, K., Kjeldsen, M., Edvinsson, L., Jansen, I., Olesen, J. (1989). Effect of neurokinin A on human temporal muscle blood flow. *Peptides* 10(5): 921–924.
79. Sakaguchi, M., Inaishi, Y., Kashihara, Y., Kuno, M. (1991). Release of calcitonin gene-related peptide from nerve terminals in rat skeletal muscle. *J Physiol* 434:257–270.
80. McMahon, S.B., Sykova, E., Wall, P.D., Woolf, C.J., Gibson, S.J. (1984). Neurogenic extravasation and substance P levels are low in muscle as compared to skin the rat hindlimb. *Neurosci Lett* 52(3):235–240.
81. Ambalavanar, R., Moritani, M., Moutanni, A., Gangula, P., Yallampalli, C., Dessem, D. (2006). Deep tissue inflammation upregulates neuropeptides and evokes nociceptive behaviors which are modulated by a neuropeptide antagonist. *Pain* 120(1-2):53–68.
82. Sato, A., Sato, Y., Shimura, M., Uchida, S. (2000). Calcitonin gene-related peptide produces skeletal muscle vasodilation following antidromic stimulation of unmyelinated afferents in the dorsal root in rats. *Neurosci Lett* 283(2):137–140.
83. Reinert, A., Kaske, A., Mense, S. (1998). Inflammation-induced increase in the density of neuropeptide-immunoreactive nerve endings in rat skeletal muscle. *Exp Brain Res* 121(2):174–180.
84. Carleson, J., Lundeberg, T., Appelgren, B. (2004). Muscle and brain changes of calcitonin gene-related peptide in experimentally induced unilateral rat masseter myositis. *J Orofac Pain* 18(3):246–252.
85. Mense, S. (1996). Group III and IV receptors in skeletal muscle: are they specific or polymodal? *Prog Brain Res* 113:83–100.
86. De Stefano, R., Selvi, E., Villanova, M., Frati, E., Manganelli, S., Franceschini, E., Biasi, G., Marcolongo, R. (2000). Image analysis quantification of substance P immunoreactivity in the trapezius muscle of patients with fibromyalgia and myofascial pain syndrome. *J Rheumatol* 27(12):2906–2910.
87. Shah, J.P., Danoff, J.V., Desai, M.J., Parikh, S., Nakamura, L.Y., Phillips, T.M., Gerber, L.H. (2008). Biochemicals associated with pain and inflammation are elevated in sites near to and remote from active myofascial trigger points. *Arch Phys Med Rehabil* 89(1):16–23.
88. Russell, I.J. (1998). Advances in fibromyalgia: possible role for central neurochemicals. *Am J Med Sci* 315(6):377–384.
89. Ambalavanar, R., Dessem, D., Moutanni, A., Yallampalli, C., Yallampalli, U., Gangula, P., Bai, G. (2006). Muscle inflammation induces a rapid increase in cal-

citonin gene-related peptide (CGRP) mRNA that temporally relates to CGRP immunoreactivity and nociceptive behavior. *Neuroscience* 143(3):875–884.

90. Schaible, H.G. (2007). Peripheral and central mechanisms of pain generation. *Handb Exp Pharmacol* 177:3–28.
91. Calza, L., Pozza, M., Zanni, M., Manzini, C.U., Manzini, E., Hokfelt, T. (1998). Peptide plasticity in primary sensory neurons and spinal cord during adjuvant-induced arthritis in the rat: an immunocytochemical and in situ hybridization study. *Neuroscience* 82(2):575–589.
92. Hong, S.K., Han, J.S., Min, S.S., Hwang, J.M., Kim, Y.I., Na, H.S., Yoon, Y.W., Han, H.C. (2002). Local neurokinin-1 receptor in the knee joint contributes to the induction, but not maintenance, of arthritic pain in the rat. *Neurosci Lett* 322(1):21–24.
93. Saxler, G., Loer, F., Skumavc, M., Pfortner, J., Hanesch, U. (2007). Localization of SP- and CGRP-immunopositive nerve fibers in the hip joint of patients with painful osteoarthritis and of patients with painless failed total hip arthroplasties. *Eur J Pain* 11(1):67–74.
94. Sato, J., Segami, N., Kaneyama, K., Yoshimura, H., Fujimura, K., Yoshitake, Y. (2004). Relationship of calcitonin gene-related peptide in synovial tissues and temporomandibular joint pain in humans. *Oral Surg Oral Med Oral Pathol Oral Radiol Endod* 98(5):533–540.
95. Shinoda, M., Honda, T., Ozaki, N., Hattori, H., Mizutani, H., Ueda, M., Sugiura, Y. (2003). Nerve terminals extend into the temporomandibular joint of adjuvant arthritic rats. *Eur J Pain* 7(6):493–505.
96. Szadek, K.M., Hoogland, P.V., Zuurmond, W.W., de Lange, J.J., Perez, R.S. (2008). Nociceptive nerve fibers in the sacroiliac joint in humans. *Reg Anesth Pain Med* 33(1):36–43.
97. Storer, R.J., Akerman, S., Goadsby, P.J. (2004). Calcitonin gene-related peptide (CGRP) modulates nociceptive trigeminovascular transmission in the cat. *Br J Pharmacol* 142(7):1171–1181.
98. Olesen, J., Diener, H.C., Husstedt, I.W., Goadsby, P.J., Hall, D., Meier, U., Pollentier, S., Lesko, L.M. (2004). Calcitonin gene-related peptide receptor antagonist BIBN 4096 BS for the acute treatment of migraine. *N Engl J Med* 350(11):1104–1110.
99. Ho, T.W., Mannix, L.K., Fan, X., Assaid, C., Furtek, C., Jones, C.J., Lines, C.R., Rapoport, A.M. (2008). Randomized controlled trial of an oral CGRP receptor antagonist, MK-0974, in acute treatment of migraine. *Neurology* 70(16): 1304–1312.
100. Recober, A., Russo, A.F. (2007). Olcegepant, a non-peptide CGRP1 antagonist for migraine treatment. *IDrugs* 10(8):566–574.
101. Link, A.S., Kuris, A., Edvinsson, L. (2008). Treatment of migraine attacks based on the interaction with the trigemino-cerebrovascular system. *J Headache Pain* 9(1):5–12.
102. Doods, H., Arndt, K., Rudolf, K., Just, S. (2007). CGRP antagonists: unravelling the role of CGRP in migraine. *Trends Pharmacol Sci* 28(11):580–587.
103. Goadsby, P.J. (2007). Recent advances in understanding migraine mechanisms, molecules and therapeutics. *Trends Mol Med* 13(1):39–44.
104. Edvinsson, L., Petersen, K.A. (2007). CGRP-receptor antagonism in migraine treatment. *CNS Neurol Disord Drug Targets* 6(4):240–246.

105. Benemei, S., Nicoletti, P., Capone, J.A., Geppetti, P. (2007). Pain pharmacology in migraine: focus on CGRP and CGRP receptors. *Neurol Sci* 28(Suppl. 2): S89–S93.

106. Durham, P.L. (2004). CGRP-receptor antagonists–a fresh approach to migraine therapy? *N Engl J Med* 350(11):1073–1075.

107. Hill, R.G., Oliver, K.R. (2007). Neuropeptide and kinin antagonists. *Handb Exp Pharmacol* 177:181–216.

108. Matsuka, Y., Neubert, J.K., Maidment, N.T., Spigelman, I. (2001). Concurrent release of ATP and substance P within the guinea pig trigeminal ganglia in vivo. *Brain Res* 915:248–255.

109. Takeda, M., Tanimoto, T., Nasu, M., Ikeda, M., Kadoi, J., Matsumoto, S. (2005). Activation of NK1 receptor of trigeminal root ganglion via substance P paracrine mechanism contributes to the mechanical allodynia in the temporomandibular joint inflammation in rats. *Pain* 116(3):375–385.

110. Zhang, S.H., Sun, Q.X., Seltzer, Z., Cao, D.Y., Wang, H.S., Chen, Z., Zhao, Y. (2008). Paracrine-like excitation of low-threshold mechanoceptive C-fibers innervating rat hairy skin is mediated by substance P via NK-1 receptors. *Brain Res Bull* 75(1):138–145.

111. Lennerz, J.K., Ruhle, V., Ceppa, E.P., Neuhuber, W.L., Bunnett, N.W., Grady, E.F., Messlinger, K. (2008). Calcitonin receptor-like receptor (CLR), receptor activity-modifying protein 1 (RAMP1), and calcitonin gene-related peptide (CGRP) immunoreactivity in the rat trigeminovascular system: differences between peripheral and central CGRP receptor distribution. *J Comp Neurol* 507(3): 1277–1299.

112. Natura, G., von Banchet, G.S., Schaible, H.G. (2005). Calcitonin gene-related peptide enhances TTX-resistant sodium currents in cultured dorsal root ganglion neurons from adult rats. *Pain* 166(3):194–204.

113. Anderson, L.E., Seybold, V.S. (2004). Calcitonin gene-related peptide regulates gene transcription in primary afferent neurons. *J Neurochem* 91(6):1417–1429.

114. Fabbretti, E., D'Arco, M., Fabbro, A., Simonetti, M., Nistri, A., Giniatullin, R. (2006). Delayed upregulation of ATP P2X3 receptors of trigeminal sensory neurons by calcitonin gene-related peptide. *J Neurosci* 26(23):6163–6171.

115. Ambalavanar, R., Moritani, M., Dessem, D. (2005). Trigeminal P2X3 receptor expression differs from dorsal root ganglion and is modulated by deep tissue inflammation. *Pain* 117(3):280–291.

116. Shinoda, M., Ozaki, N., Sugiura, Y. (2008). Involvement of ATP and its receptors on nociception in rat model of masseter muscle pain. *Pain* 134(1-2):148–157.

117. Segond Von Banchet, G., Petersen, M., Schaible, H.G. (1999). Expression of neurokinin-1 receptors on cultured dorsal root ganglion neurons from the adult rat. *Neuroscience* 90:677–684.

118. Dray, A., Pinnock, R.D. (1982). Effects of substance P on adult rat sensory ganglion neurones in vitro. *Neurosci Lett* 33(1):61–66.

119. Quirion, R., van, R.D., Dumont, Y., St-Pierre, S., Fournier, A. (1992). Characterization of CGRP1 and CGRP2 receptor subtypes. *Ann N Y Acad Sci* 657:88–105.

120. Arulmani, U., Maassenvandenbrink, A., Villalon, C.M., Saxena, P.R. (2004). Calcitonin gene-related peptide and its role in migraine pathophysiology. *Eur J Pharmacol* 500(1-3):315–330.

121. Poyner, D.R. (1997). Molecular pharmacology of receptors for calcitonin-gene-related peptide, amylin and adrenomedullin. *Biochem Soc Trans* 25(3): 1032–1036.

122. Conner, A.C., Simms, J., Barwell, J., Wheatley, M., Poyner, D.R. (2007). Ligand binding and activation of the CGRP receptor. *Biochem Soc Trans* 35(Pt 4): 729–732.

123. McLatchie, L.M., Fraser, N.J., Main, M.J., Wise, A., Brown, J., Thompson, N., Solari, R., Lee, M.G., Foord, S.M. (1998). RAMPs regulate the transport and ligand specificity of the calcitonin-receptor-like receptor. *Nature* 393(6683):333–339.

124. Mallee, J.J., Salvatore, C.A., LeBourdelles, B., Oliver, K.R., Longmore, J., Koblan, K.S., Kane, S.A. (2002). Receptor activity-modifying protein 1 determines the species selectivity of non-peptide CGRP receptor antagonists. *J Biol Chem* 277(16):14294–14298.

125. Zhang, Z., Winborn, C.S., Marquez de, P.B., Russo, A.F. (2007). Sensitization of calcitonin gene-related peptide receptors by receptor activity-modifying protein-1 in the trigeminal ganglion. *J Neurosci* 27(10):2693–2703.

126. Evans, B.N., Rosenblatt, M.I., Mnayer, L.O., Oliver, K.R., Dickerson, I.M. (2000). CGRP-RCP, a novel protein required for signal transduction at calcitonin gene-related peptide and adrenomedullin receptors. *J Biol Chem* 275(40): 31438–31443.

127. Ma, W., Chabot, J.G., Powell, K.J., Jhamandas, K., Dickerson, I.M., Quirion, R. (2003). Localization and modulation of calcitonin gene-related peptide-receptor component protein-immunoreactive cells in the rat central and peripheral nervous systems. *Neuroscience* 120(3):677–694.

128. Ye, Z., Wimalawansa, S.J., Westlund, K.N. (1999). Receptor for calcitonin gene-related peptide: localization in the dorsal and ventral spinal cord. *Neuroscience* 92(4):1389–1397.

129. Van der Schueren, B.J., Rogiers, A., Vanmolkot, F.H., Van, H.A., Depre, M., Kane, S.A., De, L., I, Sinclair, S.R., de Hoon, J.N. (2008). Calcitonin gene-related peptide 8-37 antagonizes capsaicin-induced vasodilation in the skin: evaluation of a human in vivo pharmacodynamic model. *J Pharmacol Exp Ther* 325(1):248–255.

130. Wu, D., Eberlein, W., Rudolf, K., Engel, W., Hallermayer, G., Doods, H. (2000). Characterisation of calcitonin gene-related peptide receptors in rat atrium and vas deferens: evidence for a [Cys(Et)(2, 7)]hCGRP-preferring receptor. *Eur J Pharmacol* 400(2-3):313–319.

131. Hershey, J.C., Corcoran, H.A., Baskin, E.P., Salvatore, C.A., Mosser, S., Williams, T.M., Koblan, K.S., Hargreaves, R.J., Kane, S.A. (2005). Investigation of the species selectivity of a nonpeptide CGRP receptor antagonist using a novel pharmacodynamic assay. *Regul Pept* 127(1-3):71–77.

132. Fischer, M.J., Koulchitsky, S., Messlinger, K. (2005). The nonpeptide calcitonin gene-related peptide receptor antagonist BIBN4096BS lowers the activity of neurons with meningeal input in the rat spinal trigeminal nucleus. *J Neurosci* 25(25):5877–5883.

133. Kopp, S. (1998). The influence of neuropeptides, serotonin, and interleukin 1beta on temporomandibular joint pain and inflammation. *J Oral Maxillofac Surg* 56(2): 189–191.

134. Todd, A.J., Puskar, Z., Spike, R.C., Hughes, C., Watt, C., Forrest, L. (2002). Projection neurons in lamina I of rat spinal cord with the neurokinin 1 receptor are selectively innervated by substance p-containing afferents and respond to noxious stimulation. *J Neurosci* 22(10):4103–4113.
135. Mantyh, P.W., DeMaster, E., Malhotra, A., Ghilardi, J.R., Rogers, S.D., Mantyh, C.R., Liu, H., Basbaum, A.I., Vigna, S.R., Maggio, J.E. (1995). Receptor endocytosis and dendrite reshaping in spinal neurons after somatosensory stimulation. *Science* 268(5217):1629–1632.
136. Marshall, G.E., Shehab, S.A., Spike, R.C., Todd, A.J. (1996). Neurokinin-1 receptors on lumbar spinothalamic neurons in the rat. *Neuroscience* 72(1):255–263.
137. Duffy, R.A. (2004). Potential therapeutic targets for neurokinin-1 receptor antagonists. *Expert Opin Emerg Drugs* 9(1):9–21.
138. Snider, R.M., Constantine, J.W., Lowe, J.A., III, Longo, K.P., Lebel, W.S., Woody, H.A., Drozda, S.E., Desai, M.C., Vinick, F.J., Spencer, R.W. (1991). A potent nonpeptide antagonist of the substance P (NK1) receptor. *Science* 251(4992): 435–437.
139. Radhakrishnan, V., Henry, J.L. (1991). Novel substance P antagonist, CP-96,345, blocks responses of cat spinal dorsal horn neurons to noxious cutaneous stimulation and to substance P. *Neurosci Lett* 132(1):39–43.
140. Yamamoto, T., Yaksh, T.L. (1991). Stereospecific effects of a nonpeptidic NK1 selective antagonist, CP-96,345: antinociception in the absence of motor dysfunction. *Life Sci* 49(26):1955–1963.
141. Rupniak, N.M., Carlson, E., Boyce, S., Webb, J.K., Hill, R.G. (1996). Enantioselective inhibition of the formalin paw late phase by the NK1 receptor antagonist L-733,060 in gerbils. *Pain* 67(1):189–195.
142. Cellier, E., Fayolle, C., Hipskind, P.A., Iyengar, S., Couture, R. (1996). Peripheral effects of three novel non-peptide tachykinin NK1 receptor antagonists in the anaesthetized rat. *Eur J Pharmacol* 318(2-3):377–385.
143. Iyengar, S., Hipskind, P.A., Gehlert, D.R., Schober, D., Lobb, K.L., Nixon, J.A., Helton, D.R., Kallman, M.J., Boucher, S., Couture, R., Li, D.L., Simmons, R.M. (1997). LY303870, a centrally active neurokinin-1 antagonist with a long duration of action. *J Pharmacol Exp Ther* 280(2):774–785.
144. Cahill, C.M., Coderre, T.J. (2002). Attenuation of hyperalgesia in a rat model of neuropathic pain after intrathecal pre- or post-treatment with a neurokinin-1 antagonist. *Pain* 95(3):277–285.
145. Phebus, L.A., Johnson, K.W., Stengel, P.W., Lobb, K.L., Nixon, J.A., Hipskind, P.A. (1997). The non-peptide NK-1 receptor antagonist LY303870 inhibits neurogenic dural inflammation in guinea pigs. *Life Sci* 60(18):1553–1561.
146. Goldstein, D.J., Wang, O., Todd, L.E., Gitter, B.D., DeBrota, D.J., Iyengar, S. (2000). Study of the analgesic effect of lanepitant in patients with osteoarthritis pain. *Clin Pharmacol Ther* 67(4):419–426.
147. Goldstein, D.J., Offen, W.W., Klein, E.G., Phebus, L.A., Hipskind, P., Johnson, K.W., Ryan, R.E., Jr. (2001). Lanepitant, an NK-1 antagonist, in migraine prevention. *Cephalalgia* 21(2):102–106.
148. Sindrup, S.H., Graf, A., Sfikas, N. (2006). The NK1-receptor antagonist TKA731 in painful diabetic neuropathy: a randomised, controlled trial. *Eur J Pain* 10(6):567–571.

149. Hill, R. (2000). NK1 (substance P) receptor antagonists - why are they not analgesic in humans? *Trend Pharm Sci* 21:244–246.

150. Urban, L.A., Fox, A.J. (2000). NK1 receptor antagonists–are they really without effect in the pain clinic? *Trends Pharmacol Sci* 21(12):462–464.

151. Goldstein, D.J., Wang, O., Gitter, B.D., Iyengar, S. (2001). Dose-response study of the analgesic effect of lanepitant in patients with painful diabetic neuropathy. *Clin Neuropharmacol* 24(1):16–22.

152. Block, G.A., Rue, D., Panebianco, D.E.A. (1998). The substance P receptor antagonist L-754,030 (MK-0869) is ineffective in the treatment of postherpatic neuralgia. *Neurology* 4:A225.

153. Chizh, B.A., Gohring, M., Troster, A., Quartey, G.K., Schmelz, M., Koppert, W. (2007). Effects of oral pregabalin and aprepitant on pain and central sensitization in the electrical hyperalgesia model in human volunteers. *Br J Anaesth* 98(2):246–254.

154. Patel, L., Lindley, C. (2003). Aprepitant–a novel NK1-receptor antagonist. *Expert Opin Pharmacother* 4(12):2279–2296.

155. Warr, D. (2006). The neurokinin1 receptor antagonist aprepitant as an antiemetic for moderately emetogenic chemotherapy. *Expert Opin Pharmacother* 7(12): 1653–1658.

156. Olver, I., Shelukar, S., Thompson, K.C. (2007). Nanomedicines in the treatment of emesis during chemotherapy: focus on aprepitant. *Int J Nanomedicine* 2(1):13–18.

CHAPTER 16

Role of Somatostatin and Somatostatin Receptors in Pain

UJENDRA KUMAR

Faculty of Pharmaceutical Sciences, University of British Columbia

Content

16.1 INTRODUCTION

It has been almost 35 years since somatostatin (SST) was first discovered in hypothalamic extract and was identified as a growth hormone inhibitory peptide [1]. Since then, enormous progress has been made to understand the basic biology of SST in different target tissues and the pathophysiology of several diseases. In the central nervous system, SST is widely distributed in a region-specific manner and plays an important role as a neurotransmitter and

Peripheral Receptor Targets for Analgesia: Novel Approaches to Pain Management, Edited by Brian E. Cairns

neuromodulator. SST occurs naturally in two biologically active forms: SST-14 and SST-28, and is produced by the cells in the brain, pancreas, stomach, and intestine. SST acts at multiple targets to produce a wide variety of biological effects consistent with its distribution throughout the body. It is a multifunctional neuropeptide that, in addition to inhibiting the release of growth hormone from the anterior pituitary, has also been shown to regulate exocrine secretion and to modulate neurotransmission and cell proliferation [1–3]. It is now well accepted that the diverse biological effects of SST are intimately associated with its ability to inhibit two critical cell processes, that is, secretion and cell proliferation. The biological functions of SST are mediated by five different receptor subtypes, somatostatin receptors 1–5 (SSTR1–5), which belong to the family of G protein-coupled receptors (GPCRs). All somatostatin receptor (SSTR) subtypes have been well characterized pharmacologically. SSTR1–5 were initially mapped by autoradiographic detection for their mRNA expression [4–11]. Recently, receptor-specific antibodies against the individual SSTRs have been used to study their expression in the central nervous system [12–25]. Clinically, SST has become a powerful tool in several pathophysiological conditions; this chapter specifically focuses on the basic understanding of this novel peptide and its receptors in the biology of pain.

16.2 PROCESSING OF SST

SST, like many other protein hormones, is derived from a precursor protein, preprosomatostatin (PPSST), which is cleaved into two active forms, SST-14 and SST-28, which exert its biological effects in target tissues [26–27]. Both peptides are produced in variable amounts in different SST-producing cells and act as neurotransmitters or as paracrine/autocrine regulators in different target tissues. PPSST molecules were first characterized in the early 1980s followed by structural elucidation of rat somatostatin (rSST) and human somatostatin (hSST) in 1984. Interestingly, rat and human PPSST molecules are virtually identical, differing in only four amino acids. PPSST molecules (116 amino acids) are synthesized as precursors in ribosomes in the rough endoplasmic reticulum. Upon translation, PPSST is rapidly cleaved in the lumen of the endoplasmic reticulum by a signal peptidase to prosomatostatin (PSST; 92 amino acids, 10 kDa). PSST is subsequently transported to the trans-Golgi network (TGN) through the Golgi stacks where it is sorted to clathrin-coated (regulated SST processing) or non-clathrin-coated (constitutive SST processing) vesicles. During sorting, constitutive versus regulated processing may occur via a sorting receptor (e.g., membrane-bound carboxypeptidase E) or via the formation of aggregates; in the case of PSST, this process most likely requires a sorting signal sequence. To this end, the region Pro^5 to Gln^{12} has been shown to be important for PSST sorting to regulate SST processing with Leu^7 and Leu^{11} being critical residues within this signal [28–29].

16.3 EXPRESSION OF SST AND SSTRs IN THE PAIN REGULATORY PATHWAY

SST is widely distributed in the central nervous system in a region-specific manner, suggesting its important role outside of the hypothalamus. Direct evidence for a role of SST in pain processing comes from the expression of SST-like immunoreactivity in pathways involved in pain processing and regulation. SST, in addition to being one of the most important inhibitory neurotransmitters in the central nervous system, is also expressed in sensory and sympathetic neurons in the periphery and exerts inhibitory actions on nociception and some other molecular components of inflammatory processes [30]. SST-like immunoreactivity is found in the dorsal horn of cervical and lumbar regions of the spinal cord where it is confined in a laminar distribution that includes laminae I, II, and III. SST is also highly expressed by motor neurons in the ventral horn (Figure 16.1). In higher brain centers, SST is not only present in the hypothalamus, which is thought to play a role in the emotional response to pain, but has also been located in sensory regions of the thalamus that are important in the processing of nociceptive input. SST is highly expressed in different nuclei of the hypothalamus including the posterior hypothalamus, arcuate neucleus, periventricular nucleus, and median eminence. In the hypothalamus, SST is also colocalized with SSTR1–4 receptors in a receptor-specific manner [25]. In rodents as well as in humans, the posterior hypothalamus appears to contribute also to the modulation of nociceptive pain.

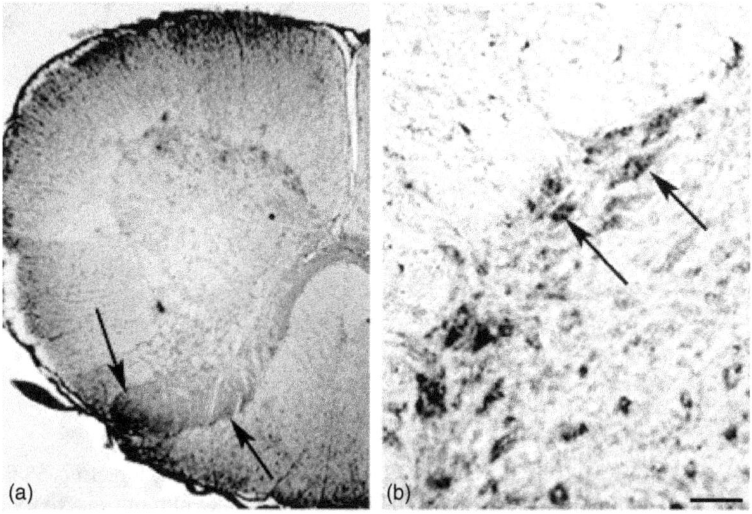

FIGURE 16.1. Photomicrographs illustrating somatostatin-like immunoreactivity in rat spinal cord are shown. The arrows indicate somatostatin-positive motor neurons in the ventral horn and somatostatin-positive immunoreactivity in the SG. SG, substantia gelatinosa. Scale bar = 50 μm (a) and 10 μm (b).

The peripheral and central distribution of SSTR subtypes is comparable to the distribution of SST. Of potential relevance to pain processing, SSTRs are found on the spinal cord dorsal root ganglion (DRG) that also express the transient receptor potential vanilloid 1 (TRPV1) receptor [31,32]. Motor neurons in the ventral horn of the spinal cord are positive for SSTR1–SSTR4 but do not express SSTR5 (Figure 16.2). In addition to certain brain regions and the spinal cord, SSTR subtypes are also found in the trigeminal sensory nucleus (Figure 16.3) in a receptor-specific manner [33,34]. In addition to

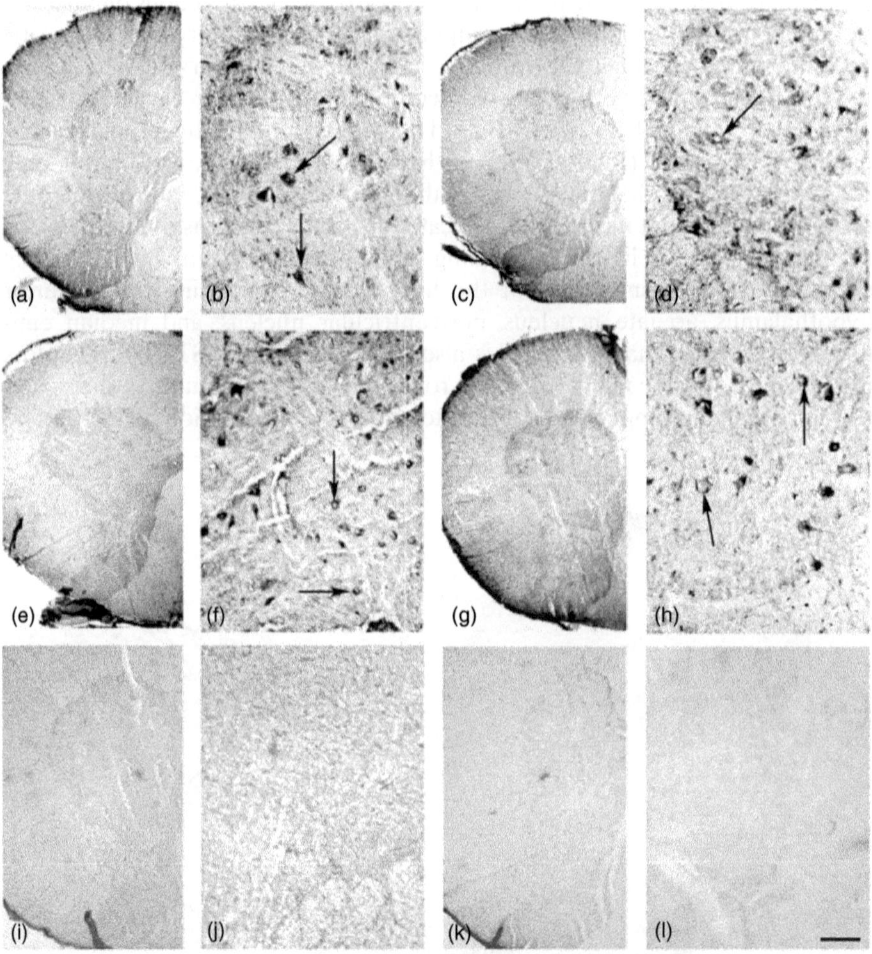

FIGURE 16.2. Low and high magnification photomicrographs depicting SSTR-like immunoreactivity in rat spinal cord are shown. SSTR1–4-like immunoreactivity is well expressed in motor neurons of the ventral horn (panels a–h). SSTR5-like immunoreactivity is virtually absent in the spinal cord (panels i and j). The arrows indicate neurons positive for SSTRs. Nonspecific staining in the absence of primary antibodies is shown (panels k and l). Scale bar = 50 μm.

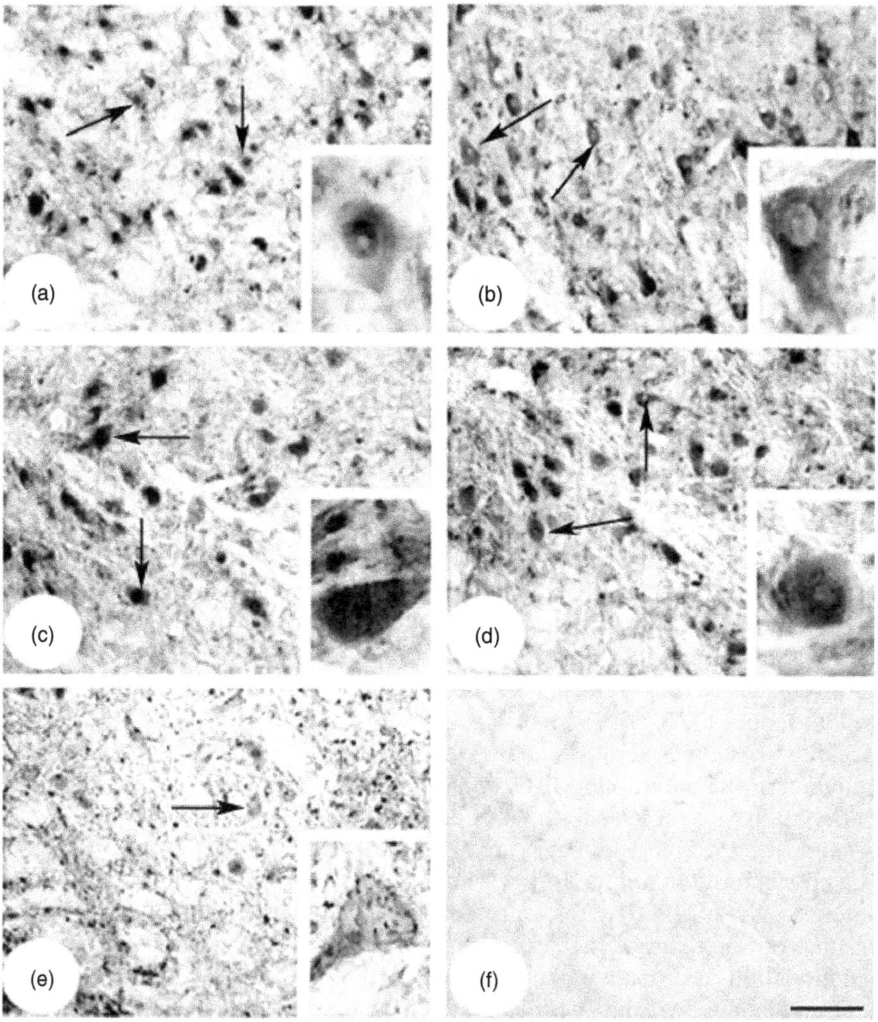

FIGURE 16.3. Photomicrographs illustrate somatostatin receptor-like immunoreactivity in the trigeminal nucleus of the rat brain stem (panels a–e). All five receptor subtypes are expressed in receptor-specific manner. The arrows indicate neurons positive for somatostatin receptors. High magnification photographs are shown in the inset for each receptor subtypes. Nonspecific staining in the absence of primary antibodies is shown (panel f). Scale bar = 10 μm.

SSTR protein expression, mRNA for all SSTR subtypes except SSTR5 have been shown [31,35]. Of the SSTRs, SSTR1 and SSTR4 are the most commonly identified receptors associated with the anti-inflammatory as well as analgesic effects of SST.

In addition to spinal cord and brainstem regions, SST and SSTRs are widely expressed in different parts of the human and rat brains. The regional localization is unique for each receptor subtype. SSTR1 and SSTR2 are highly enriched in the cortex, whereas in the hippocampus, SSTR2 and SSTR3 are predominantly expressed. In the striatum, SSTR1 is significantly expressed. The level of SSTR2 and SSTR3 expression is similar. SSTR4 along with neurons is also expressed in glial cells, predominantly in the striatum, hippocampus, and hypothalamus. In comparison, SSTR5 is sparsely distributed through out the striatum; the neuronal population expressing SSTR5 was many fold less than neuronal populations that express the other SSTRs. In the cortex, the striatum, and the hippocampus, SSTR-like immunoreactivity mainly occurs in perikarya, dendrites, and nerve fibers. Within rats, there have been no comparative studies showing the distribution of SSTR subtypes in the brain; however, the distributional patterns of individual SSTR subtypes have been shown in a regionally specific manner in human and rat brains [23,36–40].

16.4 PHARMACOLOGY OF SSTRs

The identification of high-affinity plasma membrane SSTRs was first described in 1978 using the rat pituitary GH_4C_1 cell line by whole-cell binding analysis [41]. Using the mRNA from human islets, the first two SSTRs were cloned and termed SSTR1 and SSTR2 [42]. The sequences of the remaining SSTRs were soon elucidated (SSTR3, SSTR4, and SSTR5) as identified in human and rodent tissues [3,43,44]. SSTRs range in size from 356 to 391 amino acid residues and have an overall sequence identity of 39–57%, whereas diversity is confined in the amino- and C-terminal segments [45]. Several putative phosphorylation recognition sites have been identified in the C-terminus and in the second and third intracellular loops (ILs) for protein kinase A, protein kinase C, and calmodulin kinase II for all human somatostatin receptors (hSSTRs). Interestingly, hSSTR3 is the only hSSTR that does not contain a cysteine residue downstream of the seventh transmembrane domain for purposes of palmitylation and hence membrane anchoring; however, it does possess an unusually long C-terminus, which may be a characteristic of its unique signaling properties [46]. Several postsynaptic density-95/disks large/ZO-1 (PDZ) interacting proteins have been discovered, specific to each of the five subtypes, presumably implicated in the chaperoning, scaffolding, and transport of SSTRs [47].

16.5 DEVELOPMENT OF SSTR LIGANDS

All five hSSTR subtypes bind SST-14 and SST-28 with nanomolar affinity; the exception is hSSTR5, which binds SST-28 with a 5- to 10-fold higher affinity than SST-14. The first U.S. Food and Drug Administration (FDA)-approved SST analogue, SMS 201-995 (octreotide, Sandostatin®), is an octapeptide. BIM 23014 (lanreotide) is another analogue of SST that has been more recently developed. Both lanreotide and octreotide exhibit high-affinity binding to SSTR2 and intermediate binding to SSTR3 and SSTR5. RC160 (vapreotide), an SST analogue with similar binding affinities to SSTR2, SSTR3, and SSTR5 like lanreotide and octreotide but with moderate affinity to SSTR4, was also introduced [45]. In an attempt to reduce size but to maintain metabolic stability, a cyclohexapeptide, MK-678 (seglitide), was developed and shows slightly higher affinity and selectivity for SSTR2 than for SSTR3 or SSTR5. The analogue Des-AA^{1,2,5}[D-Trp^{8} IAMP^{9}] SST (SCH-275) was reported to have high affinity for SSTR1 and moderate affinity for SSTR4 [3,48]. Recently, a highly potent and stable cyclohexapeptide, SOM230, designed by Novartis, has been demonstrated to have a high affinity for SSTR1, SSTR2, SSTR3, and SSTR5 [49,50]. SOM230 is effective in regulating pituitary control in rats, in dogs, and in monkeys and in human patients with acromegaly and Cushing's disease [49–52]. A breakthrough in SST agonist design came when the Merck Research Group constructed subtype-selective nonpeptide agonists through combinatorial chemistry [53]. Of the five nonpeptide agonists, three of the compounds, L-797,591, L-779,976, and L-803,087 display high selectivity and low nanomolar binding affinity for SSTR1, SSTR2, and SSTR4, respectively. The compound L-796,778 binds to SSTR3 with approximately 50-fold selectivity, while the SSTR5 subtype agonist, L-817,818, also displays selectivity for SSTR1.

There is some evidence that activation of SSTRs may prove to be efficacious in the treatment of inflammatory pain. The compound TT-232 is a high-affinity SSTR4 agonist that has anti-inflammatory, antiproliferative, as well as antinociceptive actions under certain experimental conditions, but lacks effects on endocrinological function. Surprisingly, TT-232 also has no effect on gastric hormone release or gastric secretion, which is one of the most characteristics features of SST. The antinociceptive/anti-inflammatory properties of TT-232 appear to be due to its action on capsaicin-sensitive sensory nerve endings to inhibit the release of proinflammatory neuropeptides such as substance P and calcitonin gene-related peptide (CGRP). It is theorized that SST released from activated capsaicin-sensitive fibers may function as a natural anti-inflammatory through the activation of SSTR4 [54–57]. Selective SSTR4 receptor-specific agonists reduce pain behavior and nociceptive activity induced by capsaicin administration, while blockade of SSTRs increases capsaicin-induced pain behavior and nociceptive activity, which suggest a modulatory role of SST in this pain model. These data strongly suggest that SSTR4 is a potential target in pain treatment or management.

The first SST peptide antagonist developed, CYN-154806, a cyclic octapeptide, displayed high affinity for SSTR2 but exhibited intermediate affinity for SSTR5 [58,59]. Unfortunately, follow-up studies demonstrated near full agonism at all SSTRs in a cyclic adenosine monophosphate (cAMP) accumulation assay [60]. In addition, other octapeptide antagonists, BIM 23056, BIM 23627, and BIM 23454, selected for their preferential binding to SSTR5 and SSTR2, respectively, showed partial affinities for the other SSTR subtypes to various degrees [61]. The first high-affinity nonpeptide antagonist was designed for SSTR3 and has a greater than 1000-fold selectivity for this receptor [62]. An SSTR1 nonpeptide antagonist, SRA880, was recently characterized *in vitro* to have modest selectivity of up to 100-fold [63]. The use of these receptor-specific antagonists for pain relief has not been reported.

16.6 SSTR SIGNALING

The signal transduction pathway of SSTRs is rather complex; however, for the most part, it begins by activation of G proteins. Binding of SSTRs by SST ligands modulates the activity of several key enzymes, including adenylate cyclase, phosphotyrosine phosphatases (PTPases) and mitogen-activated protein kinase (MAPK) along with changes in intracellular levels of calcium and potassium ions, as typified by activation of calcium and potassium channels, including the regulation of the sodium/proton antiporter. [3,64–67]. The type of signal that prevails is dependent on several factors such as the SSTR subtype(s) expressed, signaling elements, SSTR internalization, desensitization, and/or receptor cross talk.

The ability of SST to block regulated secretion from various cell types is typified in part by its effects on the synthesis and release of two important mediators, cAMP and calcium, respectively. Adenylate cyclase was the first effector enzyme to be identified as regulated by SSTRs [68]. All five SSTR subtypes are negatively coupled to this enzyme through activation of a pertussis toxin (PTX)-sensitive $G\alpha_i$ proteins, a property observed in various cell types [69]. In an attempt to elucidate the most relevant G protein subtypes involved in SSTR-mediated inhibition of adenylate cyclase, the subtypes $G\alpha_{i1}$, $G\alpha_{i2}$, and $G\alpha_{i3}$ were identified, as determined by targeted disruption using either antiserum or G protein antisense plasmids [70–72]. SSTRs are coupled to several types of potassium channels that include the delayed rectifier, inward rectifier, ATP-sensitive potassium channels, and large-conductance calcium-activated BK channels [73]. The G protein subtype $G\alpha_{i3}$ and possibly its $\beta\gamma$ dimer are implicated in potassium channel regulation [74]. SSTRs have also been shown to directly modulate high-voltage-dependent calcium channels via $G\alpha_{o2}$ [75,76]. SSTRs may also inhibit calcium currents by activation of cyclic guanosine monophosphate (cGMP) protein kinase, through the induction of cGMP to regulate channel phosphorylation [77]. Aside from regulating channels to control ion flux, SSTRs have also been shown to couple to Na^+/H^+ exchangers (NHEs) [78–80] to modulate such features as cell adhesion, migration, and proliferation [81]. SSTR1 was the first subtype shown to specifically regulate NHE-1, decreasing the extracellular acidification rate (ECAR) when transfected in either fibroblast LTK- or HEK-293 cells [82]. It was later determined that SSTR3 and SSTR4 also contribute to this effect, but not SSTR2 and SSTR5 [78].

SSTRs activate a number of phosphatases that have been implicated in cell growth [65–67,83]. For instance, the SH2 domain containing tyrosine phosphatases SHP-1 and SHP-2, which play a role in cell growth and differentiation, is known to be recruited by various SSTR subtypes. Both phosphatases are rapidly recruited to the membrane of breast cancer cells upon stimulation with SST [84]. More specifically, SHP-1 has been demonstrated to coprecipitate with SSTR2 in a constitutive manner, suggesting its importance in the formation of signaling complexes [85,86]. Furthermore, the activation of SHP-1 was shown to be highly dependent on the recruitment of SHP-2 through phosphorylation of tyrosine residues present at the C-terminal portion of the receptor, implying the importance of both phosphatases in SSTR signaling [87]. In addition to tyrosine phosphatases, the activation of serine/threonine phosphatases has also been demonstrated to be recruited by SSTRs. Modulation of N- and L-type calcium and potassium channels has been shown to be dependent on the activation of phosphatase 2A (PP2A) and calcineurin (PP2B) in several cell types such as sympathetic neurons, pancreatic alpha cells, and pituitary tumor cells. Evidence on the importance of PP2B recruitment by SSTR activation comes from studies on the regulation of neurotransmitter release and exocytosis in sympathetic neurons and in pancreatic alpha cells, respectively [88].

One important recently identified SSTR signaling pathway involves MAPKs [45,52,65,66,83,89]. SSTR-mediated activation [90,91] or inhibition [92–96] of MAPKs has been demonstrated to be mediated by PTPases. For example, the activation of SSTR5 inhibits MAPKs by the activation of a cGMP-dependent pathway when expressed in CHO-K1 cells [97]. In addition to PTPases, recruitment of phosphoinositide-3 kinase has also been shown as fundamental in the activation of MAPKs in a receptor- and species-specific manner [91,98,99].

16.7 SST AND PAIN TREATMENT

Potential clinical uses of SST in the treatment of pain are emerging. An SST-mediated analgesic effect has been demonstrated in animal as well as in human studies. SST and its analogues have been used successfully for pain management specifically in cases where opioids have failed. SST treatment has been proven highly effective, for instance, in the case of pituitary tumor as well as in proliferative pain [100]. SST analogues display analgesic properties, such as relief of headache, and morphine-sparing effects on postoperative and neoplastic pain. SST or analogues, for example, OCT, when applied to the spinal cord, also block pain in cancer patients [101,102]. SST or octreotide (OCT) administration by any route exerts an antagonistic effect in many other pain conditions, such as bone pain, rheumatoid pain, migraine, visceral pain, as well as intractable nonmalignant pain [103]. This broad spectrum of analgesia has been observed even in certain pain conditions where opioid receptor agonists have been ineffective, suggesting that SST could be used to modulate pain. However, the potential use of spinally administered SST in the management of pain is limited because of concentration-dependent damage to the spinal cord, which includes nucleolysis of the dorsal horn, pyknotic neurons, inflammation, and focal demyelination upon intrathecal administration [103–105]. Importantly, these side effects occurring upon epidural or intrathecal administration have not been seen once SSTR is administered peripherally [103]. Additionally, the rapid degradation of SST itself is one of the most problematic limits to its clinical use. These problems have limited the use of SST to the treatment of severe intractable pain.

Part of the analgesic effect of SST is mediated through a peripheral mechanism that appears to be due to an action of this peptide on peripheral nociceptors. SST, when applied locally, is devoid of any side effects, which are frequently seen in case of systemic administration or intrathecal administration of this agent. In addition, a few studies have also shown that nociceptive behavior is enhanced in control or in a formalin-administered animal upon local administration of SST antagonists or SST antibodies in rats [103]. This suggests that peripherally administered SST may offer a potential advantage when therapeutic benefits versus potential adverse effects of this agent are compared. Most importantly, SST or its analogues have been shown to produce an analgesic effect when applied locally.

The mechanism whereby SST modulates pain appears to involve both central and peripheral actions. An inhibitory action of SST on nociceptive neurons in spinal cord has also been suggested [106]. As far as a peripheral mechanism, one hypothesis is that SST enhances opioid peptide release from immune cells during the inflammatory process. Intravenous, but not epidural injection of SST produces analgesia that can be blocked by the opioid receptor antagonist naloxone [106]. As discussed in Chapter 13, opioids can act peripherally to mediate analgesia. Immune cells have also been shown to produce or to release SST under inflammatory and several other pathophysiological conditions. Further evidence to support the concept that SST functions as an anti-inflammatory and antinociceptive agent is manifested by its role on the sensory afferent nerve terminals and the inhibition of neurotransmitter release [107,108]. Although the exact molecular mechanism involving SST and SSTR subtypes in pain relief is not well understood yet, it has been shown that SST acts on DRG neurons to decrease Ca^{2+} channel conductance [45,65,109]. As previously reported, Ca^{2+} channel inactivation might potentially interfere with the release of some excitatory peptides [65]. SST is also known to block forskolin-stimulated arachidonic acid release via inhibiting cAMP and activating K conductance that also support the role of SSTR to Ca^{2+} channel inactivation [45]. These observations suggest that inactivation of Ca^{2+} channels by SST might play an important role in decreasing nociceptor response to noscious mechanical and thermal stimulation.

16.8 SST, INFLAMMATION, AND PAIN

Inflammation is often an important component of pathological pain. Cytokines, which serve in an autocrine, paracrine, as well as endocrine manner, are intimately associated with the initiation of inflammatory pain. In the central nervous system, induction of SST gene expression in response to tissue damage is mediated in large part through the release of cytokines from glial cells, which stimulate SST secretion and steady-state mRNA accumulation [3]. Microglia and astrocytes produce a number of cytokines in response to many different forms of neuronal injuries [26]. In cultured neuronal cells, some of the inflammatory cytokines stimulate the release of SST [110]. Chief among these are the inflammatory cytokines interleukin (IL)-1, tumor necrosis factor (TNF)-α, and IL-6. There is now considerable evidence that these inflammatory cytokines as well as other members of the growth factor–cytokine family, for example, growth hormone and insulin growth factor 1, are potent inducers of neuronal SST secretion and synthesis [110–114]. IL-1, TNF-α, and IL-6 have been shown to stimulate SST gene expression and peptide secretion from cultured rat brain cells [110,111]. The IL-1 effect is seen with doses as low as 10^{-11} M and is dose dependent up to a maximally effective dose of 10^{-9} M. TNF-α has a slightly lower potency but shows synergism with IL-1 [111]. Basic fibroblast growth factor, which shares sequence homology with IL-1, also augments SST function [113]. Finally, IL-6 has been shown to be trophic for SST neurons [111]. The immediate postreceptor events linking the inflammatory cytokines to gene activation are unclear but appear to involve MAPK and α-casein kinase [115].

It is presently unknown whether SST-positive neurons express receptors for IL-1, TNF-α, and IL-6. Most importantly, the presence of SST in immune cells, such as macrophages, supports the idea that SST may play a critical role in modulating inflammation. For example, OCT attenuates the release of inflammatory mediators from isolated guinea pig bladder and also provides significant symptomatic improvement in patients suffering from refractory rheumatoid arthritis (RA) [116,117]. The clinical manifestation of inflammatory pain is associated with increased response to mechanical stimulation, which is further increased by leukocyte migration to the inflamed tissue. Additional support to connect SST with inflammation and pain has emerged from studies on glial cell line-derived neurotrophic factor (GDNF). Exogenous GDNF exerts anti-inflammatory as well as antihyperanalgesic effects in animals, and these effects of GDNF are blocked by the SST antagonist cyclo-somatostatin (c-SOM) [118]. Most importantly, in the absence of SST, there is no anti-inflammatory role of GDNF, whereas GDNF exerts an anti-inflammatory effect by inducing SST release from nerve fibers that are also positive for GDNF receptors [118].

SST also inhibits neurogenic inflammation. As mentioned above, it is believed that SST is released from capsaicin-sensitive primary sensory neurons and inhibits the release of proinflammatory peptides such as substance P and CGRP. During neurogenic inflammation, SST release is coincident with the release of substance P and CGRP, and it is possible that the relative level of SST to proinflammatory peptides determines the magnitude of pain and edema during inflammation [34]. SST has also been reported to function as an antagonist to SP, and this effect is associated to modulate neurogenic inflammation and pain perception as well [119]. Further, the use of OCT for endocrine treatment symptomatically might suggest that it is possible to use it as a local treatment for inflammatory pain [117,120].

16.9 ROLE OF SST IN THE TREATMENT OF RA

RA is a chronic autoimmune disease and is characterized by the presence of synovitis [117]. RA is accompanied by inflammation in joint tissue due to the production of cytokines. In RA, gradual destruction of the joint is frequently seen, which is mainly attributed to angiogenesis. The administration of SST and SSTR agonists into the knee joint improves the pain of RA [121,122]. In RA patients, the presence of SSTR subtypes has also been reported in lymphocytes, in macrophages, as well as in synovial tissues [123–126]. SSTR4 seems to be a potential target in the development of new drugs. For example, the SSTR4-selective agonist TT-232 has been shown to block neurogenic inflammation and to protect against cartilage and bone destruction normally observed with Freud's adjuvant induced model of RA. Furthermore, the analgesic effect of another SSTR4-specific agonist, J-2156, has been shown in acute and chronic models of pain in mice [57]. The recently discovered neuropeptide cortistatin, a relative of SST, has many pharmacological and functional properties similar to SST, although it also has some distinct properties. Like SST, cortistatin has been shown to be beneficial in the treatment of arthritis because it reduces the severity of collagen-induced arthritis secondary to a downregulation of inflammation in a mouse model of RA [127].

16.10 CONCLUSION

At this stage, there is no doubt that SSTR subtypes can be used as a potential target for the development of novel anti-inflammatory drugs. In certain pain conditions such as joint pain and certain cancer pains, SST has some clinical usefulness; however, the molecular mechanism underlying the analgesic effect of this peptide is still unknown. Peripheral administration rather than central administration of SST and its analogues may decrease untoward side effects that occur with systemic administration of SST for pain treatment. Most importantly, the activation of specific SSTR subtypes might play an important role not only to suppress inflammatory pain but also to decrease side effects normally seen with other analgesic drugs. One important approach for delineating the biological response and the clinical implication of individual SSTR subtypes in pain processing will be the use SSTR gene knockout mice. Certain precautions are warranted in the interpretation of data from these knockout mice because SSTR subtypes functionally interact with each other as well as with other GPCRs as heterodimers, and compensatory mechanism in the lack of one subtype might play an important role.

ACKNOWLEDGMENT

This work was supported by grants from the Canadian Institute for Health Research (MOP-6196 and MOP-74465). UK is a senior scholar of the Michael Smith Foundation for Health Research.

REFERENCES

1. Brazeau, P., Vale, W., Burgus, R., Ling, N., Butcher, M., Rivier, J., Guillemin, R. (1973). Hypothalamic polypeptide that inhibits the secretion of immunoreactive pituitary growth hormone. *Science* 179:77–79.
2. Lamberts, S.W., van der Lely, A.J., de Herder, W.W., Hofland, L.J. (1996). Somatostatin analogs: future directions. *Metabolism* 45:104–106.
3. Patel, Y.C. (1997). Molecular pharmacology of somatostatin receptor subtypes. *J Endocrinol Invest* 20:348–367.
4. Epelbaum, J., Tapia Arancibia, L., Kordon, C., Enjalbert, A. (1982). Characterization, regional distribution, and subcellular distribution of 125I-Tyr1-somatostatin binding sites in rat brain. *J Neurochem* 38:1515–1523.
5. Tran, V.T., Uhl, G.R., Perry, D.C., Manning, D.C., Vale, W.W., Perrin, M.H., Rivier, J.E., Martin, J.B., Snyder, S.H. (1984). Autoradiographic localization of somatostatin receptors in rat brain. *Eur J Pharmacol* 101:307–309.
6. Leroux, P., Quirion, R., Pelletier, G. (1985). Localization and characterization of brain somatostatin receptors as studied with somatostatin-14 and somatostatin-28 receptor radioautography. *Brain Res* 347:74–84.
7. Reubi, J.C., Maurer, R. (1985). Autoradiographic mapping of somatostatin receptors in the rat central nervous system and pituitary. *Neuroscience* 15:1183–1193.
8. Uhl, G.R., Tran, V., Snyder, S.H., Martin, J.B. (1985). Somatostatin receptors: distribution in rat central nervous system and human frontal cortex. *J Comp Neurol* 240:288–304.
9. Raynor, K., Reisine, T. (1989). Analogs of somatostatin selectively label distinct subtypes of somatostatin receptors in rat brain. *J Pharmacol Exp Ther* 251: 510–517.
10. Krantic, S., Martel, J.C., Weissmann, D., Pujol, J.F., Quirion, R. (1990). Quantitative radioautographic study of somatostatin receptors heterogeneity in the rat extrahypothalamic brain. *Neuroscience* 39:127–137.
11. Martin, J.L., Chesselet, M.F., Raynor, K., Gonzales, C., Reisine, T. (1991). Differential distribution of somatostatin receptor subtypes in rat brain revealed by newly developed somatostatin analogs. *Neuroscience* 41:581–593.
12. Dournaud, P., Boudin, H., Schonbrunn, A., Tannenbaum, G.S., Beaudet, A. (1998). Interrelationships between somatostatin sst2A receptors and somatostatin-containing axons in rat brain: evidence for regulation of cell surface receptors by endogenous somatostatin. *J Neurosci* 18(3):1056–1071.
13. Schindler, M., Sellers, L.A., Humphrey, P.P., Emson, P.C. (1997). Immunohistochemical localization of the somatostatin SST2(A) receptor in the rat brain and spinal cord. *Neuroscience* 76:225–240.

14. Helboe, L., Stidsen, C.E., Moller, M. (1998). Immunohistochemical and cytochemical localization of the somatostatin receptor subtype sst1 in the somatostatinergic parvocellular neuronal system of the rat hypothalamus. *J Neurosci* 18: 4938–4945.

15. Hervieu, G., Emson, P.C. (1998). The localization of somatostatin receptor 1 (sst1) immunoreactivity in the rat brain using an N-terminal specific antibody. *Neuroscience* 85:1263–1284.

16. Handel, M., Schulz, S., Stanarius, A., Schreff, M., Erdtmann-Vourliotis, M., Schmidt, H., Wolf, G., Hollt, V. (1999). Selective targeting of somatostatin receptor 3 to neuronal cilia. *Neuroscience* 89:909–926.

17. Helboe, L., Hay-Schmidt, A., Stidsen, C.E., Moller, M. (1999). Immunohistochemical localization of the somatostatin receptor subtype 2 (sst2). in the central nervous system of the golden hamster (*Mesocricetus auratus*). *J Comp Neurol* 405:247–261.

18. Schindler, M., Humphrey, P.P., Lohrke, S., Friauf, E. (1999). Immunohistochemical localization of the somatostatin sst2 (b) receptor splice variant in the rat central nervous system. *Neuroscience* 90:859–874.

19. Stroh, T., Kreienkamp, H.J., Beaudet, A. (1999). Immunohistochemical distribution of the somatostatin receptor subtype 5 in the adult rat brain: predominant expression in the basal forebrain. *J Comp Neurol* 412:69–82.

20. Selmer, I.S., Schindler, M., Humphrey, P.P., Emson, P.C. (2000). Immunohistochemical localization of the somatostatin sst(4) receptor in rat brain. *Neuroscience* 98:523–533.

21. Schreff, M., Schulz, S., Handel, M., Keilhoff, G., Braun, H., Pereira, G., Klutzny, M., Schmidt, H., Wolf, G., Hollt, V. (2000). Distribution, targeting, and internalization of the sst4 somatostatin receptor in rat brain. *J Neurosci* 20:3785–3797.

22. Schulz, S., Handel, M., Schreff, M., Schmidt, H., Hollt, V. (2000). Localization of five somatostatin receptors in the rat central nervous system using subtype-specific antibodies. *J Physiol (Paris)* 94:259–264.

23. Kumar, U. (2005). Expression of somatostatin receptor subtypes (SSTR1-5) in Alzheimer's disease brain: an immunohistochemical analysis. *Neuroscience* 134: 525–538.

24. Stroh, T., Sarret, P., Tannenbaum, G.S., Beaudet, A. (2006). Immunohistochemical distribution and subcellular localization of the somatostatin receptor subtype 1 (sst1) in the rat hypothalamus. *Neurochem Res* 31:247–257.

25. Kumar, U. (2007). Colocalization of somatostatin receptor subtypes (SSTR1-5) with somatostatin, NADPH-diaphorase (NADPH-d), and tyrosine hydroxylase in the rat hypothalamus. *J Comp Neurol* 504:185–205.

26. Patel, Y.C., Srikant, C.B. (1997). Somatostatin receptors. *Trends Endocrinol Metab* 8:398–405.

27. Mouchantaf, R., Kumar, U., Sulea, T., Patel, Y.C. (2001). A conserved ?-helix at the amino terminal segment of prosomatostatin serves as a sorting signal for the regulated secretory pathway. *J Biol Chem* 276:26308–26316.

28. Patel, Y.C., Galanopoulou, A.S., Rabbani, S.N., Liu, J.L., Ravazzola, M., Amherdt, M. (1997). Somatostatin-14, somatostatin-28, and prosomatostatin[1-10] are independently and efficiently processed from prosomatostatin in the constitutive

secretory pathway in islet somatostatin tumor cells (1027B2). *Mol Cell Endocrinol* 131:183–194.

29. Mouchantaf, R., Watt, H.L., Suela, T., Seidah, N.G., Alturaihi, H., Patel, Y.C., Kumar, U. (2004). Prosomatostatin is proteolytically processed at the amino terminal segment by subtilase SKI-1. *Regul Pept* 120:133–140.
30. Elekes, K., Helyes, Z., Kereskai, L., Sandor, K., Pinter, E., Pozsgai, G., Tekus, V., Banvolgyi, A., Nemeth, J., Szuts, T., Keri, G., Szolcsanyi, J. (2008). Inhibitory effects of synthetic somatostatin receptor subtype 4 agonists on acute and chronic airway inflammation and hyperreactivity in the mouse. *Eur J Pharmacol* 578:313–322.
31. Bar, K.J., Schurigt, U., Scholze, A., Segond Von Banchet, G., Stopfel, N., Brauer, R., Halbhuber, K.J., Schaible, H.G. (2004). The expression and localization of somatostatin receptors in dorsal root ganglion neurons of normal and monoarthritic rats. *Neuroscience* 127:197–206.
32. Carlton, S.M., Zhou, S., Du, J., Hargett, G.L., Ji, G., Coggeshall, R.E. (2004). Somatostatin modulates the transient receptor potential vanilloid 1 (TRPV1) ion channel. *Pain* 110:616–627.
33. Hokfelt, T., Elde, R., Johansson, O., Luft, R., Nilsson, G., Arimura, A. (1976). Immunohistochemical evidence for separate populations of somatostatin-containing and substance P-containing primary afferent neurons in the rat. *Neuroscience* 1:131–136.
34. Tessler, A., Himes, B.T., Gruber-Bollinger, J., Reichlin, S. (1986). Characterization of forms of immunoreactive somatostatin in sensory neuron and normal and deafferented spinal cord. *Brain Res* 370:232–240.
35. Pan, H.L., Wu, Z.Z., Zhou, H.Y., Chen, S.R., Zhang, H.M., Li, D.P. (2008). Modulation of pain transmission by G-protein-coupled receptors. *Pharmacol Ther* 117:141–161.
36. Dournaud, P., Gum, Y.Z., Schonbrunn, A., Mazella, J., Tannenbaum, G.S., Beaudet, A. (1996). Localization of the somatostatin receptor SST2A in rat brain using a specific anti-peptide antibody. *J Neurosci* 16(14):4468–4478.
37. Hervieu, G., Emson, P.C. (1998). The localization of somatostatin receptor 1 (sst1) immunoreactivity in the rat brain using an N-terminal specific antibody. *Neuroscience* 85:1263–1284.
38. Hervieu, G., Emson, P.C. (1999). Visualisation of somatostatin receptor sst(3) in the rat central nervous system. *Brain Res Mol Brain Res* 71(2):290–303.
39. Selmer, I.S., Schindler, M., Humphrey, P.P., Emson, P.C. (2000). Immunohistochemical localization of the somatostatin sst(4) receptor in rat brain. *Neuroscience* 98(3):523–233.
40. Stroh, T., Kreienkamp, H.J., Beaudet, A. (1999). Immunohistochemical distribution of the somatostatin receptor subtype 5 in the adult rat brain: predominant expression in the basal forebrain. *J Comp Neurol* 412(1):69–82.
41. Schonbrunn, A., Tashjian, H., Jr. (1978). Characterization of functional receptors for somatostatin in rat pituitary cells in culture. *J Biol Chem* 253:6473–6483.
42. Yamada, Y., Post, S.R., Wang, K., Tager, H.S., Bell, G.I., Seino, S. (1992). Cloning and functional characterization of a family of human and mouse somatostatin receptors expressed in brain, gastrointestinal tract, and kidney. *Proc Natl Acad Sci U S A* 89:251–255.

43. Patel, Y.C., Greenwood, M.T., Panetta, R., Demchyshyn, L., Niznik, H. Srikant, C.B. (1995). The somatostatin receptor family. *Life Sci* 57:1249–1265.

44. Patel, Y.C., Greenwood, M., Panetta, R., Hukovic, N., Grigorakis, S., Robertson, L.A., Srikant, C.B. (1996). Molecular biology of somatostatin receptor subtypes. *Metabolism* 45:31–38.

45. Patel, Y.C. (1999). Somatostatin and its receptor family. *Front Neuroendocrinol* 20:157–198.

46. Sharma, K., Patel, Y.C., Srikant, C.B. (1999). C-terminal region of human somatostatin receptor 5 is required for induction of Rb and G1 cell cycle arrest. *Mol Endocrinol* 13:82–90.

47. Kreienkamp, H.J., Liew, C.W., Bachner, D., Mameza, M.G., Soltau, M., Quitsch, A., Christenn, M., Wente, W., Richter, D. (2004). Physiology of somatostatin receptors: From genetics to molecular analysis. In: Srikant, C.B. (ed.)., *Somatostatin*. Norwell, MA: Kluwer Academic Publishers, pp. 185–202.

48. Liapakis, G., Hoeger, C., Rivier, J., Reisine, T. (1996). Development of a selective agonist at the somatostatin receptor subtype sstr1. *J Pharmacol Exp Ther* 276: 1089–1094.

49. Bruns, C., Lewis, I., Briner, U., Meno-Tetang, G., Weckbecker, G. (2002). SOM230: a novel somatostatin peptidomimetic with broad somatotropin release inhibiting factor (SRIF) receptor binding and a unique antisecretory profile. *Eur J Endocrinol* 146:707–716.

50. Weckbecker, G., Briner, U., Lewis, I., Bruns, C. (2002). SOM230: a new somatostatin peptidomimetic with potent inhibitory effects on the growth hormone/insulin-like growth factor-I axis in rats, primates, and dogs. *Endocrinology* 143: 4123–4130.

51. Labeur, M., Theodoropoulou, M., Sievers, C., Paez-Pereda, M., Castillo, V., Arzt, E., Stalla, G.K. (2006). New aspects in the diagnosis and treatment of Cushing disease. *Front Horm Res* 35:169–178.

52. Weckbecker, G., Lewis, I., Albert, R., Schmid, H.A., Hoyer, D., Bruns, C. (2003). Opportunities in somatostatin research: biological, chemical and therapeutic aspects. *Nat Rev Drug Discov* 2:999–1017.

53. Rohrer, S.P., Birzin, E.T., Mosley, R.T., Berk, S.C., Hutchins, S.M., Shen, D.M., Xiong, Y., Hayes, E.C., Parmar, R.M., Foor, F., Mitra, S.W., Degrado, S.J., Shu, M., Klopp, J.M., Cai, S.J., Blake, A., Chan, W.W., Pasternak, A., Yang, L., Patchett, A.A., Smith, R.G., Chapman, K.T., Schaeffer, J.M. (1998). Rapid identification of subtype-selective agonists of the somatostatin receptor through combinatorial chemistry. *Science* 282:737–740.

54. Helyes, Z., Szabo, A., Nemeth, J., Jakab, B., Pinter, E., Banvolgyi, A., Kereskai, L., Keri, G., Szolcsanyi, J. (2004). Antiinflammatory and analgesic effects of somatostatin released from capsaicin-sensitive sensory nerve terminals in a Freund's adjuvant-induced chronic arthritis model in the rat. *Arthritis Rheum* 50: 1677–1685.

55. Than, M., Nemeth, J., Szilvassy, Z., Pinter, E., Helyes, Z., Szolcsanyi, J. (2000). Systemic anti-inflammatory effect of somatostatin released from capsaicin-sensitive vagal and sciatic sensory fibres of the rat and guinea-pig. *Eur J Pharmacol* 399:251–258.

56. Szolcsanyi, J., Bolcskei, K., Szabo, A., Pinter, E., Petho, G., Elekes, K., Borzsei, R., Almasi, R., Szuts, T., Keri, G., Helyes, Z. (2004). Analgesic effect of TT-232, a heptapeptide somatostatin analogue, in acute pain models of the rat and the mouse and in streptozotocin-induced diabetic mechanical allodynia. *Eur J Pharmacol* 498:103–109.

57. Sándor, K., Elekes, K., Szabó, A., Pintér, E., Engström, M., Wurster, S., Szolcsányi, J., Helyes Z. (2006). Analgesic effects of the somatostatin sst4 receptor selective agonist J-2156 in acute and chronic pain models. *Eur J Pharmacol* 539(1-2): 71–75.

58. Bass, R.T., Buckwalter, B.L., Patel, B.P., Pausch, M.H., Price, L.A., Strnad, J., Hadcock, J.R. (1996). Identification and characterization of novel somatostatin antagonists. *Mol Pharmacol* 50:709–715.

59. Feniuk, W., Jarvie, E., Luo, J., Humphrey, P.P. (2000). Selective somatostatin sst(2) receptor blockade with the novel cyclic octapeptide, CYN-154806. *Neuropharmacology* 39:1443–1450.

60. Nunn, C., Langenegger, D., Hurth, K., Schmidt, K., Fehlmann, D., Hoyer, D. (2003). Agonist properties of putative small-molecule somatostatin sst2 receptor-selective antagonists. *Eur J Pharmacol* 465:211–218.

61. Tulipano, G., Soldi, D., Bagnasco, M., Culler, M.D., Taylor, J.E., Cocchi, D., Giustina, A. (2002). Characterization of new selective somatostatin receptor subtype-2 (sst2) antagonists, BIM-23627 and BIM-23454. Effects of BIM-23627 on GH release in anesthetized male rats after short-term high-dose dexamethasone treatment. *Endocrinology* 143:1218–1224.

62. Poitout, L., Roubert, P., Contour-Galcera, M.O., Moinet, C., Lannoy, J., Pommier, J., Plas, P., Bigg, D., Thurieau, C. (2001). Identification of potent non-peptide somatostatin antagonists with sst(3) selectivity. *J Med Chem* 44:2990–3000.

63. Hoyer, D., Nunn, C., Hannon, J., Schoeffter, P., Feuerbach, D., Schuepbach, E., Langenegger, D., Bouhelal, R., Hurth, K., Neumann, P., Troxler, T., Pfaeffli, P. (2004). SRA880, in vitro characterization of the first non-peptide somatostatin sst(1) receptor antagonist. *Neurosci Lett* 361:132–135.

64. Barnett, P. (2003). Somatostatin and somatostatin receptor physiology. *Endocrine* 20:255–264.

65. Moller, L.N., Stidsen, C.E., Hartmann, B., Holst, J.J. (2003). Somatostatin receptors. *Biochim Biophys Acta* 1616:1–84.

66. Olias, G., Viollet, C., Kusserow, H., Epelbaum, J., Meyerhof, W. (2004). Regulation and function of somatostatin receptors. *J Neurochem* 89:1057–1091.

67. Patel, Y.C., Liu, J.L., Galanopoulou, A.S., Papachristou, D.N. (1999). Production, action, and degradation of somatostatin. In: Jefferson, L.S., Cherrington, A.D. (eds.). *The Handbook of Physiology, The Endocrine Pancreas and Regulation of Metabolism.* New York: Oxford University Press, pp. 267–302.

68. Patel, Y.C., Greenwood, M.T., Warszynska, A., Panetta, R., Srikant, C.B. (1994). All five cloned human somatostatin receptors (hSSTR1-5) are functionally coupled to adenylyl cyclase. *Biochem Biophys Res Commun* 198:605–612.

69. Meyerhof, W. (1998). The elucidation of somatostatin receptor functions: a current view. *Rev Physiol Biochem Pharmacol* 133:55–108.

70. Gu, Y.Z., Schonbrunn, A. (1997). Coupling specificity between somatostatin receptor sst2A and G proteins: isolation of the receptor-G protein complex with a receptor antibody. *Mol Endocrinol* 11:527–537.
71. Liu, Y.F., Jakobs, K.H., Rasenick, M.M., Albert, P.R. (1994). G protein specificity in receptor-effector coupling. Analysis of the roles of G0 and Gi2 in GH4C1 pituitary cells. *J Biol Chem* 269:13880–13886.
72. Tallent, M., Reisine, T. (1992). Gi alpha 1 selectively couples somatostatin receptors to adenylyl cyclase in pituitary-derived AtT-20 cells. *Mol Pharmacol* 41: 452–455.
73. Akopian, A., Johnson, J., Gabriel, R., Brecha, N., Witkovsky, P. (2000). Somatostatin modulates voltage-gated K(+) and Ca(2+) currents in rod and cone photoreceptors of the salamander retina. *J Neurosci* 20:929–936.
74. Takano, K., Yasufuku-Takano, J., Teramoto, A., Fujita, T. (1997). Gi3 mediates somatostatin-induced activation of an inwardly rectifying K^+ current in human growth hormone-secreting adenoma cells. *Endocrinology* 138:2405–2409.
75. Ikeda, S.R., Schofield, G.G. (1989). Somatostatin blocks a calcium current in rat sympathetic ganglion neurones. *J Physiol* 409:221–240.
76. Kleuss, C., Hescheler, J., Ewel, C., Rosenthal, W., Schultz, G., Wittig, B. (1991). Assignment of G-protein subtypes to specific receptors inducing inhibition of calcium currents. *Nature* 353:43–48.
77. Meriney, S.D., Gray, D.B., Pilar, G.R. (1994). Somatostatin-induced inhibition of neuronal Ca^{2+} current modulated by cGMP-dependent protein kinase. *Nature* 369:336–339.
78. Lin, C.Y., Varma, M.G., Joubel, A., Madabushi, S., Lichtarge, O., Barber, D.L. (2003). Conserved motifs in somatostatin, D2-dopamine, and alpha 2B-adrenergic receptors for inhibiting the Na-H exchanger, NHE1. *J Biol Chem* 278:15128–15135.
79. Smalley, K.S., Feniuk, W., Humphrey, P.P. (1998). Differential agonist activity of somatostatin and L-362855 at human recombinant sst4 receptors. *Br J Pharmacol* 125:833–841.
80. Ye, W.Z., Mathieu, S., Marteau, C. (1999). Somatostatin inhibits the Na^+/H^+ exchange activity of rat hepatocytes in short term primary culture. *Cell Mol Biol (Noisy-le-grand)* 45:1183–1189.
81. Putney, L.K., Denker, S.P., Barber, D.L. (2002). The changing face of the Na^+/H^+ exchanger, NHE1: structure, regulation, and cellular actions. *Annu Rev Pharmacol Toxicol* 42:527–552.
82. Hou, C., Gilbert, R.L., Barber, D.L. (1994). Subtype-specific signaling mechanisms of somatostatin receptors SSTR1 and SSTR2. *J Biol Chem* 269:10357–10362.
83. Csaba, Z., Dournaud, P. (2001a). Cellular biology of somatostatin receptors. *Neuropeptides* 35:1–23.
84. Srikant, C.B., Shen, S.H. (1996). Octapeptide somatostatin analog SMS 201-995 induces translocation of intracellular PTP1C to membranes in MCF-7 human breast adenocarcinoma cells. *Endocrinology* 137:3461–3468.
85. Hortala, M., Ferjoux, G., Estival, A., Bertrand, C., Schulz, S., Pradayrol, L., Susini, C., Clemente, F. (2003). Inhibitory role of the somatostatin receptor SST2 on the intracrine-regulated cell proliferation induced by the 210-amino acid fibroblast growth factor-2 isoform: implication of JAK2. *J Biol Chem* 278:20574–20581.

86. Lopez, F., Esteve, J.P., Buscail, L., Delesque, N., Saint-Laurent, N., Theveniau, M., Nahmias, C., Vaysse, N., Susini, C. (1997). The tyrosine phosphatase SHP-1 associates with the sst2 somatostatin receptor and is an essential component of sst2-mediated inhibitory growth signaling. *J Biol Chem* 272:24448–24454.

87. Ferjoux, G., Lopez, F., Esteve, J.P., Ferrand, A., Vivier, E., Vely, F., Saint-Laurent, N., Pradayrol, L., Buscail, L., Susini, C. (2003). Critical role of Src and SHP-2 in sst2 somatostatin receptor-mediated activation of SHP-1 and inhibition of cell proliferation. *Mol Biol Cell* 14:3911–3928.

88. Gromada, J., Hoy, M., Buschard, K., Salehi, A., Rorsman, P. (2001). Somatostatin inhibits exocytosis in rat pancreatic alpha-cells by G(i2).-dependent activation of calcineurin and depriming of secretory granules. *J Physiol* 535:519–532.

89. Bousquet, C., Puente, E., Buscail, L., Vaysse, N., Susini, C. (2001). Antiproliferative effect of somatostatin and analogs. *Chemotherapy* 47(Suppl. 2):30–39.

90. Florio, T., Yao, H., Carey, K.D., Dillon, T.J., Stork, P.J. (1999). Somatostatin activation of mitogen-activated protein kinase via somatostatin receptor 1 (SSTR1).. *Mol Endocrinol* 13:24–37.

91. Lahlou, H., Saint-Laurent, N., Esteve, J.P., Eychene, A., Pradayrol, L., Pyronnet, S., Susini, C. (2003). sst2 Somatostatin receptor inhibits cell proliferation through Ras-, Rap1-, and B-Raf-dependent ERK2 activation. *J Biol Chem* 278:39356–39371.

92. Cattaneo, M.G., Scita, G., Vicentini, L.M. (1999). Somatostatin inhibits PDGF-stimulated Ras activation in human neuroblastoma cells. *FEBS Lett* 459:64–68.

93. Dent, P., Wang, Y., Gu, Y.Z., Wood, S.L., Reardon, D.B., Mangues, R., Pellicer, A., Schonbrunn, A., Sturgill, T.W. (1997). S49 cells endogenously express subtype 2 somatostatin receptors which couple to increase protein tyrosine phosphatase activity in membranes and down-regulate Raf-1 activity in situ. *Cell Signal* 9:539–549.

94. Douziech, N., Calvo, E., Coulombe, Z., Muradia, G., Bastien, J., Aubin, R.A., Lajas, A., Morisset, J. (1999). Inhibitory and stimulatory effects of somatostatin on two human pancreatic cancer cell lines: a primary role for tyrosine phosphatase SHP-1. *Endocrinology* 140:765–777.

95. Florio, T., Arena, S., Thellung, S., Iuliano, R., Corsaro, A., Massa, A., Pattarozzi, A., Bajetto, A., Trapasso, F., Fusco, A., Schettini, G. (2001). The activation of the phosphotyrosine phosphatase eta (r-PTP eta). is responsible for the somatostatin inhibition of PC Cl3 thyroid cell proliferation. *Mol Endocrinol* 15:1838–1852.

96. Florio, T., Morini, M., Villa, V., Arena, S., Corsaro, A., Thellung, S., Culler, M.D., Pfeffer, U., Noonan, D.M., Schettini, G., Albini, A. (2003a). Somatostatin inhibits tumor angiogenesis and growth via somatostatin receptor-3-mediated regulation of endothelial nitric oxide synthase and mitogen-activated protein kinase activities. *Endocrinology* 144:1574–1584.

97. Cordelier, P., Esteve, J.P., Bousquet, C., Delesque, N., O'Carroll, A.M., Schally, A.V., Vaysse, N., Susini, C., Buscail, L. (1997). Characterization of the antiproliferative signal mediated by the somatostatin receptor subtype sst5. *Proc Natl Acad Sci U S A* 94:9343–9348.

98. Smalley, K.S., Feniuk, W., Sellers, L.A., Humphrey, P.P. (1999). The pivotal role of phosphoinositide-3 kinase in the human somatostatin sst(4). receptor-mediated

stimulation of p44/p42 mitogen-activated protein kinase and extracellular acidification. *Biochem Biophys Res Commun* 263:239–243.

99. Sellers, L.A., Alderton, F., Carruthers, A.M., Schindler, M., Humphrey, P.P. (2000). Receptor isoforms mediate opposing proliferative effects through gbetagamma-activated p38 or Akt pathways. *Mol Cell Biol* 20:5974–5985.
100. Williams, G., Ball, J., Bloom, S., Joplin, G.F. (1986). Improvement in headache associated with prolactinoma during treatment with a somatostatin analogue: an "N of 1" study. *N Engl J Med* 315:1166–1167.
101. Mollenholt, P., Rawal, N., Gordh, T., Jr., Olsson, Y. (1994). Intrathecal and epidural somatostatin for patients with cancer. Analgesic effects and postmortem neuropathologic investigations of spinal cord and nerve roots. *Anesthesiology* 81:534–542.
102. Penn, R.D., Paice, J.A., Kroin, J.S. (1992). Octreotide: a potent new non-opiate analgesic for intrathecal infusion. *Pain* 49(1):13–19.
103. Carlton, S.M., Du, J., Davidson, E., Zhou, S., Coggeshall, R.E. (2001). Somatostatin receptors on peripheral primary afferent terminals: inhibition of sensitized nociceptors. *Pain* 90:233–244.
104. Gaumann, D.M., Yaksh, T.L., Post, C., Wilcox, G.L., Rodriguez, M. (1989). Intrathecal somatostatin in cat and mouse studies on pain, motor behavior, and histopathology. *Anesth Analg* 68(5):623–632.
105. Gaumann, D.M., Yaksh, T.L. (1988). Adrenal and intestinal secretion of catecholamines and neuropeptides during splanchnic artery occlusion shock. *Circ Shock* 26(4):391–407.
106. Bentoin, F., Ardid, D., Herbet, A., Aumaitre, O., Kemeny, J.L., Duchene-Marullaz, P., Lavarenne, J., Eschalier, A. (1994). Evidence for a central long-lasting antinociceptive effect of vapreotide, an analog of somatostatin, involving an opioidergic mechanism. *J Pharmacol Exp Ther* 269:7–14.
107. Green, P.G., Basbaum, A.I., Levine, J.D. (1992). Sensory neuropeptide interactions in the production of plasma extravasation in the rat. *Neuroscience* 50:745–749.
108. Pinter, E., Helyes, Z., Szolcsanyi, J. (2006). Inhibitory effect of somatostatin on inflammation and nociception. *Pharmacol Ther* 112:440–456.
109. Polo-Parada, L., Pilar, G. (1999). Kappa- and mu-opioids reverse the somatostatin inhibition of Ca^{2+} currents in ciliary and dorsal root ganglion neurons. *J Neurosci* 19:5213–5227.
110. Scarborough, D.E., Lee, S.L., Dinarello, C.A., Reichlin, S. (1989). Interleukin 1 stimulates somatostatin biosynthesis in primary cultures of fetal rat brain. *Endocrinology* 124:549–551.
111. Scarborough, D.E. (1990). Somatostatin regulation by cytokines. *Metabolism* 39:108–111.
112. Rogers, K.V., Vician, L., Stein, R.A., Clifton, D.K. (1988). The effect of hypophysectomy and growth hormone administration on preprosomatostatin mRNA in the periventricular nucleus of the rat hypothalamus. *Endocrinology* 122:586–591.
113. Zeytin, F.N., Rusk, S.F., De Lellis, R. (1988). Growth hormone releasing factor and fibroblast growth factor regulate somatostatin gene expression. *Endocrinology* 122:1133–1136.
114. Lopez-Fernandez, J., Sanchez-Franco, F., Yelasco, B., Tolon, R.M., Pazos, F., Cacicedo, L. (1996). Growth hormone induces somatostatin and insulin like

growth factor I gene expression in the cerebral hemispheres of aging rats. *Endocrinology* 137:4384–439.

115. Saklatvala, J., Davis, W., Guesdon, F. (1996). Interleukin 1 (IL-1) and tumour necrosis factor (TNF) signal transduction. *Philos Trans R Soc Lond B Biogr Sci* 351:151–157.
116. Pawlak, M., Schmidt, R.F. (2004). Octreotide, a somatostatin analogue, attenuates movement evoked discharges of fine afferent units from inflamed knee joints of rats. *Neurosci Lett* 361:180–183.
117. Paran, D., Elkayam, O., Mayo, A., Paran, H., Amit, M., Yaron, M., Caspi, D. (2001). A pilot study of a long acting somatostatin analogue for the treatment of refractory rheumatoid arthritis. *Ann Rheum Dis* 60:888–891.
118. Malcangio, M. (2003). GDNF and somatostatin in sensory neurones. *Curr Opin Pharmacol* 3:41–45.
119. Kolasinski, S.L., Haines, K.A., Siegel, E.L., Cronstein, B.N., Abramson, S.B. (1992). Neuropeptides and inflammation. A somatostatin analog as a selective antagonist of neutrophil activation by substance P. *Arthritis Rheum* 35(4):369–375.
120. Fioravanti, A., Govoni, M., La Montagna, G., Perpignano, G., Tirri, G., Trotta, F., Bogliolo, A., Ciocci, A., Mauceri, M. T., Marcolongo, R. (1995). Somatostatin 14 and joint inflammation: evidence for intraarticular efficacy of prolonged administration in rheumatoid arthritis. *Drugs Exp Clin Res* 21:97–103.
121. Matucci-Cerinic, M., Marabini, S. (1998). Somatostatin treatment for pain in rheumatoid arthritis: a double blind versus placebo study in knee involvement. *Med Sci Res* 16:233–234.
122. Silveri, F., Morosini, P., Brecciaroli, D., Cervini, C. (1994). Intra-articular injection of somatostatin in knee osteoarthritis: clinical results and IGF-1 serum levels. *Int J Clin Pharmacol Res* 14(2):79–85.
123. Reichlin, S. (1993). Neuroendocrine-immune interaction. *N Engl J Med* 329:1246–1253.
124. Fais, S., Annibale, B., Boirivant, M., Santoro, A., Pallone, F., Delle Fave, G. (1991). Effect of somatostatin on human intestinal lamina propria lymphocytes. Modulation of lymphocyte activation. *J Neuroimmunol* 31:211–219.
125. Van Hagen, P.M., Markusse, H.M., Lamberts, S.W., Kwekkeboom, D.J., Reubi, J.C., Krenning, E.P. (1994). Somatostatin receptor imaging. The presence of somatostatin receptors in rheumatoid arthritis. *Arthritis Rheum* 37:1521–1527.
126. Takeba, Y., Suzuki Ntakeno, M., Asai, T., Tsuboi, S., Hoshino, T., Sakane, T. (1997). Modulationn of sinovial cell function by somatostatin in patients with rheumatoid arthritis. *Arthritis Rheum* 40:2128–2138.
127. Gonzalez-Ray, E., Chorny, A., Del Moral, R.G., Varela, N., Delgado, M. (2007). Therapeutic effect of cortistatin on experimental arthritis by downregulating inflammatory and Th1 response. *Ann Rheum Dis* 66:582–588.

CHAPTER 17

Cytokines (Tumor Necrosis Factor, Interleukins) and Prostaglandins

PER ALSTERGREN

Department of Dental Medicine, Karolinska Institutet

Content

Peripheral Receptor Targets for Analgesia: Novel Approaches to Pain Management, Edited by Brian E. Cairns

17.1 INTRODUCTION TO CYTOKINES

Cytokines are small and pleiotropic extracellular peptides with redundant effects that mediate potent stimulatory or inhibitory effects in, for example, immunity and inflammation. All nucleated cells are capable of synthesizing cytokines, which are produced de novo in response to immune stimuli, and most cell types respond to them. Cytokines generally act at very low concentrations during short periods of time in an autocrine or paracrine manner, although additional endocrine effects have been described for some cytokines [1,2].

Originally identified as being important in host reactions to disease and infection by mediating inflammatory processes and immune responses, it is now apparent that cytokines are involved in most physiological processes, including modulation of repair and remodeling of damaged tissue. For the most part, however, cytokines are produced and released during inflammation. Cytokines are often produced in a cascade, as one cytokine stimulates its target cells to make additional cytokines. Even so, the complex interconnectivity and dynamics of cytokine biology might be better visualized as a network within a cascade where cytokines can act independently, additively, or synergistically [3]. The central role of tumor necrosis factor (TNF) within the proinflammatory cytokine network is now conclusively established [4].

Cytokine-mediated inflammation induces gene products usually not produced while in a healthy state. In addition to cytokines like TNF, interleukin-1 (IL-1), and interleukin-6 (IL-6), these gene products include phospholipase A2, cyclooxygenase-2 (COX-2), and inducible nitric oxide synthase, chemokines, and endothelial adhesion factors. TNF and IL-1 are particularly effective in initiating and stimulating the expression of these genes [5]. There is, on the other hand, a simultaneous production and release of anti-inflammatory cytokines like IL-4, IL-10, and IL-13 that block or suppress the intensity of this cascade as an endogenous control of the net cytokine effects [2]. In inflammatory conditions, a dramatic increase in cytokine production can be seen at the same time as the balance between the cytokine production and its control is disturbed [6]. Indeed, it appears that the balance of proinflammatory cytokines and their endogenous control mediators (anti-inflammatory cytokines, soluble or decoy receptors, and antagonists) is at least as important as the absolute levels of individual cytokines [7].

Cytokines have been extensively studied in immune reactions and inflammation, but less so regarding their specific and distinct roles in pain. The relation between cytokines and pain is probably better understood by placing it in a broader context as a part of an immune reaction or inflammation. In fact, most, if not all, models to study hyperalgesia or pain facilitation induce release of proinflammatory cytokines [8].

This chapter will focus on the contribution of peripheral effects of cytokines and their peripheral receptors on pain. As mentioned above, the available knowledge about peripheral cytokines and pain is, however, limited in general with the possible exception of the cytokines TNF, IL-1, and IL-6, which will be discussed in detail below.

17.2 PERIPHERAL CYTOKINE MODULATION OF PAIN

Peripheral cytokines are believed to peripherally influence or modulate pain in a complex manner on several levels:

(1) direct effects on nociceptors via cell-surface receptors,
(2) indirect effects on nociceptors via stimulation of local production of other cytokines and mediators with nociceptive effects,
(3) pain/hyperalgesia as a part of the illness response, and
(4) the cholinergic anti-inflammatory pathway.

17.2.1 Direct Effects on Nociceptive Fibers via Cell-Surface Receptors

Peripheral nociceptive neurons express receptors for various cytokines. When stimulated, these receptors may influence nerve fiber depolarization and conductivity as well as apoptosis and gene expression of factors important for nociceptive signaling in the neuron [2]. There is now evidence for a role of proinflammatory cytokines not only in inflammatory pain but also in neuropathic pain [9,10].

17.2.2 Indirect Effects on Nociceptors via Stimulation of Local Production of Other Cytokines and Mediators with Nociceptive Effects

In inflammatory responses, the release of hyperalgesic mediators seems to be secondary to the release of proinflammatory cytokines. TNF and IL-1β rapidly induce synthesis and release of other nociceptive mediators such as IL-1, IL-6, bradykinin, and prostaglandins as well as themselves. This has to be taken into account when discussing the contribution of these cytokines to pain; that is, these cytokines exert both direct effects as well as indirect effects [8]. In addition, many cytokines also influence systemic and central pain-related mechanisms besides local sensitization of nociceptors.

17.2.3 Pain/Hyperalgesia as a Part of the Illness Response

Besides local effects, cytokines also cause or modulate a wide array of changes called the "illness response," which follow immune activation by inflammation, injury, or infection. The illness responses promote survival for the organism and include physiological, behavioral, endocrine, and neural changes like fever, increased sleep, decreased activity and social interaction, and decreased food and water intake, changes that also form a part of chronic pain. Generalized reduction of pain thresholds and exaggerated pain responses, that is, hyperalgesia, are also aspects of the illness response [8,11–13].

The illness response occurs due to the release of proinflammatory cytokines, especially TNF, IL-1β, and IL-6. Peripheral administration of these cytokines can create the entire illness response. Once proinflammatory cytokines are released in the periphery, illness responses are produced as a result of signals reaching specific centers in the brain. It is now clear that peripherally released proinflammatory cytokines activate certain peripheral nerves with vagal sensory afferent nerves being most relevant. Once activated, these peripheral nerves communicate with the brain to induce and maintain the illness response, including pain and hyperalgesia [14–16].

Work by Watkins and coworkers on animal models has demonstrated that IL-1β produces hyperalgesia following either intraperitoneal or intracerebroventricular injection. In contrast, IL-1β delivered intrathecally does not affect pain response. Liver macrophages, that is, Kupffer cells, appear to be critically involved in this process and relay signals to the brain via hepatic vagal afferents. Both TNF and IL-1β appear to be critical mediators of this kind of hyperalgesia, whereas prostaglandins do not appear to be involved. Taken together, substances classically thought of as products of the immune system may dynamically enhance pain response via actions either on the hepatic vagus or at central sites [17].

17.3 THE CHOLINERGIC ANTI-INFLAMMATORY PATHWAY

Health requires that cytokine production is balanced and only low levels of some cytokines are required to maintain homeostasis. In most inflammatory disease, a dramatic increase in cytokine production can be seen at the same time as the balance between the cytokine production and its control is disturbed [6]. Endogenous cytokine control mechanisms include anti-inflammatory cytokines, soluble receptors with anti-inflammatory effects, decoy receptors, cytokine antagonists, and autoantibodies [2]. In addition, a novel neuronal cholinergic anti-inflammatory pathway exerting peripheral cytokine control has recently been demonstrated [18]. As described in more detail above, sensory fibers traveling with the vagus nerve transmit information to the brain that is both necessary and sufficient for initiating generalized hyperalgesia, fever, and other responses to injury or infection [8,19]. In the central nervous system, these inflammatory signals activate a neural loop that elicits an efferent response in the vagus that suppresses cytokine production in the periphery in order to control the net effects of the cytokines. This mechanism of endogenous cytokine control is now termed the *cholinergic anti-inflammatory pathway* [20]. This pathway functions as a fast, reflex-like anti-inflammatory mechanism controlled by brain networks [18] and seems to be mediated by the vagus nerve. Activation causes downregulation of peripheral cytokine production by the reticuloendothelial system (e.g., liver and spleen) and redirection of leukocyte trafficking away from the periphery [21].

Efferent stimulation of the vagus nerve has been shown to inhibit TNF release and cytokine activities as well as to improve outcome of, for example, experimental arthritis [22,23]. Mice exposed to endotoxin have an unbalanced and excessive cytokine response if they are deficient in vagus nerve activity. Moreover, vagus nerve stimulation significantly inhibits peripheral cytokine release in wild-type mice [24]. Vagus nerve stimulation has been studied in at least two models of experimental arthritis. Stimulation of the vagus nerve in animals subjected to carrageenan-induced paw swelling inhibits the local production of cytokines [25]. Vagus nerve stimulation of mice in a model of subcutaneous inflammation caused by injecting carrageenan into an air pouch inhibits recruitment of polymorphonuclear leukocytes to the inflammatory zone [26]. As the vagus nerve does not signal directly to either the paw or the subcutaneous tissues, it is likely that the reduction in inflammation observed following vagus nerve stimulation in these models is attributable to downregulation of cytokine production by the reticuloendothelial system and redirection of leukocyte trafficking away from the periphery [21]. This indicates that vagus nerve-derived signals provide tonic or continuous neurological modulation of peripheral cytokine synthesis, controlling the magnitude of the immune response.

The major vagus nerve neurotransmitter is acetylcholine and it has been found to be responsible for inhibition of cytokine synthesis [24,27,28]. Macrophages and other cytokine-producing cells express acetylcholine receptors that, when stimulated, inhibit cytokine synthesis [24,27].

17.4 EICOSANOIDS

Eicosanoids (from the Greek word *eicosa*, i.e., 20) comprise prostaglandins, thromboxanes and leukotrienes. Prostaglandins are lipid mediators with 20 carbon atoms and are produced from arachidonic acid, an essential fatty acid. Prostaglandins have diverse and potent biological autocrine or paracrine effects on almost all organs and are primarily involved in inflammation-related vasodilation. Other effects are, for example, sensitization of nociceptors, initiation and maintenance of cytokine production, platelet aggregation, and fever. Prostaglandins synergize with other proinflammatory mediators such as histamine and bradykinin to increase their inflammatory effects [29].

Figure 17.1 shows a schematic overview of the cytokines TNF, IL-1β, and IL-6, as well as their receptors.

17.5 TNF

17.5.1 Ligands

TNF exists in both a soluble (17 kD) and a cell-bound, transmembrane form (tmTNF, 26 kD), and it is primarily produced in response to various inflammatory stimuli.

The main physiological role of TNF is activation of the first-line reaction to microbial, viral, and mechanical stress. TNF rapidly induces synthesis of other mediators such as IL-1, IL-6, and prostaglandins. TNF is not considered to be produced by normal cells but rather by cells stimulated by, for example, neoplastic or infectious disease [30]. TNF is synthesized by a wide variety of different cell types like macrophages and monocytes, T cells, B cells, astrocytes, fibroblasts, basophils, mast cells, NK cells, Kupffer cells, smooth muscle cells, epidermal cells, and several cancer tumor forms. About 45% of small dorsal root ganglion neurons also express TNF, suggesting it may also be released by peripheral afferent fibers [31–33]. TNF production is induced by immune-potentiating cytokines such as IL-1, IL-2, IL-6, and interferons, complement system components, immune complexes, as well as lipopolysaccarides (LPS) from bacterial cell walls. Indeed, almost all stressful and inflammatory stimuli have been shown to induce TNF release, including UV light and X-rays. Interestingly, TNF can also upregulate its own synthesis [2]. Several agents also downregulate TNF expression, for example, inhibitors of prostaglandin synthesis (salicylate), glucocorticoids, and endogenous immunosuppressive cytokines like IL-4, IL-10, IL-11, and IL-13 [34].

TNF is released from cells as a soluble cytokine after being enzymatically cleaved from its cell-bound precursor tmTNF by the TNF-converting enzyme. Both the soluble TNF and the cell-surface-bound tmTNF are biologically active, and the relative amounts of each are collectively determined by the inducing stimuli, the cell types involved, the activation status of the cells, the amounts of active TNF-converting enzyme, and the amounts of natural TNF-converting enzyme inhibitors such as the tissue inhibitor of metalloproteinase-3 [35].

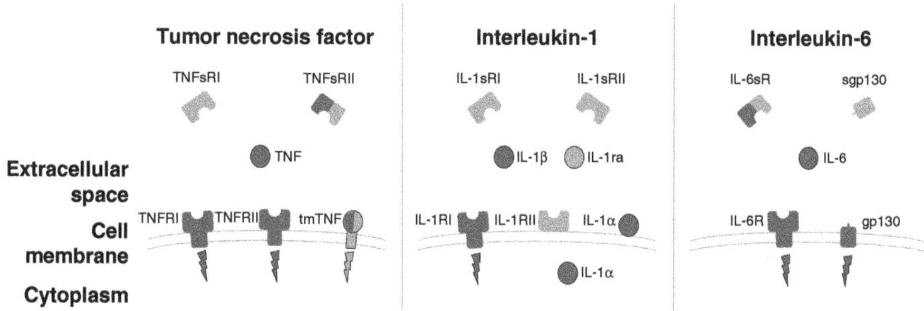

FIGURE 17.1. Endogenous ligands and receptors for tumor necrosis factor (TNF), interleukin-1β (IL-1β), and interleukin-6 (IL-6). In this figure, the red color represents proinflammatory effects and the green color represents anti-inflammatory effects.

TNF elicits proinflammatory effects by binding to and activating two cell-surface-bound receptors, the TNF receptor I (TNFRI) and the TNF receptor II (TNFRII). These receptors can also be found as soluble receptors, TNFsRI and TNFsRII, in the extracellular space and circulation where they have anti-inflammatory effects by binding to and inactivating TNF. The two TNF receptors have similar binding affinities for TNF, but the kinetics by which TNF binds to and releases from the two receptors differ. Binding of TNF to TNFRI is nearly irreversible, whereas TNFRII shows a highly reversible binding with a 30-fold faster dissociation rate than TNFRI. The TNFsRII may therefore also function as a ligand passer with proinflammatory effects by binding to and transferring TNF to the cell-bound TNFsRI. TNF is also present as a transmembrane protein (tmTNF) with proinflammatory effects upon receptor binding in cell-to-cell contact signaling. Interestingly, TNFsRI and TNFsRII as well as several TNF blockers may bind to tmTNF and may trigger reverse signaling through tmTNF, which elicits anti-inflammatory effects like suppression of cytokine production in the cell.

There are three subtypes of IL-1: the agonists IL-1α and IL-1β, as well as an endogenous receptor antagonist, IL-1ra. Most of the IL-1α remains intracellularly or on the surface of the cell membrane, while IL-1β is transported out of the cell. IL-1ra competes with IL-1α and IL-1β for receptor binding but has an anti-inflammatory character because it does not elicit a biological response. There are two IL-1 receptors: IL-1RI with low/high affinity for IL-1β/IL-1ra and IL-1RII with high/low affinity for IL-1β/IL-1ra. IL-1RII causes no signal transduction when stimulated and is therefore considered as a "decoy receptor." Soluble IL-1RI (IL-1sRI) and soluble IL-1RII (IL-1sRII) are present in the extracellular space and circulation, and together with the IL-1ra and the inactive form of the receptor, the soluble IL-1 receptors modulate the effects of IL-1.

After synthesis, IL-6 is transported out of the cell. A soluble form of the IL-6 receptor (IL-6sR) can be found in the extracellular space and circulation after it is shed from the membrane-bound version of the protein or by synthesis from an alternatively spliced mRNA. The cell-surface-bound IL-6R consists of two subunits: IL-6sR and the transmembrane protein gp130. On cells expressing IL-6R, IL-6 binds to IL-6R and this complex then associates with gp130, which induces signaling. gp130 is expressed by all cells in the body, whereas IL-6R is mainly expressed by hepatocytes, neutrophils, monocytes/macrophages, and some lymphocytes. Besides IL-6 binding to IL-6R, an additional model of IL-6 modulation of cell function exists. The IL-6 and IL-6sR complex binds to the cell-bound gp130 and may thus stimulate cells that express gp130 but not IL-6R. This mechanism is named IL-6 trans-signaling. The agonistic properties of the IL-6–IL-6sR complex are counteracted by a soluble form of gp130 (sgp130), which prevents signaling through membrane-bound gp130. See color insert.

17.5.2 Receptors

Biological responses to TNF are mediated by ligand binding via two structurally distinct transmembrane receptors: the type I receptor with a molecular mass of 55–60 kDa (TNFRI) and the 75- to 80-kDa type II receptor (TNFRII). The TNFRI is present on all cell types except erythrocytes, whereas the TNFRII is mainly expressed by cells of the immune system and on endothelial cells. Most cells have a receptor density of approximately 1000 receptors per cell, but some cells might have up to 5000 receptors per cell [36].

The cytoplasmic domains of both receptors differ to a large extent, but both lack enzymatic activity. However, activation of the receptors recruits intracellular proteins that in turn initiate intracellular signaling. The receptors primarily modulate activation of the transcription factor nuclear factor kappa B (NF-κB), which controls a large number of inflammatory genes, as well as caspase-8- and caspase-3-dependent apoptosis. Regarding pain mechanisms, stimulation of TNFRI leads to induction of NF-κB, c-fos, and IL-6, and prostaglandin E_2 (PGE_2) synthesis as well as stimulation of phospholipase A2. On the other hand, TNFRII stimulation induces NF-κB and IL-6 [36].

During chronic and acute inflammatory conditions, the concentrations of both receptors increase dramatically. The TNF receptors are upregulated by a number of factors including glucocorticoids, interferons, leukotriene B_4, IL-2, IL-6 and IL-4 and LPS [34]. So far, there is no report of differential regulation by one type of TNF receptor over another. There is also very little known about the regulation of TNF receptor at the transcription, translation, or post-translation levels [36].

Both TNF receptors are subject to proteolytic cleavage by matrix metalloproteases. The TNF-converting enzyme, the enzyme that causes the release of TNF, is also involved in this cleavage where the extracellular portion is released from the cell surface. This cleavage is increased in response to inflammatory signals such as TNF ligand–receptor binding. The soluble receptors have been found in blood, urine, cerebral spinal fluid, and synovial fluid in patients, and the levels of these receptors increase during inflammation or infection [37,38]. The soluble forms of both receptors, TNFsRI and TNFsRII, are primarily believed to be endogenous inhibitors of TNF bioactivity by binding to TNF and by removal of TNF from the site of its release [38]. Indeed, a dimer of TNFsRII is today an approved pharmaceutical drug (etanercept, Enbrel®) in many countries for treatment of chronic and general inflammatory diseases like rheumatoid arthritis (RA) and psoriatic arthritis [39,40].

The two TNF receptors have similar binding affinities for TNF, but the kinetics by which TNF binds to and releases from the two receptors differ. Binding of TNF to TNFRI is nearly irreversible, whereas TNFRII shows a highly reversible binding with a 30-fold faster dissociation rate than TNFRI [41]. The different TNF binding properties may indicate that the two receptor types have different primary functions. Indeed, shedding of the cellular receptors, their increased plasma concentrations in inflammation, and their retained ability to bind TNF has led to the hypothesis that the soluble TNF receptors may serve either as natural antagonists or as delivery peptides (ligand passers) for circulating TNF, depending upon their relative concentrations. In this sense, TNFRII may serve as a ligand passer, that is, as a means to deliver or to pass TNF to TNFRI for signaling when concentrations of TNF are low. In fact, the primary inflammatory responses to soluble 17-kD TNF, *in vivo*, are mediated by TNFRI rather than by TNFRII signaling [42]. The principal ligand for TNFRI has therefore been proposed to be the secreted form of TNF, whereas cell-associated TNF has been suggested as the primary signaling ligand for TNFRII, implying that TNFRII contributes to the local TNF response in tissues as occurs in RA. Along these same lines, overexpression of human TNFRII has been demonstrated to induce an exaggerated inflammatory response in several organs [36].

TNF-mediated cell signaling gains additional complexity from the distinct signaling pathways mediated not only through TNFRI and TNFRII but also through tmTNF because tmTNF can function as a ligand as well as a receptor. Interestingly, binding by TNF receptors, or even TNF antagonists, to tmTNF can induce reverse signaling through this cell-surface-bound ligand. Reverse signaling by tmTNF may by this means trigger cytokine suppression or apoptosis [43–45], but knowledge regarding the *in vivo* functional significance of tmTNF-mediated reverse signaling is still lacking.

17.6 IL-1

17.6.1 Ligands

IL-1 has a molecular weight of 17 kDa and is mainly derived from macrophages and T cells. So far, three subtypes of IL-1 have been identified; two agonists with strong proinflammatory effects, IL-1α and IL-1β, as well as an IL-1 receptor antagonist, IL-1ra. Most of the IL-1α remains intracellularly or on the surface of the cell membrane where it functions more as an autocrine messenger rather than as an extracellular mediator, while most IL-1β is transported out of the cell where it acts locally or enters the blood circulation [46]. Indeed, both have been shown to be involved in inflammatory reactions, but only IL-1β has been found in synovial fluid from patients with RA [47]. IL-1ra competes with IL-1α and IL-1β for receptor binding and is produced in substantially higher concentrations than IL-1β during inflammation. IL-1ra does not elicit a biological response when coupled to an IL-1 receptor and has therefore anti-inflammatory character [1].

IL-1α and IL-1β are produced as 31-kDa precursors, and processing of pro-IL-1α and pro-IL-1β to the mature forms of IL-1α and IL-1β requires specific cellular proteases, calpain for IL-1α and the IL-1β-converting enzyme for IL-1β. IL-1ra is not produced as a proform but is readily transported out of the cells [46]. On inflammatory stimulus, cells rapidly start to produce large amounts of pro-IL-1α, pro-IL-1β, and IL-1ra and release IL-1β and IL-1ra. The inflammatory process causes an increased local IL-1ra release but during active inflammation probably in insufficient amounts to inhibit the strong proinflammatory effects of IL-1β [1].

IL-1 induces several inflammatory events, that is, activation of lymphocytes and stimulation of cytokine, prostaglandin, and collagenase release from connective tissue cells, but it is also involved in hyperalgesia and pain. In addition, it has systemic effects by stimulating the production and release of C-reactive protein, eliciting fever and the illness response [48].

17.6.2 Receptors

There are two IL-1 receptors identified: IL-1RI with low/high affinity for IL-1β/IL-1ra and IL-1RII with high/low affinity for IL-1β/IL-1ra. When stimulated, IL-1RI elicits a biological response in the cell, whereas IL-1RII causes no signal transduction and is therefore considered as a decoy receptor [46].

17.6.3 IL-1 Receptor I

The extracellular domain of the IL-1RI is an 80-kDa immunoglobulin (Ig)-like receptor, whereas the cytoplasmic portion contains a Toll-like protein [49]. IL-1RI is found predominantly on T cells, endothelial cells, epithelial cells, fibroblasts, hepatocytes, and dendritic cells [2]. Primary cells usually express less than 200 IL-1RI per cell and sometimes less than 50 per cell [50].

Signal transduction requires the formation of a heterodimer of IL-1RI with IL-1R accessory protein [46]. Following binding of either IL-1α or IL-1β to the IL-1RI, the IL-1R accessory protein forms a complex with IL-1/IL-1RI. This high-affinity complex then results in signal transduction. Lacking a second binding site, IL-1ra binds primarily to IL-1RI but does not trigger a biological response because the IL-1R accessory protein will not form the required complex with IL-1/IL-1RI, and thus no signal is transduced. Stimulation of the receptor eventually leads to activation of the transcription factor NF-κB, among others [51,52]. In turn, genes encoding pro- and anti-inflammatory cytokines as well as enzymes involved in inflammation like COX-2, phospholipase A2, and nitric oxide synthase are upregulated [1]. Mice deficient in IL-1RI show no abnormal phenotype in health and exhibit normal homeostasis [53,54].

There is also a soluble form of this receptor, IL-1sRI, which is released from the cell surface by proteolytic cleavage. It comprises only the extracellular part of IL-1RI and has anti-inflammatory effects by binding to and thereby blocking IL-1 from reaching cell-bound IL-1RI receptors. The rank of affinities for the IL-1sRI is remarkably different for each of the three IL-1 molecules. The rank for the three IL-1 ligands binding to IL-1sRI is IL-1ra > IL-1α > IL-1β [2].

17.6.4 IL-1 Receptor II

IL-1RII is primarily expressed on monocytes, macrophages, neutrophils, and B lymphocytes. The IL-1sRII is a decoy receptor in that it lacks a cytoplasmic portion capable if signaling and its primary ligand, IL-1β, preferably binds to this receptor rather than to the signaling receptor IL-1sRI. The extracellular domain of IL-1sRII is structurally related to those of IL-1RI, but binding of IL-1β to IL-1RII is nearly irreversible due to the long disassociation rate, approximately 2 hours [55,56].

Similar to soluble receptors for TNF and IL-1RI, the extracellular domains of the type II IL-1R are found as soluble molecules. IL-1sRII has been demonstrated in the circulation and urine of healthy subjects and in inflammatory synovial and other pathologic body fluids [55,57,58]. It is likely that as cell-bound IL-1RII increases, there is a comparable increase in soluble forms [59]. The induction of release of the IL-1sRII decoy receptor is probably an early event in inflammation to limit the cascade [2]. For example, chemoattractants as well as bacterial LPS cause rapid shedding of the IL-1sRII [60]. However, unlike soluble TNF receptors, it is unknown whether the soluble form of IL-1RII acts as a carrier for IL-1 and prolongs its half-life in the circulation.

17.6.5 IL-1 Receptor Accessory Protein

Similar to the IL-1RI and IL-1RII, a soluble form of the IL-1R accessory protein exists, but this form seems to be a truncated protein without a transmembrane region and it is not formed by proteolytic cleavage. The effect or role of this soluble accessory protein is, however, unclear because it does not bind IL-1β [61].

17.7 IL-6

17.7.1 Ligands

IL-6 is a protein of 186 amino acids with a molecular weight of 21–28 kDa that is synthesized as a precursor protein of 212 amino acids. IL-6 can be produced and released by nearly all, if not all, nucleated cells, but the main sources are macrophages, fibroblasts, and endothelial cells [62].

Traditionally, IL-6 is considered to be a regulator of acute-phase responses and a lymphocyte stimulatory factor [63]. IL-6 plays a pivotal role in chronic disease, where it regulates both local inflammatory events and associated systemic symptoms such as fever and induction of acute-phase reactants [64].

17.7.2 Receptors

The IL-6 receptor (IL-6R) consists of two subunits: the extracellular portion, an 80-kDa transmembrane glycoprotein that binds IL-6 with low affinity, and the gp130, a 130-kDa transmembrane glycoprotein [62]. On target cells, IL-6 first binds to the IL-6R. The complex of IL-6 and IL-6R then associates with the signal-transducing membrane protein gp130, thereby inducing signaling. gp130 is expressed by all cells in the body, whereas IL-6R is mainly expressed by hepatocytes, neutrophils, monocytes/macrophages, and some lymphocytes [63].

A naturally occurring soluble form of the IL-6R (IL-6sR) has been found in various body fluids. This soluble form of IL-6R is generated by two independent mechanisms: shedding of the membrane-bound protein by proteolytic cleavage and translation from an alternatively spliced mRNA [62].

Besides IL-6 binding to cell-bound IL-6R to cause biological responses in target cells, an additional model of IL-6–IL-6R modulation of cell function has been described. The IL-6 and IL-6sR complex may in fact bind to the cell-bound gp130 and thereby stimulate cells that express gp130 but not the cell-bound IL-6R. This mechanism is named IL-6 trans-signaling [62] and enables IL-6 to influence cells different from those that are modulated by IL-6 coupling to cell-bound IL-6R. IL-6 may thereby elicit distinct functions in gp130-expressing cells [64]. T cells, many neural cells, smooth muscle cells, and endothelial cells, among others, do not express cell-bound IL-6R, but they are remarkably responsive to IL-6 but only in the presence of IL-6sR [62,64].

The agonist properties of the sIL-6R are counteracted by a soluble form of gp130 (sgp130), which circulates at relatively high levels (100–300 ng/mL) in human sera. This naturally occurring antagonist prevents signaling through membrane-bound gp130 by binding to the IL-6/sIL-6R complex. Indeed, the course of a murine model of monoarthritic antigen-induced arthritis can be blocked by this protein, which suggests a possible future therapeutic potential of sgp130 [62,64].

17.8 PROSTAGLANDINS

17.8.1 Ligands

Prostaglandins are synthesized de novo from membrane-released arachidonic acid by most cells when cells are activated by mechanical trauma or by specific cytokine, growth factor, and other stimuli. Prostaglandins exert their pharmacological actions on target cells in close proximity as both an inflammatory mediator released at the site of tissue inflammation and neuromodulators that alter neuronal excitability and synaptic processing [29].

The cellular level of arachidonic acid is closely regulated by phospholipases, that is, enzymes that control arachidonic acid release from membranes. Arachidonic acid is thereby released by cytosolic phospholipase A2 and is presented to prostaglandin H synthase, which is also called cyclooxygenase (COX). COX mediates the conversion of arachidonic acid into the prostaglandin precursors PGG_2 and PGH_2. PGH_2 exists as two isoforms: PGHS-1 (metabolized by cyclooxygenase-1 [COX-1]) and PGHS-2 (metabolized by COX-2) [65]. COX-1 is constitutively expressed in nearly all tissues and of particular importance for gastrointestinal protection. COX-2 is inducible by inflammatory signaling, for example, by the proinflammatory cytokines TNF and IL-Iβ, at the site of local inflammation [29,66]. In most instances, COX-1 expression is marginally affected by inflammatory stimuli. However, exceptions to the constitutive mode of COX-1 prostanoid synthesis are known; for example, both COX-1 and COX-2 are expressed in the inflamed synovia of joints [66].

Downstream metabolism of PGH_2 is from here highly cell specific. For example, microsomal PGE synthase (mPGES) is responsible for PGE_2 synthesis [67] and prostacyclin synthase is found in endothelial cells. Prostaglandins are finally released from cells by the prostaglandin transporter and potentially by other still uncharacterized transporters [68].

17.8.2 Receptors

There are at least nine known prostaglandin receptor forms in mouse and man, and some of these can be found in splice variants [69]. Most of the prostaglandin receptors are localized at the plasma membrane, although some are situated at the nuclear envelope [70].

Four of the receptor subtypes bind PGE_2: EP1–EP4, and two bind PGD_2: DP1 and DP2. The ligand for the receptor FP is PGF_2 and for IP it is PGI_2 (Table 17.1) [71,72]. All four EP receptor subtypes are expressed in subsets of primary sensory neurons and recognize PGE_2 but differ in their pharmacology and responses to various PGE analogues [66]. The prostaglandin receptors are G protein-coupled receptors with seven transmembrane regions with the exception of DP2. The receptors IP, DP1, EP2, and EP4 signal through Gs proteins that increase intracellular cyclic adenosine monophosphate (cAMP). The EP2 receptor is also linked to Gs protein but primarily activates adenylyl cyclase that, in turn, causes an increase in sensory neuron excitability [73]. The receptors EP1 and FP act through Gq-mediated increases in intracellular calcium, and the EP3 receptor couples to Gi and decreases cAMP formation.

TABLE 17.1. PGE_2 and PGI_2 Receptors Involved in Pain Sensitization.

Receptor	G Protein Coupling	Expression on Primary Sensory Neurons
EP1	Gq	Yes, including their spinal terminals.
EP2	Gs	Possibly.
EP3 (A–D)	A: Gi; B: Gs; C: Gs; D: Gi, Gs, Gq	Yes, including their spinal terminals.
EP4	Gs	Yes.
IP	Gs	Yes.

Besides exerting most of their action through G protein-coupled receptors, prostaglandins also bind to nuclear peroxisome proliferator-activated receptors. There is, however, no evidence so far for an involvement of these receptors in the nociceptive effects of prostaglandins [66].

17.9 EVIDENCE FOR THE ROLE OF THESE MEDIATORS AND THEIR RECEPTORS IN CUTANEOUS AND DEEP TISSUE-MEDIATED PAIN

17.9.1 TNF

Most proinflammatory cytokines rapidly induce synthesis and release of other nociceptive mediators as well as themselves. In addition to local sensitization of nociceptors, many cytokines also influence systemic and central pain-related mechanisms. These direct and indirect contributions of cytokines to pain have to be considered when discussing the relation between cytokines and pain [8].

17.9.1.1 Experimental Findings. Peripheral TNF signaling is involved in nociceptive responses including hyperalgesia [8,74,75]. Local TNF administration evokes spontaneous activity in afferent C- and Aδ-nerve fibers that results in low-grade nociceptive input, contributing to central sensitization [74,76]. Indeed, peripheral TNF induces a mechanical hyperalgesia with rapid onset (<30 minutes) when administered subcutaneously. It appears to result from sensitization of cutaneous C-fibers and to be associated with signs of local inflammation and increased levels of inflammatory mediators, for example, prostaglandins [33,77]. For example, intraplantar injection of TNF in rats reduced mechanical nociceptive thresholds in a prostaglandin-dependent process [74].

TNF is involved in several animal models of arthritis [77]. Subcutaneous administration of the TNF inhibitor etanercept decreased mechanical hyperalgesia when administered prior to induction of arthritis by injection of complete Freund's adjuvance into the rat knee joint [78]. In contrast to its effects on cutaneous and articular tissues, injection of TNF into the rat gastrocnemius muscle induced prolonged mechanical sensitization but without significant muscle inflammation or recruitment of inflammatory cells, although it was associated with increased tissue levels of PGE_2, calcitonin gene-related peptide, and nerve growth factor [79].

The effects of TNF associated with experimental hyperalgesia have been shown to be dependent on TNFRI [80], and it has been shown that nonneurally derived TNF directly acts via TNFRI on primary afferent neurons to produce hyperalgesia [81]. Indeed, TNFRI neutralizing antibodies as well as antisense RNA against TNFRI, but not antibodies toward TNFRII, can reduce experimentally induced hyperalgesia [80].

TNFRI and TNFRII immunoreactivity has been found in dorsal root ganglion [79,81]. The expression of TNFRI RNA in rat dorsal root ganglion seems to be not restricted to presumed nociceptive neurons in the dorsal root ganglion, which actually implies a broader role of TNF in primary sensory functions than nociception alone [81].

At the site of nerve injury, cytokines seem to orchestrate the pathophysiological events. Cytokine synthesis is directly related to the temporal course of the many events involved in neuropathic pain, events that can be considered as neuroimmunological responses to tissue injury. These responses can be modulated with anti-inflammatory cytokine therapy to reduce both nerve injury and pain. The relationship between TNF and nerve injury has been of increasing interest because TNF has been implicated in the pathogenesis of multiple sclerosis, HIV-associated neurological disease, and peripheral demyelinating neuropathies [82]. TNF is released into the local environment after nerve injury and has been found to be very important for initiation and maintenance of neuropathic pain. After nerve injury, TNF increases in the peripheral nerve itself, its dorsal root ganglia, and in the spinal cord [83]. On the other hand, inhibition of TNF reduces hyperalgesia in animal models of neuropathic pain, for example, chronic constriction injury and partial nerve transection [84,85]. Regarding TNF receptors, both receptors are upregulated in the peripheral nerve and in the dorsal root ganglion after nerve injury [86–88]. TNFRI, but not TNFRII, seems to mediate thermal hyperalgesia and mechanical allodynia after sciatic nerve injury in mice [80], which is in line with an upregulation of TNFRI following experimental nerve lesion [86,87]. Blocking TNF and TNFRI with neutralizing antibodies decreases hyperalgesia, whereas blocking TNFRII has no such effect [80], indicating a more prominent role for TNFRI in neuropathic pain. In mice deficient of TNFRI, thermal hyperalgesia does not develop after nerve injury, whereas a reduction in mechanical and cold allodynia can be seen in mice deficient of TNFRI or TNFRII [83].

Experimental cutaneous hyperalgesia can also be caused by systemic administration of TNF. Intraperitoneal TNF produces a dose-dependent hyperalgesia by inducing release of IL-1β that activates subdiaphragmatic vagal afferents [8].

17.9.1.2 Clinical Findings. In humans, intradermal or intramuscular injection of TNF causes a dose-dependent local cutaneous erythema and edema within 2 hours of injection, although it is still unclear whether these injections also result in pain or local sensitization [89].

TNF has been detected in the synovium and the synovial fluid from patients with RA [90] and in patients with other inflammatory diseases such as psoriatic arthritis, pelvospondylitis, and reactive arthritis [91,92]. TNF has also been found in the synovial fluid of patients with internal derangement of the temporomandibular joint (TMJ) [93] as well as in patients with unspecified TMJ disorders [94]. Synovial fluid TNF levels have been shown to be significantly higher in individuals with TMJ pain than in those without such pain including pain upon mandibular movement [92]. In addition, synovial fluid TNF levels have been associated with tenderness to palpation of the TMJ, which corresponds to sensitization of afferent nerves in the synovial tissues and in tissues surrounding the TMJ. As can then be expected, TNF levels in synovial fluid and plasma appear to be predictive for the treatment response to intra-articular administration of glucocorticoid into the TMJ. A high pretreatment level of TNF in the TMJ synovial fluid was found to be a positive predictor for TMJ pain relief after intra-articular administration of glucocorticoid [90]. The pain relief after treatment was associated with reduction of synovial fluid TNF. It is thus quite likely that TNF is involved in the modulation of joint pain.

Patients with RA have circulating levels of soluble TNFRs that are higher than those observed in patients with osteoarthritis or non-RA inflammatory arthritis [95]. In RA, but not in osteoathritis, both TNFRI and TNFRII are strongly expressed in the synovium with the majority being TNFRI [96].

Insufficient systemic endogenous control of TNF, as estimated by the plasma level of TNFsRII, contributes to TMJ pain in RA [38]. In that study, low plasma level of TNFsRII was associated with low pressure pain threshold in patients with elevated plasma TNF.

The role of cytokines in muscle pain is largely unknown. However, pro-inflammatory cytokines such as TNF have been been associated with muscle pathology, for example, inflammatory myopathies [97] and fibromyalgia [98]. TNF and IL-1β levels are elevated in microdialysates from the trapezius muscle with myofascial trigger points in patients with idiopathic cervical pain compared to healthy controls [99]. Elevated levels of TNF, IL-1β, and IL-6 in plasma have been associated with more pronounced upper-body symptoms in patients with musculoskeletal disorders from overuse [100]. In a study of delayed-onset muscle soreness in healthy males, administration of the TNF blocker etanercept did not affect the muscle soreness itself, but the muscle strength improved more rapidly [101], suggesting that muscle soreness is not modulated by TNF. An additional systemic response may be evoked by cytokines released into the blood from the injured muscle tissue where circulating cytokines like TNF, IL-1β, and IL-6 may stimulate a global response of widespread tissue sensitization [48].

17.9.2 IL-1

17.9.2.1 Experimental Findings. IL-1β is capable of decreasing nociceptive thresholds in peripheral tissues by direct excitatory and sensitizing action on nociceptive fibers [102]. Jeanjean and coworkers [103] showed that intraplantar injections of IL-1β in rats were able to sensitize nociceptors by a long-term increase of neuronal synthesis and axonal transport of substance P as well as its release. In chronic inflammation, this effect could increase the sensitivity to stimuli by peripheral neurogenic inflammation.

Injection of IL-1β into one paw in rats evokes a dose-dependent hyperalgesia in both the ipsilateral and the contralateral paws, except for very low doses that solely produce hyperalgesia in the injected paw. This shows that IL-1β influences hyperalgesia both by local effect in the paw as well as by systemic effects. The hyperalgesia in the injected paw could be attenuated by COX inhibitors, suggesting that IL-1β evokes local hyperalgesia via stimulation of COX products as prostaglandins [104]. Intraperitoneal injection of IL-1β induces a generalized hyperalgesia, and one mechanism by which peripheral IL-1β causes a generalized hyperalgesia is via actions on the hepatic vagus nerve that elicit afferent signaling to the brain [18,104].

In mice overexpressing TNF, a rheumatoid arthritis-like disease develops. Treatment with blocking antibodies to IL-1RI prevents the onset of disease [105], indicating a pathophysiologcal role for IL-1RI in an inflammatory disease with pain as one of its hallmarks.

17.9.2.2 Clinical Findings. IL-1β is undetectable in TMJ synovial fluid from healthy individuals, while patients with polyarthritides have significantly higher such concentrations [106]. The IL-1β found in the synovial fluid of the TMJ from patients with inflammatory disorder seems to originate from local production because the correlation between plasma and synovial fluid levels is poor and the synovial fluid level is substantially higher than the plasma level. The synovial fluid level of IL-1β in human knees also shows a poor correlation to the plasma level and has accordingly been found to correlate more with local disease activity, for example, as measured by the Ritchie score (joint tenderness), than with systemic disease activity [107].

High level of IL-1β in the synovial fluid from the arthritic TMJ is associated with resting pain, tenderness to digital palpation, and a decreased pressure pain tolerance [108]. Patients with high synovial fluid IL-1ra and low IL-1β concentrations show a more rapid resolution of arthritis, including pain variables, and the balance between synovial fluid IL-1β and IL-1ra concentrations seems to determine the progression of the inflammatory process [76]. Indeed, high TMJ synovial fluid level of IL-1ra in TMJ synovial fluid has been found to be associated with few or no painful mandibular movements [58]. High level of IL-1ra in TMJ synovial fluid was associated with few or no painful mandibular movements, perhaps due to receptor binding and inhibition of IL-1β [58].

IL-1sRI and IL-1sRII are present in the extracellular matrix and blood both in healthy individuals and in patients with inflammatory disorders. Elevated levels of especially IL-1sRII are found in plasma and synovial fluid of patients with inflammatory joint disease [55]. However, RA patients seropositive for the rheumatoid factor seem to have lower plasma concentrations of IL-1sRII than seronegative patients, indicating a deficient systemic control of the effects of IL-1β [58]. Upregulation of these soluble receptors has anti-inflammatory effects per se [1], but these anti-inflammatory effects are often insufficient to completely inhibit the very strong proinflammatory effects of elevated IL-1β levels, especially during high inflammatory activity.

17.9.3 IL-6

17.9.3.1 Experimental Findings. Sensory neurons express receptors for cytokines including IL-6, and nociceptive effects of peripheral cytokines have been reported in behavioral studies [109]. IL-6 plus IL-6sR induces thermal hyperalgesia on rat skin [110], and IL-6sR alone or in combination with IL-6 was shown to rapidly sensitize cutaneous nociceptors to noxious heat [111], indicating a prompt action of IL-6 on sensory neurons.

IL-6 influences responses of unmyelinated knee joint afferents to mechanical stimulation *in vivo* as the response of C-fibers increases slowly after local application of IL-6 to a normal knee joint. This increase can be prevented by coapplication of sgp130. However, application of sgp130 after establishment of IL-6-induced sensitization does not reverse the enhanced responses. In the inflamed knee, local application of IL-6sR causes an increase in responses to mechanical stimuli, whereas local application of sgp130 does not reduce the response rate. Thus, IL-6 and its receptor signaling are important factors in the generation of mechanical hypersensitivity under arthritic conditions [112].

17.9.3.2 Clinical Findings. IL-6 is found more frequently in the synovial fluid from patients with TMJ pain than in healthy controls, and high IL-6 levels are associated with pain [113]. IL-6 is significantly raised in RA and the plasma level of IL-6 was reduced after systemic administration of infliximab in parallel with a reduction of global joint pain intensity [114]. In an arthroscopic study of TMJ internal derangements, IL-6 showed the closest correlation with the degree of synovitis [93].

IL-6sR has the potential to regulate both local and systemic IL-6-mediated response. For example, IL-6sR is present in plasma of healthy individuals, but elevated levels of this soluble receptor can be observed in numerous disease states [115], and pain in fibromyalgia is associated with high levels of sgp130 and IL-6sR in serum [116].

17.9.4 Prostaglandins

A consistent finding throughout most studies is that prostanoid receptor-deficient mice exhibit normal baseline nociceptive behavior. Responses to acute thermal and mechanical stimulation seem to be more or less indistinguishable from responses in wild-type mice, indicating that prostaglandins are not required for acute nociception and that they do not exert a tonic influence on the nociceptive system [117–119].

Subcutaneous infusion of PGE_1, PGE_2, and PGI_2 causes pronounced hyperalgesia [120,121]. EP receptor-deficient mice show reduced responses in the writhing test [122] and reduced peripheral pain sensitization after subcutaneous injection of mustard oil [118]. However, recent data support involvement of both PGI_2 by IP and PGE_2 by EP1 receptors in pain [123–125]. Indeed, a selective monoclonal antibody against the EP receptor inhibited carageenan-induced paw hyperalgesia in rats to the same extent as indomethacin, further implicating the EP receptor in pain. Prostaglandins elicit a hyperalgesic response to touch by sensitizing the free end of pain neurons in peripheral inflammation. For example, PGE_2 contributes to human visceral pain hypersensitivity via actions on the EP1 receptor [126]. Hyperalgesia induced by

PGE_2 is reduced by about 50% in EP1 receptor-deficient mice, and PGI_2-induced thermal hyperalgesia is completely abolished in mice deficient of the capsaicin or IP receptor [118].

A possible contribution of the EP2, EP3, and EP4 receptor subtypes to peripheral pain sensitization different from that of EP1 is less well characterized. However, the EP3 and EP4 subtypes have been studied to a limited extent. The EP3 receptor, which is coupled to stimulatory G proteins and is predominantly expressed in dorsal root ganglion neurons [127], seems to contribute to peripheral hyperalgesia because proinflammatory agents induce both the expression of COX-2 and of EP3 receptors [117]. The EP4 receptor seems to contribute to chronic inflammation in animal models [128,129], but *in vivo* evidence for a direct involvement in pain sensitization is still missing.

Following partial sciatic nerve ligation, PGE_2 seems to be overproduced in the injured nerve where EP1–EP4 receptors are upregulated [130]. Three weeks after induction of a chronic constriction injury model of neuropathic pain in rats, mechanical hyperalgesia will develop on the operated side and a doubling of EP1 and EP4 expression on infiltrating macrophages and Schwann cells compared to the sham-operated side can be observed. Prostaglandins thus seem to be involved in the pathogenesis of neuropathic pain, and Schwann cells may be involved in the modulation of these mediators in response to nerve injury [131].

Consistent with the existence of only a single IP receptor, the pronociceptive effects of PGI_2 are completely absent in IP –/– mice tested in the mouse writhing test or after subcutaneous injection, supporting an important peripheral contribution of PGI_2 to nociceptive sensitization. Due to the short-lasting writhing test, this effect of PGI_2 should be primarily peripherally mediated [118,119].

Other potential targets of peripheral prostaglandins are tetrodotoxin-resistant Na^+ channels (Nav1.8), which are specifically expressed in primary nociceptors [132]. PGE_2 shifts the voltage dependence of this channel to more hyperpolarized values [133]. Indeed, Nav1.8-deficient mice develop inflammatory hyperalgesia with a certain delay [134], which would be consistent with a contribution of this channel to PGE_2-induced inflammatory pain.

17.10 SPECIFIC ANTAGONISTS THAT TARGET THESE RECEPTORS

17.10.1 Cytokines

There is no clinically available specific antagonist that targets TNF receptors [135]. There are, on the other hand, three TNF antagonists registered today in the United States and in the European Union: infliximab, etanercept, and adalimumab (Table 17.2) for the treatment of RA and other cytokine-related diseases. In addition, there are ongoing clinical trials covering two other TNF blockers: certolizumab pegol (certolizumab) and golimumab (Table 17.2 as

TABLE 17.2. Overview of Pharmacological, Biochemical, and Mechanistic Profiles of Tumor Necrosis Factor (TNF) Antagonists.

	Infliximab	Adalumimab	Golimumab	Certolizumab	Etanercept
Brand name	Remicade	Humira	ND	ND	Enbrel
Class	Monoclonal antibody	Monoclonal antibody	Monoclonal antibody	Monoclonal antibody fragment	Fc fusion protein
Structure	Chimeric mouse/human	Human IgG1	Human IgG1	PEGylated human IgG1 Fab	Human TNFRII
Molecular weight, kDa	150	150	150	95	150
Administration	i.v.	s.c.	s.c.	s.c.	s.c.
Plasma half-life, days	8–10	10–20	7–20	14	4
Specificity	TNF	TNF	TNF	TNF	TNF/LT
TNF ligands	TNF, tmTNF	TNF, tmTNF	TNF, tmTNF	TNF, tmTNF	TNF, tmTNF
TNF neutralization	Strong	Strong	ND	Strong	Strong
tmTNF binding	Strong	Strong	ND	Strong	Moderate
tmTNF neutralization	Strong	Strong	ND	Strong	Moderate
Reverse signaling (cytokine expression)	Strong	Strong	ND	Strong	Weak–moderate

ND, not determined/no data available; IgG, immunoglobulin G; i.v., intravenous; LT, lymphotoxin; PEGylated, polyethylene glycol polymer chained molecules; s.c., subcutaneous; tmTNF, cell-surface-bound transmembrane TNF.

well as http://clinicaltrials.gov/ and http://www.who.int/). However, only very little public knowledge is available regarding the *in vivo* effects of certolizumab and golimumab. These TNF blockers may also initiate reverse signaling through tmTNF with anti-inflammatory effects as a result, but the potential clinical significance for this mechanism is not understood yet.

All these TNF blockers bind TNF with high specificity. An overview of the properties of the TNF antagonists mentioned above is presented in Table 17.2, which illustrates their similarities and differences. Infliximab, adalimumab, and golimumab are full-length, bivalent IgG monoclonal antibodies capable of complement fixation and Fc receptor binding, whereas certolizumab is a monovalent Fab1 antibody fragment covalently linked to polyethylene glycol that lacks effector functions because it has no Fc region. Infliximab is a chimeric protein containing ~25% mouse-derived amino acids and ~75% human-derived amino acids. Certolizumab is a humanized protein containing amino acid sequences derived from a mouse anti-TNF monoclonal antibody. The hinge region of certolizumab is modified and covalently linked to polyethylene glycol to enhance solubility and half-life *in vivo*. Adalimumab and golimumab are fully human monoclonal antibodies. Etanercept is a genetically engineered fusion protein composed of a dimer of the extracellular portions of human TNFRII fused to the Fc portion of human IgG1.

Anakinra, a recombinant version of the endogenous soluble receptor antagonist IL-1ra, is available for treatment of, for example, RA. Anakinra is mildly to moderately effective and is well tolerated in patients with active RA when used as monotherapy or in combination with methotrexate. Inhibiting IL-1 synthesis or activity with the use of anakinra has proved to be an effective approach to treatment of RA, including pain, especially in patients resistant to or with declining treatment effects by infliximab, adalumimab, or etanercept [136].

Regarding IL-6, one molecule in development is tocilizumab, a humanized antihuman IL-6R antibody. Tocilizumab has been shown to compete for both the membrane-bound and the soluble forms of the human IL-6R, thus inhibiting the binding of IL-6 to its receptors and thereby its proinflammatory activity.

17.10.2 Prostaglandins

All prostaglandin receptors are pharmacologically feasible targets, in principle, and for many of them, more or less specific ligands have been developed [68]. Table 17.3 shows examples of such compounds. Most of the conventional compounds exhibit no absolute selectivity [137]. For example, 17-phenyl-PGE_2, which is used as an EP1 agonist in many analyses, binds to EP3 with a better affinity than that to EP1 and to FP with a reasonable affinity as well. The considerable cross-reactivity for these conventional prostaglandin analogues is probably a result of the fact that they have not been selected due to their specific binding assays. Recently, a new generation of compounds that

TABLE 17.3. Degree of Inhibition of PGE_2 and PGI_2 Receptors for Conventional Prostaglandin Analogues and Examples of More Specific Compounds.

	Prostaglandin Receptors				
	EP1	EP2	EP3	EP4	IP
Conventional analogues					
Iloprost	+++	+	+++	+	+++
Carbacyclin	–	+	+++	+	++
17-Phenyl-PGE_2	+++	–	+++	+	–
EP1 antagonist					
ONO-8711	+++	+	+	–	–
ONO-8713	+++	+	+	–	–
EP4 antagonist					
AH23848	–	–	–	++	–
EP agonists					
ONO-AE1-259	–	+++	–	–	–
ONO-AE-248	–	+	+++	+	–
ONO-AE-329	–	+	+	+++	–

Adapted from Narumiya S., Fitzgerald, G.A. (2001). Genetic and pharmacological analysis of prostanoid receptor function. *J Clin Invest* 108:25–30.
–, no inhibition; +/++/+++, mild/moderate/strong inhibition.

are highly selective for each receptor has been reported (Table 17.3). These compounds exert pharmacological actions consistent with the phenotypes of mice deficient in the corresponding receptor [138].

Regarding pain, administration of the EP4 antagonist AH23848 ((4Z)-7-[(rel-1S,2S,5R)-5-((1,1′-biphenyl-4-yl)methoxy)-2-(4-morpholinyl)-3-oxocyclopentyl]-4-heptenoic acid) attenuates inflammation-induced thermal and mechanical behavioral hypersensitivity, without changing basal pain sensitivity. AH23848 also reduces the PGE_2-mediated sensitization of capsaicin-evoked currents in dorsal root ganglion neurons *in vitro*. EP4 may thus be a potential target for pharmacological treatment of inflammatory pain [139].

Mechanically evoked pain is thought to be prostaglandin receptor-mediated to a certain extent. Peripheral administration of the selective EP1 antagonist ONO-8711 inhibits surgical incision-induced mechanical hyperalgesia [140].

17.11 CURRENT OR POTENTIAL TREATMENT OF PAIN

Even today, pain is a major medical problem. There are still therapeutic difficulties in many patients to manage moderate to severe pain, especially chronic pain, despite all available pharmaceutical treatment options. Targeting cytokine or prostaglandin receptors for specific treatment of pain is promising, but this approach is not clinically available today and seems to require substantial development and trial before it may be considered an option. Given that, both the use of receptor agonists and antagonists as well as the administration route may be of importance. It is not unlikely, for example, that gene therapy to enhance the local expression of anti-inflammatory mediators like the decoy receptor IL-1RII will be a future option.

17.11.1 Cytokine Receptors

There is today only one approved treatment with a specific cytokine receptor antagonist for clinical use: anakinra (IL-1ra). However, anakinra is approved for treatment of RA and not for specific treatment of pain, although pain is certainly an important aspect of RA. On the other hand, several anti-TNF drugs such as infliximab, etanercept, and adalimumab are now available for the treatment of RA (Table 17.2) [135]. The clinical efficacy profiles, including reduction of pain, for infliximab, etanercept, and adalimumab, have been extensively reviewed in detail elsewhere (see, e.g., Reference 4]. Infliximab and adalimumab have very similar efficacy profiles and are highly efficacious in RA, psoriasis, psoriatic arthritis, ankylosing spondylitis, and Crohn's disease. Etanercept differs from infliximab and adalimumab primarily in the lack of efficacy of etanercept in granulomatous diseases such as Crohn's disease, Wegener's granulomatosis, and sarcoidosis. In addition, although etanercept has efficacy comparable to infliximab and adalimumab in RA, etanercept may be less efficacious than infliximab or adalimumab in psoriasis.

Despite the revolutionary improvements in RA treatment with the introduction of anticytokine therapy, about a third of the patients do not respond to anticytokine treatment or still experience symptoms from a single or a few joints [141]. This suggests, in turn, a significant influence by non-TNF-modulated inflammatory mechanisms in the nonresponders. Accordingly, more than a third of patients with TMJ pain did not respond to systemic infliximab treatment within 24 weeks, and treatment failure was associated with high circulating levels of IL-1β or rheumatoid factor [142]. Because the major pathology takes place in the synovial tissues, intra-articular administration of cytokine blockers could be a future possibility to obtain recovery of severely affected single joints. Indeed, there are some recent positive reports with single intra-articular infliximab injections in patients with RA or ankylosing spondylitis [143,144]. There is also one case report of the use of multiple intra-articular infliximab injections. In that report, the clinical and radiographic course of TMJ involvement in a patient with severe TMJ symptoms from psoriatic arthritis resistant to both systemic infliximab and intra-articular glucocorticoid was presented. The patient received multiple intra-articular infliximab injections every sixth week for 36 weeks, and the TMJ symptoms improved after the first bilateral intra-articular infliximab injections but even more so after the second set of injections. A considerable improvement remained for the 36 weeks studied [145].

Regarding neurogenic pain, there are some indications that administration of TNF blocker to the site of inflammation or injury may be effective to alleviate pain. A study using multiple perineural injections of etanercept, a dimer of TNFsRII, to treat postamputation pain indicated significant pain reductions in five out of six soldiers with residual limb pain and phantom pain. Residual pain at rest and with activity, phantom limb pain, functional capacity, and psychological well-being were improved after 3 months [146].

An emerging area of interest regarding TNF antagonists focuses on the functional outcomes of their interactions with tmTNF. Current evidence suggests that these drugs have dual functions as antagonists that block tmTNF interactions with TNFRI/TNFRII and as agonists by initiating reverse signaling through tmTNF. Reverse signaling through tmTNF has been shown *in vitro* to induce cytokine suppression and endotoxin resistance, suggesting that a similar mechanism may be operative in RA and in other diseases during TNF antagonist therapy. With regard to their tmTNF antagonist activities, infliximab, adalimumab, and certolizumab seem to have comparable activity when compared directly [147].

Anakinra, that is, recombinant IL-1ra, has been available since 2001 and is indicated for moderately to severely active RA (Table 17.2). A large double-blind, placebo-controlled multicenter phase three trial of IL-1ra in 472 patients with RA has been reported [148]. The patients had active and severe RA and were recruited into a 24-week course of therapy and were divided into a placebo group and into three IL-1ra groups. Three doses of IL-1ra administered subcutaneously were used: 30, 75, and 150 mg/day for 24 weeks. At entry, age, sex, disease duration, and percentage of patients with rheumatoid factor and joint bone erosions were similar in each of the groups. After 24 weeks, 43% of the patients receiving 150 mg/day of IL-1ra met the American College of Rheumatology criteria for response (the primary outcome measure), and a number of clinically relevant improvements were seen in, for example, the number of tender joints and pain score on a visual analog scale.

Short-term clinical trials of tocilizumab, a monoclonal antibody to IL-6R, in RA and in juvenile arthritis have demonstrated acceptable safety and significant efficacy [149,150]. Results from a double-blind randomized and placebo-controlled clinical trial of tocilizumab on 359 RA patients with previously inadequate response to methotrexate showed that infusions of tocilizumab every fourth week produce marked and dose-related improvements in RA disease activity and clinically significant improvement of various pain measures [151].

17.11.2 Prostaglandin Receptors

Highly specific prostaglandin receptor antagonists useful for *in vivo* testing have been lacking for a long time and are in many cases still not available [66]. Prostaglandin receptors are, however, potential targets for novel and potentially better tolerated analgesics.

The clinical potential of selective prostaglandin receptor agonists and antagonists is intriguing, specifically when compared to selective inhibitors of COX-2 or to traditional nonsteroidal anti-inflammatory drugs such as aspirin. Aspirin inhibits both COX isozymes but preferentially targets COX-1 when used in low doses [152]. Low-dose aspirin is effective in the prevention of myocardial infarction and stroke but can still result in gastric toxicity. COX-2 inhibitors like celecoxib theoretically bypass the consequences of inhibiting COX-1-dependent prostanoids relevant to homeostatic functions, such as hemostasis and gastric cytoprotection. However, although COX-2 is typically induced by inflammatory stimuli, its products may also be protective in some tissues or organs. COX-2 appears to be the predominant source of PGI_2 formation by the normal vasculature [122]. In addition to its role as a vasodilator and platelet inhibitor, PGI_2 appears to be important in protecting cardiomyocytes from oxidant stress. Likewise, COX-2 products appear to mediate the late phase of cardiac preconditioning [153]. There are some indications that PGI_2 and PGE_2 are not only the dominant mediators for inflammatory pain but that their inhibition is also responsible for the known side effects of COX inhibitors. Gastrointestinal and cardiovascular side effects are of particular importance, and it cannot be excluded that new unwanted effects could arise from the targeting of a single EP receptor. For example, EP2 receptors exert inhibitory control on the proliferation of lymphocytes. Blockade of EP2 receptors might hence promote the progression of autoimmune diseases. Appropriate levels of PGI_2 synthesis and IP receptors should indeed reduce the risk of unwanted cardiovascular effects, and targeting of a single EP receptor could potentially further reduce unwanted effects including gastrointestinal toxicity. This might, however, be achieved at the expense of reduced analgesic efficacy.

In contrast to deletion of COX-2 or, indeed, both COX isozymes, deletion of prostaglandin receptors, with the exception of EP4, has not been associated with serious problems during development or in the perinatal period, and the mature animals appear normal under physiological conditions. A combination of pharmacological and genetic approaches may be needed to elucidate the different effects of receptor antagonism or of COX inhibition [154].

REFERENCES

1. Dinarello, C.A. (1996). Biologic basis for interleukin-1 in disease. *Blood* 87: 2095–2147.
2. Dinarello, C.A., (2009). Immunological and inflammatory functions of the interleukin-1 family. *Annu Rev Immunol* 27:519–550.
3. Koenders, M.I., Joosten, L.A., van den Berg, W.B. (2006). Potential new targets in arthritis therapy: interleukin (IL)-17 and its relation to tumour necrosis factor and IL-1 in experimental arthritis. *Ann Rheum Dis* 65(Suppl. 3):iii29–iii33.

4. Tracey, D., Klareskog, L., Sasso, E.H., Salfeld, J.G., Tak, P.P. (2008). Tumor necrosis factor antagonist mechanisms of action: a comprehensive review. *Pharmacol Ther* 117:244–279.
5. Schutze, S., Machleidt, T., Kronke, M. (1992). Mechanisms of tumor necrosis factor action. *Semin Oncol* 19:16–24.
6. Jouvenne, P., Vannier, E., Dinarello, C.A., Miossec, P. (1998). Elevated levels of soluble interleukin-1 receptor type II and interleukin-1 receptor antagonist in patients with chronic arthritis: correlations with markers of inflammation and joint destruction. *Arthritis Rheum* 41:1083–1089.
7. Kopp, S., Sommer, C. (2007). Inflammatory mediators in temporomandibular joint pain. In: Türp, J.C., Sommer, C., Hugger, A (eds). *The Puzzle of Orofacial Pain. Integrating Research into Clinical Management*. Vol. 15. Basel: Karger, pp. 28–43.
8. Watkins, L.R., Maier, S.F., Goehler, L.E. (1995). Immune activation: the role of pro-inflammatory cytokines in inflammation, illness responses and pathological pain states. *Pain* 63:289–302.
9. DeLeo, J.A., Colburn, R.W., Nichols, M., Malhotra, A. (1996). Interleukin-6-mediated hyperalgesia/allodynia and increased spinal IL-6 expression in a rat mononeuropathy model. *J Interferon Cytokine Res* 16:695–700.
10. DeLeo, J.A., Colburn, R.W., Rickman, A.J. (1997). Cytokine and growth factor immunohistochemical spinal profiles in two animal models of mononeuropathy. *Brain Res* 759:50–57.
11. Hart, B.L. (1988). Biological basis of the behavior of sick animals. *Neurosci Biobehav Rev* 12:123–137.
12. Kent, S., Bluthe, R.M., Kelley, K.W., Dantzer, R. (1992). Sickness behavior as a new target for drug development. *Trends Pharmacol Sci* 13:24–28.
13. Maier, S.F., Wiertelak, E.P., Martin, D., Watkins, L.R. (1993). Interleukin-1 mediates the behavioral hyperalgesia produced by lithium chloride and endotoxin. *Brain Res* 623:321–324.
14. Ban, E., Haour, F., Lenstra, R. (1992). Brain interleukin 1 gene expression induced by peripheral lipopolysaccharide administration. *Cytokine* 4:48–54.
15. Gatti, S., Bartfai, T. (1993). Induction of tumor necrosis factor-alpha mRNA in the brain after peripheral endotoxin treatment: comparison with interleukin-1 family and interleukin-6. *Brain Res* 624:291–294.
16. Laye, S., Bluthe, R.M., Kent, S., Combe, C., Medina, C., Parnet, P., Kelley, K., Dantzer, R. (1995). Subdiaphragmatic vagotomy blocks induction of IL-1 beta mRNA in mice brain in response to peripheral LPS. *Am J Physiol* 268: R1327–R1331.
17. Watkins, L.R., Wiertelak, E.P., Goehler, L.E., Smith, K.P., Martin, D., Maier, S.F. (1994). Characterization of cytokine-induced hyperalgesia. *Brain Res* 654:15–26.
18. Tracey, K.J. (2007). Physiology and immunology of the cholinergic antiinflammatory pathway. *J Clin Invest* 117:289–296.
19. Hansen, M.K., O'Connor, K.A., Goehler, L.E., Watkins, L.R., Maier, S.F. (2001). The contribution of the vagus nerve in interleukin-1beta-induced fever is dependent on dose. *Am J Physiol* 280:R929–R934.
20. Tracey, K.J. (2002). The inflammatory reflex. *Nature* 420:853–859.

21. Huston, J.M., Ochani, M., Rosas-Ballina, M., Liao, H., Ochani, K., Pavlov, V.A., Gallowitsch-Puerta, M., Ashok, M., Czura, C.J., Foxwell, B., Tracey, K.J., Ulloa, L. (2006). Splenectomy inactivates the cholinergic antiinflammatory pathway during lethal endotoxemia and polymicrobial sepsis. *J Exp Med* 203:1623–1628.

22. Bernik, T.R., Friedman, S.G., Ochani, M., DiRaimo, R., Susarla, S., Czura, C.J., Tracey, K.J. (2002). Cholinergic antiinflammatory pathway inhibition of tumor necrosis factor during ischemia reperfusion. *J Vasc Surg* 36:1231–1236.

23. De Jonge, W.J., The, F.O., van der Zanden, E.P., van den Wijngaard, R.M., Boeckxstaens, G.E. (2005). Inflammation and gut motility; neural control of intestinal immune cell activation. *J Pediatr Gastroenterol Nutr* 41(Suppl. 1):S10–S11 .

24. Wang, H., Yu, M., Ochani, M., Amella, C.A., Tanovic, M., Susarla, S., Li, J.H., Wang, H., Yang, H., Ulloa, L., Al-Abed, Y., Czura, C.J., Tracey, K.J. (2003). Nicotinic acetylcholine receptor alpha7 subunit is an essential regulator of inflammation. *Nature* 421:384–388.

25. van Westerloo, D.J., Giebelen, I.A., Florquin, S., Bruno, M.J., Larosa, G.J., Ulloa, L., Tracey, K.J., van der Poll, T. (2006). The vagus nerve and nicotinic receptors modulate experimental pancreatitis severity in mice. *Gastroenterology* 130: 1822–1830.

26. Saeed, R.W., Varma, S., Peng-Nemeroff, T., Sherry, B., Balakhaneh, D., Huston, J., Tracey, K.J., Al-Abed, Y., Metz, C.N. (2005). Cholinergic stimulation blocks endothelial cell activation and leukocyte recruitment during inflammation. *J Exp Med* 201:1113–1123.

27. Borovikova, L.V., Ivanova, S., Zhang, M., Yang, H., Botchkina, G.I., Watkins, L.R., Wang, H., Abumrad, N., Eaton, J.W., Tracey, K.J. (2000). Vagus nerve stimulation attenuates the systemic inflammatory response to endotoxin. *Nature* 405: 458–462.

28. Wang, H., Liao, H., Ochani, M., Justiniani, M., Lin, X., Yang, L., Al-Abed, Y., Wang, H., Metz, C., Miller, E.J., Tracey, K.J., Ulloa, L. (2004). Cholinergic agonists inhibit HMGB1 release and improve survival in experimental sepsis. *Nat Med* 10:1216–1221.

29. Funk, C.D. (2001). Prostaglandins and leukotrienes: advances in eicosanoid biology. *Science* 294:1871–1875.

30. Feldmann, M., Brennan, F.M., Williams, R.O., Cope, A.P., Gibbons, D.L., Katsikis, P.D., Maini, R.N. (1992). Evaluation of the role of cytokines in autoimmune disease: the importance of TNF alpha in rheumatoid arthritis. *Prog Growth Factor Res* 4:247–255.

31. Darnay, B.G., Aggarwal, B.B. (1999). Signal transduction by tumour necrosis factor and tumour necrosis factor related ligands and their receptors. *Ann Rheum Dis* 58(Suppl. 1):I2–I13.

32. Schafers, M., Sorkin, L.S., Geis, C., Shubayev, V.I. (2003). Spinal nerve ligation induces transient upregulation of tumor necrosis factor receptors 1 and 2 in injured and adjacent uninjured dorsal root ganglia in the rat. *Neurosci Lett* 347:179–182.

33. Sommer, C., Kress, M. (2004). Recent findings on how proinflammatory cytokines cause pain: peripheral mechanisms in inflammatory and neuropathic hyperalgesia. *Neurosci Lett* 361:184–187.

34. Aggarwal, B.B., Natarajan, K. (1996). Tumor necrosis factors: developments during the last decade. *Eur Cytokine Netw* 7:93–124.

35. Smookler, D.S., Mohammed, F.F., Kassiri, Z., Duncan, G.S., Mak, T.W., Khokha, R. (2006). Tissue inhibitor of metalloproteinase 3 regulates TNF-dependent systemic inflammation. *J Immunol* 176:721–725.

36. Aggarwal, B.B., Samanta, A., Feldmann, M. (2000). TNF Receptors. In: Oppenheim, J.J., Feldmann, M., Durum, S.K., Hirano, T., Vilcek, J., Nicola, N.A. (eds.). *Cytokine Reference*. Burlington, MA: Academic Press, pp. 1619–1632.

37. Engelmann, H., Aderka, D., Rubinstein, M., Rotman, D., Wallach, D. (1989). A tumor necrosis factor-binding protein purified to homogeneity from human urine protects cells from tumor necrosis factor toxicity. *J Biol Chem* 264: 11974–11980.

38. Alstergren, P., Kopp, S. (2006). Insufficient endogenous control of tumor necrosis factor-alpha contributes to temporomandibular joint pain and tissue destruction in rheumatoid arthritis. *J Rheumatol* 33:1734–1739.

39. Moreland, L.W., Schiff, M.H., Baumgartner, S.W., Tindall, E.A., Fleischmann, R.M., Bulpitt, K.J., Weaver, A.L., Keystone, E.C., Furst, D.E., Mease, P.J., Ruderman, E.M., Horwitz, D.A., Arkfeld, D.G., Garrison, L., Burge, D.J., Blosch, C.M., Lange, M.L., McDonnell, N.D., Weinblatt, M.E. (1999). Etanercept therapy in rheumatoid arthritis. A randomized, controlled trial. *Ann Intern Med* 130:478–486.

40. Weinblatt, M.E., Kremer, J.M., Bankhurst, A.D., Bulpitt, K.J., Fleischmann, R.M., Fox, R.I., Jackson, C.G., Lange, M., Burge, D.J. (1999). A trial of etanercept, a recombinant tumor necrosis factor receptor: Fc fusion protein, in patients with rheumatoid arthritis receiving methotrexate. *N Engl J Med* 340:253–259.

41. Grell, M., Wajant, H., Zimmermann, G., Scheurich, P. (1998). The type 1 receptor (CD120a) is the high-affinity receptor for soluble tumor necrosis factor. *Proc Natl Acad Sci U S A* 95:570–575.

42. Ksontini, R., MacKay, S.L., Moldawer, L.L. (1998). Revisiting the role of tumor necrosis factor alpha and the response to surgical injury and inflammation. *Arch Surg* 133:558–567.

43. Eissner, G., Kirchner, S., Lindner, H., Kolch, W., Janosch, P., Grell, M., Scheurich, P., Andreesen, R., Holler, E. (2000). Reverse signaling through transmembrane TNF confers resistance to lipopolysaccharide in human monocytes and macrophages. *J Immunol* 164:6193–6198.

44. Harashima, S., Horiuchi, T., Hatta, N., Morita, C., Higuchi, M., Sawabe, T., Tsukamoto, H., Tahira, T., Hayashi, K., Fujita, S., Niho, Y. (2001). Outside-to-inside signal through the membrane TNF-alpha induces E-selectin (CD62E) expression on activated human CD4+ T cells. *J Immunol* 166:130–136.

45. Eissner, G., Kolch, W., Scheurich, P. (2004). Ligands working as receptors: reverse signaling by members of the TNF superfamily enhance the plasticity of the immune system. *Cytokine Growth Factor Rev* 15:353–366.

46. Dinarello, C.A. (1994). The biological properties of interleukin-1. *Eur Cytokine Netw* 5:517–531.

47. Ruschen, S., Lemm, G., Warnatz, H. (1989). Spontaneous and LPS-stimulated production of intracellular IL-1 beta by synovial macrophages in rheumatoid arthritis is inhibited by IFN-gamma. *Clin Exp Immunol* 76:246–251.

48. Barbe, M.F., Barr, A.E. (2006). Inflammation and the pathophysiology of work-related musculoskeletal disorders. *Brain Behav Immun* 20:423–429.
49. Gay, N.J., Keith, F.J. (1991). Drosophila Toll and IL-1 receptor. *Nature* 351: 355–356.
50. Shirakawa, F., Tanaka, Y., Ota, T., Suzuki, H., Eto, S., Yamashita, U. (1987). Expression of interleukin 1 receptors on human peripheral T cells. *J Immunol* 138:4243–4248.
51. Muegge, K., Williams, T.M., Kant, J., Karin, M., Chiu, R., Schmidt, A., Siebenlist, U., Young, H.A., Durum, S.K. (1989). Interleukin-1 costimulatory activity on the interleukin-2 promoter via AP-1. *Science* 246:249–251.
52. Muegge, K., Vila, M., Gusella, G.L., Musso, T., Herrlich, P., Stein, B., Durum, S.K. (1993). Interleukin 1 induction of the c-jun promoter. *Proc Natl Acad Sci U S A* 90:7054–7058.
53. Horai, R., Asano, M., Sudo, K., Kanuka, H., Suzuki, M., Nishihara, M., Takahashi, M., Iwakura, Y. (1998). Production of mice deficient in genes for interleukin (IL)-1alpha, IL-1beta, IL-1alpha/beta, and IL-1 receptor antagonist shows that IL-1beta is crucial in turpentine-induced fever development and glucocorticoid secretion. *J Exp Med* 187:1463–1475.
54. Zheng, H., Fletcher, D., Kozak, W., Jiang, M., Hofmann, K.J., Conn, C.A., Soszynski, D., Grabiec, C., Trumbauer, M.E., Shaw, A. (1995). Resistance to fever induction and impaired acute-phase response in interleukin-1 beta-deficient mice. *Immunity* 3:9–19.
55. Arend, W.P., Malyak, M., Smith, M.F., Jr., Whisenand, T.D., Slack, J.L., Sims, J.E., Giri, J.G., Dower, S.K. (1994). Binding of IL-1 alpha, IL-1 beta, and IL-1 receptor antagonist by soluble IL-1 receptors and levels of soluble IL-1 receptors in synovial fluids. *J Immunol* 153:4766–4774.
56. Dower, S.K., Fanslow, W., Jacobs, C., Waugh, S., Sims, J.E., Widmer, M.B. (1994). Interleukin-I antagonists. *Ther Immunol* 1:113–122.
57. Jakobsson, P.J., Thoren, S., Morgenstern, R., Samuelsson, B. (1999). Identification of human prostaglandin E synthase: a microsomal, glutathione-dependent, inducible enzyme, constituting a potential novel drug target. *Proc Natl Acad Sci U S A* 96:7220–7225.
58. Alstergren, P., Benavente, C., Kopp, S. (2003). Interleukin-1beta, interleukin-1 receptor antagonist, and interleukin-1 soluble receptor II in temporomandibular joint synovial fluid from patients with chronic polyarthritides. *J Oral Maxillofac Surg* 61:1171–1178.
59. Giri, J.G., Newton, R.C., Horuk, R. (1990). Identification of soluble interleukin-1 binding protein in cell-free supernatants. Evidence for soluble interleukin-1 receptor. *J Biol Chem* 265:17416–17419.
60. Penton-Rol, G., Orlando, S., Polentarutti, N., Bernasconi, S., Muzio, M., Introna, M., Mantovani, A. (1999). Bacterial lipopolysaccharide causes rapid shedding, followed by inhibition of mRNA expression, of the IL-1 type II receptor, with concomitant up-regulation of the type I receptor and induction of incompletely spliced transcripts. *J Immunol* 162:2931–2938.
61. Greenfeder, S.A., Nunes, P., Kwee, L., Labow, M., Chizzonite, R.A., Ju, G. (1995). Molecular cloning and characterization of a second subunit of the interleukin 1 receptor complex. *J Biol Chem* 270:13757–13765.

62. Matsuda, T., Hirano, T. (2000). IL-6. In: Oppenheim, J.J., Feldmann, M., Durum, S. C., Hirano, T., Vilcek, J., Nicola, N.A. (eds.). *Cytokine Reference*. Burlington, MA: Academic Press, pp. 537–563.
63. Jones, S.A., Rose-John, S. (2002). The role of soluble receptors in cytokine biology: the agonistic properties of the sIL-6R/IL-6 complex. *Biochim Biophys Acta* 1592:251–263.
64. Hirano, T., Fukada, T. (2000). IL-6 ligand and receptor family. In: Oppenheim, J.J., Feldmann, M., Durum, S.C., Hirano, T., Vilcek, J., Nicola, N.A. (eds.). *Cytokine Reference*. Burlington, MA: Academic Press, pp. 523–535.
65. Smith, W.L., DeWitt, D.L., Garavito, R.M. (2000). Cyclooxygenases: structural, cellular, and molecular biology. *Annu Rev Biochem* 69:145–182.
66. Zeilhofer, H.U. (2007). Prostanoids in nociception and pain. *Biochem Pharmacol* 73:165–174.
67. Schuster, V.L. (1998). Molecular mechanisms of prostaglandin transport. *Annu Rev Physiol* 60:221–242.
68. Narumiya, S., FitzGerald, G.A. (2001). Genetic and pharmacological analysis of prostanoid receptor function. *J Clin Invest* 108:25–30.
69. Bhattacharya, M., Peri, K.G., Almazan, G., Ribeiro-da-Silva, A., Shichi, H., Durocher, Y., Abramovitz, M., Hou, X., Varma, D.R., Chemtob, S. (1998). Nuclear localization of prostaglandin E2 receptors. *Proc Natl Acad Sci U S A* 95: 15792–15797.
70. Hirai, H., Tanaka, K., Yoshie, O., Ogawa, K., Kenmotsu, K., Takamori, Y., Ichimasa, M., Sugamura, K., Nakamura, M., Takano, S., Nagata, K. (2001). Prostaglandin D2 selectively induces chemotaxis in T helper type 2 cells, eosinophils, and basophils via seven-transmembrane receptor CRTH2. *J Exp Med* 193:255–261.
71. Monneret, G., Gravel, S., Diamond, M., Rokach, J., Powell, W.S. (2001). Prostaglandin D2 is a potent chemoattractant for human eosinophils that acts via a novel DP receptor. *Blood* 98:1942–1948.
72. Okuse, K. (2007). Pain signalling pathways: from cytokines to ion channels. *Int J Biochem Cell Biol* 39:490–496.
73. Cunha, F.Q., Poole, S., Lorenzetti, B.B., Ferreira, S.H. (1992). The pivotal role of tumour necrosis factor alpha in the development of inflammatory hyperalgesia. *Br J Pharmacol* 107:660–664.
74. Junger, H., Sorkin, L.S. (2000). Nociceptive and inflammatory effects of subcutaneous TNFalpha. *Pain* 85:145–151.
75. Sorkin, L.S., Xiao, W.H., Wagner, R., Myers, R.R. (1997). Tumour necrosis factor-alpha induces ectopic activity in nociceptive primary afferent fibres. *Neuroscience* 81:255–262.
76. Cunha, T.M., Verri, W.A., Jr., Silva, J.S., Poole, S., Cunha, F.Q., Ferreira, S.H. (2005). A cascade of cytokines mediates mechanical inflammatory hypernociception in mice. *Proc Natl Acad Sci U S A* 102:1755–1760.
77. Inglis, J.J., Nissim, A., Lees, D.M., Hunt, S.P., Chernajovsky, Y., Kidd, B.L. (2005). The differential contribution of tumour necrosis factor to thermal and mechanical hyperalgesia during chronic inflammation. *Arthritis Res Ther* 7:R807–R816.
78. Schafers, M., Svensson, C.I., Sommer, C., Sorkin, L.S. (2003). Tumor necrosis factor-alpha induces mechanical allodynia after spinal nerve ligation by activation of p38 MAPK in primary sensory neurons. *J Neurosci* 23:2517–2521.

79. Sommer, C., Schmidt, C., George, A. (1998). Hyperalgesia in experimental neuropathy is dependent on the TNF receptor 1. *Exp Neurol* 151:138–142.
80. Li, Y., Ji, A., Weihe, E., Schafer, M.K. (2004). Cell-specific expression and lipopolysaccharide-induced regulation of tumor necrosis factor alpha (TNFalpha) and TNF receptors in rat dorsal root ganglion. *J Neurosci* 24:9623–9631.
81. Pollock, J., McFarlane, S.M., Connell, M.C., Zehavi, U., Vandenabeele, P., MacEwan, D.J., Scott, R.H. (2002). TNF-alpha receptors simultaneously activate Ca^{2+} mobilisation and stress kinases in cultured sensory neurones. *Neuropharmacology* 42:93–106.
82. Myers, R.R., Wagner, R., Sorkin, L.S. (1999). Hyperalgesic actions of cytokines on peripheral nerves. In: Watkins, L.R., Maier, S.F. (eds.). *Cytokines and Pain*. Basel: Birkhäuser Verlag, pp. 133–157.
83. Vogel, C., Stallforth, S., Sommer, C. (2006). Altered pain behavior and regeneration after nerve injury in TNF receptor deficient mice. *J Peripher Nerv Syst* 11:294–303.
84. Sommer, C., Lindenlaub, T., Teuteberg, P., Schafers, M., Hartung, T., Toyka, K.V. (2001). Anti-TNF-neutralizing antibodies reduce pain-related behavior in two different mouse models of painful mononeuropathy. *Brain Res* 913:86–89.
85. Sommer, C., Schafers, M., Marziniak, M., Toyka, K.V. (2001). Etanercept reduces hyperalgesia in experimental painful neuropathy. *J Peripher Nerv Syst* 6:67–72.
86. Shubayev, V.I., Myers, R.R. (2000). Upregulation and interaction of TNFalpha and gelatinases A and B in painful peripheral nerve injury. *Brain Res* 855:83–89.
87. Schafers, M., Lee, D.H., Brors, D., Yaksh, T.L., Sorkin, L.S. (2003). Increased sensitivity of injured and adjacent uninjured rat primary sensory neurons to exogenous tumor necrosis factor-alpha after spinal nerve ligation. *J Neurosci* 23:3028–3038.
88. George, A., Buehl, A., Sommer, C. (2005). Tumor necrosis factor receptor 1 and 2 proteins are differentially regulated during Wallerian degeneration of mouse sciatic nerve. *Exp Neurol* 192:163–166.
89. Bhushan, M., Cumberbatch, M., Dearman, R.J., Andrew, S.M., Kimber, I., Griffiths, C.E. (2002). Tumour necrosis factor-alpha-induced migration of human Langerhans cells: the influence of ageing. *Br J Dermatol* 146:32–40.
90. Fredriksson, L., Alstergren, P., Kopp, S. (2006). Tumor necrosis factor-alpha in temporomandibular joint synovial fluid predicts treatment effects on pain by intra-articular glucocorticoid treatment. *Mediators Inflamm* 2006(6):1–7.
91. Partsch, G., Steiner, G., Leeb, B.F., Dunky, A., Broll, H., Smolen, J.S. (1997). Highly increased levels of tumor necrosis factor-alpha and other proinflammatory cytokines in psoriatic arthritis synovial fluid. *J Rheumatol* 24:518–523.
92. Nordahl, S., Alstergren, P., Kopp, S. (2000). Tumor necrosis factor-alpha in synovial fluid and plasma from patients with chronic connective tissue disease and its relation to temporomandibular joint pain. *J Oral Maxillofac Surg* 58:525–530.
93. Sandler, N.A., Buckley, M.J., Cillo, J.E., Braun, T.W. (1998). Correlation of inflammatory cytokines with arthroscopic findings in patients with temporomandibular joint internal derangements. *J Oral Maxillofac Surg* 56:534–43; discussion 543–544.
94. Takahashi, T., Kondoh, T., Fukuda, M., Yamazaki, Y., Toyosaki, T., Suzuki, R. (1998). Proinflammatory cytokines detectable in synovial fluids from patients with

temporomandibular disorders. *Oral Surg Oral Med Oral Pathol Oral Radiol Endod* 85:135–141.

95. Roux-Lombard, P., Punzi, L., Hasler, F., Bas, S., Todesco, S., Gallati, H., Guerne, P.A., Dayer, J.M. (1993). Soluble tumor necrosis factor receptors in human inflammatory synovial fluids. *Arthritis Rheum* 36:485–489.
96. Deleuran, B.W., Chu, C.Q., Field, M., Brennan, F.M., Mitchell, T., Feldmann, M., Maini, R.N. (1992). Localization of tumor necrosis factor receptors in the synovial tissue and cartilage-pannus junction in patients with rheumatoid arthritis. Implications for local actions of tumor necrosis factor alpha. *Arthritis Rheum* 35:1170–1178.
97. Lundberg, I.E. (2000). The role of cytokines, chemokines, and adhesion molecules in the pathogenesis of idiopathic inflammatory myopathies. *Curr Rheumatol Rep* 2:216–224.
98. Wallace, D.J., Linker-Israeli, M., Hallegua, D., Silverman, S., Silver, D., Weisman, M.H. (2001). Cytokines play an aetiopathogenetic role in fibromyalgia: a hypothesis and pilot study. *Rheumatology (Oxford)* 40:743–749.
99. Shah, J.P., Phillips, T.M., Danoff, J.V., Gerber, L.H. (2005). An in vivo microanalytical technique for measuring the local biochemical milieu of human skeletal muscle. *J Appl Physiol* 99:1977–1984.
100. Carp, S.J., Barbe, M.F., Winter, K.A., Amin, M., Barr, A.E. (2007). Inflammatory biomarkers increase with severity of upper-extremity overuse disorders. *Clin Sci (Lond)* 112:305–314.
101. Rice, T.L., Chantler, I., Loram, L.C. (2007). Neutralization of muscle tumour necrosis factor alpha does not attenuate exercise-induced muscle pain but does improve muscle strength in healthy male volunteers. *Br J Sports Med* 42:758–762.
102. Fukuoka, H., Kawatani, M., Hisamitsu, T., Takeshige, C. (1994). Cutaneous hyperalgesia induced by peripheral injection of interleukin-1 beta in the rat. *Brain Res* 657:133–140.
103. Jeanjean, A.P., Moussaoui, S.M., Maloteaux, J.M., Laduron, P.M. (1995). Interleukin-1 beta induces long-term increase of axonally transported opiate receptors and substance P. *Neuroscience* 68:151–157.
104. Ferreira, S.H., Lorenzetti, B.B., Bristow, A.F., Poole, S. (1988). Interleukin-1 beta as a potent hyperalgesic agent antagonized by a tripeptide analogue. *Nature* 334:698–700.
105. Probert, L., Plows, D., Kontogeorgos, G., Kollias, G. (1995). The type I interleukin-1 receptor acts in series with tumor necrosis factor (TNF) to induce arthritis in TNF-transgenic mice. *Eur J Immunol* 25:1794–1797.
106. Alstergren, P., Kopp, S., Theodorsson, E. (1999). Synovial fluid sampling from the temporomandibular joint: sample quality criteria and levels of interleukin-1 beta and serotonin. *Acta Odontol Scand* 57:16–22.
107. Rooney, M., Symons, J.A., Duff, G.W. (1990). Interleukin 1 beta in synovial fluid is related to local disease activity in rheumatoid arthritis. *Rheumatol Int* 10:217–219.
108. Alstergren, P., Ernberg, M., Kvarnstrom, M., Kopp, S. (1998). Interleukin-1beta in synovial fluid from the arthritic temporomandibular joint and its relation to pain, mobility, and anterior open bite. *J Oral Maxillofac Surg* 56:1059–1065; discussion 1066.

109. Chichorro, J.G., Lorenzetti, B.B., Zampronio, A.R. (2004). Involvement of bradykinin, cytokines, sympathetic amines and prostaglandins in formalin-induced orofacial nociception in rats. *Br J Pharmacol* 141:1175–1184.

110. Obreja, O., Biasio, W., Andratsch, M., Lips, K.S., Rathee, P.K., Ludwig, A., Rose-John, S., Kress, M. (2005). Fast modulation of heat-activated ionic current by proinflammatory interleukin 6 in rat sensory neurons. *Brain* 128:1634–1641.

111. Obreja, O., Schmelz, M., Poole, S., Kress, M. (2002). Interleukin-6 in combination with its soluble IL-6 receptor sensitises rat skin nociceptors to heat, in vivo. *Pain* 96:57–62.

112. Brenn, D., Richter, F., Schaible, H.G. (2007). Sensitization of unmyelinated sensory fibers of the joint nerve to mechanical stimuli by interleukin-6 in the rat: an inflammatory mechanism of joint pain. *Arthritis Rheum* 56:351–359.

113. Shinoda, C., Takaku, S. (2000). Interleukin-1 beta, interleukin-6, and tissue inhibitor of metalloproteinase-1 in the synovial fluid of the temporomandibular joint with respect to cartilage destruction. *Oral Dis* 6:383–390.

114. Kopp, S., Alstergren, P., Ernestam, S., Nordahl, S., Morin, P., Bratt, J. (2005). Reduction of temporomandibular joint pain after treatment with a combination of methotrexate and infliximab is associated with changes in synovial fluid and plasma cytokines in rheumatoid arthritis. *Cells Tissues Organs* 180:22–30.

115. Scheller, J., Rose-John, S. (2006). Interleukin-6 and its receptor: from bench to bedside. *Med Microbiol Immunol* 195:173–183.

116. Maes, M., Libbrecht, I., Van Hunsel, F., Lin, A.H., De Clerck, L., Stevens, W., Kenis, G., de Jongh, R., Bosmans, E., Neels, H. (1999). The immune-inflammatory pathophysiology of fibromyalgia: increased serum soluble gp130, the common signal transducer protein of various neurotrophic cytokines. *Psychoneuroendocrinology* 24:371–383.

117. Reinold, H., Ahmadi, S., Depner, U.B., Layh, B., Heindl, C., Hamza, M., Pahl, A., Brune, K., Narumiya, S., Muller, U., Zeilhofer, H.U. (2005). Spinal inflammatory hyperalgesia is mediated by prostaglandin E receptors of the EP2 subtype. *J Clin Invest* 115:673–679.

118. Moriyama, T., Higashi, T., Togashi, K., Iida, T., Segi, E., Sugimoto, Y., Tominaga, T., Narumiya, S., Tominaga, M. (2005). Sensitization of TRPV1 by EP1 and IP reveals peripheral nociceptive mechanism of prostaglandins. *Mol Pain*. Available at http://www.molecularpain.com/content/1/1/3.

119. Murata, T., Ushikubi, F., Matsuoka, T., Hirata, M., Yamasaki, A., Sugimoto, Y., Ichikawa, A., Aze, Y., Tanaka, T., Yoshida, N., Ueno, A., Oh-ishi, S., Narumiya, S. (1997). Altered pain perception and inflammatory response in mice lacking prostacyclin receptor. *Nature* 388:678–682.

120. Ferreira, S.H. (1986). Prostaglandins, pain, and inflammation. *Agents Actions Suppl* 19:91–98.

121. Ferreira, S.H., Lorenzetti, B.B. (1996). Intrathecal administration of prostaglandin E2 causes sensitization of the primary afferent neuron via the spinal release of glutamate. *Inflamm Res* 45:499–502.

122. Stock, J.L., Shinjo, K., Burkhardt, J., Roach, M., Taniguchi, K., Ishikawa, T., Kim, H.S., Flannery, P.J., Coffman, T.M., McNeish, J.D., Audoly, L.P. (2001). The prostaglandin E2 EP1 receptor mediates pain perception and regulates blood pressure. *J Clin Invest* 107:325–331.

123. Narumiya, S., Sugimoto, Y., Ushikubi, F. (1999). Prostanoid receptors: structures, properties, and functions. *Physiol Rev* 79:1193–1226.

124. Nguyen, M., Camenisch, T., Snouwaert, J.N., Hicks, E., Coffman, T.M., Anderson, P.A., Malouf, N.N., Koller, B.H. (1997). The prostaglandin receptor EP4 triggers remodelling of the cardiovascular system at birth. *Nature* 390:78–81.

125. Vasquez, E., Bar, K.J., Ebersberger, A., Klein, B., Vanegas, H., Schaible, H.G. (2001). Spinal prostaglandins are involved in the development but not the maintenance of inflammation-induced spinal hyperexcitability. *J Neurosci* 21: 9001–9008.

126. Sarkar, S., Hobson, A.R., Hughes, A., Growcott, J., Woolf, C.J., Thompson, D.G., Aziz, Q. (2003). The prostaglandin E2 receptor-1 (EP-1) mediates acid-induced visceral pain hypersensitivity in humans. *Gastroenterology* 124:18–25.

127. Southall, M.D., Vasko, M.R. (2001). Prostaglandin receptor subtypes, EP3C and EP4, mediate the prostaglandin E2-induced cAMP production and sensitization of sensory neurons. *J Biol Chem* 276:16083–16091.

128. McCoy, J.M., Wicks, J.R., Audoly, L.P. (2002). The role of prostaglandin E2 receptors in the pathogenesis of rheumatoid arthritis. *J Clin Invest* 110:651–658.

129. Honda, T., Segi-Nishida, E., Miyachi, Y., Narumiya, S. (2006). Prostacyclin-IP signaling and prostaglandin E2-EP2/EP4 signaling both mediate joint inflammation in mouse collagen-induced arthritis. *J Exp Med* 203:325–335.

130. Ma, W., Eisenach, J.C. (2003). Intraplantar injection of a cyclooxygenase inhibitor ketorolac reduces immunoreactivities of substance P, calcitonin gene-related peptide, and dynorphin in the dorsal horn of rats with nerve injury or inflammation. *Neuroscience* 121:681–690.

131. Woodhams, P.L., MacDonald, R.E., Collins, S.D., Chessell, I.P., Day, N.C. (2007). Localisation and modulation of prostanoid receptors EP1 and EP4 in the rat chronic constriction injury model of neuropathic pain. *Eur J Pain* 11:605–613.

132. Akopian, A.N., Souslova, V., England, S., Okuse, K., Ogata, N., Ure, J., Smith, A., Kerr, B.J., McMahon, S.B., Boyce, S., Hill, R., Stanfa, L.C., Dickenson, A.H., Wood, J.N. (1999). The tetrodotoxin-resistant sodium channel SNS has a specialized function in pain pathways. *Nat Neurosci* 2:541–548.

133. Gold, M.S., Reichling, D.B., Shuster, M.J., Levine, J.D. (1996). Hyperalgesic agents increase a tetrodotoxin-resistant Na^+ current in nociceptors. *Proc Natl Acad Sci U S A* 93:1108–1112.

134. Kerr, B.J., Souslova, V., McMahon, S.B., Wood, J.N. (2001). A role for the TTX-resistant sodium channel Nav 1.8 in NGF-induced hyperalgesia, but not neuropathic pain. *Neuroreport* 12:3077–3080.

135. Nash, P.T., Florin, T.H. (2005). Tumour necrosis factor inhibitors. *Med J Aust* 183:205–208.

136. Furst, D.E. (2004). Anakinra: review of recombinant human interleukin-I receptor antagonist in the treatment of rheumatoid arthritis. *Clin Ther* 26:1960–1975.

137. Kiriyama, M., Ushikubi, F., Kobayashi, T., Hirata, M., Sugimoto, Y., Narumiya, S. (1997). Ligand binding specificities of the eight types and subtypes of the mouse prostanoid receptors expressed in Chinese hamster ovary cells. *Br J Pharmacol* 122:217–224.

138. Shinomiya, S., Naraba, H., Ueno, A., Utsunomiya, I., Maruyama, T., Ohuchida, S., Ushikubi, F., Yuki, K., Narumiya, S., Sugimoto, Y., Ichikawa, A., Oh-ishi, S. (2001).

Regulation of TNFalpha and interleukin-10 production by prostaglandins I(2) and E(2): studies with prostaglandin receptor-deficient mice and prostaglandin E-receptor subtype-selective synthetic agonists. *Biochem Pharmacol* 61:1153–1160.

139. Lin, C.R., Amaya, F., Barrett, L., Wang, H., Takada, J., Samad, T.A., Woolf, C.J. (2006). Prostaglandin E2 receptor EP4 contributes to inflammatory pain hypersensitivity. *J Pharmacol Exp Ther* 319:1096–1103.
140. Omote, K., Kawamata, T., Nakayama, Y., Kawamata, M., Hazama, K., Namiki, A. (2001). The effects of peripheral administration of a novel selective antagonist for prostaglandin E receptor subtype EP(1), ONO-8711, in a rat model of postoperative pain. *Anesth Analg* 92:233–238.
141. Maini, R.N., Taylor, P.C. (2000). Anti-cytokine therapy for rheumatoid arthritis. *Annu Rev Med* 51:207–229.
142. Kopp, S., Alstergren, P., Ernestam, S., Nordahl, S., Bratt, J. (2006). Interleukin-1beta influences the effect of infliximab on temporomandibular joint pain in rheumatoid arthritis. *Scand J Rheumatol* 35:182–188.
143. Bokarewa, M., Tarkowski, A. (2003). Local infusion of infliximab for the treatment of acute joint inflammation. *Ann Rheum Dis* 62:783–784.
144. Conti, F., Priori, R., Chimenti, M.S., Coari, G., Annovazzi, A., Valesini, G., Signore, A. (2005). Successful treatment with intraarticular infliximab for resistant knee monarthritis in a patient with spondylarthropathy: a role for scintigraphy with 99mTc-infliximab. *Arthritis Rheum* 52:1224–1226.
145. Alstergren, P., Larsson, P.T., Kopp, S. (2008). Successful treatment with multiple intra-articular injections of infliximab in a patient with psoriatic arthritis. *Scand J Rheumatol* 37:155–157.
146. Dahl, E., Cohen, S.P. (2008). Perineural injection of etanercept as a treatment for postamputation pain. *Clin J Pain* 24:172–175.
147. Kirchner, S., Holler, E., Haffner, S., Andreesen, R., Eissner, G. (2004). Effect of different tumor necrosis factor (TNF) reactive agents on reverse signaling of membrane integrated TNF in monocytes. *Cytokine* 28:67–74.
148. Bresnihan, B., Alvaro-Gracia, J.M., Cobby, M., Doherty, M., Domljan, Z., Emery, P., Nuki, G., Pavelka, K., Rau, R., Rozman, B., Watt, I., Williams, B., Aitchison, R., McCabe, D., Musikic, P. (1998). Treatment of rheumatoid arthritis with recombinant human interleukin-1 receptor antagonist. *Arthritis Rheum* 41:2196–2204.
149. Yokota, S., Miyamae, T., Imagawa, T., Katakura, S., Kurosawa, R., Mori, M. (2005). Clinical study of tocilizumab in children with systemic-onset juvenile idiopathic arthritis. *Clin Rev Allergy Immunol* 28:231–238.
150. Yokota, S., Imagawa, T., Mori, M., Miyamae, T., Aihara, Y., Takei, S., Iwata, N., Umebayashi, H., Murata, T., Miyoshi, M., Tomiita, M., Nishimoto, N., Kishimoto, T. (2008). Efficacy and safety of tocilizumab in patients with systemic-onset juvenile idiopathic arthritis: a randomised, double-blind, placebo-controlled, withdrawal phase III trial. *Lancet* 371:998–1006.
151. Maini, R.N., Taylor, P.C., Szechinski, J., Pavelka, K., Broll, J., Balint, G., Emery, P., Raemen, F., Petersen, J., Smolen, J., Thomson, D., Kishimoto, T., CHARISMA Study Group. (2006). Double-blind randomized controlled clinical trial of the interleukin-6 receptor antagonist, tocilizumab, in European patients with rheuma-

toid arthritis who had an incomplete response to methotrexate. *Arthritis Rheum* 54:2817–2829.

152. Malmberg, A.B., Yaksh, T.L. (1992). Antinociceptive actions of spinal nonsteroidal anti-inflammatory agents on the formalin test in the rat. *J Pharmacol Exp Ther* 263:136–146.
153. Tominaga, M., Caterina, M.J., Malmberg, A.B., Rosen, T.A., Gilbert, H., Skinner, K., Raumann, B.E., Basbaum, A.I., Julius, D. (1998). The cloned capsaicin receptor integrates multiple pain-producing stimuli. *Neuron* 21:531–543.
154. Narumiya, S., FitzGerald, G.A. (2001). Genetic and pharmacological analysis of prostanoid receptor function. *J Clin Invest* 108:25–30.

CHAPTER 18

Neurotrophic Factors and Pain

PETER SVENSSON

Department of Clinical Oral Physiology, School of Dentistry, University of Aarhus; Department of Oral and Maxillofacial Surgery, Aarhus University Hospital; Orofacial Pain Laboratory, Center for Sensory-Motor Interaction, Aalborg University

Content

18.1 INTRODUCTION

In this chapter, the evidence for the role of the neurotrophic factors and receptor mechanisms in cutaneous and deep tissue-mediated nociception and pain will be reviewed. Moreover, the specific agonists/antagonists that target these receptors and current or potential treatment of pain based on the role of these receptors in pain transduction that would involve both peripheral and/or central mechanisms will be discussed. A detailed description of the signaling pathways in the nervous system is beyond the scope of this chapter and the reader is referred to several comprehensive reviews, for example, References 1–5.

Peripheral Receptor Targets for Analgesia: Novel Approaches to Pain Management, Edited by Brian E. Cairns

18.2 OVERVIEW OF RECEPTOR MECHANISMS

Neurotrophins, as the name implies ("neuron nourishing"), play a decisive role for neuronal differentiation, survival, growth, and apoptosis, but research over the last couple of decades has provided good evidence that they also act as potent modulators of nociceptive transmission [4,6,7]. Neurotrophins are a family of related proteins and can be divided into five main types (Table 18.1). In addition to these neurotrophins, also the so-called glial cell line-derived neurotrophic factor (GDNF) has been identified. Neurotrophic factor-3 and neurotrophic factor-4/5 do not appear to be strong modulators of nociceptive processing, and neurotrophic factor-6 does not exist in humans; therefore, only nerve growth factor (NGF), brain-derived neurotrophic factor (BDNF), and GDNF and their receptors will be considered in the following text.

All neurotrophins are synthesized as proforms of approximately 30 kDa and are cleaved to a mature form of 13 kDa. NGF exists in two forms: a 7S (s = sedimentation coefficient) and a 2.5S [4]. The precursors of NGF are processed inside the cell (sensory neurons as well as keratinocytes, fibroblasts, mast cells) by furin or prohormone convertase or extracellularly by plasmin or matrix metalloproteinases (MMP3/MMP7) to produce the mature neurotrophin [3]. Pro-NGF is packaged into constitutive vesicles before secretion from sympathetic and sensory target organs. Pro-BDNF is mainly packaged into regulated secretory pathway vesicles, processed, and secreted in an activity-dependent manner [3].

Besides the biological effects of NGF and BDNF, it also appears that pro-NGF and pro-BDNF can activate distinct transduction pathways and can have independent biological activity, for example, cell death by apoptosis, facilitation of the late phase of long-term potentiation, and depression [4].

The neurotrophic receptors are differentially expressed in the peripheral and central nervous system. All neurotrophins bind to the low-affinity transmembrane receptor p75, and each of the neurotrophins bind with high affinity to one of the tyrosine kinase (trk) family of transmembrane receptors (Table 18.1). For further details of the structure of the receptors, the reader can consult Allen and Dawbarn [3]. Thus, NGF exerts its biological effects by acting on both the high-affinity trkA receptor and the low-affinity receptor p75. These receptors are commonly expressed on sensory neurons including

TABLE 18.1. Overview of the Neurotrophin Family.

Neurotrophins	High-Affinity Receptors
Nerve growth factor (NGF)	trkA
Brain-derived neurotrophic factor (BDNF)	trkB
Neurotrophic factor-3	trkC (and trkA)
Neurotrophic factor-4/5	trkB
Neurotrophic factor-6 (nonhuman)	

trkA, B, C, tyrosine kinase receptors.

nociceptive cells but seem to vary depending on tissue and location. For example, trkA receptors on trigeminal ganglion neurons have been reported to range between 4% and 70% [8]. Preliminary findings indicate that up to about 70% of trigeminal ganglion neurons projecting from the masseter (jaw closer) muscle express trkA and p75 receptors [9] (Figure 18.1), which is in marked contrast to the spinal system where only about 4% of tibialis muscle dorsal root ganglion neurons express the trkA receptor [10]. Interestingly, these neurotrophic receptors are coexpressed with peripheral N-methyl-D-aspartate (NMDA) receptors (NR2B subtype) in approximately 45% of the masseter ganglion neurons, indicating the potential for receptor interactions [9]. Peripheral NMDA receptors have, indeed, been implicated in deep tissue nociception, mechanical sensitization, as well as reflex mechanisms [11–18] (see Chapter 8). Also, BDNF can modulate the responsiveness of sensory (nociceptive) neurons by potentiation of postsynaptic NMDA receptors, that is, central sensitization [4].

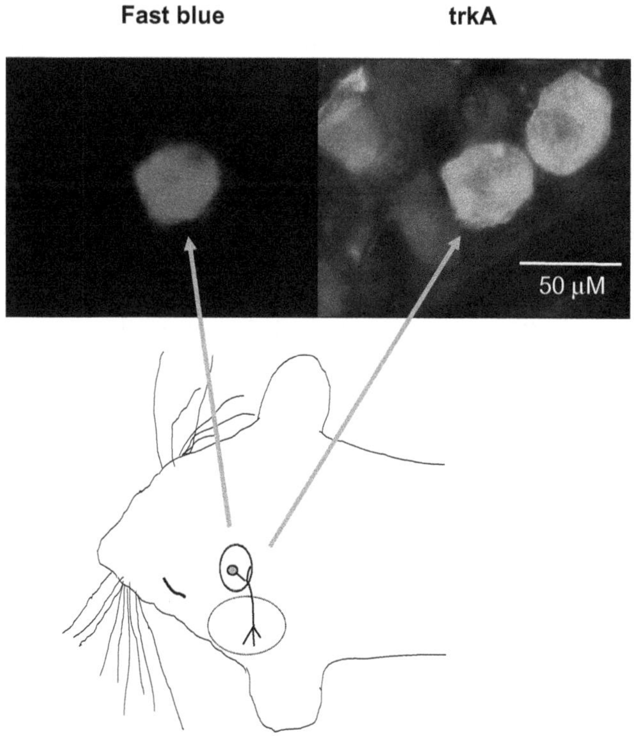

FIGURE 18.1. Fast Blue dye (1.5%, 10 mL) injected into the masseter muscle was used to identify trigeminal ganglion neurons that innervate the rat masseter muscle. Immunohistochemistry was used to label the expression of trkA receptors on these masseter ganglion neurons [9]. See color insert.

NGF binding to the trkA receptors causes receptor activation and dimerization, which results in transautophosphorylation and activation of intracellular signaling cascades like extracellular signal-regulated kinase (ERK), ras–raf mitogen-activated protein kinase (MAPK), phosphatidylinositol 3-kinase (PI3K), and phospholipase Cγ (PLC-γ) pathways to rapidly affect changes in downstream receptor function as well as to initiate slower alterations in receptor expression [1,4,19,20]. In terms of pain, one of the consequences of the cascade of intracellular events affecting the sensitivity of the neurons is peripheral sensitization. Furthermore, the NGF-mediated mechanisms also involve a slow (hours–days) retrograde transportation of internalized trkA–neurotrophin complex that contributes to gene expression and may have transcriptional control over the neuron and be associated with upregulation of sensory neuropeptides and neuromodulators such as calcitonin gene-related peptide (CGRP), substance P, BDNF, as well as receptors like transient receptor potential vanilloid 1 (TRPV1) and purinergic receptors of ATP (P2X3), and ion channels, for example, tetrodotoxin-sensitive and tetrodotoxin-resistant sodium channels (TTX and TTXr) [4,5]. Recently, it has been shown that NGF participates in a functional upregulation of the transient receptor potential ankyrin repeat 1 (TRPA1) channel in trigeminal ganglion neurons [21]. The authors suggested that the increased activities of TRPA1 could play an important role in the development of hyperalgesia following nerve and tissue injury in the orofacial region [21].

In contrast to NGF, which has widespread and significant biological effects in the peripheral nervous system, BDNF appears to be mainly involved in the central modulation of pain [4,7]. Thus, BDNF is constitutively synthesized by a subset of dorsal root ganglion cells and trigeminal ganglion cells [4,22]. BDNF is upregulated by peripheral inflammation and an NGF-dependent mechanism, which also appears to be susceptible to estrogen levels [23]. Activation of the ERK signaling pathway is one of the downstream effects of BDNF and contributes to its pronociceptive characteristics [4]. Thus, as previously mentioned, BDNF is able to potentiate the NMDA receptors in spinal cord neurons leading to central sensitization. A recent study demonstrated that experimentally inflamed skin had significantly higher levels of NGF, but not BDNF, when compared to noninflamed human skin; however, acute activation of nociceptors in the inflamed skin was associated with elevated levels of BDNF [24], further supporting the suggestion that BDNF plays an important role in neuronal sensitization [24,25]. Animal studies have also provided evidence that direct injections of BDNF into rat paw lead to thermal hyperalgesia as indicated by both behavioral and electrophysiological techniques [26]. However, the magnitude of such direct effects of BDNF on thermal sensitivity is significantly smaller than the effects of NGF [26].

It should also be mentioned that another member of the neurotrophin family, GDNF, has attracted interest particularly in relation to neuropathic pain. GDNF-related ligands include neurturin and artemin, which act on the complex c-Ret proto-oncogene receptor trk and coreceptor GDNF receptor

(GFRα1-4) [27]. For example, GDNF has been shown to be upregulated following nerve injury, and in animal models, GDNF has been shown to possess neuroprotective effects [28]. Direct administration of GDNF, neurturin, and artemin in rat hind paws also produced acute thermal hyperalgesia lasting up to 4 hours, suggesting that the GDNF family participates in the regulation of thermal nociceptors in inflammatory states [29]. Thus, GDNF may play an important role in various types of pain conditions, but the clinical use may unfortunately be hampered by unacceptable side effects [27].

In the following three paragraphs, the evidence for a specific role of neurotrophins for nociception and pain will be reviewed with a particular emphasis on muscle tissue in animal, human, experimental, and clinical studies.

18.3 EVIDENCE FROM ANIMAL STUDIES

Essentially, two different lines of experiments have bolstered the suggestion that NGF is critically involved in nociceptive transmission. One line of research has consistently shown that different types of tissue injury and manipulation (e.g., cutaneous injections of carrageenan, complete Freund adjuvant, incisions) lead to an increase in endogenous levels of NGF associated with C-fiber sensitization and thermal and mechanical hyperalgesia [4,7]. Also, constriction of the trigeminal nerve (infraorbital nerve) is associated with elevated levels of NGF and mechanical sensitization [30]. Many of these studies have also demonstrated that anti-NGF techniques lead to analgesia [4]. For example, intraperitoneal administration of a monoclonal antibody against endogenous NGF was able to attenuate nociceptive behavior in rats after a plantar incision [31]. The observations of increases in endogenous levels of NGF are evident in various models of inflammatory muscle and joint pain as well as several other conditions such as arthritis, bone cancer, spinal cord injury, disk herniation, and bladder inflammation [4].

Another experimental approach has been to administer exogenous NGF. In mice, subcutaneous injection of NGF-evoked mechanical hyperalgesia 6–7 hours after administration and thermal hyperalgesia 15 minutes after administration [32,33]. Injection of NGF into mouse muscle tissue evoked secondary hyperalgesia (assumed to reflect a central mechanism) and a dose-dependent decrease in mechanical nociceptive threshold after 24 hours, which lasted for 5 days [34]. Other studies in animal preparations with intramuscular injections of NGF into the cervical muscles have shown long-lasting facilitatory effects on the jaw-opening reflex [35]. Direct administration of NGF into neck muscles is also associated with distinct patterns of c-fos expression as a potential marker of nociceptive processing in the mesencephalic periaqueductal gray, medullary lateral reticular nucleus, and laminae I and II of the cervical spinal horn C1-C3 [36]. Interestingly, intramuscular administration of NGF and ATP activates different muscle nociceptive afferent fibers and pathways, which may be of importance to understand the complexity of neck muscle pain and tension-type headaches [37]. The peripheral effects of NGF could possibly lead to plastic changes in nociceptive synaptic transmission and could subsequently involve a process of central sensitization. The initiator of this central sensitization may be due to NGF-evoked excitation of nociceptive C-fibers, which has been reported to occur upon intramuscular injection of NGF into the rat gastrocnemius-soleus muscle [38]. Thus, Hoheisel et al. [38] found a robust activation of 10 out of 28 C-fibers in the gastrocnemius-soleus muscle of rats but no significant changes in C-fiber discharges in response to fixed mechanical stimuli, which indicates a lack of mechanical sensitization in these fibers. In contrast to this finding in C-fibers, another recent study showed that injection of NGF into jaw-closing muscles does not evoke significant discharge in Aδ-fibers in either male or female rats [39] (Figure 18.2a). However, the differential activation of nociceptive muscle afferent fibers is, in fact, in accordance with the observations from Ellrich and Makowska [37]. Intracellular recordings of dorsal horn neurons have shown that about half of the neurons do not react to injection of NGF into the rat gastrocnemius-soleus muscle, although about 25% of the neurons respond with excitatory postsynaptic potentials (EPSPs), and 20% of the neurons show both EPSPs and action potentials [40]. This pattern of neuronal response was suggested by the authors to be sufficient to induce a sensitization of central nociceptive neurons. Injections of NGF into another spinal muscle, the multifidus muscle in rats, have been shown to be associated with increased responsiveness of the neurons with inputs from the low back [41]. In the trigeminal system, we have recently found that within 1 hour of injection of human NGF into the rat masseter muscle, the mechanical threshold of Aδ-fibers decreases in female rats, which may suggest that females are particularly sensitive to elevated levels of NGF [39]. We have replicated this finding in another blinded and controlled study clearly demonstrating peripheral sensitization of Aδ-fibers from the masseter muscle in rats [9] (Figure 18.2b). Although there may be a coexpression of p75, trkA, and NMDA receptors on masseter trigeminal ganglion neurons, there seems to be no additional effects of NGF-induced mechanical sensitization on a subsequent glutamate injection in terms of evoked discharges or magnitude of mechanical sensitization [9]. NGF directly injected into the temporomandibular joint (TMJ) does not provoke spontaneous nociceptive behaviors in rats, but prior sensitization of the TMJ with the inflammatory substance carrageenan leads to a significant increase in spontaneous nociception [42]. A curious observation is that rat NGF is unable to activate or sensitize Aδ-fibers from the masseter muscle, whereas human NGF has consistent and profound effects [9,39]. This observation raises the question about species differences in the biological effects of NGF and possibly other neurotrophins.

In summary, the animal studies have convincingly shown that endogenous levels of NGF increase in response to tissue injury (inflammation) or nerve injury (neuropathic pain) and are associated with measures of nociceptive activity and behavior. Experimental models with administration of exogenous NGF have suggested direct activation of C-fibers in spinal muscles but no activation of Aδ-fibers in jaw-closing muscles in addition to a pronounced and longer-lasting (hours) mechanical sensitization.

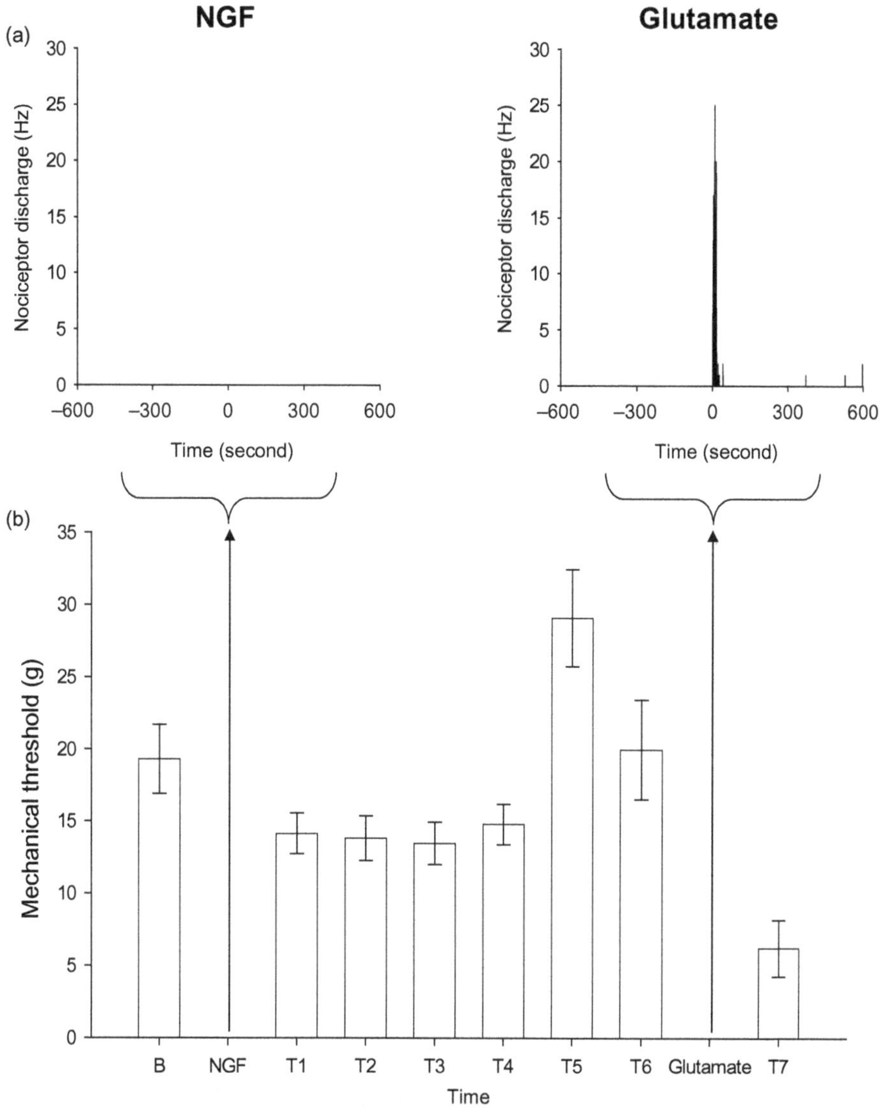

FIGURE 18.2. The peristimulus histograms in (a) illustrate evoked masseter muscle nociceptor discharge, and the vertical bar charts in (b) illustrate masseter muscle nociceptor mechanical threshold before and after injection of nerve growth factor (NGF) and a subsequent injection, 3.5 hours later, of glutamate. (a) Prior to injection of substances into the masseter muscle, this nociceptor did not exhibit spontaneous discharge. Injection of NGF did not evoke any discharge in this nociceptor; however, injection of glutamate evoked a robust initial discharge in this nociceptor, and continued sporadic discharge for 10 minutes postinjection. The average (± standard error of the mean) baseline (b) mechanical threshold of this nociceptor was calculated from 10 consecutive threshold determinations at 1-minute intervals. After injection of NGF, mean mechanical threshold was determined by the same method every 30 minutes (T1–T6). Injection of NGF lowered mechanical threshold in this nociceptor for 2 hours. At the end of 3 hours and after injection of glutamate, the mechanical threshold was reassessed (T7). The injection of glutamate had a more profound effect on the mechanical threshold of this nociceptor than NGF.

18.4 EVIDENCE FROM HUMAN EXPERIMENTAL STUDIES

As NGF is intimately related to development and maintenance of sympathetic and sensory neurons, a study in the early 1990s set out to examine the safety and pharmacokinetics of the administration of exogenous NGF to healthy human volunteers ($n = 45$) under the premise of testing the potential use of NGF to treat and to prevent peripheral and central nervous system diseases [43]. Interestingly, a series of side effects were noted after intravenous administration of 1.0 μg/kg beginning with diffuse myalgias about 60–90 minutes after infusion. These muscle pain symptoms appeared to peak around 4–6 hours after the injection but lasted for up to 1 week. Furthermore, the subjects reported pain in the masseter muscle that increased during chewing, sore throats, and pain on eye movements. Also, with subcutaneous administration of 1.0 μg/kg NGF, mild, diffuse myalgias developed in addition to an injection-site hyperalgesia to both touch and heat [43]. None of the subjects exposed to NGF administration reported any spontaneous pain or needed to take analgesics for the hyperalgesia, and all side effects resolved completely [43]. A subsequent study extended the findings from Petty et al. [43] and examined the effects of 1- to 3-μg subcutaneous NGF in healthy volunteers ($n = 16$) [44]. None of the subjects reported spontaneous pain, but it was a consistent finding that subjects developed localized tenderness to compression around the injection site. Careful analysis of somatosensory function revealed allodynia to pressure stimuli and reduced heat pain thresholds, but no effects on vibratory or cold sensitivity. The observed changes in somatosensory function were found 3 hours after the NGF injections and lasted for some subjects up to 3 weeks [44]. The authors noted that this onset probably was too rapid to reflect uptake of NGF by nociceptive terminals, retrograde transportation, and upregulation of central pain modulators [44].

More recently, we have shown that direct administration of small doses (5 μg) into the masseter muscle of healthy male subjects ($n = 12$) is associated with a prolonged period (2 weeks) of increased sensitivity to mechanical pressure stimuli and chewing-evoked pain [45]. These features were speculated to mimic the clinical symptoms of myofascial temporomandibular disorders (TMDs), which are characterized by pain on palpation of the jaw muscles and pain on jaw movements [46,47]. However, TMD predominately affects women [46], so in a follow-up study, we employed the same methodology with a single bolus injection of 5 μg in 0.2 mL (~0.1 μg/kg) into healthy female volunteers ($n = 14$) [47]. Also, this study demonstrated a consistent and long-lasting increase in mechanical sensitivity (allodynia and hyperalgesia) in the NGF-injected masseter muscle and pain associated with jaw functions but without spontaneous pain or any systemic side effects. An indirect comparison of the maximum decrease in pressure pain thresholds (PPTs) 1 day after the NGF injection in women ($66.3 \pm 4.2\%$) to the data in men ($39.4 \pm 6.7\%$) indicated a significantly greater amount of sensitization in women compared with men [45,47].

The time course of these sensitization effects could provide some insight into the underlying mechanisms. In the first study in men [45], the mechanical sensitivity was assessed 1 hour after NGF injections and indicated no allodynia or hyperalgesia, whereas the second study in women [47] found significant decreases in PPTs (mechanical allodynia) and pressure pain tolerance levels (PPTOLs—hyperalgesia) 3 hours after the NGF injections consistent with the observations from Dyck et al. [44]. Thus, this mechanical sensitization effect is probably mediated by a peripheral mechanism because we have found that NGF also sensitizes masseter muscle Aδ-fibers within 1–3 hours after injection into the rat masseter muscle [39,47]. However, the possibility remains that increases in mechanical sensitivity observed after 1 day are due, at least in part, to a central mechanism involving upregulation of sensory neuropeptides and neuromodulators such as CGRP, substance P, BDNF, receptors like TRPV1 and P2X3, and ion channels such as TTX and TTXr [4]. However, indirect evidence of NGF-induced central pain mechanisms comes from another recent study [48]. In a double-blind placebo-controlled study of the spatial distribution of muscle hyperalgesia over time (immediately after; 3 hours; 1, 4, 7, and 21 days) after NGF (5 μg) was injected into the tibialis anterior muscle of both healthy women ($n = 10$) and men ($n = 10$), an area of mechanical hyperalgesia was observed locally at the site of injection 3 hours after injection of NGF, which expanded both proximally and distally on the following day and subsided on day 4. In this study, there were no sex-related differences in the magnitude or spread of mechanical hyperalgsia [48], but the expansion of muscle hyperalgesia to distant areas was taken as an indication that central mechanisms are involved.

Very recently, we addressed another hypothesis that NGF-induced mechanical sensitization of muscle tissue could be associated with changes in vibration sense and stretch reflex sensitivity as well as with facilitation of glutamate-evoked pain responses [49]. We performed a double-blind, randomized and placebo-controlled study on 14 healthy men with two sessions. In one session, the subjects received an injection of NGF (5 μg) into the masseter muscle, and in a control session, the subjects received an injection of buffered isotonic saline (0.9%). The subjects assessed their pain intensity on a 0- to 10-cm visual analog scale (VAS) for 15 minutes after the injections. PPTs, vibration sense, and jaw stretch reflexes were recorded at baseline and 1, 2, 3, and 24 hours postinjection. The sensitivity to injections of glutamate into the masseter muscle (1 M, 0.2 mL) was assessed after 24 hours. The results from this study showed that NGF did not cause more pain than isotonic saline, but significantly reduced PPTs 1, 2, 3, and 24 hours postinjection, whereas isotonic saline had no effects on PPTs. Overall, these effects are consistent with the previously mentioned studies [45,47,48]. The injection of glutamate after 24 hours was associated with reduced PPTs in both sessions, but the PPTs remained lower in the NGF-pretreated masseter than in the control masseter [49]. Ratings of vibratory stimuli and the normalized amplitude of the jaw stretch reflex were not affected by the NGF-induced sensitization; however, after glutamate injection, a significant increase in the stretch reflex was observed in the injected masseter muscle in both sessions in accordance with previous studies [13]. There were no significant differences in the perceived pain intensity of the glutamate injection between the masseter muscle pretreated with NGF or control, although the glutamate-evoked pain drawing areas were larger for the NGF-pretreated masseter muscle. In conclusion, this study confirmed that masseter muscle injection of NGF is associated with a distinct and prolonged sensitization to mechanical stimuli, but without an effect on large-diameter mechanoreceptive and muscle spindle afferent fibers [49]. The additional challenge of the NGF-pretreated muscle with glutamate did not indicate a conspicuous sensitization to noxious chemical stimuli despite the coexpression of NR2B receptors with trkA and p75 receptors [9]. Finally, a human experimental study assessed the influence of NGF on delayed onset muscle soreness (DOMS) in the trapezius muscle as well as the temporal summation of pressure pain during hyperalgesia induced by NGF and DOMS in 10 healthy volunteers [50]. The soreness intensity to muscle contraction significantly increased at 3 and 24 hours in both shoulders and subsided at day 7 consistent with a decrease in PPTs. Interestingly, the NGF-injected side had higher pain ratings during temporal summation compared with the contralateral side 1 day after injections. The authors concluded that intramuscular administration of NGF exacerbated the DOMS responses and facilitated temporal summation, but no definite conclusions could be made with respect to peripheral or central sensitization mechanisms [50]. It seems inevitable that further studies in animals will be required to separate the peripheral versus the central component of NGF-induced mechanical sensitization.

An intriguing finding in all the human studies that have tested the effects of different types of administration (intravenous, subcutaneous, intramuscular) of NGF is the consistent lack of spontaneous pain reports [43–50]. Combined, these findings suggest that NGF in itself does not activate a sufficient number of nociceptive afferent fibers necessary for a conscious sensation of pain and that volume effects of the injected solution play a minor role. Nevertheless, exogenous administration of NGF is able to trigger biological effects to initiate a robust and longer-lasting sensitization of mechanical (and thermal heat) stimuli in healthy volunteers (Figure 18.3).

18.5 EVIDENCE FROM CLINICAL PAIN CONDITIONS

Increased levels of NGF have been implicated in various inflammatory pain conditions such as pancreatitis, prostatitis, and cystitis [51–53]. Also, in degenerative disorders of human intervertebral disks, expression of NGF and BDNF can be found [54]. However, animal studies have also provided evidence that injection of NGF does not lead to overt inflammation as assessed by plasma extravasation in rat masseter muscles [39]. This is a marked difference from other animal models of myositis such as injection of complete Freund adju-

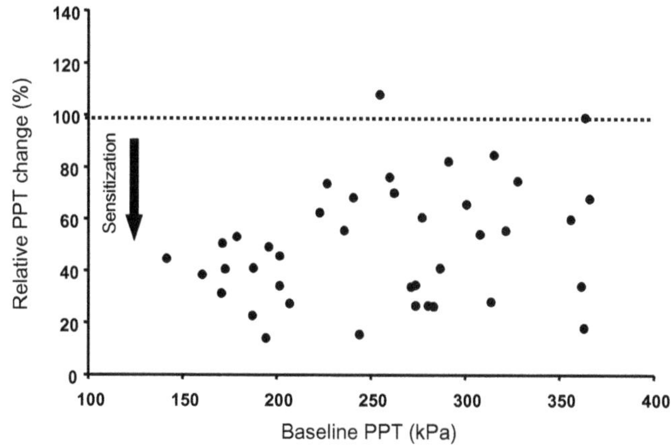

FIGURE 18.3. The scatter plot demonstrates the consistent mechanical sensitization 1 day after intramuscular injection of NGF into the masseter muscle in healthy subjects. Sensitization is expressed as relative changes (%) of the PPT at baseline. There are no relationships between baseline PPTs and degree of mechanical sensitization (Spearman correlation coefficient: $R = 0.256, p = 0.111$). Data from Svensson, P., Cairns, B.E., Wang, K., Arendt-Nielsen, L. (2003). Injection of nerve growth factor into human masseter muscle evokes long-lasting mechanical allodynia and hyperalgesia. *Pain* 104:241–247; Svensson, P., Castrillon, E., Cairns, B.E. (2008). NGF-evoked masseter muscle sensitization and perturbation of jaw motor function in healthy women. *J Orofac Pain* 22:340–348; and Svensson, P., Wang, K., Arendt-Nielsen, L., Cairns, B.E. (2008). Effects of NGF-induced muscle sensitization on proprioception and nociception. *Exp Brain Res* 189:1–10. $n = 40$.

vant, mustard oil, or formalin (see, e.g., References 55–57). Increased concentrations of NGF have furthermore been found in the cerebrospinal fluid in patients with headache [58,59] and in patients with fibromyalgia [60,61]. Recently, a hypothesis was proposed to explain fibromyalgia based on the concept that trauma or infections could be the initial triggering factors and NGF a key mediator in terms of phenotypic changes in sympathetic fibers and generation of neuroplasticity [62].

A recent study used biopsies from the painful tongue mucosa in patients with burning mouth syndrome and found increased markers of NGF on the immunostained nerve fibers as well as on basal epithelial cells compared to control subjects [63]. The authors proposed that selective NGF blockers could be considered a new therapy for BMS patients. This proposal is in line with a recent review by Dray and Read [27], who suggested that anti-NGF monoclonal antibody therapy could be an attractive approach with the potential for long-lasting pain effects without compromising physiological nociception. One phase I study could demonstrate reduced pain and improved mobility in osteoarthritis with the use of a humanized anti-NGF monoclonal antibody [64]. However, the approach to supply exogenous NGF to promote neuronal survival and regeneration in, for example, diabetic neuropathy has not been successful so far [65]. More studies will obviously be needed to determine the analgesic and beneficial effects of such manipulations with NGF and other neurotrophic factors.

18.6 NEUROTROPHIC FACTORS AS MODELS OF CLINICAL PAIN?

So far, the majority of studies have focused on the effects of NGF and relatively little is known with regard to BDNF, which may have multiple effects on the central nervous system function not just in terms of pain. For example, a recent study highlighted the significance of different haplotypes of BDNF for a healthy subject's ability to learn novel motor tasks [66]. We have recently provided evidence that capsaicin-evoked pain on the tongue significantly interfered with the subject's performance during a novel tongue-protrusion task and with the associated motor-evoked potentials, indicating perturbation of cortical neuroplasticity [67]. One possibility would be to link genotyping of BDNF with experimental pain studies and motor learning; however, the underlying mechanisms are unlikely to be explained by peripheral events.

We have suggested that intramuscular injection of NGF could be used as a model to study, for example, myofascial TMD [47]. One reason is the highly consistent finding in myofascial TMD patients that PPTs in the masseter muscles are decreased compared to matched controls [68–70]. Epidemiological data strongly suggest that women are at higher risk than men to develop a TMD problem and, in particular, the use of oral contraceptives seems to be an additional risk factor [71–73]. Recently, it was shown that manipulation of the estradiol levels in healthy women was associated with distinct differences in regional increases in baseline μ-opioid receptor availability *in vivo* and activation of endogenous opioid neurotransmission during experimental pain [74]. This finding suggests a role of estrogen in modulating endogenous opioid neurotransmission and psychophysical measures of experimental jaw muscle pain and is in accordance with the clinical literature demonstrating that low levels of estrogen during the menstrual cycle are associated with small but significant increases in TMD pain [72]. Stohler [75] was the first to consider a potential sex-related link between NGF and myofascial TMD. Data from animal studies have, indeed, suggested that estrogens modulate the responsiveness of cells in the dorsal root ganglion that binds NGF and expresses NGF receptor genes [76–78]. Andersen et al. [48] did not find sex-related differences in the magnitude of sensitization following NGF injections into a leg muscle; however, the women were tested in a period of the menstrual cycle with presumed low levels of estrogen. Further studies will be needed to test the association between NGF and estrogens in larger sample sizes and with more pronounced variations in sex hormone levels.

Levels of NGF or analysis of trkA receptor distribution and density has not yet been performed in TMD pain patients but could provide direct evidence of the potential role of neurotrophic factors in chronic pain conditions without clinical indications of inflammation. Another important point is that NGF injections are associated with significant perturbations of normal jaw motor function such as chewing and yawning. This sensory-motor interaction is also supported by studies of the jaw-opening reflex in animals exposed to NGF injections into the cervical muscles [35]. Although the pain scores following a chewing task are low, they consistently indicate that chewing after intramuscular injection of NGF leads to higher pain scores in accordance with clinical reports [79–81]. It is therefore proposed that intramuscular administration of NGF is an interesting model or proxy of TMD-like pain without an inflammatory component and could be used to obtain more insight into the mechanisms of mechanical sensitization of deep nociceptive afferent fibers in the craniofacial region. In addition, other musculoskeletal pain conditions could be considered [37,50].

18.7 CONCLUSIONS

The role of neurotrophins for regulation of nociception and pain has been firmly established in the literature [4,5]. NGF is a key mediator of tissue-injury pain and neuropathic pain and regulates sensory neuron excitability. Several human studies have also demonstrated the potential to use NGF as an experimental model of musculoskeletal pain disorders because of the consistent and pronounced sensitization to mechanical stimuli and interference with normal motor function. Specific antagonism of NGF appears to be a promising therapeutic target. NGF also interacts with BDNF, which contributes to central sensitization effects. BDNF is also associated with learning and memory, which interferes with pain, pointing toward new lines of research. Finally, GDNF is a significant player in, for example, peripheral nerve injuries. An understanding of polymorphisms of neurotrophins and their receptors and the development of specific receptor antagonists may be a fruitful research avenue for pain researchers.

REFERENCES

1. Kaplan, D.R., Miller, F.D. (2000). Neurotrophin signal transduction in the nervous system. *Curr Opin Neurobiol* 10:381–391.
2. Dawbarn, D., Allen, S.J. (2003). Neurotrophins and neurodegeneration. *Neuropathol Appl Neurobiol* 29:211–230.
3. Allen, S.J., Dawbarn, D. (2006). Clinical relevance of the neurotrophins and their receptors. *Clin Sci (Lond)* 110:175–191.
4. Pezet, S., McMahon, S.B. (2006). Neurotrophins: mediators and modulators of pain. *Ann Rev Neurosci* 29:507–538.
5. McMahon, S.B., Bennett, D.L.H., Bevan, S. (2006). Inflammatory mediators and modulators of pain. In: McMahon, S.B., Koltzenburg, M. (eds.). *Textbook of Pain*. Philadelphia: Elsevier Churchill Livingstone, pp. 49–72.

6. Apfel, S.C. (2000). Neurotrophic factors and pain. *Clin J Pain* 16:S7–S11.
7. Bennett, D.L.H. (2001). Neurotrophic factors: important regulators of nociceptive function. *Neuroscientist* 7:13–17.
8. Shinoda, M., Honda, T., Ozaki, N., Hattori, H., Mizutani, H., Ueda, M., Sugiura, Y. (2003). Nerve terminals extend into the temporomandibular joint of adjuvant arthritic rats. *Eur J Pain* 7:493–505.
9. Svensson, P., Wang, M., Dong, X.D., Kumar, U., Cairns, B.E. (2008). Human nerve growth factor (NGF) sensitizes masseter muscle nociceptors. In: *Abstracts of the 12th World Congress on Pain*. Seattle, WA: IASP Press, p. 66.
10. Lu, J., Zhou, X.F., Rush, R.A. (2001). Small primary sensory neurons innervating epidermis and viscera display differential phenotype in the adult rat. *Neurosci Res* 41:355–363.
11. Cairns, B.E., Hu, J.W., Arendt-Nielsen, L., Sessle, B.J., Svensson, P. (2001). Sex-related differences in human pain perception and rat afferent discharge evoked by injection of glutamate into the masseter muscle. *J Neurophysiol* 86:782–791.
12. Cairns, B.E., Svensson, P., Wang, K., Hupfeld, S., Graven-Nielsen, T., Sessle, B.J., Berde, C.B., Arendt-Nielsen, L. (2003). Activation of peripheral NMDA receptors contributes to human pain and rat afferent fiber discharge evoked by injection of glutamate into the masseter muscle. *J Neurophysiol* 90:2098–2105.
13. Cairns, B.E., Wang, K., Hu, J.W., Sessle, B.J., Arendt-Nielsen, L., Svensson, P. (2003). The effect of glutamate-evoked masseter muscle pain on the human jaw-stretch reflex differs in men and women. *J Orofac Pain* 17:317–325.
14. Cairns, B.E., Svensson, P., Wang, K., Castrillon, E., Hupfeld, S., Sessle, B.J., Arendt-Nielsen, L. (2006). Ketamine attenuates glutamate-induced mechanical sensitization of the masseter muscle in human males. *Exp Brain Res* 169:467–472.
15. Svensson, P., Cairns, B.E., Wang, K., Hu, J.W., Graven-Nielsen, T., Arendt-Nielsen, L., Sessle, B.J. (2003). Glutamate-induced sensitization of pressure pain thresholds in human masseter muscle. *Pain* 101:221–227.
16. Dong, X.D., Mann, M.K., Kumar, U., Svensson, P., Arendt-Nielsen, L., Hu, J.W., Sessle, B.J., Cairns, B.E. (2007). Sex-related differences in NMDA-evoked rat masseter muscle afferent discharge result from estrogen-mediated modulation of peripheral NMDA receptor activity. *Neuroscience* 146:822–832.
17. Cairns, B.E. (2007). The influence of gender and sex steroids on craniofacial nociception. *Headache* 47:319–324.
18. Castrillon, E.E., Cairns, B.E., Ernberg, M., Wang, K., Sessle, B.J., Arendt-Nielsen, L., Svensson, P. (2007). Effect of a peripheral NMDA receptor antagonist on glutamate-evoked masseter muscle pain and mechanical sensitization in women. *J Orofac Pain* 21:216–224.
19. Chao, M.V., Hempstead, B.L. (1995). p75 and Trk: a two-receptor system. *Trends Neurosci* 18:321–326.
20. Chao, M.V. (2003). Neurotrophins and their receptors: a convergence point for many signaling pathways. *Neuroscience* 4:299–309.
21. Diogenes, A., Akopian, A.N., Hargreaves, K.M. (2007). NGF up-regulates TRPA1: implications for orofacial pain. *J Dental Res* 86:550–555.
22. Buldyrev, I., Tanner, N.M., Hsieh, H.Y., Dodd, E.G., Nguyen, L.T., Balkowiec, A. (2006). Calcitonin gene-related peptide enhances release of native brain-derived

neurotrophic factor from trigeminal ganglion neurons. *J Neurochem*, 99, 1338–1350.

23. Allen, A.L., McCarson, K.E. (2005). Estrogen increases nociception-evoked brain-derived neurotrophic factor gene expression in the female rat. *Neuroendocrinology* 81:193–199.
24. Paterson, S., Schmelz, M., McGlone, F., Turner, G., Rukwied, R. (2009). Facilitated neurotrophin release in sensitized human skin. *Eur J Pain* 13:399–405.
25. Cho, H.J., Kim, J.K., Zhou, X.F., Rush, R.A. (1997). Increased brain-derived neurotrophic factor immunoreactivity in rat dorsal root ganglia and spinal cord following peripheral inflammation. *Brain Res* 764:269–272.
26. Shu, X.Q., Llinas, A., Mendell, L.M. (1999). Effects of trkB and trkC neurotrophin receptor agonists on thermal nociception: a behavioral and electrophysiological study. *Pain* 80:463–470.
27. Dray, A., Read, S.J. (2007). Arthritis and pain. Future targets to control osteoarthritis pain. *Arthritis Res Ther* 9:1–14.
28. Sah, D.W., Ossipov, M.H., Rossomando, A., Silvian, L., Porreca, F. (2005). New approaches for the treatment of pain: the GDNF family of neurotrophic growth factors. *Curr Top Med Chem* 5:577–583.
29. Malin, S.A., Molliver, D.C., Koerber, H.R., Cornuet, P., Frye, R., Albers, K.M., Davis, B.M. (2006). Glial cell line-derived neurotrophic factor family members sensitize nociceptors in vitro and produce thermal hyperalgesia in vivo. *J Neurosci* 26:8588–8599.
30. Anderson, L.C., Rao, R.D. (2001). Interleukin-6 and nerve growth factor levels in peripheral nerve and brainstem after trigeminal nerve injury in the rat. *Arch Oral Biol* 46:633–640.
31. Banik, R.K., Subieta, A.R., Wu, C., Brennan, T.J. (2005). Increased nerve growth factor after rat plantar incision contributes to guarding behavior and heat hyperalgesia. *Pain* 117:68–76.
32. Lewin, G.R., Mendell, L.M. (1993). Nerve growth factor and nociception. *Trends Neurosci* 16:353–359.
33. Lewin, G.R., Ritter, A.M., Mendell, L.M. (1993). Nerve growth factor-induced hyperalgesia in the neonatal and adult rat. *J Neurosci* 13:2136–2148.
34. Hathway, G.J., Fitzgerald, M. (2006). Time course and dose-dependence of nerve growth factor-induced secondary hyperalgesia in the mouse. *J Pain* 7:57–61.
35. Makowska, A., Panfil, C., Ellrich, J. (2005). Nerve growth factor injection into semispinal neck muscle evokes sustained facilitation of the jaw-opening reflex in anesthetized mice – possible implications for tension-type headache. *Exp Neurol* 191:301–309.
36. Panfil, C., Makowska, A., Ellrich, J. (2006). Brainstem and cervical spinal cord Fos immunoreactivity evoked by nerve growth factor injection into neck muscles in mice. *Cephalalgia* 26:128–135.
37. Ellrich, J., Makowska, A. (2007). Nerve growth factor and ATP excite different neck muscle nociceptors in anaesthetized mice. *Cephalalgia* 27:1226–1235.
38. Hoheisel, U., Unger, T., Mense, S. (2005). Excitatory and modulatory effects of inflammatory cytokines and neurotrophins on mechanosensitive group IV muscle afferents in the rat. *Pain* 114:168–176.

39. Mann, M.K., Dong, X.D., Svensson, P., Cairns, B.E. (2006). Influence of intramuscular nerve growth factor injection on the response properties of rat masseter muscle afferent fibers. *J Orofac Pain* 20:325–336.
40. Hoheisel, U., Unger, T., Mense, S. (2007). Sensitization of rat dorsal horn neurons by NGF-induced subthreshold potentials and low-frequency activation. A study employing intracellular recordings in vivo. *Brain Res* 1169:34–43.
41. Taguchi, T., Hoheisel, U., Mense, S. (2008). Dorsal horn neurons having input from low back structures in rats. *Pain* 138:119–129.
42. Pelegrini-da-Silva, A., Oliveira, M.C., Parada, C.A., Tambeli, C.H. (2008). Nerve growth factor acts with the beta2-adrenoceptor to induce spontaneous nociceptive behavior during temporomandibular joint inflammatory hyperalgesia. *Life Sci* 83:780–785.
43. Petty, B.G., Cornblath, D.R., Adornato, B.T., Chaudhry, V., Flexner, C., Wachsman, M., Sinicropi, D., Burton, L.E., Peroutka, S.J. (1994). The effect of systemically administered recombinant human nerve growth factor in healthy human subjects. *Ann Neurol* 36:244–246.
44. Dyck, P.J., Peroutka, S., Rask, C., Burton, E., Baker, M.K., Lehman, K.A., Gillen, D.A., Hokanson, J.L., O'Brien, P.C. (1997). Intradermal recombinant human nerve growth factor induces pressure allodynia and lowered heat-pain threshold in humans. *Neurology* 48:501–505.
45. Svensson, P., Cairns, B.E., Wang, K., Arendt-Nielsen, L. (2003). Injection of nerve growth factor into human masseter muscle evokes long-lasting mechanical allodynia and hyperalgesia. *Pain* 104:41–247.
46. Dworkin, S.F., LeResche, L. (1992). Research diagnostic criteria for temporomandibular disorders: review, criteria, examinations and specifications, critique. *J Craniomandib Disord Fac Oral Pain* 6:301–355.
47. Svensson, P., Castrillon, E., Cairns, B.E. (2008). NGF-evoked masseter muscle sensitization and perturbation of jaw motor function in healthy women. *J Orofac Pain* 22:340–348.
48. Andersen, H., Arendt-Nielsen, L., Svensson, P., Danneskiold-Samsøe, B., Graven-Nielsen, T. (2008). Spatial and temporal aspects of muscle hyperalgesia induced by nerve growth factor in humans. *Exp Brain Res* 191:371–382.
49. Svensson, P., Wang, K., Arendt-Nielsen, L., Cairns, B.E. (2008). Effects of NGF-induced muscle sensitization on proprioception and nociception. *Exp Brain Res* 189:1–10.
50. Nie, H., Madeleine, P., Arendt-Nielsen, L., Graven-Nielsen, T. (2008). Temporal summation of pressure pain during muscle hyperalgesia evoked by nerve growth factor and eccentric contractions. *Eur J Pain* Aug 16. Epub ahead of print.
51. Lowe, E.M., Anand, P., Terenghi, G., Williams-Chestnut, R.E., Sinicropi, D.V., Osborne, J.L. (1997). Increased nerve growth factor levels in the urinary bladder of women with idiopathic sensory urgency and interstitial cystitis. *Brit J Urol* 79:572–577.
52. Friess, H., Zhu, Z.W., di Mola, F.F., Kulli, C., Graber, H.U., Andren-Sandberg, A., Zimmermann, A., Korc, M., Reinshagen, M., Buchler, M.W. (1999). Nerve growth factor and its high-affinity receptor in chronic pancreatitis. *Ann Surg* 230: 615–624.

53. Miller, L.J., Fischer, K.A., Goralnick, S.J., Litt, M., Burleson, J.A., Albertsen, P., Kreutzer, D.L. (2002). Nerve growth factor and chronic prostatitis/chronic pelvic pain syndrome. *Urology* 59:603–608.

54. Purmessur, D., Freemont, A.J., Hoyland, J.A. (2008). Expression and regulation of neurotrophins in the nondegenerate and degenerate human intervertebral disc. *Arthritis Res Ther* 10(4):R99. Epub Aug 27.

55. Hu, J.W., Sessle, B.J., Raboisson, P., Dallel, R., Woda, A. (1992). Stimulation of craniofacial muscle afferents induces prolonged facilitatory effects in trigeminal nociceptive brain-stem neurones. *Pain* 48:53–60.

56. Watanabe, M., Tanaka, E., Nishi, M., Iwabe, T., Hattori, Y., Suemune, S., Tanne, K. (2002). Expression of c-Fos-like immunoreactive neurons in the supratrigeminal region in the rat following noxious stimulation of the orofacial tissues. *Neurosci Lett* 335:99–102.

57. Sugiyo, S., Takemura, M., Dubner, R., Ren, K. (2005). Trigeminal transition zone/rostral ventromedial medulla connections and facilitation of orofacial hyperalgesia after masseter inflammation in rats. *J Comp Neurol* 493:510–523.

58. Saldanha, G., Hongo, J., Plant, G., Acheson, J., Levy, I., Anand, P. (1999). Decreased CGRP, but preserved Trk A immunoreactivity in nerve fibres in inflamed human superficial temporal arteries. *J Neurol Neurosurg Psychiatr* 66:390–392.

59. Sarchielli, P., Alberti, A., Floridi, A., Gallai, V. (2001). Levels of nerve growth factor in cerebrospinal fluid of chronic daily headache patients. *Neurology* 57: 132–134.

60. Giovengo, S.L., Russell, I.J., Larson, A.A. (1999). Increased concentrations of nerve growth factor in cerebrospinal fluid of patients with fibromyalgia. *J Rheumatol* 26:1564–1569.

61. Sarchielli, P., Mancini, M.L., Floridi, A., Coppola, F., Rossi, C., Nardi, K., Acciarresi, M., Pini, L.A., Calabresi, P. (2007). Increased levels of neurotrophins are not specific for chronic migraine: evidence from primary fibromyalgia syndrome. *J Pain* 8:737–745.

62. Martinez-Lavin, M., Solano, C. (2009). Dorsal root ganglia, sodium channels, and fibromyalgia sympathetic pain. *Med Hyp* 72:64–66.

63. Yilmaz, Z., Renton, T., Yiangou, Y., Zakrzewska, J., Chessell, I.P., Bountra, C., Anand, P. (2007). Burning mouth syndrome as a trigeminal small fibre neuropathy: increased heat and capsaicin receptor TRPV1 in nerve fibres correlates with pain score. *J Clin Neurosci* 14:864–871.

64. Lane, N., Webster, L., Shiao-Ping, L., Gray, M., Hefti, F., Walicke, P. (2005). RN624 (anti-NGF) improves pain and function in subjects with moderate knee osteoarthritis: a phase I study. *Arthritis Rheum* 52:S461.

65. Apfel, S.C., Schwartz, S., Adornato, B.T., Freeman, R., Biton, V., Rendell, M., Vinik, A., Giuliani, M., Stevens, J.C., Barbano, R., Dyck, P.J. (2000). Efficacy and safety of recombinant human nerve growth factor in patients with diabetic polyneuropathy: a randomized controlled trial. rhNGF Clinical Investigator Group. *J Am Med Assoc* 284:2215–2221.

66. Kleim, J.A., Chan, S., Pringle, E., Schallert, K., Procaccio, V., Jimenez, R., Cramer, S.C. (2006). BDNF val66met polymorphism is associated with modified experience-dependent plasticity in human motor cortex. *Nat Neurosci* 9:735–737.

67. Boudreau, S., Romaniello, A., Wang, K., Svensson, P., Sessle, B.J., Arendt-Nielsen, L. (2007). The effects of intra-oral pain on motor cortex neuroplasticity associated with short-term novel tongue-protrusion training in humans. *Pain* 132:169–178.
68. Svensson, P., Arendt-Nielsen, L., Nielsen, H., Larsen, J.K. (1995). Effect of chronic and experimental jaw muscle pain on pressure-pain thresholds and stimulus-response curves. *J Orofac Pain* 9:347–356.
69. Maixner, W., Fillingim, R., Sigurdsson, A., Kincaid, S., Silva, S. (1998). Sensitivity of patients with painful temporomandibular disorders to experimentally evoked pain: evidence for altered temporal summation of pain. *Pain* 76:71–81.
70. Sarlani, E., Grace, E.G., Reynolds, M.A., Greenspan, J.D. (2004). Evidence for up-regulated central nociceptive processing in patients with masticatory myofascial pain. *J Orofac Pain* 18:41–55.
71. LeResche, L., Saunders, K., Von Korff, M.R., Barlow, W., Dworkin, S.F. (1997). Use of exogenous hormones and risk of temporomandibular disorder pain. *Pain* 69:153–160.
72. LeResche, L., Mancl, L., Sherman, J.J., Gandara, B., Dworkin, S.F. (2003). Changes in temporomandibular pain and other symptoms across the menstrual cycle. *Pain* 106:253–261.
73. Warren, M.P., Fried, J.L. (2001). Temporomandibular disorders and hormones in women. *Cells Tissues Organs* 169:187–192.
74. Smith, Y.R., Stohler, C.S., Nichols, T.E., Bueller, J.A., Koeppe, R.A., Zubieta, J.K. (2006). Pronociceptive and antinociceptive effects of estradiol through endogenous opioid neurotransmission in women. *J Neurosci* 26:5777–5785.
75. Stohler, C.S. (1997). Masticatory myalgias. Emphasis on the nerve growth factor - estrogen link. *Pain Forum* 6:176–180.
76. Sohrabji, F., Miranda, R.C., Toran-Allerand, C.D. (1994). Estrogen differentially regulates estrogen and nerve growth factor receptor mRNAs in adult sensory neurons. *J Neurosci* 14:459–471.
77. Scoville, S.A., Bufton, S.M., Liuzzi, F.J. (1997). Estrogen regulates neurofilament gene expression in adult female rat dorsal root ganglion neurons. *Exp Neurol* 146:596–599.
78. Liuzzi, F.J., Scoville, S.A., Bufton, S.M. (1999). Effects of short-term estrogen replacement on trkA mRNA levels in axotomized dorsal root ganglion neurons. *Exp Neurol* 159:433–440.
79. Dao, T.T., Lund, J.P., Lavigne, G.J. (1994). Pain responses to experimental chewing in myofascial pain patients. *J Dent Res* 73:1163–1167.
80. Gavish, A., Winocur, E., Menashe, S., Halachmi, M., Eli, I., Gazit, E. (2002). Experimental chewing in myofascial pain patients. *J Orofac Pain* 16:22–28.
81. Karibe, H., Goddard, G., Gear, R.W. (2003). Sex differences in masticatory muscle pain after chewing. *J Dent Res* 82:112–116.

PART III

DELIVERY SYSTEMS

CHAPTER 19

Topical and Systemic Drug Delivery Systems for Targeted Therapy

URS O. HÄFELI and AMIT KALE
Faculty of Pharmaceutical Sciences, The University of British Columbia

Content

Peripheral Receptor Targets for Analgesia: Novel Approaches to Pain Management, Edited by Brian E. Cairns

19.1 INTRODUCTION

The most effective drugs in the fields of pain management and pain treatment are opioids. As with all highly active drugs, however, their use produces not only the desired effect of pain amelioration but also toxicities and side effects. The side effects include nausea, constipation, and central nervous system (CNS) depression or excitation. CNS depression is more common than excitation and leads to drowsiness, lightheadedness, euphoria or dysphoria, and confusion. The less commonly observed CNS excitation side effects include hyperalgesia (extreme sensitivity to pain), myoclonus (involuntary jerking of muscles), or, in rare cases, seizures. Some less common side effects of opioids are urinary retention, respiratory depression, pruritus, and miosis. Most of these side effects can be managed well, for example, by administering the antiemetic drug metoclopramide for the treatment/prevention of nausea and by using oral laxatives, suppositories, or enemas for the treatment of constipation. Such additional drug interventions for the prevention of side effects would be rendered unnecessary if these side effects could be kept to a minimum, an outcome that is possible when opioids are delivered only to where they are needed.

Although early attempts at targeted drug delivery were described by the Roman scholar Pliny the Elder (23–79 AD) and by the Greek speculative scientist Thales of Miletus (ca. 624–547 BC), it was not until 1900 that drug targeting became a clearly stated concept. In that year, Paul Ehrlich spoke about his "search for the magic bullet" in his Croonian lecture before the Royal Society [1]. He was looking for a cure for syphilis and some 9 years later found it with his synthesis of salvarsan. Salvarsan proved to be amazingly effective because it targeted only the bacterial intruder in patients and spared all other cells. For these two reasons, it quickly became the most prescribed drug ever until the advent of penicillin in the 1940s. Salvarsan demonstrates how packaging of the active component arsenic into the organic arsenical compound arsphenamine can reduce undesired systemic side effects by being specifically targeted toward the syphilis-causing bacteria.

In principle, drug targeting can be achieved by physical or biological means [2,3]. The physical means of drug targeting include the direct application of a drug into the target tissue (the diseased area) via one of the many different methods to be discussed in this chapter. A more indirect application of physical means includes passive drug targeting in which the drug itself, or the drug bound to a nano- or microsized carrier, spontaneously accumulates in areas with leaky vasculature (e.g., tumors) with the help of the enhanced permeability and retention (EPR) effect [4]. The reasons for this accumulation are blood flow and tissue pressures, as well as accumulation of drugs based on abnormal pH values [5] and/or temperatures [6] in the pathological zone. Another more recent physical means of drug delivery is the combination of an active drug with a magnetically responsive carrier, the result of which is then directed, accumulated, and held in the target tissue with the help of externally applied magnetic fields [7]. Overall, the aim of employing physical means in drug targeting is to gain improved control over the fate of the drug.

Biological means of drug targeting refer to the use of drugs with a natural affinity for body tissues, most advantageously for the diseased tissue of interest. Not all drugs have this natural affinity and therefore constructs must be engineered to fill the gap. Most often, the drug is directly connected to specific "vector" molecules or ligands that are able to bind to specific groups in the body and thus accumulate in the target tissue. To date, the most successful biologically targeted drug deliveries have included the use of monoclonal antibodies, peptides, and specific cell receptor ligands [8–13] either on their own or bound to pharmaceutical drug carriers. Such carriers include soluble polymers, microcapsules, microparticles, cells, cell ghosts, liposomes, and micelles [2].

It is important to understand that for both physical and biological drug targeting, simply getting the drug near the site of action may not be sufficient. To guarantee that the drug is able to bind to (pain) receptors or to pass through membranes and reach the target cells (e.g., neurons), cell compartments, or intracellular target molecules, the drug must be first released from the mentioned drug carriers. This release occurs by passive mechanisms, such as desorption or release from within microspheres, by enzymatic mechanisms, such as the chemical cleaving of ester bonds, or by physical effects, such as temperature changes or ultrasound.

The group of drug delivery systems that can be targeted both by physical and biological means is the chemical drug delivery systems which consist of a drug chemically linked to a carrier molecule. In order to be active, the chemical link between drug and carrier molecule must be broken at the time the effect is needed and the active component then released. This is often done by enzymatic means, taking advantage of abundant esterases present in the human blood and other body compartments. This so-called prodrug therapy [14,15], where a nonactive drug-carrier construct is activated in the body, might also be useful in the area of local pain treatment. It has already been successfully used for the treatment of inflammatory bowel disease with a polymeric poly(anhydride ester) linked to salicylic acid [16].

19.2 OVERCOMING THE EPIDERMAL (SKIN) BARRIER

The skin can be used both as a major target for topical drug delivery (i.e., drug delivery *to* the skin for skin treatment) and also as an access point for transdermal drug delivery (i.e., drug delivery *through* the skin, mostly for systemic drug therapy). Conceptually, the skin is the most accessible body organ, can be used for the delivery of highly potent drugs without going through the parenteral route, and has been a major target of the pharmaceutical industry's developmental efforts in recent years. At the time of this writing, 19 transdermal products are U.S. Food and Drug Administration (FDA) approved in the United States [17], generating predicted sales of more than $4.5 billion in 2008.

19.2.1 Physiology of the Skin

The skin, which in an adult covers a surface area of about 2 m^2 and constitutes about 15–20% of the total body weight, is the largest organ of the body and is made up of three layers: the epidermis, the dermis, and the subcutaneous tissue (Figure 19.1). Any drugs that are intended for the deeper skin layers must first penetrate the outermost layer of densely keratinized dead cells in the stratum corneum. Depending on its location on the body, this outermost epidural layer may be as thin as a few cells, such as on the scalp, or may be thicker than 50 cell layers, such as on the elbow. Especially for water-soluble drugs, this layer is almost impenetrable, provides an excellent barrier function between the inside of our body and the outside world, and is thus crucial in maintaining homeostasis. When using the skin as the drug target, for example, into the living part of the epidermis for vaccination purposes, into the dermis for local anesthetic or systemic drug delivery, or into the fatty subcutaneous tissue for more prolonged drug action, care must be taken to deliver the drugs into the correct skin layer (Figure 19.1) by using the right technique, such as subcutaneous, intradermal, or epidermal injection or any of the specific methods mentioned in the following paragraphs.

Skin can be both the target of drug delivery and the route of administration for systemic drug delivery through blood circulation. In the first case, topical

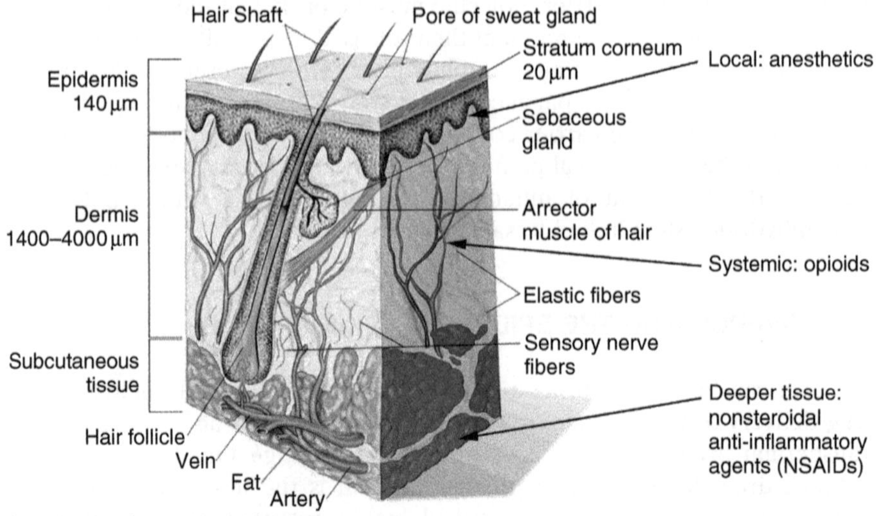

FIGURE 19.1. Anatomy and physiology of the skin with the potential targets or sites of action of selected analgesics. Modified from illustration courtesy of the American Society of Clinical Oncology.

or local dermatological delivery aims at treating diseases of the skin (e.g., allergies, psoriasis). In the second case, systemic delivery into the capillaries of the skin is useful for drugs with short half-lives and provides a continuous mode of administration, somewhat similar to that provided by an intravenous infusion. However, unlike an intravenous infusion, delivery is noninvasive and no hospitalization is required. Once absorbed, the hepatic circulation is bypassed, thus avoiding another major site of potential immediate drug degradation. Normally, only potent drugs are administered via this transdermal route because there are economic and cosmetic reasons to not exceed the patch size beyond a certain limit.

19.2.2 Skin Conditions Affecting Permeation of Active Drugs

The percutaneous absorption or deposition of the active drug applied topically on the skin surface depends on several parameters related to the inherent properties of skin itself. A summary of such factors is shown in Table 19.1.

19.3 ADVANCES IN TOPICAL AND TRANSDERMAL DRUG DELIVERY

Despite major research and development efforts in transdermal drug delivery systems, low stratum corneum permeability still limits the usefulness of topical drug delivery. To overcome this limitation, various strategic methods have been developed to increase permeation of drugs. The goal of further improvements in transdermal drug delivery systems is to increase drug flux into the skin without significantly affecting normal skin barrier function. Current technologies that attempt to increase drug flux into the skin to allow effective therapy from a reasonable sized skin area [18] can be broadly classified into passive and active approaches [19].

The passive delivery approach, sometimes called the chemical approach (Table 19.2), was conventionally based on applying drugs to the skin in ointments, creams, gels, and patches, vehicles that used diffusion as the primary method of releasing the drug. More recent developments in this area aim at enhancing the driving force of drug diffusion (thermodynamic activity) with the help of nanotechnology-based carriers such as nanoemulsions and nanogels. Not only can the vehicle be optimized toward maximized drug diffusion, but it is also possible to alter the permeability of the skin for active drugs with the help of penetration enhancers [20], supersaturated systems [21], hyaluronic acid [22], prodrugs [23–25], liposomes, and other vesicles [26–28].

The amount of drug that can be delivered with passive technologies is not sufficient for many applications because the barrier properties of the skin cannot be fundamentally changed. It is therefore often necessary to resort to the second type of approach, the active delivery approach, which acts via active mechanisms and is sometimes called the physical approach (Table 19.2). This

TABLE 19.1. Parameters Affecting Percutaneous Absorption of Active Drugs.

Biological Factors	
Age of patient	The effect of age is due to the larger surface-to-volume ratio in adults as compared with newborn infants; however, both adults and infants exhibit similar barrier functions of the skin [172,173].
Body region (site of application)	Composition and barrier properties of the stratum corneum vary at different body sites due to differences in thickness, number of cells, and, sometimes overemphasized, the density of skin appendages [174].
Moisture state of skin (hydration and occlusion)	Occlusion hydrates the keratin in corneocytes and increases the water content between adjacent intercellular lipid lamellae. For hydrophilic substances, released from an aqueous delivery device, the partition coefficient between the stratum corneum and the vehicle increases up to unity [175].
Metabolism	The viable epidermis contains several enzyme systems that catalyze processes such as oxidation, reduction, hydrolysis, or conjugation. Therefore, skin metabolism may have an additional impact on the transdermal delivery of drugs [176–178].
Disease state of skin	In general, psoriasis and other skin diseases facilitate drug delivery through the skin [179].
Species differences	The difference of skin surface lipids in different species affects the partitioning of active drugs from the vehicle to the stratum corneum [180].
Physicochemical Properties of Active Drugs and Vehicle	
Partition coefficient of active drug	For more hydrophilic molecules with low logP < 1, the transcellular route is more predominant, while the intercellular route is predominant exclusively for highly lipophilic molecules with logP > 3. For molecules with intermediate partition coefficient (logP = 1–3), both trans- and intercellular routes occur.
Molecular size of active drug	Molecular weight influences the diffusion coefficient. The larger the molecule, the lower the diffusivity. Most conventionally selected transdermal therapeutics have a narrow range of molecular weights, with the smallest being nicotine (162 Da) and the largest being oxybutinin (359 Da).
Solubility of active drug and melting point	In general, when similar drugs are compared, then the ones with better water solubility and lower melting point (less crystallinity) have the best permeation.
Ionization	The complex nature of the skin does not strictly follow the pH-partition hypothesis, which states that unionized molecules permeate more than ionized ones. Reason: Charged drugs might cross due to higher solubility and might use electrically assisted movement via shunt routes.
Drug binding	Depending on permeant (weak acid/base, ionized species, neutral molecule), varying interactions resulting from hydrogen bonding to van der Waals forces have significant to minimal effects on skin flux.
Type of formulation	The selection of the type of formulation largely affects percutaneous delivery of active drugs depending on their solubility status in the vehicle, overall charge of vehicle, and structural organization within the delivery system. For example, the transdermal flux of benzotropine in lipophilic carriers is enhanced compared to a hydrophilic vehicle [181].

TABLE 19.2. Strategies to Overcome the Stratum Corneum Barrier Function in order to Deliver Drugs Both Intra- and Transdermally.

Strategies to Overcome the Stratum Corneum Barrier		
Passive (Chemical) Approach	Active (Physical) Approach	Synergistic Approach
Formulations	Removal/bypassing of the stratum corneum	Chemical enhancers with
Vehicle systems	Skin abrasion	Iontophoresis
Supersaturation	Microneedles	Electroporation
Ion pairs and complex coacervates	Laser ablation	Ultrasound
Eutectic systems	Needleless injection	Iontophoresis with
Pharmacogel	Appendageal bypass	Electroporation
Vesicles and particles	Electrically assisted methods	Ultrasound
Microemulsions	Ultrasound/phonophoresis	Laser ablation
	Iontophoresis	Electroporation with
Prodrugs	Electrophoresis	Ultrasound
	Magnetophoresis	
Modification of the stratum corneum	Local catheterization	
Hydration	Epidural/intrathecal delivery	
Chemical enhancer to increase diffusivity increase solubility/partitioning	Magnetic drug targeting	

approach has enormously benefited from advances in precision engineering (bioengineering), computing, chemical engineering, and material sciences, all of which have helped to achieve the creation of powerful, miniaturized devices that have the ability to facilitate the generation of a desired therapeutic effect. These device-based techniques, many of them still under development, include iontophoresis, electroporation, microneedles, abrasion, needleless injection, suction, stretching, ultrasound, magnetophoresis, radiofrequency, lasers, photomechanical waves, and temperature control. Some of these techniques and their (potential) application to pain treatment are discussed in the subsequent sections.

19.3.1 Iontophoresis

Iontophoresis or iontophoretic delivery involves the application of a low-level electric current, typically $\leq 0.5\,mA/cm^2$, to enhance the percutaneous delivery of charged therapeutic drugs [29–32]. Iontophoresis uses an electrode of the same polarity as the charge on the drug to drive charged drugs into the body by electrostatic repulsion [33], utilizing the physical phenomenon of "like charges repel and opposite charges attract." In the case of the negatively charged drugs, the drug is placed between the negative electrode (cathode) and the skin for its delivery across a biological membrane, while for cationic drugs, the electrode polarities are reversed (Figure 19.2a). In both cases, the electric circuit is completed by the movement of endogenous counter ions within the skin. Generally, high voltages applied for short treatment durations (milliseconds) have been found to be most effective [34–36].

Iontophoretic drug delivery has many of the same advantages over oral and parenteral drug delivery as does the transdermal route. Specifically, it avoids first-pass effect, prevents variation in the absorption seen with oral administration, controls the rate of drug delivery, has the ability to program the drug delivery profile, and minimizes the local tissue trauma. Because iontophoresis delivers the drug to the target area without systemic exposure, it is appropriate for active drugs with (very) short biological half-lives. It delivers the active

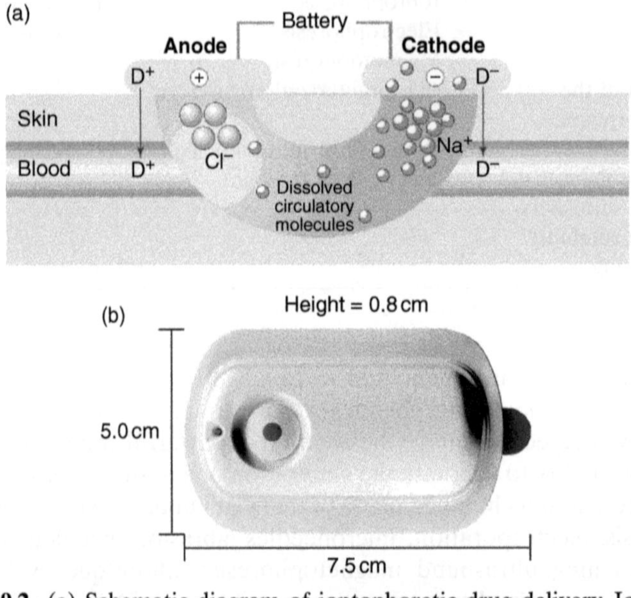

FIGURE 19.2. (a) Schematic diagram of iontophoretic drug delivery. Iontophoretic devices typically utilize anodal transport, in which the ionizable drug (D^+) is contained within the anodal compartment. A low-intensity electric current repels ionized drug molecules (D^+) from the anodal drug reservoir, driving them across the epidermis and into the subdermal tissue, where they are absorbed into the systemic circulation. Simultaneously, circulating chloride ions (Cl^-) and sodium ions (Na^+) are repelled from the cathode and anode hydrogel reservoir, respectively. Skin favors the transport of cations, which results in a net convective flow of solvent in the anode-to-cathode direction. Consequently, dissolved analytes (e.g., glucose) are also transported toward the cathode where they can be extracted and monitored. (b) A picture of the IONSYS™ device (Janssen-Cilag) with a red LED light and a button for the delivery of 40 µg fentanyl HCl per actuation.

drug directly into the bloodstream with no delay. Once the iontophoretic delivery system is turned off, the drug's effect rapidly ceases. It thus also gives the physician and patient full control over the dosing regimen, using a simple push button to activate the iontophoretic device (Figure 19.2b).

Iontophoretic delivery is affected by several factors. The first factor is the composition of the formulation and it plays an important role with respect to concentration of the drugs (an increase in concentration has been shown to increase the apparent steady-state flux of a number of drugs) [37,38]. A second factor, the pH of the donor compartment, affects the amount of ionized drug [39]. A third factor is ionic strength and the presence of co-ions (an increase in ionic strength will decrease drug delivery, as extraneous ions compete with the drug ions) [40,41]. A fourth factor is the physicochemical properties of the drugs and includes molecular size and molecular weight (MW) (transport of compounds decreases with an increase in MW under identical conditions) [42,43], charge (the sign of the charge determines the mechanism by which iontophoresis will proceed, e.g., electrorepulsion or electrorepulsion and electroosmosis), and polarity of drug (generally, the compounds that are hydrophilic are considered ideal candidates for optimum flux) [44]. A fifth factor comprises experimental conditions such as current density (a linear relationship is found between the apparent flux of a number of compounds and the applied current) [45,46], electrode material [47], and some electrical pulse parameters that include waveform, rate, and number [48]. A sixth factor is biological aspects that include variability in and among subjects, skin pH, regional blood flow [49], and skin conditions [50].

Iontophoresis is applied extensively to enhance the skin transport of a wide variety of molecules, such as molecules with different lipophilicity and size (i.e., small molecules, proteins, peptides, oligonucleotides, and even larger biopharmaceuticals) [51–53].

19.3.1.1 Iontophoresis in Pain Research. Iontophoresis is a very useful delivery technique in the area of pain relief as it provides a noninvasive means of systemic administration of a minute amount of highly active drugs [54]. It has been extensively tested in animal studies for the delivery of methadone [55] and hydromorphone [56]. In hairless rat skin, the flux of hydromorphone through the skin could be increased from 72 to 280 μg/cm^2/hour simply by adjusting the electric current from 0.1 to 0.5 mA. Control of hydromorphone flux is thus directly proportional to the applied current. In addition, the concentration of the drug in the device is proportional to the hydromorphone flux attained. From these studies, the authors conclude that it is feasible to reach therapeutically effective concentrations of hydromorphone for the management of cancer-related pain via iontophoretic administration.

In clinical trials, sodium salicylate iontophoresis has been shown to be effective in the management of hip pain [57]. Specifically, 20 patients suffering from sickle cell disorders were given conventional physiotherapy and either their regular medication or iontophoretic salicylate. The iontophoresis treatment group showed statistically significant reduction in pain intensity and improvements in the hip range of motion as compared to the control group.

In 1995, IOMED, Inc. became the first company to receive FDA approval for an iontophoretic delivery system. The system consisted of lidocaine HCl 2% and epinephrine 1:100,000 (Iontocaine® or Numby Stuff) for local dermal anesthesia. This was followed in 2004 by Vyteris (NJ, USA), which received FDA approval for its Lidosite™ topical prefilled/preprogrammed iontophoretic system for the delivery of lidocaine. Lidosite anesthetizes the skin within 10 minutes at a depth sufficient for all anticipated needlestick and dermatological procedures. Both lidocaine and lignocaine, delivered by iontophoresis, have been successfully used to prevent pain from venopuncture [58–60]. Iontophoretically delivered lidocaine was also found to be useful for decreasing the pain caused by cannulation and propofol injection [61–63].

More recently in May 2006, the FDA approved the IONSYS fentanyl HCl system from ALZA (Johnson & Johnson, NJ, USA), an iontophoretic delivery device for the treatment of postoperative pain (Figure 19.2b). The credit card-sized patch showed comparable pharmacokinetics to intravenous fentanyl infusions and is therapeutically equivalent to the standard regimen of IV morphine, the most commonly used modality for postoperative patient-controlled analgesia (PCA) [64]. The fentanyl HCl system is needle free and contains a fentanyl hydrogel that functions as an anode, a cathode composed of an inert hydrogel, microprocessor, battery, a light-emitting diode, and a drug delivery button [65]. The system is attached to the skin of the upper outer arm or chest with an adhesive backing. When the on-demand button is pressed, an imperceptible current drives the fentanyl from the hydrogel through the epidermis and into the systemic circulation.

Many more iontophoretic systems are under commercial development and include the Phoresor® device (IOMED, Inc.) [66], the Vyteris and E-TRANS devices (ALZA Corp.) [67], Dupel® from Empi, Inc., and Microphor® from Life-Tech International. Integrated iontophoretic patches are available from Travanti Pharma Inc. and IOMED, Inc., are disposable, single-use iontophoretic patches and are useful for the delivery of many charged drugs with very little additional development needed.

19.3.2 Microneedle-Based Devices

In 1976, Gerstel was the first to describe microneedles in a U.S. patent [68], but it was not until the early 1990s that microfabrication technology was developed to a level that allowed for the fabrication of microneedle systems. Microneedles are lancetlike mechanical structures with shaft widths typically between 10 and 500 μm and lengths of 30 μm to several millimeters. They are most often used to provide a pathway to the upper layers of the skin. Solid microneedles are used to abrade or to perforate the stratum corneum (the topmost about 20-μm-thick skin layer; see Figure 19.1) in order to allow topically applied drugs to reach the epidermis or to diffuse from the injection site toward the blood vessels of the dermis. Hollow microneedles additionally allow for penetration of the stratum corneum, with their lumens simultaneously providing rigid conduits for drug injection or sampling of biomolecules from the skin. Because the vast majority of nerve endings are located in the dermis, drug injection into the approximately 100-μm-thick epidermal skin layer (Figure 19.1) is painless [69].

In order to access a wider area of the skin, microneedles have been fabricated in single rows and in two-dimensional arrays. The first array of solid microneedles, the "Utah array" [70], was developed by researchers at The University of Utah and was used to record neural signals. It is currently available through Cyberkinetics, Inc. (Salt Lake City, UT, USA). The first hollow microneedles were developed by Lin et al. in 1993 [71]. Thereafter, rapid advancement in microfabrication technology led to the development of a vast variety of microneedles made primarily from silicon, metal, and more recently, polymers. Arrays of hollow silicon microneedles are already available through NanoPass Technologies Ltd. (Nes Ziona, Israel), while Theratechnologies in Montreal, Canada (supported by ALZA Corp.) is currently clinically testing its growth factor-releasing microneedle technology called Macroflux® [72].

The two main drug delivery mechanisms for the delivery of drugs by microneedles are to either dry-coat the drug on the microprojection array [73], a technique that is primarily used for intracutaneous immunizations, or to inject the drug through a hollow needle from a drug reservoir [72]. A system that is easy to implement is the use of microneedles attached directly to a syringe (Figure 19.3) [74]. A third approach of transcutaneous drug delivery with microneedles is to prepare an array of solid needles that contain the drug in a biodegradable needle matrix material, using a molding process [75]. In this approach, the encapsulated drug is released as soon as the needles start to dissolve, which occurs immediately after they have been inserted into the skin.

Successful drug delivery through microneedles into human skin has only recently been reported [69] *in vivo* using methyl nicotinate as a model drug. No standard protocols for microneedle-based transdermal administration of therapeutics have been established yet, although the technique is very promising.

19.3.3 Skin Abrasion

The abrasion technique involves either the direct disruption or removal of upper skin layers to facilitate the permeation of topically applied drugs. Some skin abrasion devices are based on techniques used by dermatologists for superficial skin resurfacing, such as microdermabrasion, which is used in the treatment of acne, scars, hyperpigmentation, and other skin blemishes as a skin rejuvenation procedure. *Microdermabrasion* partially ablates and homogenizes the skin layers. Lee et al. found an 8–24 times higher 5-fluorouracil permeation across microdermabrasion-treated skin than across intact skin [76].

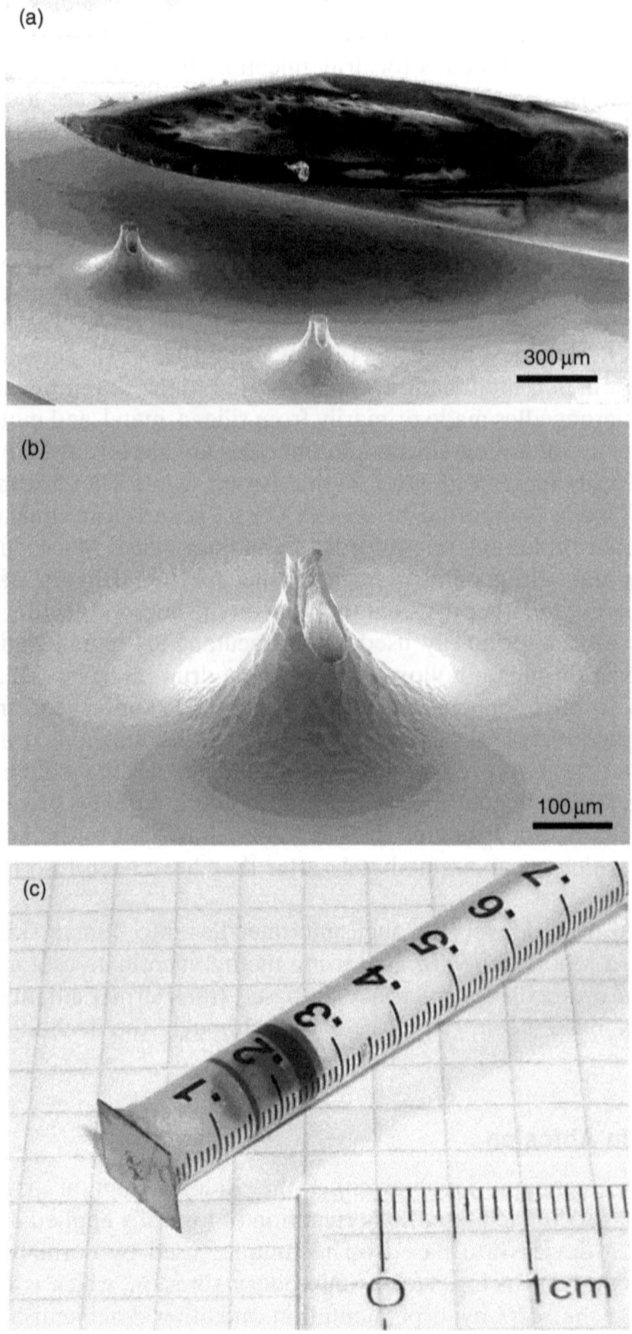

FIGURE 19.3. (a) Scanning electron microscopy image of a sharp microneedle array compared to a 25-gauge steel needle with an outer diameter of 0.53 mm. (b) Close up of one of the microneedles. (c) Potential way of using such a microneedle array connected to a normal syringe. With permission from Sivamani et al. [69].

In a similar study, microdermabrasion also enhanced the skin delivery of the hydrophilic 5-aminolevulinic acid (ALA), an enhancement of drug uptake that was not seen with the lipophilic drug clobetasol. The same group studied the effect of microdermabrasion on the enhancement of topical vitamin C delivery [77]. The flux and skin deposition of vitamin C across microdermabrasion-treated skin was approximately 20 times higher than across intact skin.

Another abrasion technique, *microscissioning*, is based on creation of microchannels in the skin through the eroding of the impermeable outer layers with sharp microscopic metal granules (Figure 19.4). It is a rapid and painless procedure and has been used *in vivo* to deliver lidocaine to the wrist of volunteers, providing complete anesthesia around the site within 3 minutes as compared to the approximately 1.5 hours required for topical application without the microconduit [78]. The authors also concluded that microscissioned microconduits can provide a minimally invasive basis for the delivery of any size molecule, and for the extraction of interstitial fluid and blood samples. Based on this technique, Carlisle Scientific is currently developing a penlike handheld device called the "microscissioner." Another company, MedPharm Ltd (Guildford, UK), has developed a novel dermal abrasion

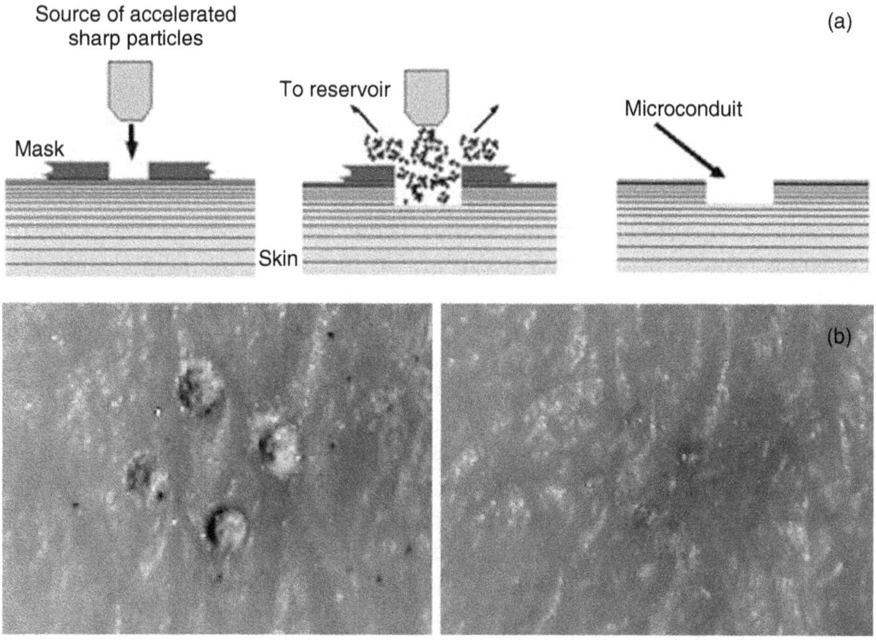

FIGURE 19.4. (a) Microscissioning produces microconduits using sharp, micron-sized, inert crystals carried by an inert gas, directed toward a mask aperture placed against the stratum corneum or the nail. (b) Four *in vivo* microconduits of 150 μm in diameter are shown on the left with abrasive particles present. On the right, the particles have been removed from the microconduits. With permission from BioMed Central [78].

device (D3S) for the delivery of a wide variety of therapeutics ranging from hydrophilic low-molecular-weight compounds to biopharmaceuticals. *In vitro* data indicate that application of the device can increase the penetration of angiotensin into the skin 100-fold compared to untreated human skin [79]. This device is noninvasive and histological studies on human skin show that the effects on the stratum corneum are reversible and nonirritating.

Microporation is another abrasive technique that utilizes a vaporization process to remove tiny areas of the stratum corneum creating microscopic pores that allow access to the underlying viable epidermis [80]. The vaporization is produced by passing a current, for a short duration (milliseconds), through an array of tiny resistive elements to the skin surface. Microporation creates micropores in the skin surface by physically removing the cells and thus alters the barrier properties of the skin for drugs. Microporation is pain free and nontraumatic as the temperature gradient does not reach the capillary loops or pain-sensing nerves in the upper dermis. Microporation technology is currently most often used to reliably and easily induce skin-directed vaccination. As an example, the reporter gene expression increased 100-fold following application of an adenoviral vector to microporated skin when compared to the same application but to intact skin [80]. Furthermore, 10- to 100-fold increases in cellular and humoral immune responses were observed thereafter.

19.3.4 Needleless Injection

Another pain-free method of administering drugs to the skin is needleless injection. This method circumvents the issues of safety, fear, and pain associated with the use of hypodermic needles. The needleless syringe comprises an elongated tubular nozzle with a rupturable membrane initially closing the passage through the nozzle. Particles of a therapeutic agent to be delivered are dispensed behind the membrane and are then blasted—with high gas pressure sufficient to burst the membrane—into the patient's skin. Different devices are available and include liquid (Ped-O-Jet, Iject, Biojector 2000, Medi-Jector, Intraject) and powder (particle mediated epidermal delivery [PMED] device formerly known as PowderJect injector) systems. The PMED device consists of a helium gas cylinder, drug powder sealed in a cassette made of plastic membrane, a specially designed convergent–divergent supersonic nozzle, and a silencer to reduce the noise associated with the rupturing of the membrane when particles are fired. The PMED device has been reported to successfully deliver testosterone, lidocaine hydrochloride and macromolecules such as calcitonin and insulin [81–83].

The most advanced application of needleless injection is the *needle-free delivery of vaccines* using a powder jet. This technique could aid in mass vaccinations by increasing the ease and speed of delivery and by offering improved safety and compliance, decreasing costs, and reducing the pain associated with vaccinations [84]. Brave et al. successfully used needle-free injection for intradermal delivery of multigene/multisubtype HIV-1 vaccine that resulted in induction of potent cellular and humoral immune responses in patients [85]. Another novel nanoparticle-based DNA vaccine delivery system was also found to enhance immune responses after intradermal injection with the needle-free jet injection device Biojector 2000 [86]. Targeting the antigen-presenting cells in the epidermis with needleless injection thus seems to work well, and even direct intracellular delivery of DNA or protein vaccines for transfection is being attempted to induce gold particle-mediated immunization [87].

19.3.5 Ultrasound (Sonophoresis or Phonophoresis)

Sonophoresis, also called phonophoresis, involves the use of ultrasonic energy to enhance the transdermal delivery of solutes. Although the exact mechanism of sonophoresis is not known, it is thought that drug absorption may involve a disruption of the stratum corneum lipids through a combination of thermal, chemical, and mechanical alterations within the skin tissue, allowing the drug to pass through the skin [18]. The enhancement induced by ultrasound is particularly significant at low frequencies of less than 100 kHz [88,89]. This so-called low-frequency sonophoresis (LFS) enhances the permeability of the skin to macromolecular drugs via induction of localized transport regions. Several therapeutic macromolecules including insulin [90–92], low-molecular-weight heparin [93], and vaccines [94] have been delivered using LFS *in vivo*. Clinical trials have been performed with several drugs including lidocaine [95] and cyclosporine [96].

The SonoPrep® device (Echo Therapeutics, Franklin, MA, USA) uses low-frequency ultrasound (55 kHz) for an average duration of 15 seconds to enhance skin permeability. This battery-operated, handheld device consists of a control unit, ultrasonic horn with control panel, a disposable coupling medium cartridge, and a return electrode [90]. Applied to the delivery of lidocaine, ultrasound seemed to disorder the lipid bilayers and increased lidocaine diffusion and uptake by 3.3-fold. In the absence of ultrasound, lidocaine diffusion in lipid bilayers of the stratum corneum is slowed to a diffusion coefficient of $50 \times 10^{-9}\,cm^2/s$ by the presence of densely packed and ordered lipid bilayers.

19.3.6 Laser Radiation

The direct and controlled exposure of skin to a laser results in the ablation of the stratum corneum without significantly damaging the underlying epidermis. Removal of the stratum corneum using this method has been shown to enhance the delivery of both lipophilic and hydrophilic drugs [97,98]. Different lasers enhance and control skin permeation differently, as has been demonstrated *in vitro* with the drug 5-fluorouracil [99]. The authors showed that an erbium-doped yttrium aluminum garnet (Er:YAG) laser partly ablated the stratum corneum and resulted in an up to 133-fold higher drug uptake than the one measured across intact skin. When a CO_2 laser was used, both stratum corneum ablation and increased temperature effects contributed to an up to 41-fold increase in 5-fluorouracil flux when higher fluencies (7.0 J/cm^2) were used. In another study, fluorescein isothiocyanate (FITC)-labeled dextran of increasing MWs (4.4, 19.4, 38.0, and 77.0 kDa) was used as the model macromolecule to investigate the skin permeation *in vitro* [97]. Dextrans of all MWs could be delivered transdermally after laser treatment. It was thought that intercellular pathways played an important role in the delivery of the dextrans. The postulated mechanisms of action were the ablation of the stratum corneum layer, photomechanical stress on intercellular regions, and alterations of the morphology and arrangement of corneocytes [97].

A handheld portable laser device has been developed by Norwood Abbey Ltd. (Victoria, Australia), which, in a study involving human volunteers, was found to reduce the onset of action of lidocaine to 3–5 minutes, while 60 minutes was required to attain a similar effect in the control group. The Norwood Abbey system has been approved by the FDA for the administration of topically applied anesthetics.

19.3.7 Magnetophoresis

Another method that might be useful to drive analgesic drugs across the skin is magnetophoresis, the process of moving particles or molecules in a viscous medium under the influence of a magnetic field [100]. Based on work by Murthy, it seems that different diamagnetic molecules, such as benzoic acid [101] and terbutaline [102], can be driven across biological barriers with the help of a magnetic field. Their system consisted of a drug-containing hydroxypropyl methyl cellulose gel, which was made into a film by applying a polyisobutylene polymer backing [102]. Control films were additionally made with or without the permeability enhancer isopropyl myristate in the gel. In a diffusion apparatus, placing a 2-mm thick magnet on the film increased the drug release about threefold over a film without the magnet. Adding the permeability enhancer resulted in a drug release similar to the release seen with a magnetic setup, both in terms of release time and amount of drug released. The authors accounted for this magnetophoretic effect by pointing to the diamagnetic properties of the drugs, explaining that these properties tend to cause "the drug escape from the applied magnetic field." Further studies, however, are needed to confirm these data and to discover the mechanistic reasons for the drug release under the influence of a magnetic field.

19.3.8 Synergistic Effects of Combination Treatments

Many of the above methods can be used in combination with each other (Table 19.2) to further enhance the uptake of drugs through the skin [103]. Although such combined approaches clearly work, the mechanisms behind their synergistic effects are often speculative. Also, the safety of the combined procedures requires additional attention as they could cause extra damage to the skin or could result in added side effects.

Combination approaches based on biological targeting can also be very useful for the treatment or prevention of pain. One recent and very elegant example is the use of QX-314 and capsaicin, which together block pain while permitting normal sensation [104]. This novel effect is based on the charged lidocaine derivative QX-314, which is not able to diffuse across membranes and thus cannot access the neuronal voltage-dependent sodium channels. When another compound, the selective transient receptor potential vanilloid 1 (TRPV1) channel activator capsaicin, was added, the large TRPV1 pores allowed the passage of QX-314, and as a result, pain was blocked. This approach is specific to sensory C-fiber neurons involved in nociception because the TRPV1 channels are restricted to that location (see Chapter 8), and thus no numbness is produced [105,106]. Applications of this combination therapy might include dentistry procedures and many other local interventions. Both drugs could be combined into a patch similar to the capsaicin patches currently used extensively in the treatment of rheumatic ailments.

It should be kept in mind that even the "simple" approach of local drug application to the skin produces not only local but also systemic effects. Systemic effects are mainly the result of transdermal uptake (Figure 19.1) of an often not insignificant percentage of the drug. Ideally, drugs used for systemic therapy should be those that are readily absorbed into the blood stream, whereas drugs used for local treatments should be those that penetrate only into the underlying deep tissue, such as the muscle tissue under viable skin. The contribution of both local and systemic effects has been explored with different nonsteroidal anti-inflammatory drugs (NSAIDs) *in vivo* by Higaki et al. [107]. Both direct penetration through the skin to the muscle as well as uptake after systemic circulation has been reported and is shown in Figure 19.5. The extent of how much of the drug stays local or gets absorbed into the

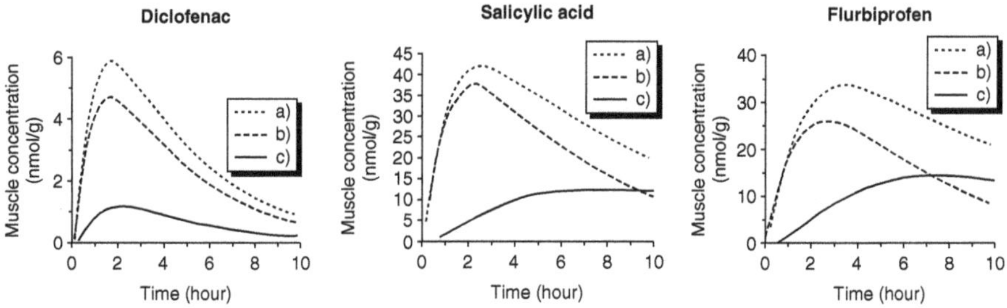

FIGURE 19.5. After dermal application, three different NSAIDs were evaluated for direct penetration and transport from systemic circulation to the muscle layer below the application site. For each drug, the a) curve indicates the total concentration that reached the target tissue; the b) curve shows the concentration due to direct penetration, and the c) curve indicates the concentration due to systemic circulation. Redrawn from Reference 107.

blood stream depends on how much of the drug in viable skin will be bound to cytosolic components, and on the balance between the unbound fraction in the skin and plasma [19]. If the unbound fraction in the skin is too large and the local effect thus becomes less important, then it might be possible to influence the system and to bind the drugs to carriers that cannot physically leave the application site. Useful carriers for such an approach are, for example, microspheres that will slowly release an encapsulated drug at the site of injection over extended time periods.

19.4 OTHER METHODS OF INCREASING LOCAL DRUG CONCENTRATION

Postoperative pain management has dramatically improved with the advent of PCA delivery. There are, however, still some issues with PCA use including premature discontinuation, resource-intensive setup and maintenance, interruptions in analgesia, and the potential for medication errors. For these reasons, pain control with preemptive analgesia and multimodal therapy has been thought to be more appropriate for some patients. Currently, the most efficient preemptive analgesia methods used in the clinic are local catheterization and epidural/intrathecal injection of therapeutic drugs.

19.4.1 Local Catheterization

Local catheterization that induces peripheral nerve blocks is especially useful in surgery on extremities [108]. Peripheral nerve blocks include perineural catheters, which are normally used for a maximum of 12–16 hours, and portable infusion pumps. The two most successful drugs for this procedure are bupivacaine and ropivacaine [109]. The intense, site-specific analgesia with local anesthetics produces fewer side effects (minimal nausea and vomiting) and leads to faster recovery and discharge, thus reducing overall healthcare costs.

19.4.2 Epidural and Intrathecal Delivery Systems

Postoperative pain management is a serious issue. Postoperative pain can be safely and effectively treated by one-time or intermittently administered bolus doses of epidural morphine and by continuous epidural infusions of opioids/local anesthetics with and without patient-controlled epidural analgesia [108]. Epidural treatments involve the insertion of a catheter into the epidural space, a narrow sleevelike area that surrounds the spinal cord, or into the intrathecal space, which contains the cerebrospinal fluid and the spinal cord. Pain-relieving drugs are then delivered through the catheter. Epidural and intrathecal analgesia are used when other methods either do not give sufficient pain relief or produce excessive adverse effects. Because the dose of drugs is much smaller than if given through a normal injection or if swallowed as a tablet, the side-effect profile for epidural and intrathecal drug delivery is much better than for these other methods.

Postoperative and postpartum pain usually lasts several days, but the injectable opioids used to treat the pain have only relatively short durations of action. To extend their action, extended-release opioid formulations have been developed. Most recently, effective postoperative analgesia was induced for 48 hours using an extended-release epidural morphine (EREM) injection [110]. EREM consists of a liposomal formulation, in particular a foam with multiple lipid vesicles containing morphine suspended in an aqueous solution. After injection, reorganization of the liposomal membrane leads to extended release of the opioid within the epidural space. Importantly, caution must be exercised with this approach because this is still a systemic drug application with serious respiratory depression as a potential side effect [108].

At the end of 2004, the FDA approved Prialt® (ziconotide intrathecal infusion; see Chapter 5) from Elan Corporation (Dublin, Ireland) for the management of severe chronic pain in patients for whom intrathecal therapy is warranted, and who do not tolerate or are refractory to other treatments, such as systemic analgesics, adjunctive therapies, or intrathecal morphine.

19.4.3 Magnetic Targeting

A more recent physical means of drug delivery involves combining a drug with a magnetically responsive carrier and directing them to, or at least accumulating them in, the target tissue with the help of magnetic fields [7]. Magnetic drug delivery by particulate carriers is a very efficient method of delivering a drug through the blood stream to a localized disease site. Very high concentrations of chemotherapeutic or radiological agents can be achieved near the target site, for example, a tumor, without any toxic effects to normal surrounding tissue (Figure 19.6).

Magnetic carriers [111] receive their magnetic responsiveness to a magnetic field from incorporated magnetic materials (magnetite, iron, nickel, cobalt) and are normally grouped according to size, starting at 4–6 nm in diameter (ferrofluids, nanospheres) up to 1–100 μm (magnetic microspheres) (Figure 19.7). Often, magnetic liposomes are also included when speaking about magnetic carriers. For biomedical applications, magnetic carriers must be water based, biocompatible, nontoxic, and nonimmunogenic. Magnetite and iron powder were the first magnetic carriers to be used *in vivo*, as contrast agents in the femoral artery [112,113]. Improved biocompatibility, however, was reached by encapsulating these magnetic components with matrix materials such as chitosan, dextran, poly(lactic acid), or albumin [7].

The only clinical application of magnetic particles currently approved by the FDA is the use of these particles as contrast agents in magnetic resonance imaging (MRI) [114]. There is, however, much ongoing research aimed at using magnetic particles as cancer-treating agents. The different approaches

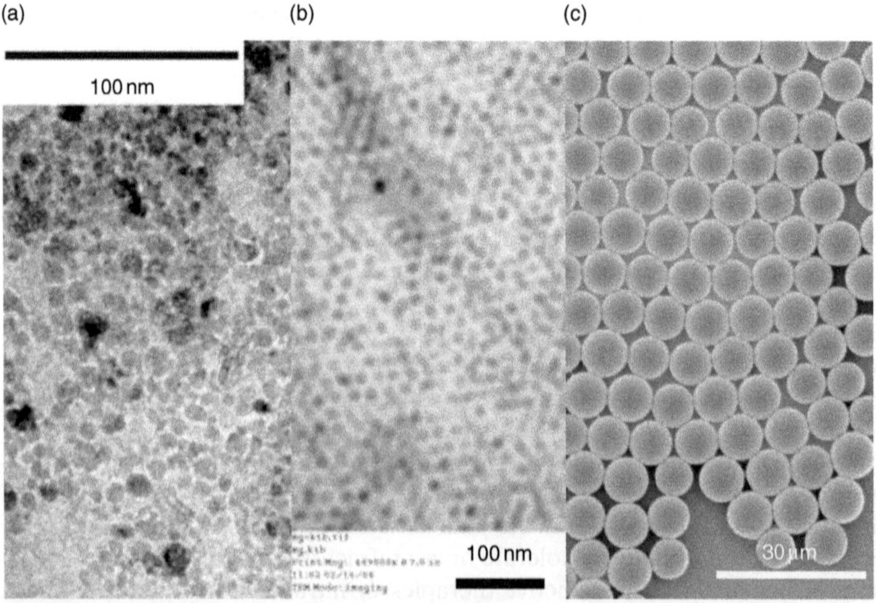

FIGURE 19.6. Magnetic nano- and microparticles made of different sizes, shapes, and materials. (a) Magnetite (Fe_3O_4) nanoparticles prepared by the most commonly used Massart method [169]. (b) Uniformly sized magnetite nanoparticles prepared by thermal decomposition of iron oleate in a high-boiling solvent [170]. (c) PLGA microspheres encapsulating nanosized magnetite particles prepared by a solvent extraction method.

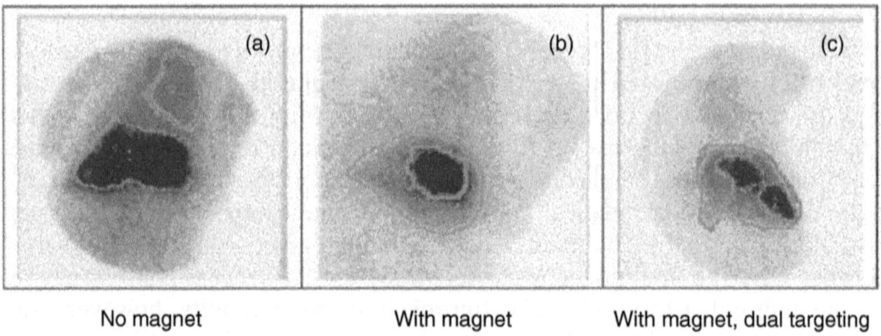

FIGURE 19.7. Principle of magnetic targeting. (a) The infusion of magnetic particles of 1–3 μm into a pig's blood supply leads to rapid liver uptake. (b) Placing a permanent NdFeB magnet above a distinct liver area (e.g., a tumor) will rapidly concentrate most of the particles. (c) The magnet can even be moved, and a secondary amount of particles can be targeted to a different area in the liver. With permission from Goodwin et al. [171]. See color insert.

undergoing testing in cancer therapy include magnetic microspheres loaded with radioactivity or chemotherapeutic drugs; they can also be used directly for magnetic fluid hyperthermia under the influence of an externally applied AC magnetic field [115], as remotely activated drug reservoirs, or for the separation of cancer cells from healthy cells, thus allowing better and side effect-free stem cell transplantation. A good source of information about magnetic carriers, including an extensive bibliography of this field, is available at http://www.magneticmicrosphere.com/.

To date, no pain-relieving drugs have been encapsulated into magnetic particles. The stage is set, however, for this to occur. Nonmagnetic poly(lactide-co-glycolide) (PLGA) microspheres with a release profile appropriate for pain-relieving drugs have been created [116]. These fentanyl-loaded microspheres slowly release the drug in a linear fashion over 2 weeks (Figure 19.8). Making these microspheres magnetic would be a straightforward procedure by adding magnetite to the polymer during the microsphere preparation [117–119]. The magnetic microspheres can then be guided to distinct target tissues or organs. Delivery of the microspheres as a whole to the brain, however, is not possible, as they are not able to cross the blood–brain barrier (BBB). For that purpose, the drug would have to be released and then independently reach the brain.

19.4.3.1 BBB. In terms of drug targeting, the BBB is a formidable obstacle to drug delivery. The BBB is defined in part by its physical structure, the junctions between the capillary endothelial cells, which are unusually tight and

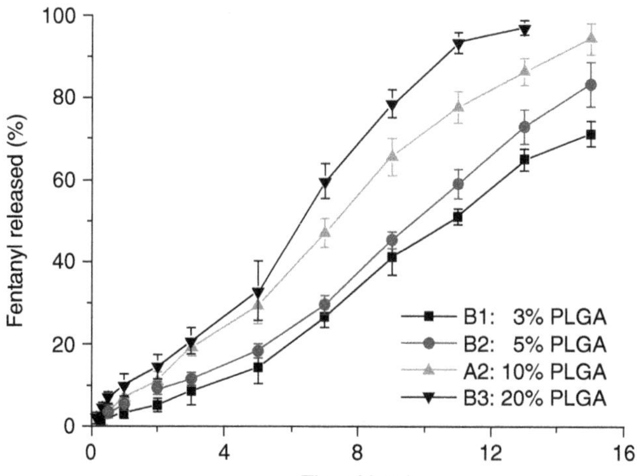

FIGURE 19.8. Effect of polymer concentration during the microsphere preparation on the fentanyl release pattern from biodegradable poly(lactide-co-glycolide) (PLGA) microspheres. Interestingly, none of the formulations showed a burst effect. With permission from Choi et al. [116].

thus completely prevent paracellular transport. A more important characteristic of the BBB, however, is the fact that it lacks the usual mechanism found in most tissues that allow drugs to be transferred across their capillary walls [120]. In particular, the mechanism of pinocytosis is completely missing. In addition, P-glycoprotein, an efflux membrane pump, actively pumps a wide range of drugs from the brain back into the blood stream. Uptake of drugs into the brain is thus normally by diffusion and depends on the MW and lipophilicity of the drug. As far as the MW limits, current research has determined that essentially no drug uptake is seen in the brain above 400Da. Because all opioids fall below this value, they generally cross the BBB well. In considering drug lipophilicity, the permeability of morphine, codeine (methylmorphine), and heroin (diacetylmorphine) with a calculated logP of 0.24, 1.14, and 1.86, respectively, illustrates well the improved delivery of more hydrophobic drugs into the brain [120]. Codeine has a BBB permeability of about 10 times that of morphine, while that of heroin is another 10 times larger. In addition to lipophilic small molecules, a few, small hydrophilic molecules such as hexose, certain amino acids, transferring, and IGF-II are known to cross the BBB by receptor-mediated drug transport [121].

For the peripheral targeting of analgesic drugs, it is possible to take advantage of the properties of the BBB and to design a drug that reaches the target tissue and spares the brain, thus avoiding any CNS side effects and toxicities. This is best illustrated by considering the drug loperamide, a phenylpiperidine derivative with a chemical structure similar to the opiate receptor agonists diphenoxylate and haloperidol [122]. Loperamide is designed to maintain the antidiarrheal activity of opiate receptor agonists, but has low oral absorption and does not cross the BBB.

There have been reports in the literature that colloids, which are 5- to 200-nm particles suspended in liquid, can pass through the BBB and might thus be useful carriers for drugs that normally cannot reach the brain [123]. In one of the reports, colloidal human serum albumin (HSA) nanoparticles filled with loperamide and conjugated with the same OX26 transferrin antibody induced significant antinociceptive effects in the tail-flick test in ICR (CD-1) mice after intravenous injection, whereas the same system with a control IgG2a antibody yielded only marginal effects [124]. This demonstrates that antibody-coupled nanoparticles are able to transport loperamide across the BBB. In another report, liposomes (which are not technically colloids, but behave similarly) coated with OX26 transferrin antibody and filled with daunomycin were shown to increase the drug concentration in the brain [125]. In a third report, it was possible to achieve central analgesia, as measured by a hot plate test, when the neuropeptides Leu-enkephalin dalargin and the Met-enkephalin kyotorphin were adsorbed to the surface of colloidal poly(butylcyanoacrylate) nanoparticles which were coated with polysorbate 80 [126]. Another group similarly showed that poly(butylcyanoacrylate) nanoparticles adsorbing loperamide and polysorbate 80 also induced analgesia, as measured by a tail-flick test [127]. The uptake mechanisms for loperamide and the peptides have yet to be fully explained, but appear to be related to the nonionic detergent, because even a simple mixture of drug and polysorbate showed a rather high brain uptake with some analgesic effect. For the other listed reports, it is not clear how colloids pass through the BBB. They may be internalized in the endothelial cells or might simply adhere to their surface, thus providing a greater concentration gradient to assist in passive diffusion.

19.4.4 Slow-Release Implants Based on Biodegradable Polymers

Biocompatible and biodegradable polymer-based controlled-release implants loaded with pain-relieving drugs (mainly opioids) have shown promising results in pain control, particularly in cancer patients. Such implants are placed subcutaneously, intrathecally, or intraspinally and then slowly release the active drug over an extended time period [128]. One such system, and a first example of a polymer-based device for the delivery of analgesic drugs, is the preparation of implantable rods containing hydromorphone, bupivacaine, or both [129]. *In vivo* studies conducted in rats showed potent, prolonged analgesia by these implants. Another example demonstrating the use of a polymer-based system consists of the preparation of microspheres from the biodegradable copolymer PLGA encapsulating bupivacaine [130]. After local subcutaneous injection into the plantar hind paw, these microspheres were shown, in the paw pressure test, to prolong analgesia while simultaneously diminishing systemic toxicity. The duration of antinociception increased from 60 to 90 minutes for a dose of 1 mg of plain bupivacaine compared to the same dose encapsulated in microspheres. Longer antinociception of 120 and 180 minutes was possible with microspheres containing 2.5 and 5.0 mg of the drug, respectively. When such doses of plain bupivacaine were used, significant systemic toxicity was induced.

There are many other examples of how polymeric implants have been used for the controlled release of fentanyl and hydromorphone. One research group showed that a single dose of intrathecal fentanyl in poly(DL-lactide) (PLA) composites produced less respiratory depression than the same dose of plain fentanyl [131]. This improved toxicity profile was due to a slow drug release from the implant. Another group prepared an ethylene vinyl acetate (EVA) copolymer disk, measuring 1.05 cm in diameter and 0.27 cm in height, which contained 50% hydromorphone by weight and was coated with poly(methyl methacrylate) [132]. This implant produced a sustained release of the drug over 4 weeks. A third group produced implants from an interpenetrating network of two biocompatible polymers, the biodegradable polyester poly(3-hydroxybutyrate-co-3-hydroxyvalerate) (PHBV) and the synthetic, nonbiodegradable poly(2-hydroxyethyl methacrylate) (PHEMA) [133]. Fentanyl was released slowly over 2 days after placing the implant in the right paw of a rat.

These examples provide only a glimpse into the enormous area of polymer-based drug delivery. For fuller information, we point the reader to recent books and reviews in the field of polymeric drug delivery systems. They encompass nanoparticles appropriate for intravascular application [134], microspheres that might be more appropriately used as depots for slow release of drugs after intramuscular or subcutaneous injection [135], polymeric films [136–138], woven or electrospun mats [139], and implants of many other shapes and sizes [140–142]. By choosing the appropriate polymer and device geometry, it is possible to adjust the drug release curve (pharmacokinetics) from zero-order release to any required shape and also from hours to days, weeks, or months for the duration of the release [6,143].

19.4.5 Lipid-Based Drug Delivery

Liposomal drug carriers constitute important vehicles for the topical delivery of pain-relieving drugs. Liposomes are phospholipid vesicles sized between 40 and several thousand micrometers. They can contain hydrophilic drugs in the aqueous core or lipophilic drugs in the phospholipid bilayer. Many liposomal formulation subtypes such as elastic liposomes, lipospheres, liposomal spray gels, transferosomes, and niosomes have shown potential to deliver a variety of analgesic drugs including anesthetics [144], anti-inflammatories [145,146], and analgesics [147]. Phospholipids, the major ingredient used to formulate liposomal systems, easily integrate with skin lipids and provide the desired hydration conditions to enhance drug penetration and localization at the site of action (i.e., in the skin layers of the target area). Liposomal bilayers fuse with multilamellar intercellular lipid layers of the stratum corneum and alter the phase transition properties of stratum corneum lipids. The enhanced permeation of liposomal incorporated drugs is thus the result of an altered physicochemical state of the skin.

The first liposomes filled with analgesic drugs were transferosomes containing 7% lidocaine or 4% tetracaine and were found to be effective for the noninvasive treatment of local pain with direct, topical drug application [148]. In Sprague Dawley rats, these dermally applied analgesic transferosomes increased the heat stimulus reaction time to greater than 70 seconds, compared to a typical reaction time of 30 seconds. The same liposome preparation was also shown to be effective in patients when tested by the pinprick method [148]. Thereafter, different companies produced similar commercially available liposomal products that include a liposomal lidocaine 4% cream (Maxilene, RGR Pharma) and a liposomal diclofenac and also a ketoprofen spray (MIKA Pharma GmbH).

Liposomal preparations are also useful in an injectable or inhalable form. As an example for the injectable form, bupivacaine lipospheres have been prepared as a parenteral sustained-release system for postoperative pain management [149]. Another type of bupivacaine-loaded liposomes was used epidurally and reached extended, complete analgesia for 11 hours in a patient suffering from pain associated with lung cancer [150]. The bupivacaine-loaded liposomes did not induce a motor blockade, although it was seen in control patients who received the free drug. Similarly, liposomal alfentanil given intrathecally to rats provided improved spinal antinociception while eliminating supraspinally mediated side effects completely [151]. An example for an inhalable fentanyl delivery system is the mixture of free and liposome-encapsulated fentanyl, which provided both rapid pain relief and extended action [152]. Specifically, the fentanyl plasma concentrations were 56% and 140% greater at 8 and 24 hours after the simple and noninvasive aerosol administration compared with the concentrations after intravenous administration.

It may be possible to make lipid-based drug delivery more specific by adding or conjugating targeting molecules to the surface of the liposomes. To date, no attempts toward this goal have been made in pain treatment but liposomes with covalently bound antibodies, so-called immunoliposomes, are well-known in the world of anticancer drug delivery [153].

19.5 ORAL DOSAGE FORMS FOR ANALGESIA

According to a report by Global Industry Analysts, Inc., the world's largest market research company, the major driving forces behind the expanding analgesics market are the aging population and the rising therapeutic benefits of drugs. Together, these factors are expected to produce a growth in demand for pain relief medications that is predicted to reach $35.5 billion by 2015. Interestingly, despite the availability of numerous analgesic products, the choice of simple over-the-counter (OTC) analgesic compounds is limited to only a handful for adults (acetaminophen or paracetamol, acetylsalicylic acid, and ibuprofen) and for children (acetaminophen or paracetamol and ibuprofen).

Most OTC and certain physician-prescribed products for pain relief are intended to immediately release the active drug after oral ingestion and thus result in rapid onset of action. Such products need to be taken frequently if the pain persists. The inconvenience associated with frequent dosing could be overcome through the use of slow-release products. Also, modified-release products have become a mainstay for the treatment of moderate to severe chronic pain. Due to the decreased dosing frequency, these products allow patients to focus on their daily activities and to get uninterrupted nights of sleep.

19.5.1 Immediate-Onset Systems

Rapid-onset pain treatment is needed for the treatment of breakthrough pain. It typically takes 0.5–2.0 hours after swallowing a tablet for an effect to manifest because the tablet must pass through the stomach to the intestines before it can be absorbed into the blood. A faster and safe way to achieve quick oral action is for the drug to be absorbed through the relatively permeable buccal mucosa. This mucosa is robust, has a rich blood supply, and is particularly well suited for the delivery of drugs that undergo significant first-pass effect in the intestines and in the liver.

The successful buccal delivery of a potent opioid is best illustrated by the fentanyl buccal tablets. The OraVescent® (Cephalon Inc., Frazer, PA, USA) drug delivery technology used in these compressed buccal tablets contains a pH-altering excipient, sodium carbonate, which provides an alkaline environment for converting the ionized fentanyl into an un-ionized, maximally absorbable form of fentanyl. Almost complete drug absorption is achieved within 15 minutes after application [154], making the buccal tablet ideal for the management of breakthrough pain in opioid-tolerant cancer patients. Buccal delivery has the faster pharmacokinetics when compared to fentanyl tablets [155]. In addition, the buccal dosage form bypasses the extensive intestinal metabolism of fentanyl and thus reaches a relative bioavailability of 50% as compared to only 30% for the tablet form [154].

19.5.2 Slow-Release Systems

Many orally ingested drugs have been formulated into extended-release tablets for the treatment of persistent pain. They typically release the active drug over 8–12 hours. Worldwide, the highest-selling such product in the pain market is OxyContin™, with the active ingredient oxycodone. In 2007, OxyContin was sold in the United States for US$1.047 billion and was thus the thirty-third best-selling drug. The following paragraphs describe the top analgesic slow-release systems on the market.

Avinza® extended-release capsules (Elan Corporation) contain morphine sulfate in both immediate- and extended-release beads that measure 1–2 mm in diameter [156]. The immediate-release component (about 10% of the total dose) helps to achieve plateau morphine concentrations within 30 minutes, and the extended-release component then maintains these plasma concentrations throughout the 24-hour dosing interval. Avinza uses SODAS™, the "Spheroidal Oral Drug Absorption System," to produce the extended-release component of the product (Figure 19.9). A sugar/starch sphere is first coated with a drug/excipient layer and then with an ammonio-methacrylate copolymer coating. The spheres are packed into a hard gelatin capsule shell that immediately dissolves after oral administration. The permeability of the ammonio-methacrylate copolymer coating becomes the rate-limiting step for the entry of gastrointestinal fluid through the polymer coating into the morphine sulphate layer. In addition to controlling the liquid flow, it is also important to control the pH of the drug environment independent of the gastrointestinal environment in order to maintain solubility and dissolution speed constant. Fumaric acid, an osmotic agent and a local pH modifier within the drug/excipient layer, plays this crucial stabilizing role in the release process of the drug.

KADIAN® sustained-release capsules (Alpharma, Bridgewater, NJ, USA) contain morphine sulfate in polymer-coated, sustained-release pellets without

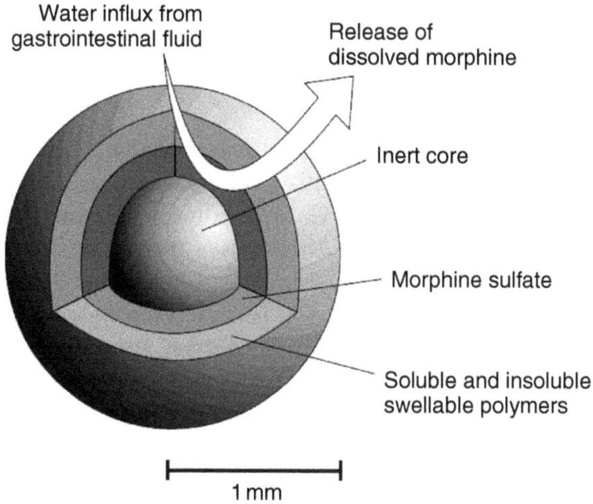

FIGURE 19.9. Sketch of the Spheroidal Oral Drug Absorption System (SODAS) technology. The gastrointestinal fluid diffuses into the core of the 1- to 2-mm large beads, dissolves the drug layer, and causes the polymer layer to swell. This swelling creates pores in the polymer coating, which then regulate the release of the dissolved drug in a rate-controlled manner.

an immediate-release component [157]. The extended-release pellets of Avinza and KADIAN share a similar general structure, but KADIAN's coating consists of an insoluble ethyl cellulose base along with polyethylene glycol (PEG) and a methacrylic acid copolymer. Though PEG and methacrylic acid copolymer are both water soluble, the water solubility of the methacrylic acid copolymer is pH dependent and increases with increasing pH. The PEG component dissolves immediately after ingestion in the stomach. As the pellets later enter and move through the intestines, the pH of the gastrointestinal (GI) environment continues to increase, and the methacrylic acid copolymer begins to dissolve and release more drug.

Oramorph® sustained-release tablets (Xanodyne Pharmaceuticals Inc., Newport, KY, USA) contain morphine sulfate in a simple matrix system instead of a polymer-coated reservoir. This design allows for easy tablet pressing after uniform blending of the drug with the hydrophilic polymer hydroxypropyl methylcellulose. After oral administration, the tablet becomes hydrated, and the cellulose matrix swells and forms a viscous gel layer. The gel layer controls both the diffusion of water into the system and the diffusion of drug out of the system. Although Oramorph controls the drug release well, patient studies have shown that the side effects are significantly larger than, for example, in transdermal fentanyl [158].

MS Contin® controlled-release tablets from Purdue Pharma L.P. (Stamford, CT, USA) contain morphine sulfate in a polymer matrix made of the hydrophilic polymer hydroxypropyl methylcellulose and the hydrophobic polymer hydroxyethyl cellulose. The drug is blended with the hydrophilic polymer, suitably hydrated with a polar solvent, and fixed with a higher aliphatic alcohol [159]. The release of drug from the tablet is controlled by the partition coefficients of the active ingredient with the hydrophilic and hydrophobic components of the formulation [160].

OxyContin controlled-release tablets (Purdue Pharma L.P.) contain oxycodone HCl that is released with a biphasic release profile. Upon dissolution of the hydrophobic ammonio-methacrylate copolymer coating, 30–40% of the drug is immediately released [161]. This causes the formation of channels in the tablet matrix [162], which in turn enhances solubility of the entrapped drug and makes it slowly diffuse through the formed channels of the matrix. The release of oxycodone is pH independent, permitting a uniform release throughout the GI tract.

Extended-release systems with opioids are not without problems, as Purdue Pharma L.P. learned in 2005. They had developed *Palladone™ extended-release capsules*, which contained hydromorphone HCl in an around-the-clock (ATC) matrix pellet formulation that provided a biphasic release of hydromorphone. Consuming ethanol while taking Palladone disrupted the modified-release mechanism of the product. Peak blood concentrations increased approximately six times with the consumption of 8 oz of a 40% (80 proof) ethanol solution and approximately two times with the consumption of 8 oz of a 4% ethanol solution [163,164]. In July 2005, the FDA advised Purdue Pharma L.P. that the risk of alcohol interaction could not be adequately managed with warnings alone. At the request of the FDA [165], Purdue suspended all marketing and sales of Palladone.

There are many more slow-release systems under development for the slow release of oral hydromorphone (ALZA Corp.), oral oxymorphone (Endo Pharmaceuticals), or a combination of oxycodon and morphine (QRxPharma). All are based on pharmaceutical technologies similar to those described above.

A different approach to extending the action of pain drugs, which does not involve the use of highly developed slow-release technology, is the chemical modification of the drug. Morphine, for example, has been glucuronated, making it into a longer-acting drug with fewer side effects (less sedation and less respiratory depression) [166]. The glucuronated morphine, however, had a slower onset of action.

19.6 OUTLOOK

The search for newer and better analgesic delivery systems and formulations is changing the face of pain management [108]. Many such systems are described in this chapter. One of the relatively mature systems is the iontophoretic patch that allows for patient-controlled drug release through the skin. Other less-mature systems include microneedles and laser abrasion. They are appropriate for analgesics that are less skin penetrating, because they can temporarily breach the stratum corneum. For some of these delivery approaches, pain-specific FDA-approved systems already exist, such as in the case of the IONSYS fentanyl iontophoretic patch. For others, the companies are providing the platform technology that can then be adapted for many different drugs. One such case is the microscissioner, an instrument that will prepare the skin for elevated drug penetration. The drug to be used can be freely chosen and must be applied in suitable concentration and form.

In order to be accepted in the healthcare system and in the marketplace, a new drug delivery system must be able to deliver sufficient drug doses to the target area and must be shown to be superior to existing conventional medicines in terms of ease of use, onset of drug action, side effects, length of action, and cost. Advantages and potential new side effects must be carefully compared and the risks calculated.

Many side effects of even the newer systems, such as transdermal systems, would be reduced if the drug could be kept away from the brain, and/or delivered in a targeted way. Drug targeting can be accomplished using organ- or tissue-specific drug delivery systems (e.g., by magnetic targeting), site-specific systems (e.g., by placing biodegradable implants or drug-releasing microspheres in a site), or process-specific systems (e.g., release of the drug from heat-sensitive liposomes in the aching tissue by inflammation-induced small temperature differences).

In the not too distant future, much more directed interventions may be possible, including the enrollment of the help of nanorobots like those described with immense imagination by Robert Freitas [167]. Such nanorobots might be made to behave like bacteria with flagellae, or fibroblasts, and could be used to repair clogged vessels, remove cancer or other cells, or perhaps even take up unwanted molecules (e.g., pain-inducing molecules) or release specific substances. It may also be possible to direct drugs on the microscopic level, not only to major organs but also to distinct organelles, such as the lysosomes, mitochondria, or chromosomes. Initial attempts to target intracellular organelles are ongoing, and success stories are beginning to appear. One example from the field of radiation oncology is directing the radiolabeled antibody trastuzumab to HER2-positive breast tumor cells [168]. Once taken up into the cells, a 13-mer peptide covalently bound to the antibody takes over and directs the construct into the nucleus, where the Auger electrons from the also attached radioisotope ^{111}In are close enough to the DNA to both arrest synthesis and repair and kill the cell [168].

More precise targeting of drugs could lead to an increase in the number of drugs available for pain treatment. Many of the highly effective drugs developed by the pharmaceutical industry are currently too toxic to be used. Packaging them into the newly developed drug delivery systems could change their toxicity profile and allow for their reevaluation in clinical trials.

The search for newer and better analgesic delivery systems also increasingly involves the application of the principles of multimodal therapy [108]. Modern medicine, and especially the field of cancer therapy, profits immensely from combination approaches in general. Sometimes, a drug or treatment alone is sufficient to eradicate cancer, but more often it is necessary to combine two or more treatment approaches to be successful. This might also prove true for analgesic drug delivery. Initial steps in this direction are currently being made. Specifically, drugs with immediate onset of action are being combined with ones that work over longer time periods (i.e., slow-release drugs). The combination of different drugs and drug delivery techniques might expand the benefits that each drug brings and might minimize the side effects of each. To rationally develop and test multimodal therapies, it would be beneficial to engage experts from many different fields, including pharmaceutics, chemistry, pharmacology, and medicine, in all stages of the development process.

REFERENCES

1. Ehrlich, P. (1900). Croonian lecture. *Proc Soc Lond Biol* 424.
2. Torchilin, V.P. (2000). Drug targeting. *Eur J Pharm Sci* 11(Suppl. 2):S81–S91.
3. Tomlinson, E. (1987). Theory and practice of site-specific drug delivery. *Adv Drug Deliv Rev* 1:87–198.
4. Gerlowski, L.E., Jain, R.K. (1986). Microvascular permeability of normal and neoplastic tissues. *Microvasc Res* 31:288–305.
5. Ulbrich, K., Subr, V. (2004). Polymeric anticancer drugs with pH-controlled activation. *Adv Drug Deliv Rev* 56:1023–1050.
6. Sershen, S., West, J. (2002). Implantable, polymeric systems for modulated drug delivery. *Adv Drug Deliv Rev* 54:1225–1235.
7. Häfeli, U.O. (2006). Magnetic nano- and microparticles for targeted drug delivery. In: Arshady, R., Kono, K. (eds.). *Smart Nanoparticles in Nanomedicine—the MML Series*, Vol. 8. London: Kentus Books, pp. 77–126.
8. Elbayoumi, T.A., Pabba, S., Roby, A., Torchilin, V.P. (2007). Antinucleosome antibody-modified liposomes and lipid-core micelles for tumor-targeted delivery of therapeutic and diagnostic agents. *J Liposome Res* 17:1–14.
9. Gupta, B., Torchilin, V.P. (2007). Monoclonal antibody 2C5-modified doxorubicin-loaded liposomes with significantly enhanced therapeutic activity against intracranial human brain U-87 MG tumor xenografts in nude mice. *Cancer Immunol Immunother* 56:1215–1223.
10. Sawant, R.M., Hurley, J.P., Salmaso, S., Kale, A., Tolcheva, E., Levchenko, T.S., Torchilin, V.P. (2006). "SMART" drug delivery systems: double-targeted pH-responsive pharmaceutical nanocarriers. *Bioconjug Chem* 17:943–949.
11. Steinhauser, I., Spankuch, B., Strebhardt, K., Langer, K. (2006). Trastuzumab-modified nanoparticles: optimisation of preparation and uptake in cancer cells. *Biomaterials* 27:4975–4983.
12. Kocbek, P., Obermajer, N., Cegnar, M., Kos, J., Kristl, J. (2007). Targeting cancer cells using PLGA nanoparticles surface modified with monoclonal antibody. *J Control Release* 120:18–26.
13. Farokhzad, O.C., Karp, J.M., Langer, R. (2006). Nanoparticle-aptamer bioconjugates for cancer targeting. *Expert Opin Drug Deliv* 3:311–324.

14. Singh, Y., Palombo, M., Sinko, P.J. (2008). Recent trends in targeted anticancer prodrug and conjugate design. *Curr Med Chem* 15:1802–1826.

15. Rautio, J., Laine, K., Gynther, M., Savolainen, J. (2008). Prodrug approaches for CNS delivery. *AAPS J* 10:92–102.

16. Erdmann, L., Campo, C., Bedell, C., Uhrich, K. (1998). Polymeric prodrugs: novel polymers with bioactive components. In: McCulloch, I., Shalaby, S.W. (eds.). *Tailored Polymeric Materials for Controlled Delivery Systems*, Vol. 709. Washington, DC: ACS, pp. 83–91.

17. Prausnitz, M.R., Langer, R. (2008). Transdermal drug delivery. *Nat Biotechnol* 26:1261–1268.

18. Naik, A., Kalia, Y.N., Guy, R.H. (2000). Transdermal drug delivery: overcoming the skin's barrier function. *Pharm Sci Technolo Today* 3:318–326.

19. Higaki, K., Amnuaikit, C., Kimura, T. (2003). Strategies for overcoming the stratum corneum: chemical and physical approaches. *Am J Drug Deliv* 1, 187–214.

20. Williams, A.C., Barry, B.W. (2004). Penetration enhancers. *Adv Drug Deliv Rev* 56:603–618.

21. Pellet, M., Raghavan, S.L., Hadgraft, J., Davis, A.F. (2003). *The Application of Supersaturated Systems to Percutaneous Drug Delivery,* 2nd ed. New York: Marcel Dekker, pp. 305–326.

22. Brown, M.B., Jones, S.A. (2005). Hyaluronic acid: a unique topical vehicle for the localized delivery of drugs to the skin. *J Eur Acad Dermatol Venereol* 19: 308–318.

23. Fang, J.Y., Leu, Y.L. (2006). Prodrug strategy for enhancing drug delivery via skin. *Curr Drug Discov Technol* 3:211–224.

24. Majumdar, S., Sloan, K.B. (2007). Synthesis and topical delivery of N-alkyl-N-alkyloxycarbonylaminomethyl prodrugs of a model phenolic drug: acetaminophen. *Int J Pharm* 337:48–55.

25. Sloan, K.B., Wasdo, S.C., Rautio, J. (2006). Design for optimized topical delivery: prodrugs and a paradigm change. *Pharm Res* 23:2729–2747.

26. Cevc, G. (2004). Lipid vesicles and other colloids as drug carriers on the skin. *Adv Drug Deliv Rev* 56:675–711.

27. Egbaria, K., Weiner, N. (1990). Liposomes as a topical drug delivery system. *Adv Drug Deliv Rev* 5:287–300.

28. Bikowski, J., Shroot, B. (2006). Multivesicular emulsion: a novel, controlled-release delivery system for topical dermatological agents. *J Drugs Dermatol* 5:942–946.

29. Alvarez-Figueroa, M.J., Araya-Silva, I., Diaz-Tobar, C. (2006). Iontophoretic transdermal delivery of haloperidol. *Pharm Dev Technol* 11:371–375.

30. Abla, N., Naik, A., Guy, R.H., Kalia, Y.N. (2006). Topical iontophoresis of valaciclovir hydrochloride improves cutaneous aciclovir delivery. *Pharm Res* 23:1842–1849.

31. Mathy, F.X., Lombry, C., Verbeeck, R.K., Preat, V. (2005). Study of the percutaneous penetration of flurbiprofen by cutaneous and subcutaneous microdialysis after iontophoretic delivery in rat. *J Pharm Sci* 94:144–152.

32. Kalia, Y.N., Naik, A., Garrison, J., Guy, R.H. (2004). Iontophoretic drug delivery. *Adv Drug Deliv Rev* 56:619–658.

33. Singh, P., Maibach, H.I. (1994). Iontophoresis in drug delivery: basic principles and applications. *Crit Rev Ther Drug Carrier Syst* 11:161–213.
34. Denet, A.R., Vanbever, R., Preat, V. (2004). Skin electroporation for transdermal and topical delivery. *Adv Drug Deliv Rev* 56:659–674.
35. Lombry, C., Dujardin, N., Preat, V. (2000). Transdermal delivery of macromolecules using skin electroporation. *Pharm Res* 17:32–37.
36. Wang, S., Kara, M., Krishnan, T.R. (1998). Transdermal delivery of cyclosporin-A using electroporation. *J Control Release* 50:61–70.
37. Thysman, S., Preat, V., Roland, M. (1992). Factors affecting iontophoretic mobility of metoprolol. *J Pharm Sci* 81:670–675.
38. Del Terzo, S., Behl, C.R., Nash, R.A. (1989). Iontophoretic transport of a homologous series of ionized and nonionized model compounds: influence of hydrophobicity and mechanistic interpretation. *Pharm Res* 6:85–90.
39. Siddiqui, O., Roberts, M.S., Polack, A.E. (1985). The effect of iontophoresis and vehicle pH on the in-vitro permeation of lignocaine through human stratum corneum. *J Pharm Pharmacol* 37:732–735.
40. Tiwari, S.B., Udupa, N. (2003). Investigation into the potential of iontophoresis facilitated delivery of ketorolac. *Int J Pharm* 260:93–103.
41. Miller, L.L., Kolaskie, C.J., Smith, G.A., Rivier, J. (1990). Transdermal iontophoresis of gonadotropin releasing hormone (LHRH) and two analogues. *J Pharm Sci* 79:490–493.
42. Green, P.G., Hinz, R.S., Cullander, C., Yamane, G., Guy, R.H. (1991). Iontophoretic delivery of amino acids and amino acid derivatives across the skin in vitro. *Pharm Res* 8:1113–1120.
43. van der Geest, R., Hueber, F., Szoka, F.C., Jr., Guy, R.H. (1996). Iontophoresis of bases, nucleosides, and nucleotides. *Pharm Res* 13:553–558.
44. Sung, K.C., Fang, J.Y., Hu, O.Y. (2000). Delivery of nalbuphine and its prodrugs across skin by passive diffusion and iontophoresis. *J Control Release* 67:1–8.
45. Hui, X., Anigbogu, A., Singh, P., Xiong, G., Poblete, N., Liu, P., Maibach, H.I. (2001). Pharmacokinetic and local tissue disposition of ^{14}C sodium diclofenac following iontophoresis and systemic administration in rabbits. *J Pharm Sci* 90:1269–1276.
46. Burnette, R.R., Marrero, D. (1986). Comparison between the iontophoretic and passive transport of thyrotropin releasing hormone across excised nude mouse skin. *J Pharm Sci* 75:738–743.
47. Phipps, J.B., Padmanabhan, R.V., Lattin, G.A. (1989). Iontophoretic delivery of model inorganic and drug ions. *J Pharm Sci* 78:365–369.
48. Banga, A.K., Bose, S., Ghosh, T.K. (1999). Iontophoresis and electroporation: comparisons and contrasts. *Int J Pharm* 179:1–19.
49. Cross, S.E., Roberts, M.S. (1995). Importance of dermal blood supply and epidermis on the transdermal iontophoretic delivery of monovalent cations. *J Pharm Sci* 84:584–592.
50. Roberts, M.S., Favretto, W.A., Meyer, A., Rechmann, M., Wongseelashote, T. (1982). Topical bioavailability of methylsalicylate. *Aust N Z J Med* 12:305–312.
51. Medi, B.M., Hoselton, S., Marepalli, R.B., Singh, J. (2005). Skin targeted DNA vaccine delivery using electroporation in rabbits. I: efficacy. *Int J Pharm* 294:53–63.

52. Regnier, V., Tahiri, A., Andre, N., Lemaitre, M., Le Doan, T., Preat, V. (2000). Electroporation-mediated delivery of 3′-protected phosphodiester oligodeoxy-nucleotides to the skin. *J Control Release* 67:337–346.
53. Regnier, V., Le Doan, T., Preat, V. (1998). Parameters controlling topical delivery of oligonucleotides by electroporation. *J Drug Target* 5:275–289.
54. Dixit, N., Bali, V., Baboota, S., Ahuja, A., Ali, J. (2007). Iontophoresis—an approach for controlled drug delivery: a review. *Curr Drug Deliv* 4:1–10.
55. Drummond, P.D., de Silva-Rossdeutscher, E. (2003). Transcutaneous iontophoresis of methadone provokes local flushing and thermal hyperalgesia. *Inflamm Res* 52:366–371.
56. Kumar, M.G., Lin, S. (2009). Transdermal iontophoresis of hydromorphone across hairless rat skin in vitro. *Pharm Dev Technol* 14(1):109–118.
57. Odebiyi, D.O., Adigun, O.T., Kehinde, M.O. (2007). Effect of sodium salicylate iontophoresis in the management of hip pain in patients with sickle cell disease. *Nig Q J Hosp Med* 17:82–86.
58. Arvidsson, S.B., Ekroth, R.H., Hansby, A.M., Lindholm, A.H., William-Olsson, G. (1984). Painless venipuncture. A clinical trial of iontophoresis of lidocaine for venipuncture in blood donors. *Acta Anaesthesiol Scand* 28:209–210.
59. Petelenz, T., Axenti, I., Petelenz, T.J., Iwinski, J., Dubel, S. (1984). Mini set for iontophoresis for topical analgesia before injection. *Int J Clin Pharmacol Ther Toxicol* 22:152–155.
60. Zempsky, W.T., Anand, K.J., Sullivan, K.M., Fraser, D., Cucina, K. (1998). Lidocaine iontophoresis for topical anesthesia before intravenous line placement in children. *J Pediatr* 132:1061–1063.
61. Sadler, P.J., Thompson, H.M., Maslowski, P., Liddle, A., Rowbotham, D.J. (1999). Iontophoretically applied lidocaine reduces pain on propofol injection. *Br J Anaesth* 82:432–434.
62. Sharpe, P., Asif, M., Victoria, A., Rowbotham, D.J. (2002). Iontophoretically applied lidocaine and the prevention of pain associated with the injection of intravenous propofol: a comparison with intravenous lidocaine. *Eur J Anaesthesiol* 19:170–172.
63. Sherwin, J., Awad, I.T., Sadler, P.J., Liddle, A.M., Rowbotham, D.J. (2003). Analgesia during radial artery cannulation: comparison of the effects of lidocaine applied by local injection or iontophoresis. *Anaesthesia* 58:474–476.
64. Mayes, S., Ferrone, M. (2006). Fentanyl HCl patient-controlled iontophoretic transdermal system for the management of acute postoperative pain. *Ann Pharmacother* 40:2178–2186.
65. Miaskowski, C. (2005). Patient-controlled modalities for acute postoperative pain management. *J Perianesth Nurs* 20:255–267.
66. Fischer, G.A. (2005). Iontophoretic drug delivery using the IOMED Phoresor system. *Expert Opin Drug Deliv* 2:391–403.
67. Mystakidou, K. (2002). E-TRANS fentanyl. ALZA. *Curr Opin Investig Drugs* 3:463–469.
68. Gerstel, M.S., Place, V.A. (1976). *Drug delivery device*. ALZA, U.S. Patent 3,964,482, issued June 22, 1976.
69. Sivamani, R.K., Stoeber, B., Wu, G.C., Zhai, H., Liepmann, D., Maibach, H. (2005). Clinical microneedle injection of methyl nicotinate: stratum corneum penetration. *Skin Res Technol* 11:152–156.

70. Campbell, P.K., Jones, K.E., Huber, R.J., Horch, K.W., Normann, R.A. (1991). A silicon-based, three-dimensional neural interface: manufacturing processes for an intracortical electrode array. *IEEE Trans Biomed Eng* 38:758–768.

71. Lin, L., Pisano, A.P., Muller, R.S. (1993). IC-processed microneedles. In: *Proceedings of the International Conference on Sensors and Actuators*. Yokohama, Japan, pp. 237–240.

72. Lin, W., Cormier, M., Samiee, A., Griffin, A., Johnson, B., Teng, C.L., Hardee, G.E., Daddona, P.E. (2001). Transdermal delivery of antisense oligonucleotides with microprojection patch (Macroflux) technology. *Pharm Res* 18:1789–1793.

73. Matriano, J.A., Cormier, M., Johnson, J., Young, W.A., Buttery, M., Nyam, K., Daddona, P.E. (2002). Macroflux microprojection array patch technology: a new and efficient approach for intracutaneous immunization. *Pharm Res* 19:63–70.

74. Stoeber, B., Liepmann, D. (2005). Arrays of hollow out-of-plane microneedles for drug delivery. *J Microelectromech Syst* 14:472–479.

75. Lee, J.W., Park, J.H., Prausnitz, M.R. (2008). Dissolving microneedles for transdermal drug delivery. *Biomaterials* 29:2113–2124.

76. Lee, W.R., Tsai, R.Y., Fang, C.L., Liu, C.J., Hu, C.H., Fang, J.Y. (2006). Microdermabrasion as a novel tool to enhance drug delivery via the skin: an animal study. *Dermatol Surg* 32:1013–1022.

77. Lee, W.R., Shen, S.C., Kuo-Hsien, W., Hu, C.H., Fang, J.Y. (2003). Lasers and microdermabrasion enhance and control topical delivery of vitamin C. *J Invest Dermatol* 121:1118–1125.

78. Herndon, T.O., Gonzalez, S., Gowrishankar, T.R., Anderson, R.R., Weaver, J.C. (2004). Transdermal microconduits by microscission for drug delivery and sample acquisition. *BMC Med* 2:12.

79. Akomeah, F.K., Martin, G.P., Muddle, A.G., Brown, M.B. (2008). Effect of abrasion induced by a rotating brush on the skin permeation of solutes with varying physicochemical properties. *Eur J Pharm Biopharm* 68:724–734.

80. Bramson, J., Dayball, K., Evelegh, C., Wan, Y.H., Page, D., Smith, A. (2003). Enabling topical immunization via microporation: a novel method for pain-free and needle-free delivery of adenovirus-based vaccines. *Gene Ther* 10:251–260.

81. Muddle, A.G., Longridge, D.J., Sweeney, P.A., Burkoth, T.L., Bellhouse, B.J. (1997). Transdermal delivery of testosterone to conscious rabbits using PowderJect (R): a supersonic powder delivery system. *Proc Int Symp Control Rel Bioact Mat* 24:713.

82. Longbridge, D.J., Sweeney, P.A., Burkoth, T.L., Bellhouse, B.J. (1998). Effects of particle size and cylinder pressure on dermal PowderJect® delivery of testosterone to conscious rabbits. *Proc Int Symp Control Rel Bioact Mat* 25:964.

83. Burkoth, T.L., Bellhouse, B.J., Hewson, G., Longridge, D.J., Muddle, A.G., Sarphie, D.F. (1999). Transdermal and transmucosal powdered drug delivery. *Crit Rev Ther Drug Carrier Syst* 16:331–384.

84. Ziegler, A.S. (2008). Needle-free delivery of powdered protein vaccines: a new and rapidly developing technique. *J Pharm Innov* 3:204–213.

85. Sandstrom, E., Nilsson, C., Hejdeman, B., Brave, A., Bratt, G., Robb, M., Cox, J., Vancott, T., Marovich, M., Stout, R., Aboud, S., Bakari, M., Pallangyo, K., Ljungberg, K., Moss, B., Earl, P., Michael, N., Birx, D., Mhalu, F., Wahren, B., Biberfeld, G.

(2008). Broad immunogenicity of a multigene, multiclade HIV-1 DNA vaccine boosted with heterologous HIV-1 recombinant modified vaccinia virus Ankara. *J Infect Dis* 198:1482–1490.

86. Cui, Z., Baizer, L., Mumper, R.J. (2003). Intradermal immunization with novel plasmid DNA-coated nanoparticles via a needle-free injection device. *J Biotechnol* 102:105–115.
87. Dean, H.J., Fuller, D., Osorio, J.E. (2003). Powder and particle-mediated approaches for delivery of DNA and protein vaccines into the epidermis. *Comp Immunol Microbiol Infect Dis* 26:373–388.
88. Mitragotri, S., Kost, J. (2004). Low-frequency sonophoresis: a review. *Adv Drug Deliv Rev* 56:589–601.
89. Merino, G., Kalia, Y.N., Guy, R.H. (2003). Ultrasound-enhanced transdermal transport. *J Pharm Sci* 92:1125–1137.
90. Kost, J., Mitragotri, S., Gabbay, R.A., Pishko, M., Langer, R. (2000). Transdermal monitoring of glucose and other analytes using ultrasound. *Nat Med* 6:347–350.
91. Lee, S., Snyder, B., Newnham, R.E., Smith, N.B. (2004). Noninvasive ultrasonic transdermal insulin delivery in rabbits using the light-weight cymbal array. *Diabetes Technol Ther* 6:808–815.
92. Park, E.J., Werner, J., Smith, N.B. (2007). Ultrasound mediated transdermal insulin delivery in pigs using a lightweight transducer. *Pharm Res* 24:1396–1401.
93. Mitragotri, S., Kost, J. (2001). Transdermal delivery of heparin and low-molecular weight heparin using low-frequency ultrasound. *Pharm Res* 18:1151–1156.
94. Tezel, A., Paliwal, S., Shen, Z., Mitragotri, S. (2005). Low-frequency ultrasound as a transcutaneous immunization adjuvant. *Vaccine* 23:3800–3807.
95. Katz, N.P., Shapiro, D.E., Herrmann, T.E., Kost, J., Custer, L.M. (2004). Rapid onset of cutaneous anesthesia with EMLA cream after pretreatment with a new ultrasound-emitting device. *Anesth Analg* 98:371–376.
96. Liu, H., Li, S., Pan, W., Wang, Y., Han, F., Yao, H. (2006). Investigation into the potential of low-frequency ultrasound facilitated topical delivery of cyclosporin A. *Int J Pharm* 326:32–38.
97. Fang, J.Y., Lee, W.R., Shen, S.C., Wang, H.Y., Fang, C.L., Hu, C.H. (2004). Transdermal delivery of macromolecules by erbium:YAG laser. *J Control Release* 100:75–85.
98. Lee, W.R., Shen, S.C., Lai, H.H., Hu, C.H., Fang, J.Y. (2001). Transdermal drug delivery enhanced and controlled by erbium:YAG laser: a comparative study of lipophilic and hydrophilic drugs. *J Control Release* 75:155–166.
99. Lee, W.R., Shen, S.C., Wang, K.H., Hu, C.H., Fang, J.Y. (2002). The effect of laser treatment on skin to enhance and control transdermal delivery of 5-fluorouracil. *J Pharm Sci* 91:1613–1626.
100. Zborowski, M. (2002). Separations based on magnetophoretic technology. *Sep Sci Technol* 37:3611–3633.
101. Murthy, S.N. (1999). Magnetophoresis: an approach to enhance transdermal drug diffusion. *Pharmazie* 54:377–379.
102. Murthy, S.N., Hiremath, S.R.R. (2001). Physical and chemical permeation enhancers in transdermal drug delivery of terbutaline sulphate. *PharmSci Tech* 2:1–5.

103. Mitragotri, S. (2000). Synergistic effect of enhancers for transdermal drug delivery. *Pharm Res* 17:1354–1359.

104. Blumberg, P.M. (2007). Lighting a backfire to quench the blaze: a combined drug approach targeting the vanilloid receptor TRPV1. *Mol Interv* 7:310–312.

105. Binshtok, A.M., Bean, B.P., Woolf, C.J. (2007). Inhibition of nociceptors by TRPV1-mediated entry of impermeant sodium channel blockers. *Nature* 449:607–610.

106. Gerner, P., Binshtok, A.M., Wang, C.F., Hevelone, N.D., Bean, B.P., Woolf, C.J., Wang, G.K. (2008). Capsaicin combined with local anesthetics preferentially prolongs sensory/nociceptive block in rat sciatic nerve. *Anesthesiology* 109: 872–878.

107. Higaki, K., Asai, M., Suyama, T., Nakayama, K., Ogawara, K., Kimura, T. (2002). Estimation of intradermal disposition kinetics of drugs: II. Factors determining penetration of drugs from viable skin to muscular layer. *Int J Pharm* 239: 129–141.

108. Polomano, R.C., Rathmell, J.P., Krenzischek, D.A., Dunwoody, C.J. (2008). Emerging trends and new approaches to acute pain management. *J Perianesth Nurs* 23:S43–S53.

109. Evans, H., Steele, S.M., Nielsen, K.C., Tucker, M.S., Klein, S.M. (2005). Peripheral nerve blocks and continuous catheter techniques. *Anesthesiol Clin North America* 23:141–162.

110. Hartrick, C.T., Hartrick, K.A. (2008). Extended-release epidural morphine (DepoDur): review and safety analysis. *Expert Rev Neurother* 8:1641–1648.

111. Horak, D., Babic, M., Mackova, H., Benes, M.J. (2007). Preparation and properties of magnetic nano- and microsized particles for biological and environmental separations. *J Sep Sci* 30:1751–1772.

112. Gilchrist, R.K., Medal, R., Shorey, W.D., Hanselman, R.C., Parrott, J.C., Taylor, C.B. (1957). Selective inductive heating of lymph nodes. *Ann Surg* 146:596–606.

113. Turner, R.D., Rand, R.W., Bentson, J.R., Mosso, J.A. (1975). Ferromagnetic silicone necrosis of hypernephromas by selective vascular occlusion to the tumor: a new technique. *J Urol* 113:455–459.

114. Tiefenauer, L.X. (2007). Magnetic nanoparticles as contrast agents for medical diagnosis. In: Vo-Dinh, T. (ed.). *Nanotechnology in Biology and Medicine: Methods, Devices, and Applications, Section D: Nanomedicine Applications D1*. Boca Raton, FL: CRC Press, Taylor and Francis, pp. 1–20.

115. Andrä, W., Häfeli, U.O., Hergt, R., Misri, R. (2007). Application of magnetic particles in medicine and biology. In: Kronmüller, H., Parkin, S. (eds.). *The Handbook of Magnetism and Advanced Magnetic Materials, 4—Novel Materials*. Chichester: John Wiley & Sons Ltd., pp. 2536–2568.

116. Choi, H.S., Seo, S.A., Khang, G., Rhee, J.M., Lee, H.B. (2002). Preparation and characterization of fentanyl-loaded PLGA microspheres: in vitro release profiles. *Int J Pharm* 234:195–203.

117. Zhao, H., Gagnon, J., Häfeli, U.O. (2007). Process and formulation variables in the preparation of injectable and biodegradable magnetic microspheres. *Biomagn Res Technol* 5:2.

118. Liu, X.Q., Kaminski, M.D., Riffle, J.S., Chen, H., Torno, M., Finck, M.R., Taylor, L.T., Rosengart, A.J. (2007). Preparation and characterization of biodegradable

magnetic carriers by single emulsion solvent evaporation. *J Magn Magn Mater* 311:84–87.

119. Jain, T.K., Labhasetwar, V., Reddy, M., Morales, M.A., Leslie-Pelecky, D.L. (2008). Biodistribution, clearance and biocompatibility of iron-oxide magnetic nanoparticles in rats. *Mol Pharm* 5:316–327.
120. Washington, N., Washington, C., Wilson, C.G. (2001). *Physiological Pharmaceutics: Barriers to Drug Absorption*. Boca Raton, FL: CRC Press.
121. Tsuji, A., Tamai, I.I. (1999). Carrier-mediated or specialized transport of drugs across the blood-brain barrier. *Adv Drug Deliv Rev* 36:277–290.
122. Baker, D.E. (2007). Loperamide: a pharmacological review. *Rev Gastroenterol Disord* 7(Suppl. 3):S11–S18.
123. Tosi, G., Costantino, L., Ruozi, B., Forni, F., Vandelli, M.A. (2008). Polymeric nanoparticles for the drug delivery to the central nervous system. *Expert Opin Drug Deliv* 5:155–174.
124. Ulbrich, K., Hekmatara, T., Herbert, E., et al. (2009). Transferrin- and transferrin-receptor-antibody-modified nanoparticles enable drug delivery across the blood-brain barrier (BBB). *Eur J Pharm Biopharm* 71: 251–256.
125. Pardridge, W.M., Buciak, J.L., Friden, P.M. (1991). Selective transport of an anti-transferrin receptor antibody through the blood-brain barrier in vivo. *J Pharmacol Exp Ther* 259:66–70.
126. Schroeder, U., Sommerfeld, P., Ulrich, S., Sabel, B.A. (1998). Nanoparticle technology for delivery of drugs across the blood-brain barrier. *J Pharm Sci* 87: 1305–1307.
127. Alyautdin, R.N., Petrov, V.E., Langer, K., Berthold, A., Kharkevich, D.A., Kreuter, J. (1997). Delivery of loperamide across the blood-brain barrier with polysorbate 80-coated polybutylcyanoacrylate nanoparticles. *Pharm Res* 14:325–328.
128. Al Malyan, M., Becchi, C., Nikkola, L., Viitanen, P., Boncinelli, S., Chiellini, F., Ashammakhi, N. (2006). Polymer-based biodegradable drug delivery systems in pain management. *J Craniofac Surg* 17:302–313.
129. Sendil, D., Bonney, I.M., Carr, D.B., Lipkowski, A.W., Wise, D.L., Hasirci, V. (2003). Antinociceptive effects of hydromorphone, bupivacaine and biphalin released from PLGA polymer after intrathecal implantation in rats. *Biomaterials* 24: 1969–1976.
130. Fletcher, D., Le Corre, P., Guilbaud, G., Le Verge, R. (1997). Antinociceptive effect of bupivacaine encapsulated in poly(D,L)-lactide-co- glycolide microspheres in the acute inflammatory pain model of carrageenin- injected rats. *Anesth Analg* 84:90–94.
131. Okuda, T., Wakita, K., Tsuchiya, N., Hatsuoka, K., Koga, Y., Kaetsu, I. (1999). Prolonged antinociceptive effect of poly (DL-lactic acid)-fentanyl composites after their intrathecal injection in rats. *Masui* 48:141–145.
132. Lesser, G.J., Grossman, S.A., Leong, K.W., Lo, H., Eller, S. (1996). In vitro and in vivo studies of subcutaneous hydromorphone implants designed for the treatment of cancer pain. *Pain* 65:265–272.
133. Keskin, D.S., Wise, D.L., Hasirci, V. (2004). Pain control via opioid analgesic-local anesthetic loaded IPNs. *Curr Drug Deliv* 1:57–64.
134. Torchilin, V.P. (2006). *Nanoparticles as Drug Carriers*. London: Imperial College Press.

135. Edlund, U., Albertsson, A.C. (2002). Degradable polymer microspheres for controlled drug delivery. *Adv Polym Sci* 157:67–112.

136. Rougeot, O., Aubry, C., Kaltsatos, V., Wehrle, P. (1997). New nonwoven controlled release device based on biodegradable or non-biodegradable polymers. *Proc Int Symp Control Rel Bioact Mater* 24:735–736.

137. Sheth, M., Kumar, R.A., Dave, V., Gross, R.A., McCarthy, S.P. (1997). Biodegradable polymer blends of PLA and PEG. *J Appl Polym Sci* 66:1495–1505.

138. Dorta, M.J., Santovena, A., Llabres, M., Farina, J.B. (2002). Potential applications of PLGA film-implants in modulating in vitro drugs release. *Int J Pharm* 248:149–156.

139. Venugopal, J., Prabhakaran, M.P., Low, S., Choon, A.T., Zhang, Y.Z., Deepika, G., Ramakrishna, S. (2008). Nanotechnology for nanomedicine and delivery of drugs. *Curr Pharm Des* 14:2184–2200.

140. Middleton, J.C., Tipton, A.J. (2000). Synthetic biodegradable polymers as orthopedic devices. *Biomaterials* 21:2335–2346.

141. Ashammakhi, N., Veiranto, M., Suokas, E., Tiainen, J., Niemela, S.M., Tormala, P. (2006). Innovation in multifunctional bioabsorbable osteoconductive drug-releasing hard tissue fixation devices. *J Mater Sci Mater Med* 17:1275–1282.

142. Wu, B.M., Borland, S.W., Giordano, R.A., Cima, L.G., Sachs, E.M., Cima, M.J. (1996). Solid free-form fabrication of drug delivery devices. *J Control Release* 40:77–87.

143. Langer, R. (1998). Drug delivery and targeting. *Nature* 392:5–10.

144. Taddio, A., Soin, H.K., Schuh, S., Koren, G., Scolnik, D. (2005). Liposomal lidocaine to improve procedural success rates and reduce procedural pain among children: a randomized controlled trial. *CMAJ* 172:1691–1695.

145. Canto, G.S., Dalmora, S.L., Oliveira, A.G. (1999). Piroxicam encapsulated in liposomes: characterization and in vivo evaluation of topical anti-inflammatory effect. *Drug Dev Ind Pharm* 25:1235–1239.

146. Singh, B., Mehta, G., Kumar, R., Bhatia, A., Ahuja, N., Katare, O.P. (2005). Design, development and optimization of nimesulide-loaded liposomal systems for topical application. *Curr Drug Deliv* 2:143–153.

147. Jain, S., Jain, N., Bhadra, D., Tiwary, A.K., Jain, N.K. (2005). Transdermal delivery of an analgesic agent using elastic liposomes: preparation, characterization and performance evaluation. *Curr Drug Deliv* 2:223–233.

148. Planas, M.E., Gonzalez, P., Rodriguez, L., Sanchez, S., Cevc, G. (1992). Noninvasive percutaneous induction of topical analgesia by a new type of drug carrier, and prolongation of local pain insensitivity by anesthetic liposomes. *Anesth Analg* 75:615–621.

149. Toongsuwan, S., Li, L.C., Erickson, B.K., Chang, H.C. (2004). Formulation and characterization of bupivacaine lipospheres. *Int J Pharm* 280:57–65.

150. Lafont, N.D., Legros, F.J., Boogaerts, J.G. (1996). Use of liposome-associated bupivacaine in a cancer pain syndrome. *Anaesthesia* 51:578–579.

151. Wallace, M.S., Yanez, A.M., Ho, R.J., Shen, D.D., Yaksh, T.L. (1994). Antinociception and side effects of liposome-encapsulated alfentanil after spinal delivery in rats. *Anesth Analg* 79:778–786.

152. Hung, O.R., Whynot, S.C., Varvel, J.R., Shafer, S.L., Mezei, M. (1995). Pharmacokinetics of inhaled liposome-encapsulated fentanyl. *Anesthesiology* 83:277–284.

153. Park, J.W., Benz, C.C., Martin, F.J. (2004). Future directions of liposome- and immunoliposome-based cancer therapeutics. *Semin Oncol* 31:196–205.

154. Brown, B.A.S., Hamed, E. (2007). OraVescent technology offers greater oral transmucosal delivery. *Drug Deliv Technol* 5:42–44.

155. Lecybyl, R., Hanna, M. (2007). Fentanyl buccal tablet: faster rescue analgesia for breakthrough pain? *Future Oncol* 3:375–379.

156. King, C.R., Khabazian, A. (2003). Avinza (morphine sulfate extended-release capsules). *Clin J Oncol Nurs* 7:458–460, 478.

157. Ross, E.L., Hahn, K. (2008). KADIAN (morphine sulfate extended-release) capsules for treatment of chronic, moderate-to-severe, nonmalignant pain. *Int J Clin Pract* 62:471–479.

158. Payne, R., Mathias, S.D., Pasta, D.J., Wanke, L.A., Williams, R., Mahmoud, R. (1998). Quality of life and cancer pain: satisfaction and side effects with transdermal fentanyl versus oral morphine. *J Clin Oncol* 16:1588–1593.

159. Leslie, S. (1986). The Contin delivery system: dosing considerations. *J Allergy Clin Immunol* 78:768–773.

160. Boroda, C., Miller, R.B., Leslie, S.T., Nicol, E.G., Thomson, I. (1973). Comparison of the bioavailability of aminophylline in a conventional base and in a continous-release base. *J Clin Pharmacol* 13:383–387.

161. Reder, R.F. (2001). Opioid formulations: tailoring to the needs in chronic pain. *Eur J Pain* 5(Suppl. A):109–111.

162. Kaplin, M., Miliman, A., Kaplan, L., Collins, M. (2004). Comparative clinical efficacy and abuse potential of oral long acting opioids in a chronic pain outpatient center. In: *Proceedings of the American Pain Society Annual Meeting*. Vancouver, BC, p. 868.

163. Murray, S., Wooltorton, E. (2005). Alcohol-associated rapid release of a long-acting opioid. *CMAJ* 173:756.

164. Darke, A.C. (2006). Controlled-release opioids and alcohol. *CMAJ* 174:352.

165. Anonymous. (2005). FDA asks Purdue Pharma to withdraw Palladone. *FDA Consum* 39:7.

166. Hanna, M.H., Elliott, K.M., Fung, M. (2005). Randomized, double-blind study of the analgesic efficacy of morphine-6-glucuronide versus morphine sulfate for postoperative pain in major surgery. *Anesthesiology* 102:815–821.

167. Freitas, R.A. (1999). *Nanomedicine, Volume I: Basic Capabilities*. Austin, TX: Landes Bioscience.

168. Costantini, D.L., Chan, C., Cai, Z., Vallis, K.A., Reilly, R.M. (2007). ^{111}In-labeled trastuzumab (Herceptin) modified with nuclear localization sequences (NLS): an Auger electron-emitting radiotherapeutic agent for HER2/neu-amplified breast cancer. *J Nucl Med* 48:1357–1368.

169. Massart, R., Cabuil, V. (1987). Synthese en milieu alcalin de magnetite colloidale. *J Chim Phys* 84:963–973.

170. Park, J., An, K., Hwang, Y., Park, J.G., Noh, H.J., Kim, J.Y., Park, J.H., Hwang, N.M., Hyeon, T. (2004). Ultra-large-scale syntheses of monodisperse nanocrystals. *Nat Mater* 3:891–895.

171. Goodwin, S., Peterson, C., Hoh, C., Bittner, C. (1999). Targeting and retention of magnetic targeted carriers (MTCs) enhancing intra- arterial chemotherapy. *J Magn Magn Mater* 194:132–139.

172. Ashton, P., Hadgraft, J., Walters, K.A. (1986). Effects of surfactants in percutaneous absorption. *Pharm Acta Helv* 61(8):228–235.

173. Roskos, K.V., Maibach, H.I., Guy, R.H. (1989). The effect of aging on percutaneous absorption in man. *J Pharmacokinet Biopharm* 17:617–630.

174. Scheuplein, R.J. (1978). *Site Variations in Diffusion and Permeability*. New York: Academic Press, pp. 1731–1752.

175. Barry, B.W. (1983). *Properties that Influence Percutaneous Absorption*. New York: Marcel Decker, pp. 127–233.

176. Bronaugh, R.L., Collier, S.W., Macpherson, S.E., Kraeling, M.E. (1994). Influence of metabolism in skin on dosimetry after topical exposure. *Environ Health Perspect* 102(Suppl. 11):71–74.

177. Kraeling, M.E., Lipicky, R.J., Bronaugh, R.L. (1996). Metabolism of benzocaine during percutaneous absorption in the hairless guinea pig: acetylbenzocaine formation and activity. *Skin Pharmacol* 9:221–230.

178. Nathan, D., Sakr, A., Lichtin, J.L., Bronaugh, R.L. (1990). In vitro skin absorption and metabolism of benzoic acid, p-aminobenzoic acid, and benzocaine in the hairless guinea pig. *Pharm Res* 7:1147–1151.

179. Roberts, M.S. (1997). Targeted drug delivery to the skin and deeper tissues: role of physiology, solute structure and disease. *Clin Exp Pharmacol Physiol* 24:874–879.

180. Sato, K., Sugibayashi, K., Morimoto, Y. (1991). Species differences in percutaneous absorption of nicorandil. *J Pharm Sci* 80:104–107.

181. Gorukanti, S.R., Li, L., Kim, K.H. (1999). Transdermal delivery of antiparkinsonian agent, benztropine. I. Effect of vehicles on skin permeation. *Int J Pharm* 192:159–172.

CHAPTER 20

Gene Therapy for Pain

MARINA MATA and DAVID J. FINK

Department of Neurology, University of Michigan School of Medicine and VA Ann Arbor Healthcare System

Content

20.1 INTRODUCTION

The safety and efficacy of a drug are conventionally considered determined by two types of specificity: the specificity of the drug for its target (receptor) and the specificity of the target in the pathogenesis of the disease process. "Off-target" effects occur as a result of insufficient specificity of either the drug for its target or the specificity of the target in the pathogenesis of the disease. For treatment of conditions of the nervous system such as pain, anatomic specificity also needs to be considered. The nervous system employs a limited repertoire of neurotransmitters, receptors, and ion channels in distinct neuroanatomic pathways to subserve different functions. Specificity of endogenous agents is achieved by synaptic release of neurotransmitters in restricted sites in the brain or in the spinal cord. Because the currently available drugs act through mechanisms that are not specific to pain-related neural pathways,

Peripheral Receptor Targets for Analgesia: Novel Approaches to Pain Management, Edited by Brian E. Cairns

off-target effects unrelated to the relief of pain often limit the maximum dose of analgesic medication that can be prescribed. For example, the potent opioid analgesic morphine administered systemically activates opioid receptors in regions of the brain unrelated to pain perception to cause somnolence, confusion, and ultimately impaired respiration. Activation by systemically administered morphine of opioid receptors in the gut and in the urinary bladder produce nausea, constipation, and urinary retention. The net result of activation of opiate receptors in non-pain-related pathways is off-target effects that often prevent the administration of a fully effective analgesic dose of the drug. These problems are not limited to opiates. Following the discovery that transient receptor potential (TRPV1) ion channels play an important role in the perception of chronic pain, pharmaceutical companies have raced to develop highly selective TRPV1 antagonists as novel analgesic agents. But TRPV1 receptors are not limited to peripheral nociceptive neurons from which they were originally isolated, and systemic administration of a selective TRPV1 antagonist results in dose-limiting hyperthermia at subanalgesic doses [1,2].

One potential strategy to avoid off-target effects of potent analgesic peptides is through selective production and release of the peptide at specific locations in nociceptive pathways. The pathways subserving acute pain perception are well established. Primary nociceptors, pseudounipolar neurons with cell bodies in the dorsal root ganglion, and axons that terminate peripherally in the skin or organs project centrally to terminate in the dorsal horn of the spinal cord in an anatomically defined (dermatomal or radicular) pattern. Second-order neurons in the dorsal horn of the spinal cord project rostrally to third-order sensory nuclei in the thalamus in addition to other mesencephalic and diencephalic nuclear groups. Thalamic neurons project to the sensory cortex to subserve discriminative aspects of pain perception, and to the limbic cortex where the affective component of the pain experience is coded. Descending pathways project from the brain stem back to the spinal dorsal horn to modulate spinal nociceptive neurotransmission.

Chronic pain differs from acute pain perception in that continuous activation of nociceptive pathways results in physiological alterations in neurotransmission ("windup," heterosynaptic central sensitization and homosynaptic long-term potentiation in the spinal cord), posttranslational modifications in neurotransmitter receptors, and voltage-gated ion channels among other proteins in components of the nociceptive pathway, and transcriptional changes in neurons and glial cells of the dorsal root ganglion, dorsal horn, and brain stem. Nonetheless, it appears that the same anatomic pathways involved in acute pain perception are involved in the perception of chronic pain and thus serve to identify potential targets for selective modulation of pain perception.

Gene therapy was first proposed as a novel method to correct inherited genetic defects [3] but to date, only one inherited condition, X-linked severe combined immunodeficiency, has been effectively treated by gene therapy [4].

Gene transfer methods, though, have been adapted for the delivery and continuous expression of bioactive peptides in the treatment of heterogeneous diseases including diseases of the nervous system. In rodent models, alteration in nociception has been achieved by gene transfer into brain nuclei (rostral agranular insular cortex [5], amygdala [6]), transduction of the meninges to result in release into the cerebrospinal fluid [7,8], direct injection of a vector into the dorsal horn of the spinal cord [9], and transduction of the dorsal root ganglia (DRG) either by injection of a vector directly into the DRG [10], into the intrathecal space [11], or into the skin [12,13].

While gene transfer to any of these sites could potentially be adapted for the treatment of patients with pain, there are advantages to targeting nociceptive neurotransmission at the first synapse in the ascending pain pathway, between the primary nociceptor and the second-order projection neuron in the dorsal horn of the spinal cord. The ability to achieve selective pain-related effects has been exploited with conventional analgesic drugs like morphine or baclofen by delivery into the cerebrospinal fluid through chronic intrathecal infusion, a route of administration that results in a 10-fold reduction in dose requirement and in a corresponding reduction in off-target adverse events at equipotent analgesic doses; this chapter will focus on that site as a target for gene transfer.

20.2 GENE TRANSFER VECTORS

There are several different methods that can be used to transfer genes. Gene transfer can be achieved through transplantation of transduced cells, but the most effective strategies use gene delivery agents (vectors) to effect genetic modification of cells in their native environment. Nonviral vectors use a variety of lipid formulations to deliver DNA to host cells. This approach is technically simpler than the development of viral vectors, and even though gene delivery is relatively inefficient, some success has been reported with intrathecal injection of liposome-encapsulated plasmids to express anti-inflammatory peptides (described below). The most potent and effective delivery vehicles are created by modification of viruses, organisms that have evolved elaborate strategies for the transfer of their genetic material into host cells. Adeno-associated virus-based vectors (AAV) and herpes simplex virus (HSV)-based vectors have shown promise in rodent models of pain and will be described in some detail.

AAV was initially discovered as a contaminant of preparations of adenovirus. Natural AAV infection is not known to cause disease and AAV-based vectors are widely used in phase 1 and phase 2 human gene transfer trials. AAV is a small (22 nm) single-stranded DNA virus that can accommodate up to 5 kb of foreign genetic sequences. AAV vectors have conventionally been propagated using a triple transfection method in which one plasmid containing packaging signals and a transgene, a second plasmid expressing the AAV *replicase* and *capsid* functions, and a third coding for the required adenovirus helper functions are cotransfected. More recently, methods involving bacterial artificial chromosomes have been developed to increase the efficiency of AAV vector production. *In vitro*, the wild-type AAV genome integrates into a specific site on chromosome 19; *in vivo*, integration is relatively inefficient and requires concatemerization of the vector genome so that it may take several weeks to achieve maximum transgene expression following vector injection. Even though wild-type AAV does not naturally infect the brain, robust transfection of neurons and glia has been demonstrated following direct intracerebral inoculation. Interestingly, different serotypes of AAV appear to demonstrate different tissue selectivity, and the AAV of serotype 8 has been reported to effectively transduce DRG neurons after intrathecal inoculation.

HSV is a naturally neurotropic virus. In natural infection of the skin or the mucous membranes, virus entry into sensory nerve endings leads to vector transport to the nerve cell body. HSV is a large double-stranded DNA virus that in its natural life cycle is spread by contact, infecting and replicating in the skin or in the mucous membrane. Viral particles released in the skin are taken up by sensory nerve terminals and are carried by retrograde axonal transport to the neuronal perikaryon in the DRG. In the DRG, wild-type virus may reenter the lytic cycle, or may alternatively establish a potentially lifelong latent state.

HSV is complex, with more than 85 genes coded in a 150-kb double-stranded DNA genome. Vectors are created from wild-type HSV by deletion of genes critical for viral replication. One class of vectors has been created by deletion of an accessory viral function (HSV thymidine kinase) that is important to virus replication in neurons and contributes to neurovirulence. Recombinant herpes viruses defective in *tk* can be propagated in unmodified monkey kidney cells in culture and are capable of replication in the skin, but are unable to replicate in the DRG and are thus forced into a pseudolatent state once the genome reaches the DRG. A second class of HSV vectors, most appropriate for human trials, has been rendered defective in essential virus genes, and thus fails to replicate in all cell types and is propagated in modified cell lines that have been engineered to provide the missing required HSV gene products from the cellular genome [14]. The immediate early (IE) HSV genes are expressed immediately on entry of the virus genome into the nucleus and include infected cell polypeptides (ICPs) ICP4 and ICP27, which are required for expression of early and late viral genes [15]. The HSV vectors moving toward human trial fail to express in addition ICP22 and ICP47, retaining only the IE gene coding for ICP0 that is required for the vector genome to remain transcriptionally active [16]. These multiply-deleted vectors are completely incapable of replication *in vivo*, but because the recombinant particles retain the targeting properties of the wild-type virus, nonreplicating recombinant vectors can be used to deliver genes from the skin to the sensory ganglion *in vivo*.

20.3 VECTOR-MEDIATED EXPRESSION OF INHIBITORY NEUROTRANSMITTERS IN PAIN

Nociceptive neurotransmission at the synapse between the primary nociceptor and second-order neurons in the dorsal horn is modulated by inhibitory neurotransmitters released from interneurons to act on presynaptic and postsynaptic receptors. Opioid peptides including enkephalin acting at the delta opioid receptor, endomorphins-1 and -2 acting at μ-opioid receptors, and gamma amino butyric acid (GABA) and glycine acting at their cognate receptors reduce pain-related signaling at the spinal level. Pohl and coworkers first showed that a *tk*-defective HSV recombinant injected subcutaneously in the paw transduces DRG neurons, resulting in expression of enkephalin in DRG [17], and Wilson and coworkers subsequently demonstrated that a similar tk^- HSV-based vector containing the human proenkephalin gene injected subcutaneously into the paw reduces hyperalgesic C-fiber responses ipsilateral to the injection [18]. Pohl then went on to demonstrate that the vector could be used to reduce pain in a model of arthritis induced by injection of complete Freund's adjuvant (CFA) in rats [19]. In addition to reducing pain-related behaviors, vector-mediated enkephalin production reduced bone and cartilage destruction in the inflamed joints, presumably related to release of enkephalin from peripheral sensory terminals innervating the joint. [19]. The investigators had previously demonstrated that enkephalin is transported bidirectionally toward the skin as well as toward the spinal cord from transduced neurons in the DRG [20].

The analgesic effects of vector inoculation are not dependent on viral replication, as a nonreplicating HSV vector deleted for both copies of the essential HSV IE gene ICP4 coding for preproenkephalin has been demonstrated to produce a similar analgesic effect in the delayed phase of the formalin model of inflammatory pain [21]. The time course of the analgesic effect, maximal at 1 week and declining over time, is consistent with the known time course of expression driven by the human cytomegalovirus immediate early promoter (HCMV IEp) inserted to drive transgene expression from this vector, and the observation that reinoculation of the vector at 4 weeks restores the analgesic effect has been interpreted as demonstrating that the animals do not develop tolerance to the vector-mediated transgene product released from synaptic terminals *in vivo*.

Expression of enkephalin in DRG achieved by subcutaneous inoculation of a nonreplicating enkephalin-expressing HSV vector has been shown to produce an analgesic effect in neuropathic pain. This effect has been demonstrated in the selective spinal nerve ligation (SNL) model of neuropathic pain, in which injection of the HSV vector 1 week after SNL results in an analgesic effect, as well as in a model of painful diabetic neuropathy created by injection of streptozotocin (STZ) in rats[22]. In the SNL model, the effect of transgene-mediated enkephalin release is additive with morphine (reducing the ED_{50} of coadministered morphine from 1.8 to 0.15 mg/kg) and persists despite the induction of tolerance to morphine [23]. The effect of enkephalin expression driven by the HCMV IEp produces an analgesic effect that persists for several weeks and is reestablished by reinoculation [23]. Similarly, in the infraorbital nerve constriction model of craniofacial pain, Pohl and colleagues have demonstrated that a tk-deleted enkephalin-expressing vector injected into the vibrissal pad produced a significant reduction in mechanical hypersensitivity on the affected side [24].

The effect of an enkephalin-expressing HSV vector has also been examined in a pancreatitis model of visceral pain, where direct injection of an enkephalin-expressing HSV vector into the pancreas attenuated evoked nocisponsive behaviors [25]. In the pancreas, enkephalin expression appeared to reduce the inflammatory response in the pancreas, analogous to the effect reported in polyarthritis [19]. In a similar fashion, injection of a nonreplicating enkephalin-expressing HSV vector into the rat bladder wall results in enkephalin expression in DRG that innervates the bladder and attenuates capsaicin-induced bladder irritation and resultant bladder hyperactivity [26,27].

Yeomans et al. have demonstrated in the primate that application of a tk-deleted HSV vector expressing enkephalin onto the dorsal surface of the foot of macaques reduces A-delta and C-fiber mediated pain-related responses [28]. Finally, in a mouse model of bone cancer pain [29], subcutaneous inoculation of the HSV vector expressing enkephalin resulted in an attenuation of spontaneous nocisponsive behaviors [30]. Taken together, these results provide proof-of-principle evidence that HSV vector-mediated delivery of enkephalin from skin inoculation can provide an analgesic effect and has set the stage for the first phase 1 trial in patients with intractable pain related to cancer, to examine the safety of HSV vector-mediated gene transfer of enkephalin, described in more detail later.

HSV-mediated expression of other inhibitory neurotransmitters has been examined in rodent models of pain. Endomorphin-2 (EM-2) (Tyr-Pro-Phe-Phe-NH2) is a highly selective μ-opioid receptor agonist [31]. Because the gene coding for endomorphin-2 has not been identified, Wolfe and colleagues constructed a tripartite synthetic gene cassette with the N terminal signal sequence of human preproenkephalin followed by a pair of endomorphin-2 coding elements, including the addition of a C-terminal glycine residue to direct amidation of the product by the widely distributed enzyme peptidylglycine α-amidating monooxygenase, flanked by dibasic cleavage sites to provide for processing and peptide liberation by cellular proteases [32]. Subcutaneous inoculation of the endomorphin-2-expressing HSV vector produces a significant reduction in both mechanical allodynia and thermal hyperalgesia in rats with neuropathic pain induced by selective L5 SNL. The effect of vector-mediated endomorphin-2 release is blocked by the highly selective μ-opioid receptor antagonist D-Phe-Cys-Tyr-D-Trp-Orn-Thr-Pen-Thr amide (CTOP). The endomorphin-2-expressing vector also produces a substantial reduction in nocifensive behaviors in the delayed phase of the formalin test and in the CFA model of inflammatory pain [33]. While vector-mediated enkephalin and endomorphin-2 expression both demonstrate statistically significant effects in neuropathic pain, the magnitude of the effect is less than complete, in agreement with the clinical observation that neuropathic pain is often relatively refractory to treatment with opiates.

GABA is the principal inhibitory neurotransmitter in the nervous system, and there is an emerging body of literature to suggest that peripheral nerve damage-related reduction in GABAergic tone in the dorsal horn of the spinal cord plays a role in the pathogenesis of neuropathic pain [34]. But similar to the case with opiate drugs, the use of GABA agonists for pain relief is limited by substantial off-target depressant central nervous system effects. A nonreplicating HSV vector coding for glutamic acid decarboxylase (GAD), the enzyme that decarboxylates glutamic acid to produce GABA, transduces neurons to produce and release GABA *in vitro* and following subcutaneous inoculation *in vivo* [35]. In the selective SNL model of neuropathic pain, subcutaneous inoculation of the GAD-expressing vector results in a substantial reduction in mechanical allodynia and thermal hyperalgesia [36], an effect that is greater in magnitude than the effect produced by either the enkephalin or endomorphin-expressing HSV vectors. The GAD-expressing HSV vector also reduces pain-related behaviors in a model of central neuropathic pain created by T13 spinal cord hemisection [35]. In the latter study, the vector-mediated analgesic effect was reversed in part by intrathecal administration of the GABA receptor antagonists, bicuculline or phaclofen, indicating that the analgesic effect of the vector is mediated by spinal GABA(A) and GABA(B) receptors.

20.4 VECTOR-MEDIATED INHIBITION OF THE SPINAL NEUROIMMUNE RESPONSE IN PAIN

In addition to the loss of inhibitory tone in the dorsal horn, a growing body of experimental evidence implicates neuroimmune activation of microglia and astrocytes in the dorsal horn in the pathogenesis of neuropathic pain [37–40]. Among the proinflammatory substances released by activated microglia and astrocytes, tumor necrosis factor alpha (TNF-α) appears to play a central role in the pathogenesis of pain, supported by observations that intraperitoneal inoculation of neutralizing antibodies directed against the p55 tumor necrosis factor receptor (TNFR) reduces thermal hyperalgesia and mechanical allodynia, and intrathecal administration of the recombinant p75 soluble tumor necrosis factor receptor (sTNFR) peptide (etanercept) reduces mechanical allodynia in a rat model of neuropathic pain [41–43]. In the spinal hemisection model of central neuropathic pain, subcutaneous inoculation of a nonreplicating HSV vector expressing the p55 sTNFR reduces the behavioral manifestations of neuropathic pain [44] concurrent with a reduction in markers of neuroimmune activation. And in the selective SNL model of neuropathic pain, subcutaneous inoculation of the p55 sTNFR-expressing HSV vector reduces behavioral manifestations of neuropathic pain while simultaneously reducing the phosphorylation of p38α, the expression of interleukin (IL)-1β, and the expression of membrane-associated TNF-α (mTNFα) in the spinal cord [45].

Interleukin-4 (IL-4) is a prototypical anti-inflammatory cytokine [46,47], and subcutaneous injection of a replication-defective HSV vector expressing IL-4 under the transcriptional control of the HSV ICP4 IE promoter [48] does not alter paw-withdrawal latency to thermal stimuli nor change the tactile threshold in normal animals, but inoculation of the vector 1 week after selective SNL reduces mechanical allodynia and reverses thermal hyperalgesia in that model of neuropathic pain. Inoculation of the vector 1 week before SNL delays, but does not ultimately prevent, the development of neuropathic pain. Similar effects have been observed using a nonreplicating HSV vector coding for the anti-inflammatory peptide interleukin (IL)-10, which reduces pain-related behaviors in the delayed phase of the formalin test [49], corresponding with a reduction in the expression of TNF-α in spinal microglia [49].

Based on the demonstration that direct intrathecal infusion of glial cell line-derived neurotrophic factor (GDNF) reduces ectopic nerve discharges and pain-related behaviors in the partial sciatic nerve injury model of neuropathic pain in rodents [50], we examined the effect of a nonreplicating GDNF-expressing HSV vector in the SNL model of neuropathic pain. Subcutaneous inoculation of the vector into the paw 1 week after SNL produced a significant antiallodynic effect [51]. Like the effects of other HSV vectors in which transgene expression is driven by the HCMV IEp, the antiallodynic effect produced by inoculation of the GDNF-expressing vector persisted for several weeks and was reestablished by reinoculation of the vector [51]. In a related approach, Pohl and colleagues have demonstrated that direct inoculation into the spinal dorsal horn of a lentiviral-based vector coding for the NF-κB repressor IκBα prevents the enhanced expression of interleukin-6 and of inducible nitric oxide synthase associated with chronic nerve constriction injury, producing prolonged antihyperalgesic and antiallodynic effects [9].

20.5 VECTOR-MEDIATED KNOCKDOWN OF GENE EXPRESSION TO TREAT CHRONIC PAIN

Recent advances in RNA technology have made it possible to reduce endogenous gene expression *in vivo*. There is substantial evidence from animal studies and human genetics that the voltage-gated sodium channel isoform $Na_V1.7$ and the peptide neurotransmitter calcitonin gene-related peptide (CGRP) play important roles in pain perception and chronic pain states. Yeomans and coworkers have reported that an HSV vector coding a sequence antisense to $Na_V1.7$ applied to the skin prevents the increase in $Na_V1.7$ expression caused by CFA injection. The effect correlates with a reduction in the development of hyperalgesia in C- and A-delta thermonociceptive tests [52].

More recently, the same group has shown that an HSV vector coding a sequence antisense to CGRP reduces CGRP expression in transduced DRG neurons with concomitant reduction in nociceptive neurotransmission *in vivo* [53].

20.6 INTRATHECAL INJECTION OF GENE TRANSFER VECTORS FOR CHRONIC PAIN

In an early study, Iadarola and coworkers injected an adenovirus vector coding for β-endorphin intrathecally to transduce meningeal cells of the pia [54]. The resulting β-endorphin secretion attenuated inflammatory hyperalgesia without affecting basal nociceptive responses [54]. Because adenoviral vectors elicit a substantial immune response of their own, subsequent studies have used other vectors. In a series of studies, Watkins and colleagues have shown that intrathecal injection of plasmid or AAV-based vectors expressing IL-10 can be used to reduce the behavioral manifestations of neuropathic pain in several different models of pain [7,8,55,56]. Robust and prolonged antiallodynic effects have been demonstrated using paired injections of plasmid alone, but the identity of the cells transduced by this approach has not yet been established.

More recently, Beutler and coworkers have shown that similar effects can be achieved by intrathecal inoculation of an AAV vector of serotype 8 expressing either β-endorphin or IL-10 [11]. In recent years, several novel serotypes including AAV serotypes 7, 8, and 9 and more than 100 other AAV variants have been isolated as DNA sequences from human or primate tissues [57], with several of these variants showing distinct tissue tropisms. Beutler and colleagues demonstrated that intrathecal injection of a serotype 8 AAV containing a green fluorescent protein (GFP) reporter transgene results in transduction of DRG neurons. The DRG lies physically at the end of root sleeves that are continuous with the intrathecal space and are thus bathed by the cerebrospinal fluid (CSF), but the infection of DRG neurons by serotype 8 AAV is distinct; serotype 2 AAV, for example, does not infect DRG neurons when administered by the same route. The magnitude of the antiallodynic effect of intrathecal injection of a serotype 8 AAV vector containing the prepro-β-endorphin gene in the SNL model of neuropathic pain is comparable to that achieved by other gene transfer methods, and the duration of pain relief is longer than that achieved by a single injection of other vectors intrathecally. The single set of experiments reported with serotype 8 AAV demonstrates several features that may be desirable for the treatment of chronic pain, but also raises important issues that will need to be explored further, including the following: (i) What is the rostrocaudal extent of transgene expression in DRG following intrathecal injection? (ii) How many genomes infect the brain (reported to be 10^{-4}, the level of transduction of DRG) and what regions of the brain are transduced? (iii) What is the effect on brain infection if the vector is injected at thoracic or higher levels of the spinal cord? (iv) Are other organs outside the nervous system (e.g., liver, pancreas, muscle, all efficiently transduced by serotype 8 AAV) infected following intrathecal injection of serotype 8 AAV? (v) Is a single injection of an AAV vector into the CSF more or less toxic than two injections of a plasmid vector by the same site?

20.7 FUTURE PROSPECTS

The preclinical studies of HSV-based vectors have advanced the furthest toward human application and, as reviewed in this chapter, have demonstrated that different genes can effectively be delivered to the DRG by subcutaneous inoculation of HSV to provide analgesic effects in different models of pain. Though comparison of different models is difficult, it would appear from published data that the most effective gene product may vary according to the type of pain being treated. Experience garnered from studies of replication-compromised HSV vectors in the treatment of patients with glioblastoma, which have not demonstrated significant toxicity [58,59], suggests that the intradermal inoculation of replication-incompetent vectors should be safe, and an Investigational New Drug (IND) application for the first phase 1 human trial of HSV was approved by the U.S. Food and Drug Administration in February 2008 to examine the well-characterized enkephalin-expressing nonreplicating HSV vector in patients with intractable pain caused by cancer. This phase 1 trial is designed to test the safety of using HSV vectors for pain gene therapy and will be carried out at the University of Michigan by one of us (DJF) with sponsorship by Diamyd Inc. Ultimately, only human trials will allow us to determine whether HSV-mediated gene transfer can be moved from rodent studies to humans to add to the armamentarium of available pain treatments.

ACKNOWLEDGMENTS

The authors were supported by grants from the Department of Veterans Affairs, the Juvenile Diabetes Research Foundation, and National Institutes of Health grants NS038850 and DK044935.

REFERENCES

1. Gavva, N.R., Treanor, J.J., Garami, A., Fang, L., Surapaneni, S., Akrami, A. et al. (2008). Pharmacological blockade of the vanilloid receptor TRPV1 elicits marked hyperthermia in humans. *Pain* 136:202–210.
2. Caterina, M.J. (2008). On the thermoregulatory perils of TRPV1 antagonism. *Pain* 136:3–4.
3. Friedmann, T., Roblin, R. (1972). Gene therapy for human genetic disease? *Science* 175:949–955.

4. Cavazzana-Calvo, M., Hacein-Bey, S., de Saint Basile, G., Gross, F., Yvon, E., Nusbaum, P. et al. (2000). Gene therapy of human severe combined immunodeficiency (SCID)-X1 disease. *Science* 288:669–672.

5. Jasmin, L., Rabkin, S.D., Granato, A., Boudah, A., Ohara, P.T. (2003). Analgesia and hyperalgesia from GABA-mediated modulation of the cerebral cortex. *Nature* 424:316–320.

6. Kang, W., Wilson, M.A., Bender, M.A., Glorioso, J.C., Wilson, S.P. (1998). Herpes virus-mediated preproenkephalin gene transfer to the amygdala is antinociceptive. *Brain Res* 792:133–135.

7. Ledeboer, A., Jekich, B.M., Sloane, E.M., Mahoney, J.H., Langer, S.J., Milligan, E.D. et al. (2007). Intrathecal interleukin-10 gene therapy attenuates paclitaxel-induced mechanical allodynia and proinflammatory cytokine expression in dorsal root ganglia in rats. *Brain Behav Immun* 21:686–698.

8. Milligan, E.D., Soderquist, R.G., Malone, S.M., Mahoney, J.H., Hughes, T.S., Langer, S.J. et al. (2006). Intrathecal polymer-based interleukin-10 gene delivery for neuropathic pain. *Neuron Glia Biol* 2:293–308.

9. Meunier, A., Latremoliere, A., Dominguez, E., Mauborgne, A., Philippe, S., Hamon, M. et al. (2007). Lentiviral-mediated targeted NF-kappaB blockade in dorsal spinal cord glia attenuates sciatic nerve injury-induced neuropathic pain in the rat. *Mol Ther* 15:687–697.

10. Xu, Y., Gu, Y., Xu, G.Y., Wu, P., Li, G.W., Huang, L.Y. (2003). Adeno-associated viral transfer of opioid receptor gene to primary sensory neurons: a strategy to increase opioid antinociception. *Proc Natl Acad Sci U S A* 100:6204–6209.

11. Storek, B., Reinhardt, M., Wang, C., Janssen, W.G., Harder, N.M., Banck, M.S. et al. (2008). Sensory neuron targeting by self-complementary AAV8 via lumbar puncture for chronic pain. *Proc Natl Acad Sci U S A* 105:1055–1060.

12. Glorioso, J.C., Fink, D.J. (2004). Herpes vector-mediated gene transfer in treatment of diseases of the nervous system. *Annu Rev Microbiol* 58:253–271.

13. Mata, M., Hao, S., Fink, D.J. (2008). Applications of gene therapy to the treatment of chronic pain. *Curr Gene Ther* 8:42–48.

14. DeLuca, N.A., McCarthy, A.M., Schaffer, P.A. (1985). Isolation and characterization of deletion mutants of herpes simplex virus type 1 in the gene encoding immediate-early regulatory protein ICP4. *J Virol* 56:558–570.

15. Roizman, B., Knipe, D.M. (2001). Herpes simplex viruses and their replication. In: Knipe, D.M., Howley, P.M. (eds.). *Fields Virology*, 4th ed. Philadelphia: Lippincott Williams & Wilkins, pp. 2399–2460.

16. Wolfe, D., Goins, W.F., Yamada, M., Moriuchi, S., Krisky, D.M., Oligino, T.J. et al. (1999). Engineering herpes simplex virus vectors for CNS applications. *Exp Neurol* 159:34–46.

17. Antunes Bras, J.M., Epstein, A.L., Bourgoin, S., Hamon, M., Cesselin, F., Pohl, M. (1998). Herpes simplex virus 1-mediated transfer of preproenkephalin A in rat dorsal root ganglia. *J Neurochem* 70:1299–1303.

18. Wilson, S.P., Yeomans, D.C., Bender, M.A., Lu, Y., Goins, W.F., Glorioso, J.C. (1999). Antihyperalgesic effects of infection with a preproenkephalin-encoding herpes virus. *Proc Natl Acad Sci U S A* 96:3211–3216.

19. Braz, J., Beaufour, C., Coutaux, A., Epstein, A.L., Cesselin, F., Hamon, M. et al. (2001). Therapeutic efficacy in experimental polyarthritis of viral-driven enkephalin overproduction in sensory neurons. *J Neurosci* 21:7881–7888.

20. Antunes bras, J., Becker, C., Bourgoin, S., Lombard, M., Cesselin, F., Hamon, M. et al. (2001). Met-enkephalin is preferentially transported into the peripheral processes of primary afferent fibres in both control and HSV1-driven proenkephalin A overexpressing rats. *Neuroscience* 103:1073–1083.

21. Goss, J.R., Mata, M., Goins, W.F., Wu, H.H., Glorioso, J.C., Fink, D.J. (2001). Antinociceptive effect of a genomic herpes simplex virus-based vector expressing human proenkephalin in rat dorsal root ganglion. *Gene Ther* 8:551–556.

22. Chattopadhyay, M., Mata, M., Fink, D.J. (2008). Continuous delta opioid receptor activation reduces neuronal voltage gated sodium channel ($Na_V1.7$) levels through activation of protein kinase C in painful diabetic neuropathy. *J Neurosci* 28:6652–6658.

23. Hao, S., Mata, M., Goins, W., Glorioso, J.C., Fink, D.J. (2003). Transgene-mediated enkephalin release enhances the effect of morphine and evades tolerance to produce a sustained antiallodynic effect. *Pain* 102:135–142.

24. Meunier, A., Latremoliere, A., Mauborgne, A., Bourgoin, S., Kayser, V., Cesselin, F. et al. (2005). Attenuation of pain-related behavior in a rat model of trigeminal neuropathic pain by viral-driven enkephalin overproduction in trigeminal ganglion neurons. *Mol Ther* 11:608–616.

25. Lu, Y., McNearney, T.A., Lin, W., Wilson, S.P., Yeomans, D.C., Westlund, K.N. (2007). Treatment of inflamed pancreas with enkephalin encoding HSV-1 recombinant vector reduces inflammatory damage and behavioral sequelae. *Mol Ther* 15:1812–1819.

26. Goins, W.F., Yoshimura, N., Phelan, M.W., Yokoyama, T., Fraser, M.O., Ozawa, H. et al. (2001). Herpes simplex virus mediated nerve growth factor expression in bladder and afferent neurons: potential treatment for diabetic bladder dysfunction. *J Urol* 165:1748–1754.

27. Yoshimura, N., Franks, M.E., Sasaki, K., Goins, W.F., Goss, J., Yokoyama, T. et al. (2001). Gene therapy of bladder pain with herpes simplex virus (HSV) vectors expressing preproenkephalin (PPE). *Urology* 57:116.

28. Yeomans, D.C., Lu, Y., Laurito, C.E., Peters, M.C., Vota-Vellis, G., Wilson, S.P. et al. (2006). Recombinant herpes vector-mediated analgesia in a primate model of hyperalgesia. *Mol Ther* 13:589–597.

29. Honore, P., Rogers, S.D., Schwei, M.J., Salak-Johnson, J.L., Luger, N.M., Sabino, M.C. et al. (2000). Murine models of inflammatory, neuropathic and cancer pain each generates a unique set of neurochemical changes in the spinal cord and sensory neurons. *Neuroscience* 98:585–598.

30. Goss, J.R., Harley, C.F., Mata, M., O'Malley, M.E., Goins, W.F., Hu, X.-P. et al. (2002). Herpes vector-mediated expression of proenkephalin reduces pain-related behavior in a model of bone cancer pain. *Ann Neurol* 52:662–665.

31. Zadina, J.E., Hackler, L., Ge, L.J., Kastin, A.J. (1997). A potent and selective endogenous agonist for the mu-opiate receptor. *Nature* 386:499–502.

32. Wolfe, D., Hao, S., Hu, J., Srinivasan, R., Goss, J., Mata, M. et al. (2007). Engineering an endomorphin-2 gene for use in neuropathic pain therapy. *Pain* 133:29–38.

33. Hao, S., Wolfe, D., Glorioso, J.C., Mata, M., Fink, D.J. (2008). Effects of transgen-mediated endomorphin-2 in inflammatory pain. *Eur J Pain* (in press).
34. Moore, K.A., Kohno, T., Karchewski, L.A., Scholz, J., Baba, H., Woolf, C.J. (2002). Partial peripheral nerve injury promotes a selective loss of GABAergic inhibition in the superficial dorsal horn of the spinal cord. *J Neurosci* 22:6724–6731.
35. Liu, J., Wolfe, D., Hao, S., Huang, S., Glorioso, J.C., Mata, M. et al. (2004). Peripherally delivered glutamic acid decarboxylase gene therapy for spinal cord injury pain. *Mol Ther* 10:57–66.
36. Hao, S., Mata, M., Wolfe, D., Glorioso, J.C., Fink, D.J. (2005). Gene transfer of glutamic acid decarboxylase reduces neuropathic pain. *Ann Neurol* 57:914–918.
37. DeLeo, J.A., Yezierski, R.P. (2001). The role of neuroinflammation and neuroimmune activation in persistent pain. *Pain* 90:1–6.
38. Watkins, L.R., Milligan, E.D., Maier, S.F. (2001). Glial activation: a driving force for pathological pain. *Trends Neurosci* 24:450–455.
39. Wieseler-Frank, J., Maier, S.F., Watkins, L.R. (2004). Glial activation and pathological pain. *Neurochem Int* 45:389–395.
40. DeLeo, J.A., Tanga, F.Y., Tawfik, V.L. (2004). Neuroimmune activation and neuroinflammation in chronic pain and opioid tolerance/hyperalgesia. *Neuroscientist* 10:40–52.
41. Sommer, C., Schmidt, C., George, A. (1998). Hyperalgesia in experimental neuropathy is dependent on the TNF receptor 1. *Exp Neurol* 151:138–142.
42. Schafers, M., Svensson, C.I., Sommer, C., Sorkin, L.S. (2003). Tumor necrosis factor-alpha induces mechanical allodynia after spinal nerve ligation by activation of p38 MAPK in primary sensory neurons. *J Neurosci* 23:2517–2521.
43. Svensson, C.I., Schafers, M., Jones, T.L., Powell, H., Sorkin, L.S. (2005). Spinal blockade of TNF blocks spinal nerve ligation-induced increases in spinal P-p38. *Neurosci Lett* 379:209–213.
44. Peng, X., Zhou, Z., Glorioso, J.C., Fink, D.J., Mata, M. (2006). Tumor necrosis factor alpha contributes to below-level neuropathic pain after spinal cord injury. *Ann Neurol* 59:843–851.
45. Hao, S., Mata, M., Glorioso, J.C., Fink, D.J. (2007). Gene transfer to interfere with TNFalpha signaling in neuropathic pain. *Gene Ther* 14:1010–1016.
46. te Velde, A.A., Huijbens, R.J., Heije, K., de Vries, J.E., Figdor, C.G. (1990). Interleukin-4 (IL-4) inhibits secretion of IL-1 beta, tumor necrosis factor alpha, and IL-6 by human monocytes. *Blood* 76:1392–1397.
47. Mijatovic, T., Kruys, V., Caput, D., Defrance, P., Huez, G. (1997). Interleukin-4 and -13 inhibit tumor necrosis factor-alpha mRNA translational activation in lipopolysaccharide-induced mouse macrophages. *J Biol Chem* 272:14394–14398.
48. Hao, S., Mata, M., Glorioso, J.C., Fink, D.J. (2006). HSV-mediated expression of interleukin-4 in dorsal root ganglion neurons reduces neuropathic pain. *Mol Pain* 2:6.
49. Zhou, Z., Peng, X., Hao, S., Fink, D.J., Mata, M. (2008). HSV-mediated transfer of interleukin-10 reduces inflammatory pain through modulation of membrane tumor necrosis factor alpha in spinal cord microglia. *Gene Ther* 15:183–190.
50. Bennett, D.L., Boucher, T.J., Armanini, M.P., Poulsen, K.T., Michael, G.J., Priestley, J.V. et al. (2000). The glial cell line-derived neurotrophic factor family receptor

components are differentially regulated within sensory neurons after nerve injury. *J Neurosci* 20:27–437.

51. Hao, S., Mata, M., Wolfe, D., Huang, S., Glorioso, J., Fink, D.J. (2003). HSV-mediated gene transfer of the glial cell derived neurotrophic factor (GDNF) provides an anti-allodynic effect in neuropathic pain. *Mol Ther* 8:367–375.
52. Yeomans, D.C., Levinson, S.R., Peters, M.C., Koszowski, A.G., Tzabazis, A.Z., Gilly, W.F. et al. (2005). Decrease in inflammatory hyperalgesia by herpes vector-mediated knockdown of $Na_V1.7$ sodium channels in primary afferents. *Hum Gene Ther* 16:271–277.
53. Tzabazis, A.Z., Pirc, G., Votta-Velis, E., Wilson, S.P., Laurito, C.E., Yeomans, D.C. (2007). Antihyperalgesic effect of a recombinant herpes virus encoding antisense for calcitonin gene-related peptide. *Anesthesiology* 106:1196–1203.
54. Finegold, A.A., Mannes, A.J., Iadarola, M.J. (1999). A paracrine paradigm for in vivo gene therapy in the central nervous system: treatment of chronic pain. *Hum Gene Ther* 10:1251–1257.
55. Milligan, E.D., Sloane, E.M., Langer, S.J., Hughes, T.S., Jekich, B.M., Frank, M.G. et al. (2006). Repeated intrathecal injections of plasmid DNA encoding interleukin-10 produce prolonged reversal of neuropathic pain. *Pain* 126:294–308.
56. Milligan, E.D., Sloane, E.M., Langer, S.J., Cruz, P.E., Chacur, M., Spataro, L. et al. (2005). Controlling neuropathic pain by adeno-associated virus driven production of the anti-inflammatory cytokine, interleukin-10. *Mol Pain* 1:9.
57. Wu, Z., Asokan, A., Samulski, R.J. (2006). Adeno-associated virus serotypes: vector toolkit for human gene therapy. *Mol Ther* 14:316–327.
58. Shand, N., Weber, F., Mariani, L., Bernstein, M., Gianella-Borradori, A., Long, Z. et al. (1999). A phase 1-2 clinical trial of gene therapy for recurrent glioblastoma multiforme by tumor transduction with the herpes simplex thymidine kinase gene followed by ganciclovir. GLI328 European-Canadian Study Group. *Hum Gene Ther* 10:2325–2335.
59. Rainov, N.G. (2000). A phase III clinical evaluation of herpes simplex virus type 1 thymidine kinase and ganciclovir gene therapy as an adjuvant to surgical resection and radiation in adults with previously untreated glioblastoma multiforme. *Hum Gene Ther* 11:2389–2401.

CHAPTER 21

Topical Analgesics

AKHLAQ WAHEED HAKIM and BRIAN E. CAIRNS
Faculty of Pharmaceutical Sciences, The University of British Columbia

Content

21.1 NONSTEROIDAL ANTI-INFLAMMATORY DRUGS (NSAIDs)

Although considered relatively safe drugs, chronic systemic administration of NSAIDs is associated with significant side effects, in particular the development of gastrointestinal ulceration, renal dysfunction, and, in sensitive individuals, the exacerbation of existing hypertension [1,2]. Topical administration of NSAIDs results in high concentrations in the skin and in deeper tissues (joint, muscle) that decrease pain with reduced systemic side effects. Recent reviews of the available literature have concluded that topical NSAIDs (Table 21.1) are more effective than placebo for acute musculoskeletal pain (sprains, sports injuries) as well as for chronic inflammatory conditions (arthritis, rheumatism) and offer significantly lower incidence of side effects [2,3].

As discussed in Chapter 4, inflammation results in the release of prostaglandins (PGs), which are thought to be partly responsible for the increased sensitivity of cutaneous, joint, and muscle afferent fibers (peripheral sensitization) [4–7]. The analgesic efficacy of NSAIDs appears to result principally from the ability of these compounds to inhibit the conversion of arachidonic acid to PGs (and perhaps also leukotrienes) at the site of tissue injury [2,8,9], thus preventing the afferent sensitization. It is clear that all currently available

Peripheral Receptor Targets for Analgesia: Novel Approaches to Pain Management, Edited by Brian E. Cairns

TABLE 21.1. Topical NSAIDs.

Drugs	Form	Therapeutic Indications	Regional Availability
Benzydamide	5% cream, 0.15% spray, 0.15% oral rinse	Pain and inflammatory conditions of mouth and throat [11–13]	Asia, North America, Europe, United Arab Emirates
Diclofenac	3% gel, 0.1% eye drops, 1.5% topical solution, foam	Musculoskeletal pain and inflammation [11–13]	Australia, Asia, Europe, North America, United Arab Emirates
Fepradinol	6% gel, 6% spray	Pain and inflammation [12]	Europe
Flufenamic acid	3.5% cream	Musculoskeletal and soft tissue pain [12]	Europe
Felbinac	3% gel	Musculoskeletal and soft tissue pain [12]	Europe
Ibuprofen	5% cream, 10% gel	Musculoskeletal pain and inflammation [12]	Australia, Asia, Europe, North America, United Arab Emirates
Isonixin	2.5% cream	Musculoskeletal pain [12]	Europe
Indomethacin	1% solution	Musculoskeletal pain and inflammation [12]	Asia
Ketoprofen	2.5% gel	Musculoskeletal pain and inflammation [11,12]	Europe, North America, United Arab Emirates
Ketorolac	0.5% eye drops	Eye pain [11–13]	Australia, Asia, Europe, North America, United Arab Emirates
Nimesulide	3% cream, foam, gel, spray	Musculoskeletal pain and inflammation [12]	Asia, Europe
Naproxan	10% gel	Musculoskeletal pain and inflammation [14]	Asia
Phenazone	5% ear drops	Pain and inflammation associated with otitis externa [12,13]	Australia, North America
Piroxicam	0.5% gel	Musculoskeletal pain and inflammation [12]	Asia, Europe, United Arab Emirates

TABLE 21.1. ***Continued***

Drugs	Form	Therapeutic Indications	Regional Availability
Phenazopyridine	Tablets	Urinary tract pain [11–13]	Asia, North America, Europe
Rofecoxib	5% ointment	Musculoskeletal pain and inflammation [14]	Asia
Triethanoleamine salicylate	10–20% cream, gel, ointment, lotion	Musculoskeletal pain [12,13]	Australia, North America

NSAIDs inhibit one or more of the isoforms of cyclooxygenase (COX), the rate-limiting enzyme involved in the conversion of arachidonic acid to PGs [2,5,8,9]. However, the analgesic properties of at least some NSAIDs, for example, topical ketorolac, appear to occur without significant alteration of tissue PG concentrations under certain conditions [10], which suggests that mechanisms other than inhibition of COX also contribute to the analgesic properties of topical NSAIDs.

21.2 RUBEFACIENTS (COUNTERIRRITANTS)

Rubefacients (Table 21.2) are used to relieve pain in muscles, joints, and tendons, although some (capsaicin, menthol) may also be used to treat cutaneous (neuropathic) pain [15]. These compounds generally produce local vasodilation and a sensation of warmth or cold when administered to the skin, but have little or no effect on deeper tissues despite their use to treat deep tissue pain [15]. They are often combined, for example, combinations of menthol and camphor, and many topical preparations will also contain methyl salicylate, a topical NSAID with irritant properties. It is thought that these compounds produce analgesic effects in deeper tissues by masking or deflecting attention away from the original source of pain.

The exact mechanism of action of many of the topical irritants remains unknown. It has been suggested that irritation of cutaneous nerve endings decreases pain in the underlying muscle or joints because they are served by the same nerves [15]. On the other hand, the mechanism of some topical irritants, such as capsaicin, is now reasonably well understood. As discussed in Chapter 8, capsaicin is known to open a nonselective cation channel, the transient receptor potential vanilloid 1 (TRPV1) receptor [16]. While it initially excites primary afferent fibers, its activation of these fibers results in a prolonged afferent desensitization that has been speculated to be mediated by an afferent phenotypic switch, whereby the affected afferent fiber decreases

TABLE 21.2. Rubefacients.

Drugs	Form	Therapeutic Indications	Regional Availability
Camphor	4–11% gel, spray, cream	Musculoskeletal pain [12]	Australia, Asia, Europe, North America, United Arab Emirates
Capsaicin	0.02% cream	Musculoskeletal and neuropathic pain [16]	Australia, Asia, Europe, North America, United Arab Emirates
Clove oil	20% gel, 5% ointment	Tooth pain [17], musculoskeletal and joint pain [12]	Australia, Asia, Europe, North America, United Arab Emirates
Ethyl nicotinate	1% gel, cream	Musculoskeletal pain and soft tissue pain [12]	Europe
Eucalyptus oil	3.0% lotion	Musculoskeletal pain [12]	Australia, Asia, Europe, North America
Glycol salicylate	2% spray, cream	Muscular and rheumatic pain [12]	Asia, North America, Europe
Menthol	5–10% gel, cream, patch	Musculoskeletal pain and soft tissue pain [12]	Australia, Asia, Europe, North America, United Arab Emirates
Methyl salicylate	30% cream	Musculoskeletal pain [12]	Australia, Asia, Europe, North America, United Arab Emirates

synthesis of excitatory peptides (e.g., substance P) or their receptors and increases synthesis of inhibitory peptides (e.g., galanin) or their receptors [16].

21.3 LOCAL ANESTHETICS

Topical local anesthetics (Table 21.3) are used in many painful conditions of the skin and oral mucosa. Topical formulations of local anesthetics are widely used in chronic conditions with minimal systemic adverse effects. Local anesthesia is induced by the ability of these drugs to block the generation and propagation of nerve impulses [18]. The mechanism of action of local anesthetics is primarily sodium channel blockade (see Chapter 3), although at the concentrations achieved clinically (and especially topically), they may also affect potassium and calcium channels [18].

21.4 INVESTIGATIONAL AGENTS

Studies have been conducted with topical agents containing compounds directed toward peripheral α2-adrenergic, N-methyl-D-aspartate (NMDA) and μ-opioid receptors (Table 21.4). Clinical evidence for the efficacy of these agents for the conditions listed in Table 21.4 is still lacking.

TABLE 21.3. Select Local Anesthetics.

Drugs	Form	Therapeutic Indication	Regional Availability
Benzocaine	20% spray, solution, 10mg lozenges	Sunburn, minor skin irritation, tooth and mucous membrane pain, sore throat [11,12,14]	Australia, Europe, North America
Butesin picrate	1% ointment	Insect bites and minor skin pain, mucous membrane pain [12]	North America
Dibucaine	0.5% cream, 1% ointment	Pain associated with sunburn, minor burns, hemorrhoids, and cuts [12]	Australia, Asia, North America, Europe, United Arab Emirates
Lidocaine	5% gel, ointment, cream, topical aerosol, spray, patch	Neuropathic pain, neuralgia, muscle and mucous membrane pain [12,13]	Australia, Asia, Europe North America, United Arab Emirates
Pramoxine	1% cream, lotion, gel, spray	Pain from insect bites, minor cuts, and hemorrhoids [12]	Europe, North America
Prilocaine	2.5% cream, 1% solution	Mucous membrane pain, surface anesthesia [12]	Australia, Europe, North America
Tetracaine	1% ointment, cream, 2% solution, 4% gel	Muscle pain [11,12,14]	Australia, Europe, North America

TABLE 21.4. Select Investigational Agents.

Drugs	Form	Potential Therapeutic Indications
Amitriptyline (tricyclic antidepressant)	2% cream	Neuropathic pain [19]
Clonidine (α2-adrenergic agonist)	0.02% cream	Neuropathic and orofacial pain [20,21]
Doxepin (tricyclic antidepressant)	5% cream	Neuropathic pain [19]
Glyceryl trinitrate	2% cream, spray	Anginal pain, neuropathic pain, osteoarthritis, vulvar pain [21]
Ketamine (NMDA receptor antagonist)	1% cream	Neuropathic pain [19]
Loperamide (μ-opioid receptor agonist)	Subcutaneous	Neuropathic pain [22]

REFERENCES

1. McQuay, H.J., Moore, R.A. (2003). Side effects of COX-2 inhibitors and other NSAIDs. In: Koltzenburg, M. (ed.). *Proceedings of the 10th World Congress on Pain*, Vol. 24. Seattle, WA: IASP Press, pp. 499–510.
2. Gotzsche, P.C. (2000). Non-steroidal anti-inflammatory drugs. *BMJ* 320: 1063–1070.
3. Moore, R.A., Tramer, M.R., Carroll, D., Wiffen, P.J., McQuay, H.J. (1998). Quantitative systematic review of topically applied non-steroidal anti-inflammatory drugs. *BMJ* 316:333–338.
4. Mense, S. (1993). Nociception from skeletal muscle in relation to clinical muscle pain. *Pain* 54:241–289.
5. Schaible, H.G., Ebersberger, A., Von Banchet, G.S. (2002). Mechanisms of pain in arthritis. *Ann N Y Acad Sci* 966:343–354.
6. Schaible, H.-G., Grubb, B.D. (1993). Afferent and spinal mechanisms of joint pain. *Pain* 55:5–54.
7. Graven-Nielsen, T., Mense, S. (2001). The peripheral apparatus of muscle pain: evidence from animal and human studies. *Clin J Pain* 17:2–10.
8. Walker, J.S. (1995). NSAID: an update on their analgesic effects. *Clin Exp Pharmacol Physiol* 22:855–860.
9. Cashman, J.N. (1996). The mechanisms of action of NSAIDs in analgesia. *Drugs* 52(Suppl. 5):13–23.
10. Gordon, S.M., Brahim, J.S., Rowan, J., Kent, A., Dionne, R.A. (2002). Peripheral prostanoid levels and nonsteroidal anti-inflammatory drug analgesia: replicate clinical trials in a tissue injury model. *Clin Pharmacol Ther* 72:175–183.
11. Anon. (2008). *AHFS Drug Information*. New York: American Society of Health System Pharmacists.
12. Anon. (2007). *Martindale: The Complete Drug Reference*. London: Pharmaceutical Press.
13. Anon. (2008). *Compendium of Pharmaceuticals and Specialties*. Ottawa: Canadian Pharmacists Association.
14. Anon. (2007). *Monthly Index of Medical Specialties*. New Delhi.
15. Moore, R.A., Derry, S., McQuay, H.J. (2008). Topical agents in the treatment of rheumatic pain. *Rheum Dis Clin North Am* 34:415–432.
16. Knotkova, H., Pappagallo, M., Szallasi, A. (2008). Capsaicin (TRPV1 agonist) therapy for pain relief: farewell or revival? *Clin J Pain* 24:142–154.
17. Alqareer, A., Alyahya, A., Andersson, L. (2006). The effect of clove and benzocaine versus placebo as topical anesthetics. *J Dent Res* 34:747–750.
18. Scholz, A. (2002). Mechanisms of (local) anaesthetics on voltage-gated sodium and other ion channels. *Br J Anaesth* 89:52–61.
19. Sawynok, J. (2003). Topical and peripherally acting analgesics. *Pharmacol Rev* 55:1–20.
20. Epstein, J.B., Grushka, M., Le, N. (1997). Topical clonidine for orofacial pain: a pilot study. *J Orofacial Pain* 11:345–352.

21. McCleane, G. (2007). Topical analgesics. *Anesthesiology Clin* 25:825–839.

22. Guan, Y., Johanak, L.M., Hartke, T.V., Shim, B., Tao, Y.X., RingKamp, M., Meyer, R.A., Raja, S.N. (2008). Peripherally acting mu—opiod receptor agonist attenuated neuropathic pain in rats after L5 spinal nerve injury. *Pain* 138:318–329.

INDEX

Peripheral Receptor Targets for Analgesia: Novel Approaches to Pain Management, Edited by Brian E. Cairns

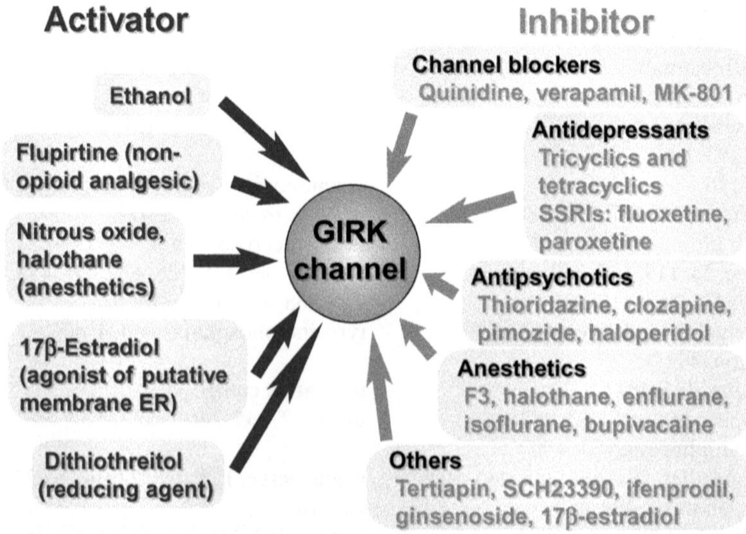

FIGURE 4.2. Various modulators of GIRK channels. Blue and red arrows show the activating and inhibiting effect on GIRK channels, respectively.

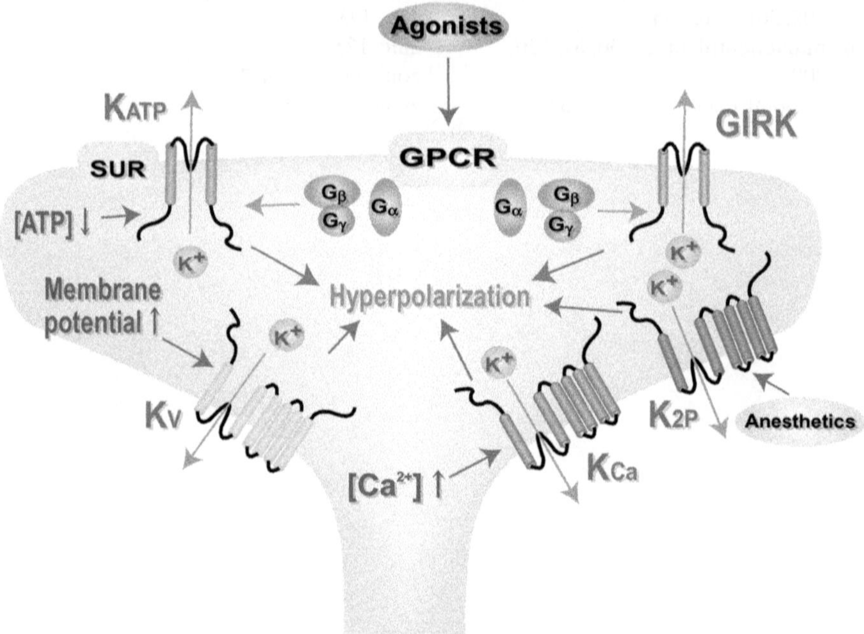

FIGURE 4.3. Schematic illustration of peripheral endogenous analgesia, focusing on major potassium channels, induced by hyperpolarization of membrane potential in the nerve terminus of the peripheral sensory neuron. GPCR, G protein-coupled receptor; SUR, sulfonylurea receptor.

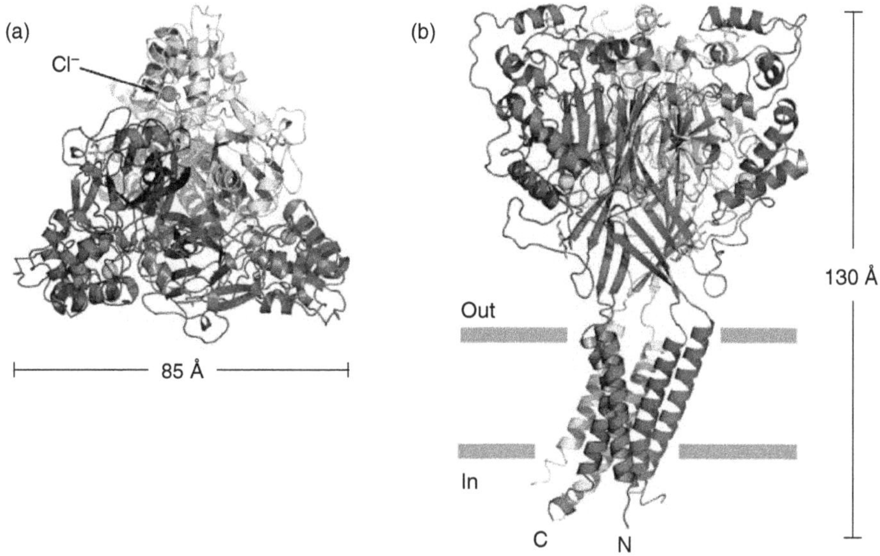

Figure 7.1. Trimeric structure of ASIC1. (a) View from the extracellular side. (b) Side view of the three subunits, viewed parallel to the membrane. Reprinted by permission from Jasti, J., Furukawa, H., Gonzales, E.B., Gouaux, E. (2007). Structure of acid-sensing ion channel 1 at 1.9 A resolution and low pH. *Nature* 449:316–323, copyright (2007), with permission from Macmillan Publishers Ltd.

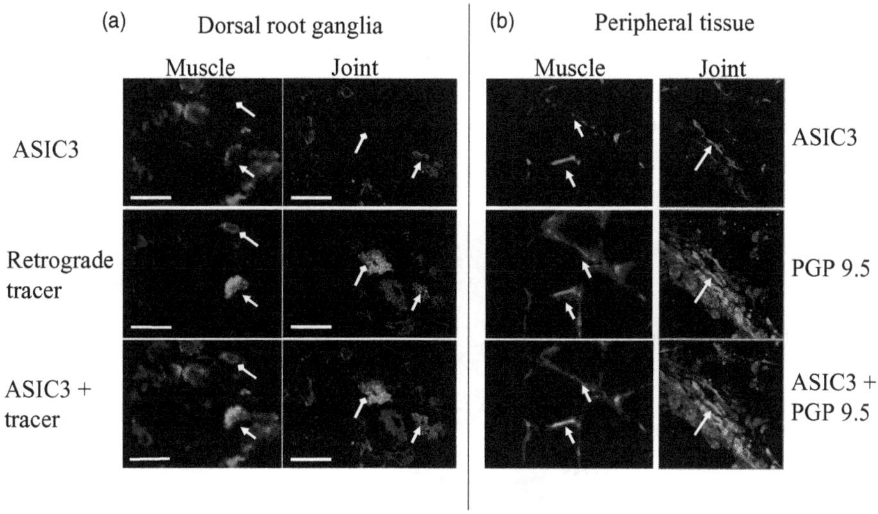

Figure 7.2. Immunohistochemical localization of ASIC3 in retrogradely labeled DRG neurons from the muscle and joint, or primary afferent fibers located within the muscle endomysium or joint synovium. (See text for full caption.)

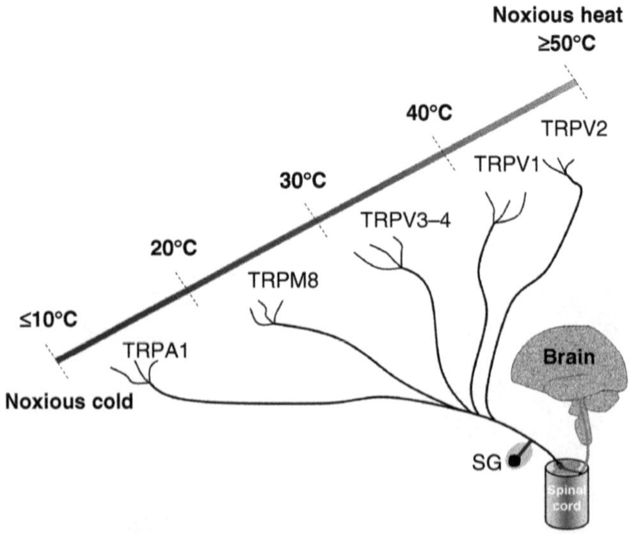

FIGURE 8.1. "ThermoTRPs" as sensors of the whole spectrum of temperatures, from painful cold (10°C) to painful heat (53°C). SG, sensory ganglia.

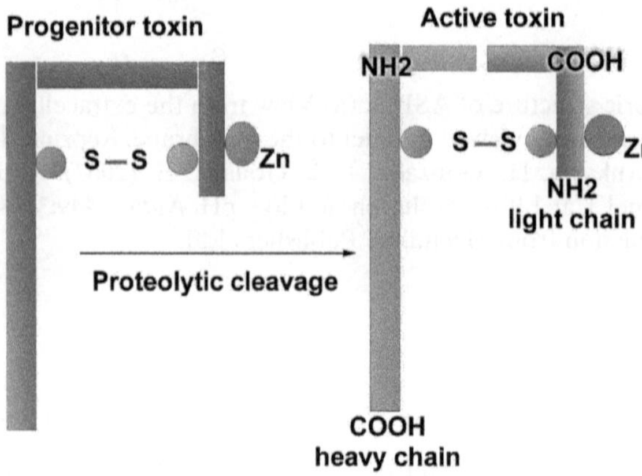

FIGURE 12.1. Botulinum toxin structure (schematic diagram) (image reprinted with permission from eMedicine.com. (See text for full caption.)

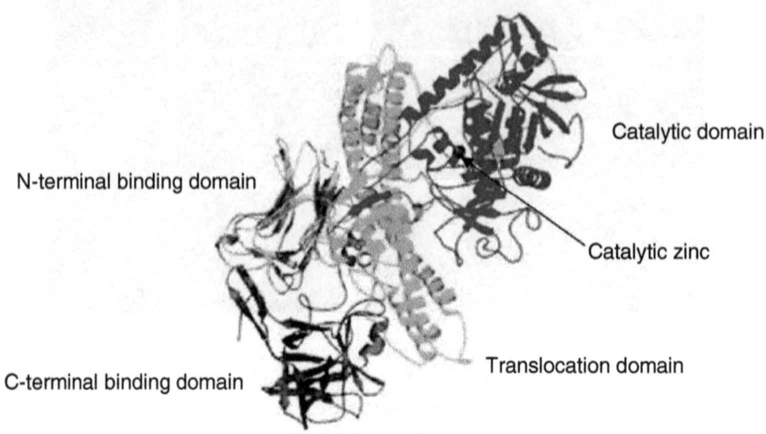

FIGURE 12.2. Domain structure of botulinum neurotoxin type A: The catalytic domain is colored blue; the translocation domain is green; the N-terminal binding subdomain is yellow, and the C-terminal binding subdomain is red. (See text for full caption.)

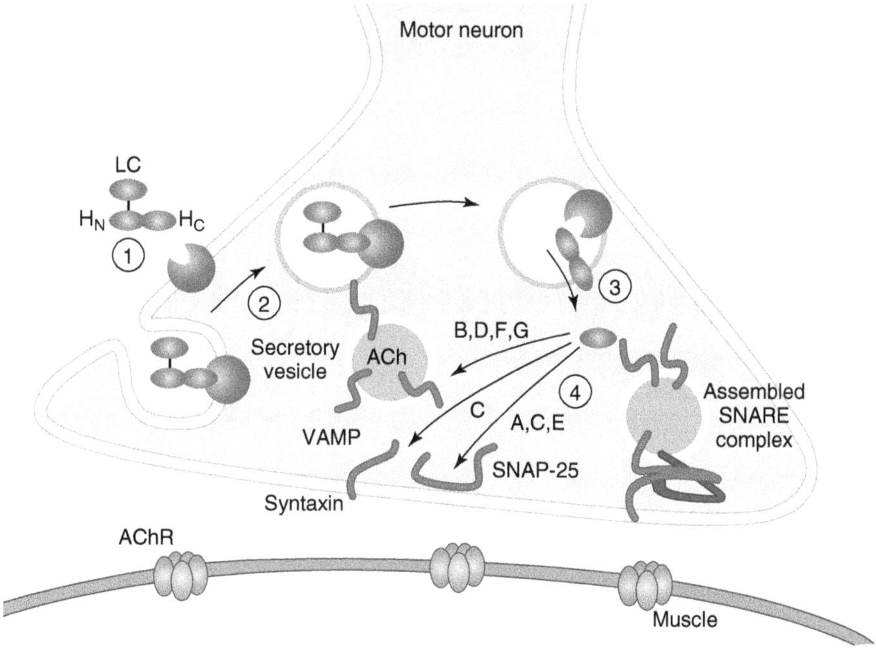

FIGURE 12.3. Biological activity of botulinum toxins at the neuromuscular junction. (See text for full caption.)

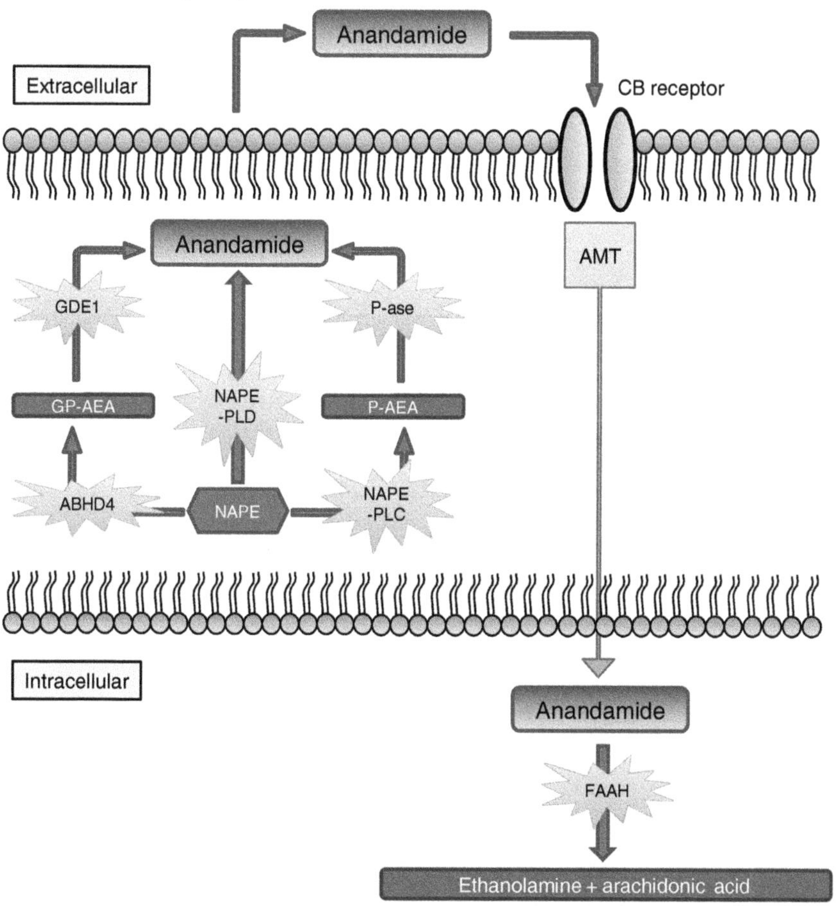

FIGURE 13.1. Biosynthesis and degradation of anandamide. (See text for full caption.)

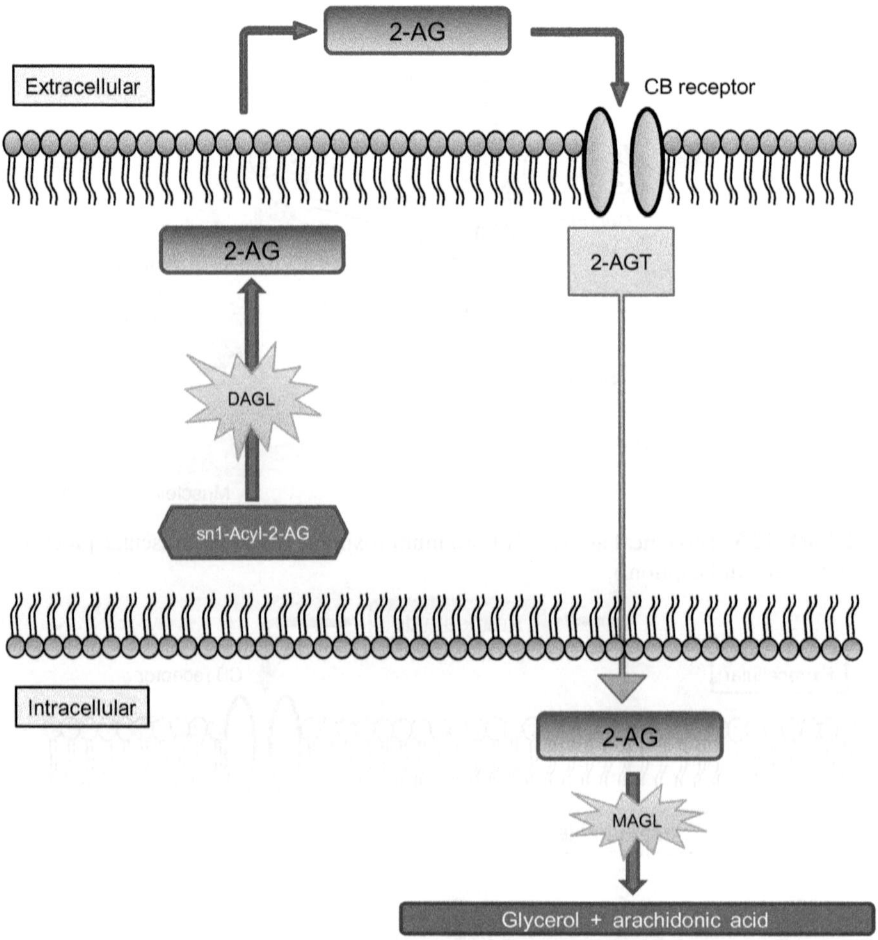

Figure 13.2. Biosynthesis and degradation of 2-acyl-glycerol (2-AG). Initially, sn1-acyl-2-arachidonoylglycerol (sn1-acyl-2-AG) is converted to 2-AG by diacylglycerol lipase (DAGL). Following cannabinoid receptor signaling, 2-AG is transported intracellularly by a 2-AG transporter (2-AGT) and is then broken down by monoacylglycerol lipase (MAGL) to produce glycerol and arachidonic acid.

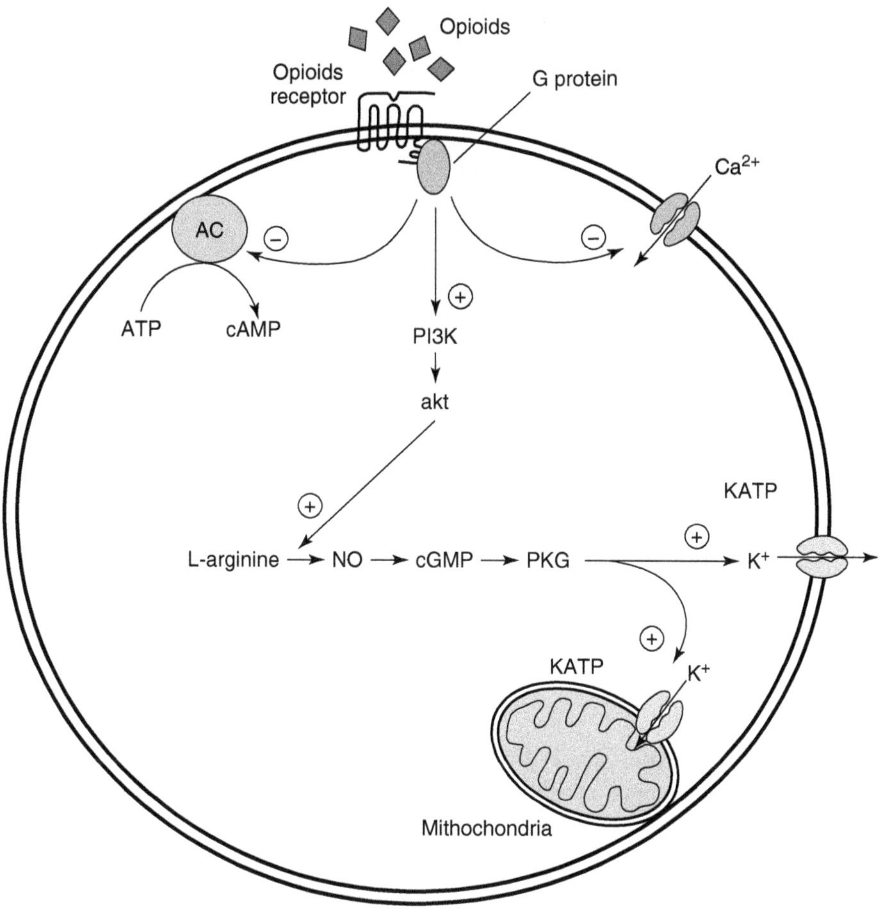

FIGURE 14.2. Proposed model for opioid receptor-mediated analgesia in the peripheral terminal of primary sensory neurons. (See text for full caption.)

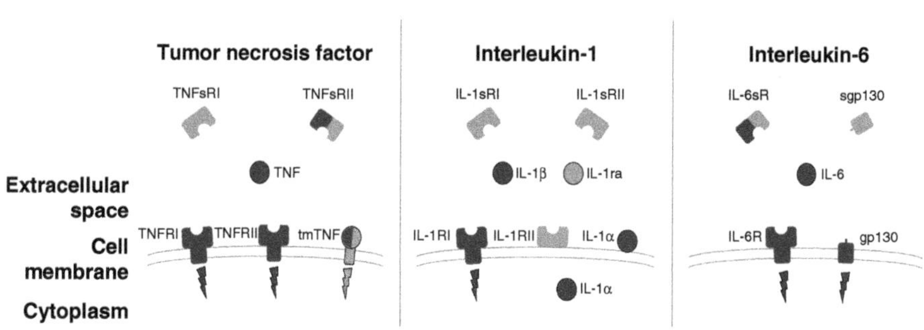

FIGURE 17.1. Endogenous ligands and receptors for tumor necrosis factor (TNF), interleukin-1β (IL-1β), and interleukin-6 (IL-6). In this figure, the red color represents proinflammatory effects and the green color represents anti-inflammatory effects. (See text for full caption.)

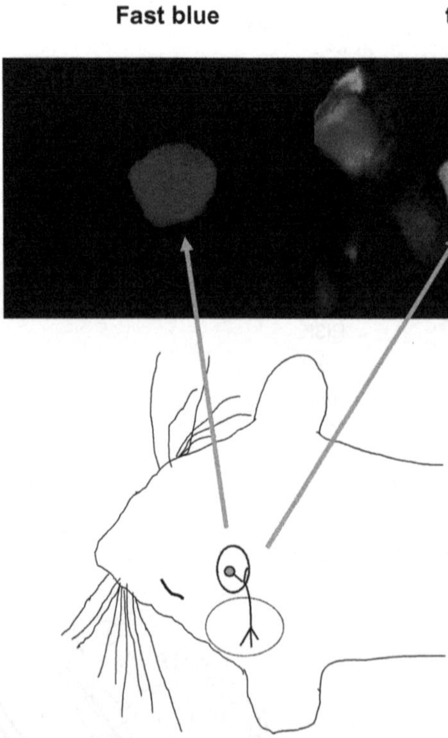

FIGURE 18.1. Fast Blue dye (1.5%, 10 mL) injected into the masseter muscle was used to identify trigeminal ganglion neurons that innervate the rat masseter muscle. Immunohistochemistry was used to label the expression of trkA receptors on these masseter ganglion neurons [9].

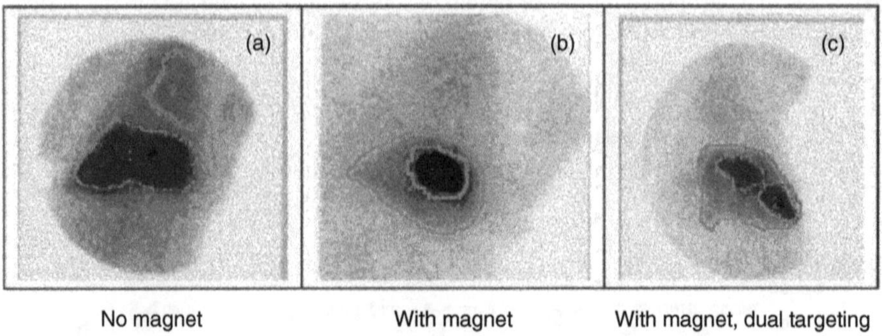

FIGURE 19.7. Principle of magnetic targeting. (a) The infusion of magnetic particles of 1–3 μm into a pig's blood supply leads to rapid liver uptake. (b) Placing a permanent NdFeB magnet above a distinct liver area (e.g., a tumor) will rapidly concentrate most of the particles. (c) The magnet can even be moved, and a secondary amount of particles can be targeted to a different area in the liver. With permission from Goodwin et al. [171].

Lightning Source UK Ltd.
Milton Keynes UK
UKHW01n0817050918
328316UK00003B/372/P

9 780470 251317